ESSENTIALS of KINESIOLOGY for the PHYSICAL THERAPIST ASSISTANT

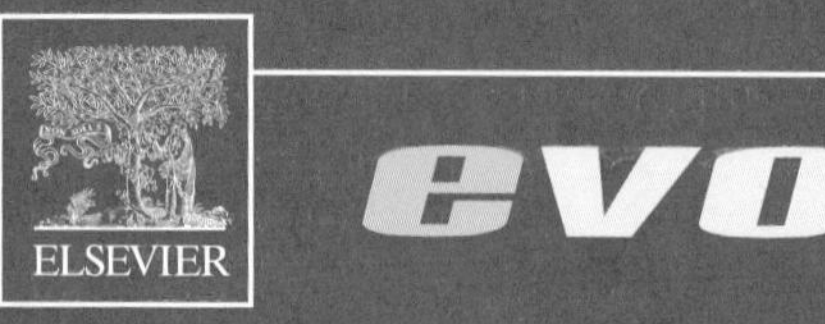

To access your Student Resources, visit:

http://evolve.elsevier.com/Mansfield/kinesiology

Evolve® Student Resources for ***Mansfield and Neumann: Essentials of Kinesiology for the Physical Therapist Assistant*** offer the following features:

Student Resources

- **Vocabulary Flashcards**
  Glossary terms and definitions are provided within a fun and interactive format to help you master the language of kinesiology.
- **Labeling Exercises**
  More than 110 of the book's images featuring anatomy and basic human movement are reproduced with interactive drag-and-drop labels for a fun and effective way to study.
- **Bibliography**
  Additional Readings within each chapter are compiled into an overall bibliography that includes Medline links to journal articles where applicable for quick and easy research.

http://evolve.elsevier.com/Mansfield/kinesiology

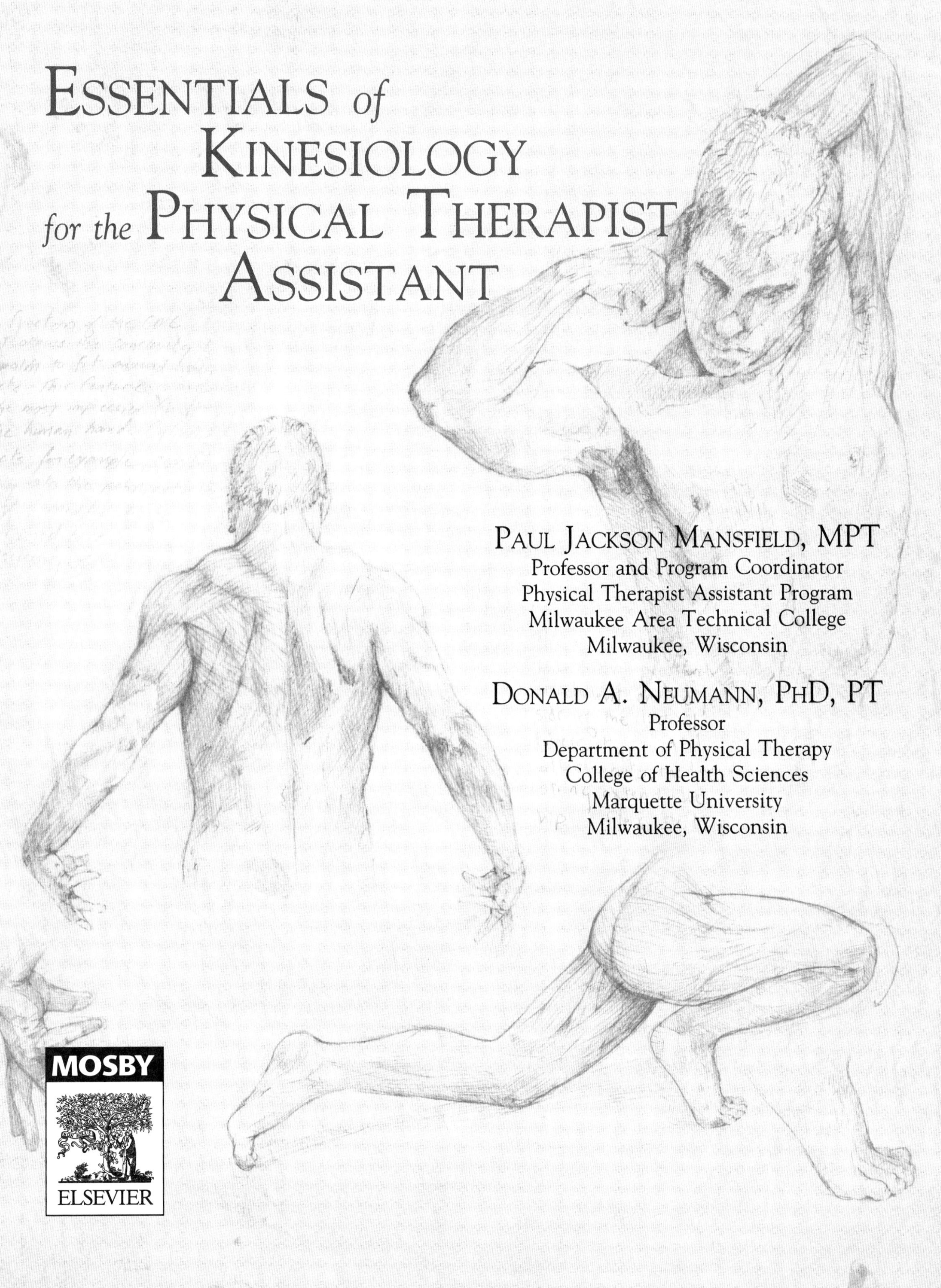

ESSENTIALS *of* KINESIOLOGY *for the* PHYSICAL THERAPIST ASSISTANT

PAUL JACKSON MANSFIELD, MPT
Professor and Program Coordinator
Physical Therapist Assistant Program
Milwaukee Area Technical College
Milwaukee, Wisconsin

DONALD A. NEUMANN, PHD, PT
Professor
Department of Physical Therapy
College of Health Sciences
Marquette University
Milwaukee, Wisconsin

MOSBY
ELSEVIER

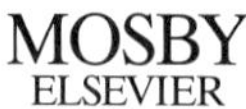
MOSBY
ELSEVIER
11830 Westline Industrial Drive
St. Louis, Missouri 63146

ESSENTIALS OF KINESIOLOGY FOR THE PHYSICAL THERAPIST ASSISTANT

ISBN: 978-0-323-03616-0

Library of Congress Control Number: 2007939688

ISBN: 978-0-323-03616-0

Vice President and Publisher: Linda Duncan
Senior Editor: Kathy Falk
Managing Editor: Kristin Hebberd
Associate Developmental Editor: Sarah Vales
Publishing Services Manager: Patricia Tannian
Senior Project Manager: Kristine Feeherty
Design Direction: Julia Dummitt

Printed in the United States of America

Last digit is the print number: 9 8 7 6 5 4 3 2

To my former patients at the spinal cord injury center, thanks for teaching me what persistence and courage really mean.
And to my wife, Heather—I love you.

PJM

To Shep Barish, PT, my first role model as a practicing Physical Therapist Assistant more than 35 years ago. His passion and respect for clinical kinesiology have left an indelible mark on my career.

DAN

PREFACE

Essentials of Kinesiology for the Physical Therapist Assistant is intended to provide students with a firm foundation of kinesiology—the study of human movement. This text focuses strongly on the structure and function of the musculoskeletal system, serving as prerequisite subject matter for all aspects of physical therapist assistant (PTA) practice. Thorough yet clear explanations of normal human movement set the stage for relevant discussions of many common compensatory strategies, treatment techniques, and abnormal movement patterns. Vivid anatomic detail of the bones, joints, supporting ligaments, and muscles is interwoven with an emphasis on clinical relevance for the PTA.

Kinesiology is the heart of physical therapy practice, regardless of the precise role of the practitioner. Furthermore, a firm understanding of kinesiology is based on a solid background in the anatomy and function of the musculoskeletal system. This knowledge sets the stage for understanding the basis for normal and abnormal movement. Only with this knowledge can the clinician clearly treat dysfunctional, labored, weakened, or painful movement.

Audience

This book is intended primarily for students in PTA programs. However, its usefulness does not end there. The text is also a valuable tool for practicing PTAs or for any student or professional seeking a clear, clinically relevant introduction to kinesiology.

Unique Author Team

By combining our experiences, we are able to offer the PTA community a comprehensive, anatomically rich, and clinically relevant textbook on kinesiology. Paul Jackson Mansfield has practiced physical therapy for 10 years and at present is the director of the physical therapist assistant program at Milwaukee Area Technical College. Mr. Mansfield also teaches extensively in the program, including courses in kinesiology, musculoskeletal anatomy, orthopedics, advanced therapeutic exercise, and neurology. These experiences have provided him with exceptional insight into the needs, clinical relevance, and methods used to effectively teach the PTA student.

Dr. Donald A. Neumann has practiced physical therapy for 30 years and is currently a professor in the physical therapy department at Marquette University. Dr. Neumann has taught kinesiology for more than 20 years and is the author of the bestselling text *Kinesiology of the Musculoskeletal System: Foundations for Physical Rehabilitation*. Once a practicing PTA himself, Dr. Neumann also understands the mission and needs of the PTA student and clinician.

Essentials of Kinesiology for the Physical Therapist Assistant represents a rich blend of the experiences from these two authors. Mr. Mansfield provides the text's direction and relevance, whereas Dr. Neumann offers a solid scientific background and years of educational experience.

Concept

Many of the illustrations used in this text are from Dr. Neumann's larger *Kinesiology* text (mentioned above). The overwhelming success of this core textbook stimulated us to write a version intended for PTAs. We have spent countless hours thoughtfully crafting the concepts behind the text to suit the specific needs of the PTA student, while working hard to maintain the beauty of the illustrations, clarity of the writing, attention to detail, and strong emphasis on clinical relevance.

Contribution to Physical Therapist Assistant Education

Anyone who has taught in a PTA program knows that the students must survive the quick (typically 2-year) journey from not knowing much about physical therapy to being able to meet and exceed the expectations placed on a newly graduated PTA. Students in this fast-paced curriculum must master the basics of human motion before moving on to more complex and layered clinical topics. We believe that for the large majority of PTA programs, kinesiology is—or can be—the foundation on which physical therapy knowledge and practice are based. It is our sincere hope that the students and educators who use this text embrace the level of knowledge and explanation we have provided and find that it supplies them with the tools they need to build and support this foundation within their own classes and programs.

Philosophical Approach

Essentials of Kinesiology for the Physical Therapist Assistant is *not* a watered-down version of kinesiology, and upon reading, you will likely agree that it pulls very few punches. It is also much more than a slimmed-down version of Dr. Neumann's larger textbook. We feel strongly that students at all levels of physical therapy education are typically gifted and very motivated to learn. To this end, the wonderful artwork and clear and relevant explanations within this textbook will help students capitalize on that motivation and make the most of their educational experience. We also hope that our high expectations for both students and educators are shared by many others and will stimulate continued growth throughout the profession. A profession grows through the strength of its education, and the education of today's PTAs needs to parallel the rapid and continued education and advancements of the entire physical therapy profession.

Organization

This textbook teaches kinesiology through a layered approach. Each chapter on a particular region of the body starts with a description of the anatomy and function of the bones. This is followed by a detailed yet clear description of the joints and related supportive tissues. Next the anatomy and actions of muscles are presented, including information on the proximal and distal attachments, actions, and innervations. Each muscle within a particular region is artfully and clearly illustrated with exceptional anatomic detail. Chapters then progress from anatomy to an explanation of the ways in which muscles and joints normally operate together and subsequently the ways in which disease or trauma can disrupt this relationship and result in abnormal movement. This sets the final stage for a description of *why* this material is relevant to the practice of physical therapy. Throughout each chapter are a number of feature boxes containing clinical examples, corollaries, and illustrations that help further bridge the gap between the classroom and clinical practice.

Chapters 1, 2, and 3 provide a solid and relevant background on the basic terminology used in kinesiology, fundamental biomechanics, joint structure, and muscle anatomy and physiology. Chapters 4 through 11 focus on the specific anatomy and kinesiologic principles of the various regions of the body—the true heart and soul of this book. Chapters 12 and 13, on the kinesiology of walking (gait) and on mastication and ventilation, respectively, round out the necessary kinesiologic foundation and also incorporate and synthesize material from many previous chapters.

Distinctive Features

- *Outstanding Artwork*: The number and quality of renderings and photographs truly set this text apart from similar books designed with the PTA student in mind.
- *Atlas-Style Muscle Presentations*: Individual muscles and groups of related muscles are presented in a unique atlas style that clearly pairs the illustration of that muscle or group with the relevant attachments, innervations, and actions. This approach serves as an effective tool for both education and clinical reference.
- *Combined Authorship*: The expertise of the authors, culled from a combined 40 years of physical therapy practice and approximately 25 years of teaching experience, provides for an authoritative and unique voice in PTA education.
- *Clinical Relevance*: This text consistently links concepts within kinesiology with the practice of physical therapy, first presenting the foundational knowledge of human motion and then layering that with clinically relevant information and features.

Learning Features

- *Colorful, Clear, and Robust Art Program*: Nearly 400 high-quality images—mostly two-color renderings—populate the book, essentially telling a story of their own and invaluably supplementing the written text.
- *Atlas-Style Muscle Presentations*: This unique layout (described above in greater detail) pairs illustrations with a consistent text format to effectively lay all the necessary information at the reader's fingertips.
- *Feature Boxes*: Both *Clinical Insight* and *Consider This* boxes supplement the content, continually linking the concepts of kinesiology with their clinical applications in the context of physical therapy.
- *Summary Boxes and Tables*: Sections of text are followed by lists or tables that summarize the main concepts presented, pulling the content together into concise and reader-friendly tools useful for study or quick reference.
- *Study Questions*: Each chapter's text presentation concludes with 20 to 30 multiple-choice and true/false practice questions that serve as a valuable self-assessment tool for exam preparation.
- *Key Terms*: Because the language of kinesiology is key to mastery of the content, chapters include a list of key words, each of which appears in boldface within the chapter in the context of its discussion.
- *Glossary*: Chapter key terms are compiled alphabetically and defined in a back-of-book glossary as a handy reference tool.

- *Learning Objectives*: Each chapter begins with a list of outcome objectives, which provides a summary of content coverage and a quick checklist for students during exam preparation.
- *Chapter Outlines*: The main levels of headings are provided on the first page of each chapter, supplying an overview of the structure or framework of the content.

Ancillary Materials

An Evolve website has been created to accompany *Essentials of Kinesiology for the Physical Therapist Assistant*. Please visit the following URL to access the wealth of information provided to supplement this text: http://evolve.elsevier.com/Mansfield/kinesiology/.

For Instructors

- *Test Bank*: Approximately 350 objective-style questions—a mixture of multiple-choice, true/false, matching, and short-answer formats—with accompanying rationales for correct responses and page-number references to where that information can be found within the book
- *PowerPoint Presentations*: Approximately 40 text slides per chapter for use in classroom lecture presentations
- *Image Collection*: Electronic version of the entire textbook art program available for download
- *Animations*: Three-dimensional animations that bring the musculoskeletal system and orthopedics to life
- *Laboratory Activities*: Interactive materials designed to accompany the core chapters on specific body regions, providing practice on identification and palpation of landmarks and muscle and motion analysis

For Students

- *Flashcards*: Key terms provided in a fun and interactive exercise for vocabulary mastery
- *Labeling Exercises*: Drag-and-drop matching of labels to images of anatomy and basic kinesiology from the textbook
- *Bibliography*: Chapter *Additional Readings* compiled into a single document with Medline links to journal articles where available for quick and easy research

We hope you find in this textbook all the information and resources you need to instruct students entering the dynamic PTA profession. We believe that if the subject matter is presented in a clear, organized, and relevant manner, there are no limits to what students can learn. This text is designed exactly on this premise.

Paul Jackson Mansfield
Donald A. Neumann

ABOUT THE AUTHORS

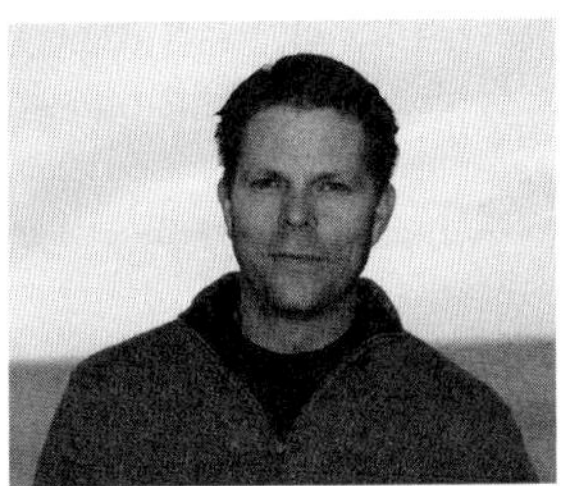

Paul Jackson Mansfield, MPT, graduated from Marquette University in 1997 with his master's degree in physical therapy. He has worked in many different fields of physical therapy, including pediatrics, orthopedics, and neurology, with an emphasis on spinal cord injury rehabilitation. Mr. Mansfield began teaching within the physical therapist assistant (PTA) program at Milwaukee Area Technical College (MATC) in 2001 and serves as the program's director. He teaches extensively within the PTA curriculum, including courses in kinesiology, musculoskeletal anatomy, orthopedics, advanced therapeutic exercise, and neurology.

For the past 3 years, Mr. Mansfield has been the curriculum director for the department of educational research and dissemination at MATC. During this time, he has taught numerous courses for faculty development that involve best-teaching practices and educational strategies based on the latest (educational) neurologic research.

Mr. Mansfield lives in Wisconsin with his wife Heather and five children. In his spare time, he enjoys coaching soccer and volleyball, drumming, and playing hockey.

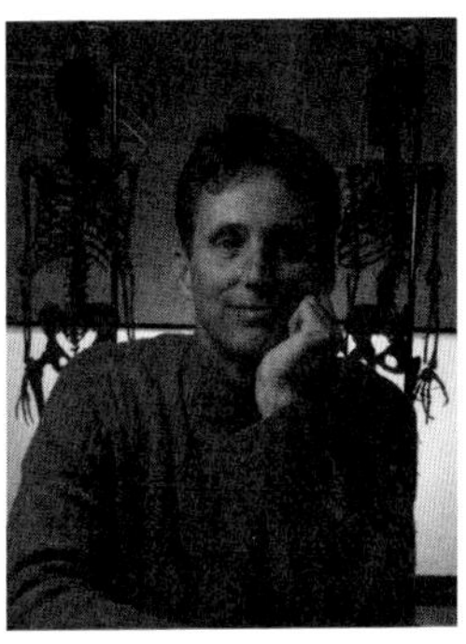

Donald A. Neumann, PhD, PT, started his career as a physical therapist assistant, earning an associate's degree of science from Miami-Dade Community College. After practicing a few years, he received a bachelor's degree of science in physical therapy from the University of Florida. After several years of clinical practice and graduate study, he received a PhD in exercise science from the University of Iowa. In 1986 Dr. Neumann joined the faculty at Marquette University, where he is currently a full professor in the physical therapy department. Dr. Neumann received the "Teacher of the Year Award" at Marquette University in 1994, and he was named by the Carnegie Foundation as "Wisconsin's College Professor of the Year" in 2006. Both awards reflect his teaching of kinesiology to physical therapy students.

Dr. Neumann has received numerous national awards from the American Physical Therapy Association, which has recognized his research, teaching, and other scholarly activity. (For details, see his web page at www.marquette.edu/chs/pt/faculty/neumann.shtml.) Over the years, Dr. Neumann's research and teaching projects have been funded by the National Arthritis Foundation and the Paralyzed Veterans of America. He is the author of *Kinesiology of the Musculoskeletal System: Foundations for Physical Rehabilitation*, published by Elsevier (2002), and serves as associate editor of the *Journal of Orthopaedic & Sports Physical Therapy*. Dr. Neumann has received three Fulbright Scholarships to teach kinesiology in Kaunas Medical University in Lithuania (2002) and in Semmelweis Medical University in Budapest, Hungary (2005 and 2006). In 2007 Dr. Neumann received an honorary doctorate from the Lithuania Academy of Physical Education in recognition of his impact on physical therapy education in Lithuania.

Dr. Neumann lives with his wife Brenda (and two dogs) in Wisconsin. His son, Donald Jr. ("Donnie"), and his stepdaughter, Megann, also live in Wisconsin. Outside work, he enjoys photography, a wide range of music, mountaineering, and paying attention to the weather.

ACKNOWLEDGMENTS

This is a welcome opportunity for me to thank a great number of people who supported the completion of this text in many different ways.

I would first like to thank Dr. Donald Neumann for his endless patience and guidance through this process. His never-ending quest for educational excellence is as contagious as it is inspirational. Don, you are the best teacher I have ever known—and now I know why.

Anyone who has undertaken a project of this magnitude knows that it cannot be done without the support of family, and for that I will be forever grateful. I would like to give a very special "thanks" to my beautiful wife, Heather, who was forced on many occasions to suffer the load of raising five children while her husband disappeared into "the cave" to write. Thanks for helping make this dream come true.

I would also like to thank my children: Rachael, Daniel, Megan, Hannah, and Beckett (who is lovingly referred to as "the book baby" for her arrival in the middle of this process). Your continuous flow of hugs, smiles, and laughs keeps the sparkle in my eyes.

My parents, Jack and Betty Mansfield, whom I credit for my love and respect of education, also deserve a great deal of thanks for pulling "grandma and grandpa duty" whenever it was needed.

Brian Axtell, who is responsible for many of the illustrations, including the front cover and the detailed muscular renderings within this text, played a significant role in developing the art that truly drove the writing.

I would also like to acknowledge my "compatriot in arms," Kathy Tomczyk Born, for her continuous assistance with running the physical therapist assistant program at Milwaukee Area Technical College.

To Kristin Hebberd and Kristine Feeherty—thank you so much for your hard work and strong commitment to making this book a great one.

A final thanks goes out to Mike Adler, Matt Mulder, Dan Peterchak, Jeff Druley, and Spencer Mayhew. Thanks for serving as my own personal think-tank and for your continuous support throughout this project.

Paul Jackson Mansfield

I thank my wife, Brenda, for her kind understanding of my commitment to writing. I also wish to thank Paul Mansfield for his extraordinary perseverance throughout the arduous process of completing this text. And finally, I thank Elisabeth Rowan-Kelly for her fantastic art, much of which continues to live on in this text.

Donald A. Neumann

CONTENTS

CHAPTER 1

Basic Principles of Kinesiology

CHAPTER OUTLINE

OBJECTIVES

- Define commonly used anatomic and kinesiologic terminology.
- Describe the common movements of the body.
- Differentiate between osteokinematic and arthrokinematic movement.
- Describe the arthrokinematic principles of movement.
- Analyze the planes of motion and axes of rotation for common motions.
- Describe how force, torque, and levers affect biomechanical movement.
- Describe the three biomechanical lever systems, and explain their advantages and disadvantages.
- Analyze how muscular lines of pull produce specific biomechanical motions.
- Explain how muscular force vectors are used to describe movement.

KEY TERMS

abduction
active movements
adduction
anatomic position
anterior
arthrokinematics
axis of rotation
caudal
center of mass
cephalad
circumduction
closed-chain motion
congruency
deep
degrees of freedom
distal
dorsiflexion
eversion
extension
external force
external moment arm
external rotation
external torque
flexion
force
frontal plane
horizontal abduction
horizontal adduction
horizontal (transverse) plane
inferior
insertion
internal force
internal moment arm
internal rotation
internal torque
inversion
kinematics
kinesiology
kinetics
lateral
leverage
line of pull
medial
midline
open-chain motion
origin
osteokinematics
passive movements
plantar flexion
posterior
pronation
prone
protraction
proximal

radial deviation
resultant force
retraction
rotation
sagittal plane
superficial
superior
supination
supine
torque
translation
ulnar deviation
vector

The origins of the word **kinesiology** are from the Greek *kinesis*, "to move," and *ology*, "to study." *Essentials of Kinesiology* serves as a guide to kinesiology by focusing on the anatomic and biomechanical interactions within the musculoskeletal system.

The primary intent of this book is to provide physical therapist assistant students and clinicians with a fundamental understanding of the kinesiology of the musculoskeletal system. A detailed review of the musculoskeletal system, including innervation, is presented as a background to the structural and functional concepts of normal and abnormal movement. The discussions within this text are intended to provide insight and provoke thoughtful dialogue about commonly used therapeutic models and treatments.

Kinematics

Kinematics is a branch of biomechanics that describes the motion of a body without regard to the forces that produce the motion. In biomechanics the word *body* is used rather loosely to describe either the entire body, particular segments such as an individual bone, or an area of the body such as the arm. In general, two types of motion exist: translation and rotation.

Translation occurs when all parts of a "body" move in the same direction as every other part. This can occur in a straight line (rectilinear motion), for example, sliding a book across a table, or a curved line (curvilinear motion), such as the arc of a ball being tossed to a friend. Figure 1-1 illustrates the curvilinear motion that occurs during walking, reflecting the normal up-and-down translation of the head as the entire body moves forward.

Rotation describes the arc of movement of a "body" about an axis of rotation. The axis of rotation is the "pivot-point" that the rotation of the body occurs about. Figure 1-2 illustrates rotation of the forearm around the axis of rotation of the elbow.

Movement of the entire human body is generally described as a translation of the body's **center of mass**, or center of gravity (Figure 1-3). An activity such as walking results from forward translation of the body's center of mass, thus the entire body. Interestingly, however, movement or translation of the entire body is powered by muscles that rotate the limbs. This concept is illustrated in Figure 1-4, which shows an individual running (anterior translation of the center of mass) as a result of muscles rotating the legs around the axis of rotation of each hip. Importantly, the functional movement of nearly all joints in the body occurs through rotation.

Regardless of the type of body movement, a movement can be classified as either active or passive. **Active movements** are generated by stimulated or "active" muscle; for example, an individual flexing his or her arm overhead is considered an active movement. **Passive movements**, on the other hand, are generated by sources other than muscular activation such as gravity, the resistance of a stretched ligament, or a push from another person. For example, if a clinician is providing the force to move

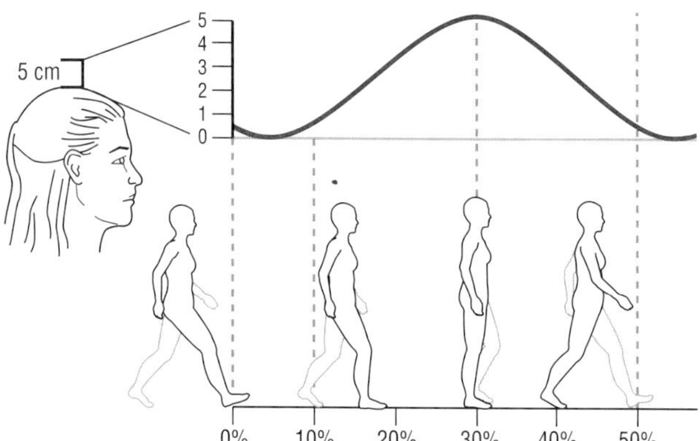

Figure 1-1 A point on the top of the head is shown translating upward and downward in a curvilinear fashion while walking. (From Neumann DA: *Kinesiology of the musculoskeletal system: foundations for physical rehabilitation*, St Louis, 2002, Mosby, Figure 1-2.)

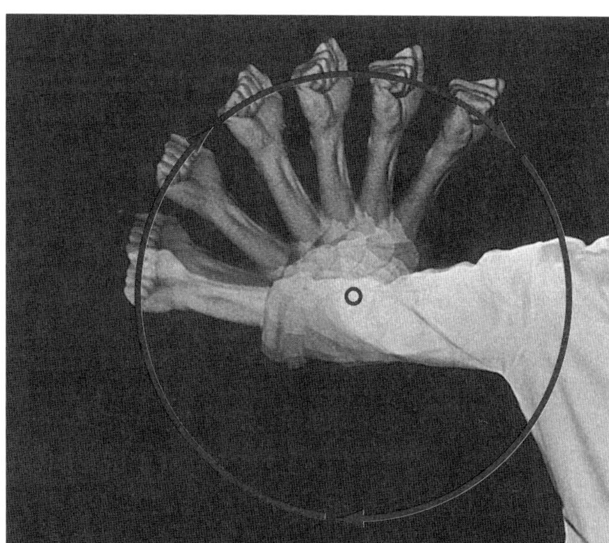

Figure 1-2 Rotation of the forearm around the axis of rotation of the elbow. (From Neumann DA: *Kinesiology of the musculoskeletal system: foundations for physical rehabilitation*, St Louis, 2002, Mosby, Figure 1-3.)

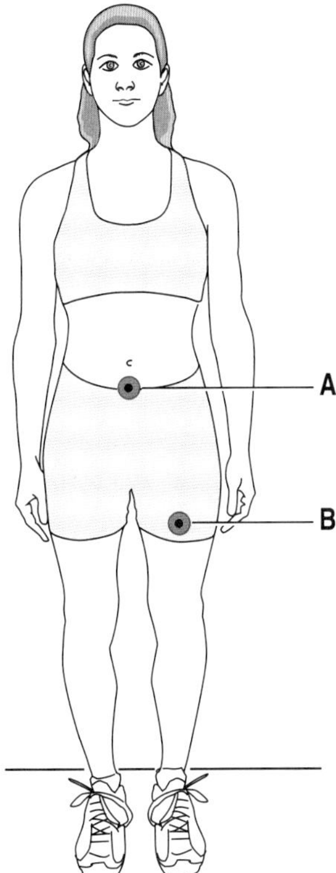

Figure 1-3 **A**, Center of mass of the entire body. **B**, Center of mass of the thigh. (From Neumann DA: *Kinesiology of the musculoskeletal system: foundations for physical rehabilitation*, St Louis, 2002, Mosby, Figure 4-1.)

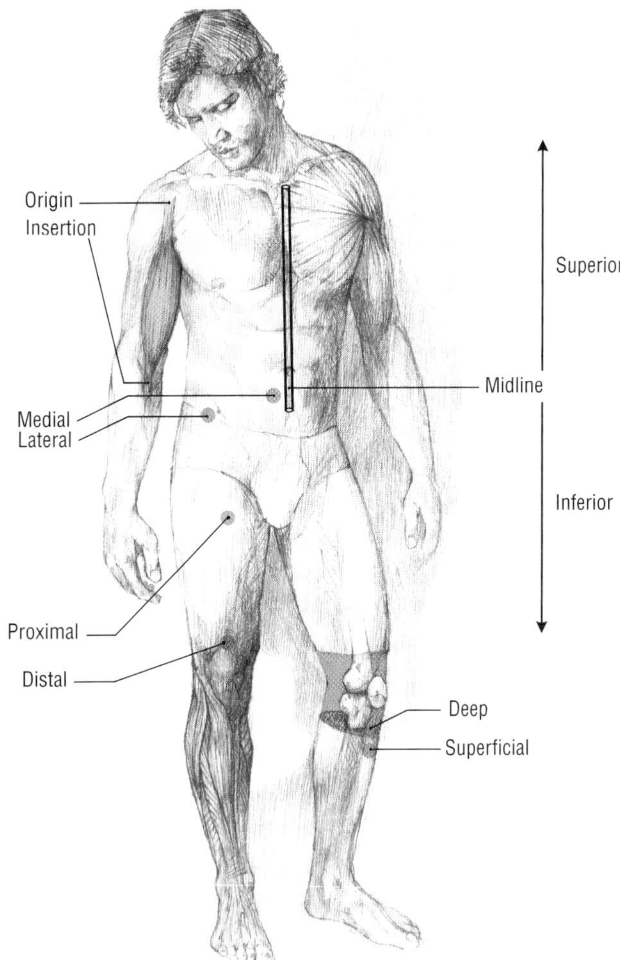

Figure 1-5 Anatomic terminology.

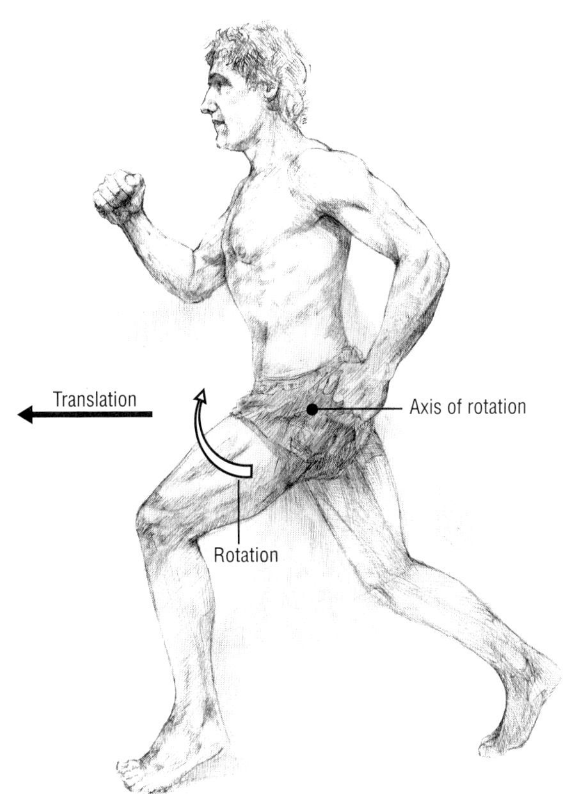

Figure 1-4 Forward translation of the body resulting from rotation of the lower extremities.

an individual's limb through various ranges of motion, it is considered a *passive* movement—thus the common clinical term passive range of motion.

Terminology

The study of kinesiology requires the use of specific terminology to describe movement, position, and location of anatomic features. Many of these terms are illustrated in Figure 1-5.

- **Anterior:** Toward the front of the body
- **Posterior:** Toward the back of the body
- **Midline:** An imaginary line that courses vertically through the center of the body
- **Medial:** Toward the midline of the body
- **Lateral:** Away from the midline of the body
- **Superior:** Above, or toward the head
- **Inferior:** Below, or toward the feet
- **Proximal:** Closer to, or toward the torso
- **Distal:** Away from the torso
- **Cephalad:** Toward the head
- **Caudal:** Toward the feet (or "tail")
- **Superficial:** Toward the surface (skin) of the body

- **Deep:** Toward the inside (core) of the body
- **Origin:** The proximal attachment of a muscle or ligament
- **Insertion:** The distal attachment of a muscle or ligament
- **Prone:** Describes the position of an individual lying face down
- **Supine:** Describes the position of an individual lying face up

Osteokinematics

PLANES OF MOTION

Osteokinematics describes the motion of bones relative to the three cardinal planes of the body: sagittal, frontal, and horizontal (Figure 1-6) (Box 1-1).

- **Sagittal plane:** Divides the body into left and right halves. Typically, flexion and extension movements occur in the sagittal plane.
- **Frontal plane:** Divides the body into front and back sections. Nearly all abduction and adduction motions occur in the frontal plane.
- **Horizontal (transverse) plane:** Divides the body into upper and lower sections. Nearly all rotational movements such as internal and external rotation of the shoulder or hip and rotation of the trunk occur in the horizontal plane.

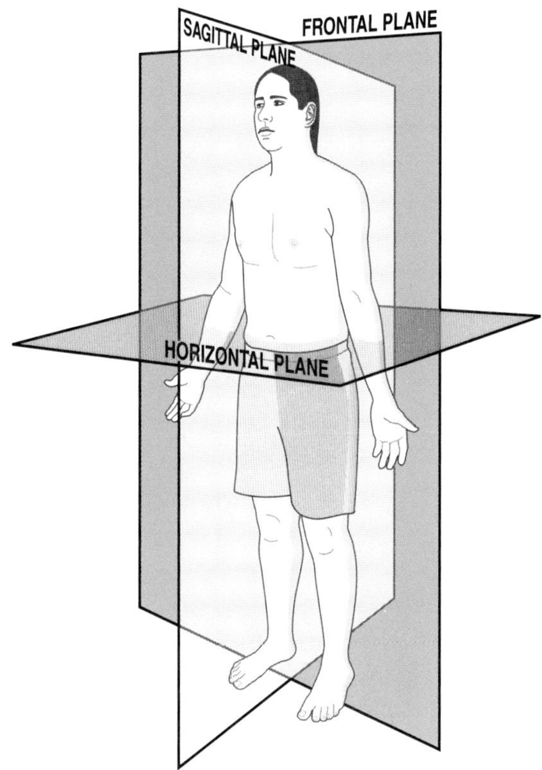

Figure 1-6 The three cardinal planes of the body are shown on an individual in the anatomic position. (From Neumann DA: *Kinesiology of the musculoskeletal system: foundations for physical rehabilitation,* St Louis, 2002, Mosby, Figure 1-4.)

ANATOMIC POSITION

The **anatomic position**, illustrated in Figure 1-6, serves as a standard reference for anatomic descriptions, axis of rotation, and planes of motion. For example, the action of a muscle is based on the assumption that it contracts with the body in the anatomic position.

AXIS OF ROTATION

The **axis of rotation** of a joint may be considered the pivot point about which joint motion occurs. Consequently, the axis of rotation is always perpendicular to the plane of motion. Traditionally, movements of the body are described as occurring about three separate axes of rotation: anterior-posterior, medial-lateral, and vertical—sometimes referred to as the longitudinal axis (Figure 1-7).

The anterior-posterior axis of rotation is oriented in an anterior-posterior direction through the convex member of the joint and allows movement to occur in the frontal plane, such as abduction and adduction of the hip.

The medial-lateral axis of rotation is oriented in an medial-lateral direction through the convex member of the joint. The medial-lateral axis of rotation allows motion to occur in the sagittal plane, for instance, flexion or extension of the elbow.

BOX 1-1

Common Osteokinematic Terms

Sagittal Plane	Frontal Plane	Horizontal Plane
• Flexion and extension • Dorsiflexion and plantar flexion • Forward and backward bending	• Abduction and adduction • Lateral flexion • Ulnar and radial deviation • Eversion and inversion	• Internal (medial) and external (lateral) rotation • Axial rotation

From Neumann DA: *Kinesiology of the musculoskeletal system: foundations for physical rehabilitation,* St Louis, 2002, Mosby, Table 1-2. Many of the terms are specific to a particular region of the body. The thumb, for example, uses different terminology.

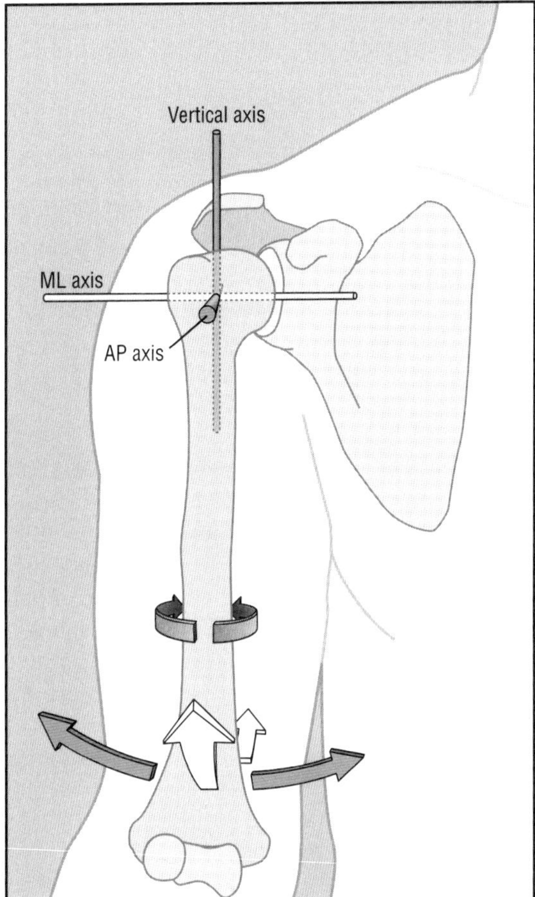

Figure 1-7 The right glenohumeral (shoulder) joint highlights the axes of rotation and associated planes of motion: Flexion and extension *(white curved arrows)* occur about a medial-lateral *(ML)* axis of rotation; abduction and adduction *(red curved arrows)* occur about an anterior-posterior *(AP)* axis of rotation; and internal and external rotation *(gray curved arrows)* occur about a vertical axis of rotation. (Modified from Neumann DA: *Kinesiology of the musculoskeletal system: foundations for physical rehabilitation*, St Louis, 2002, Mosby, Figure 1-5.)

The vertical (longitudinal) axis of rotation is oriented vertically when in the anatomic position. However, if motion occurs out of the anatomic position, it is often described as occurring about the longitudinal axis; this axis courses through the shaft of the bone. Motion about the vertical or longitudinal axis of rotation occurs in the horizontal (or transverse) plane. Typically these are called rotational movements such as rotation of the trunk when twisting side to side, or internal and external rotation of the shoulder. A summary of these axes can be found in Table 1-1.

DEGREES OF FREEDOM

Degrees of freedom refers to the number of planes of motion allowed at a joint. A joint can have 1, 2, or 3 degrees of angular freedom, corresponding to the three cardinal planes (see the earlier section on terminology). As depicted in Figure 1-7, for example, the shoulder has 3 degrees of freedom, meaning the shoulder can move freely in all three planes. The wrist, on the other hand, allows motion in two planes, so it is considered to have 2 degrees of freedom. Joints such as the elbow (humeroulnar joint) allow motion in only one plane and therefore are considered to have just 1 degree of freedom.

FUNDAMENTAL MOVEMENTS

The movements of the body have specific terminology to help describe the motion at a joint or region of the body.

Flexion and Extension

The motions of flexion and extension occur in the sagittal plane about a medial-lateral axis of rotation (Figure 1-8). Generally, **flexion** describes the motion of one bone as it approaches the flexor surface of the other bone. **Extension** is considered a movement opposite that of flexion; an approximation of the extensor surfaces of two bones.

Abduction and Adduction

Abduction describes movement of a body segment in the frontal plane, away from the midline, whereas **adduction** describes a frontal plane movement toward the midline (Figure 1-9). Exceptions to this definition occur in the hands and feet; these are described in the joint-specific chapters.

Rotation

Rotation describes the movement of a bony segment (or segments) as it spins about its longitudinal axis of rotation. For example, turning the head or turning the trunk side-to-side are considered rotational movements (Figure 1-10, A). Motions of the extremities can be further classified into internal and external rotation.

TABLE 1-1 AXES OF ROTATION AND ASSOCIATED MOVEMENTS

Axis of Rotation	Plane of Motion	Examples of Movement
Anterior-posterior	Frontal	Hip abduction-adduction Shoulder abduction-adduction
Medial-lateral	Sagittal	Elbow flexion-extension Knee flexion-extension
Vertical or longitudinal	Horizontal	Shoulder internal-external rotation Rotation of the trunk

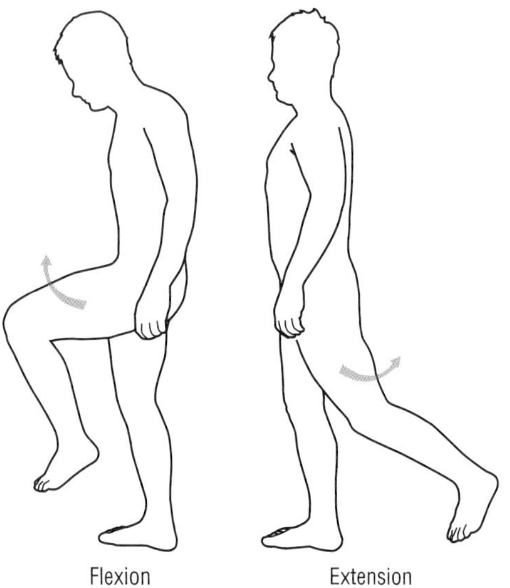

Figure 1-8 Flexion and extension.

Internal rotation describes the motion of a bony segment that results in the anterior surface of the bone rotating toward the midline. **External rotation** involves rotation of the anterior surface of a bone rotating away from the midline (Figure 1-10, *B*).

Circumduction

Circumduction describes a circular motion through two planes; therefore joints must have at least 2 degrees of freedom in order to circumduct. A general rule is that if a joint allows a circle to be "drawn in the air," the joint can circumduct (Figure 1-11).

Protraction and Retraction

Protraction describes the translation of a bone away from the midline in a plane parallel to the ground. **Retraction**, conversely, is movement of a bony segment toward the midline in a plane parallel to the ground. These terms are generally used to describe motions of the scapula or jaw (Figure 1-12).

Horizontal Adduction and Abduction

These terms generally describe motions of the shoulder in the horizontal plane (Figure 1-13). With the shoulder in an abducted position (near 90 degrees), movement of the upper extremities that results in the hands being brought together is considered **horizontal adduction**. Movement of the upper extremities away from the midline (in the horizontal plane) is considered **horizontal abduction**.

Pronation and Supination

Pronation describes a rotational movement of the forearm that results in the palm facing posteriorly (when in the anatomic position). **Supination** describes the motion of turning the palm anteriorly (Figure 1-14). Most often these motions occur with the hands in front of the body to accommodate grasping and holding types of activities, so supination is often considered turning the palm of the hand upward and pronation is considered turning the palm downward. Pronation and supination also describe complex motions of the ankle and foot and are described in detail in Chapter 11.

Radial and Ulnar Deviation

Radial and ulnar deviation describe frontal plane motions of the wrist (Figure 1-15). **Radial deviation** results in the hand moving laterally—toward the radius. **Ulnar deviation** results in the hand moving medially—toward the ulna.

Dorsiflexion and Plantar Flexion

Dorsiflexion and plantar flexion are sagittal plane motions of the ankle (Figure 1-16). **Dorsiflexion** describes the motion of bringing the foot upward, whereas **plantar flexion** describes pushing the foot downward.

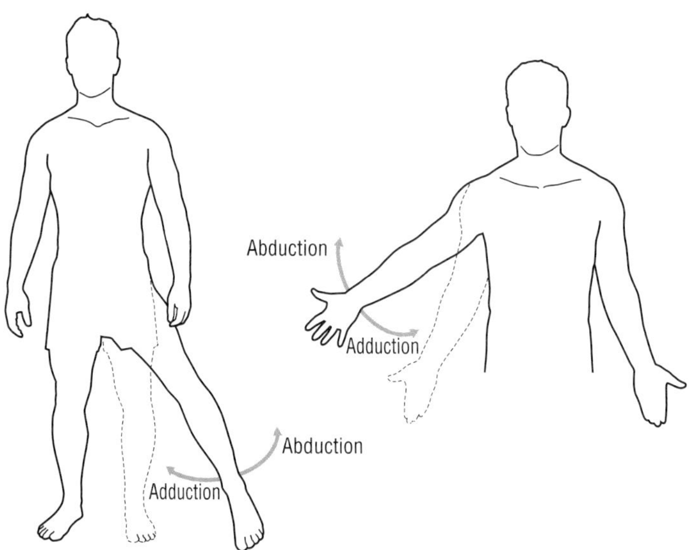

Figure 1-9 Abduction and adduction.

Inversion and Eversion

Inversion is a frontal plane motion of the foot that results in the sole of the foot facing medially; **eversion** is the opposite, resulting in the sole of the foot facing laterally (Figure 1-17).

OSTEOKINEMATICS: IT'S ALL RELATIVE

In general the articulation of two bones constitutes a joint. Movement at a joint can therefore be considered from two

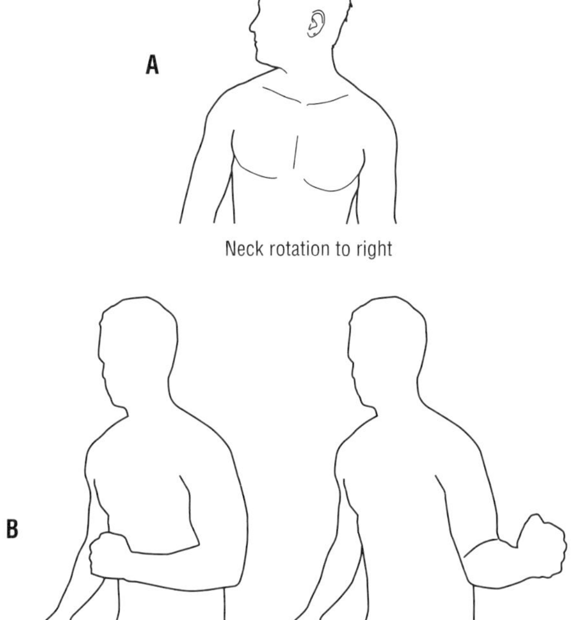

Figure 1-10 **A**, Rotation of the head and neck. **B**, Internal and external rotation of the shoulder.

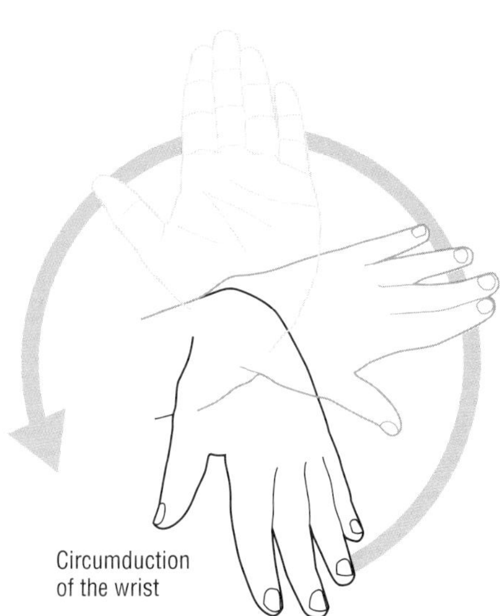

Figure 1-11 Circumduction of the wrist.

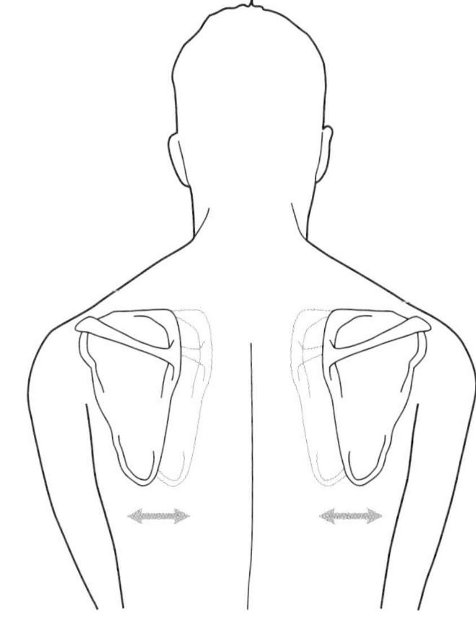

Figure 1-12 Protraction and retraction of the scapula.

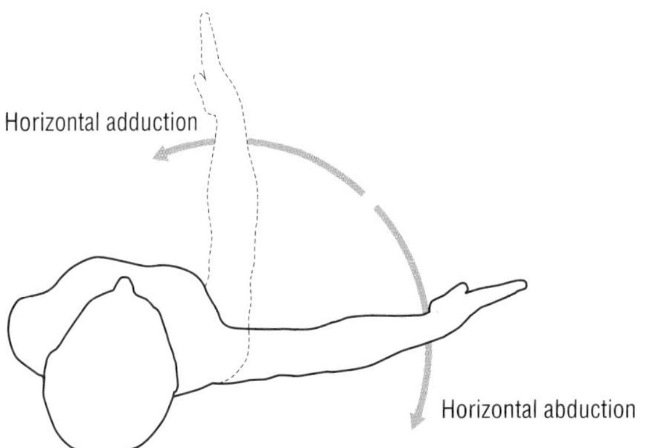

Figure 1-13 Horizontal abduction and adduction of the shoulder.

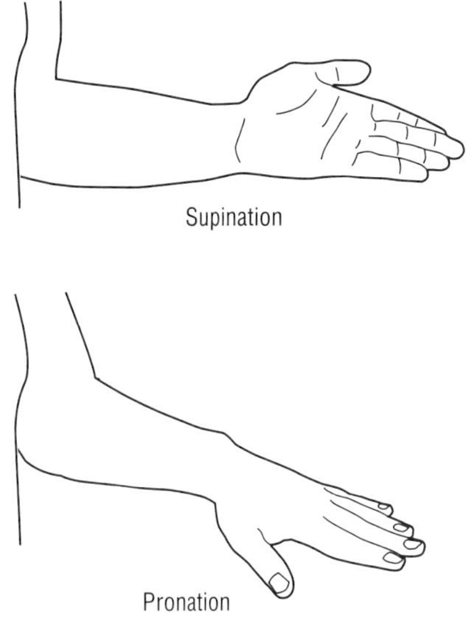

Figure 1-14 Supination and pronation of the forearm.

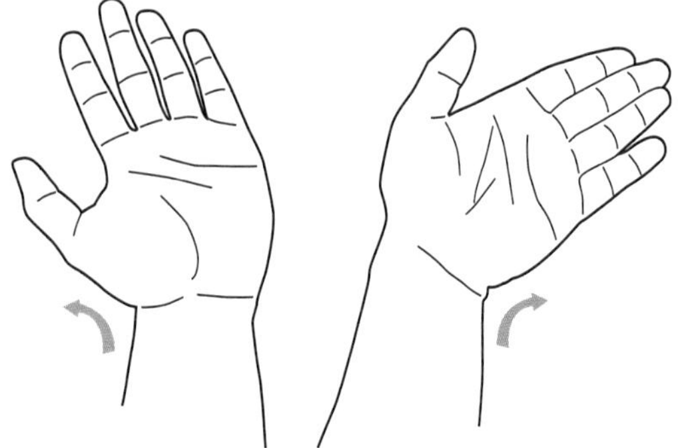

Figure 1-15 Radial and ulnar deviation of the wrist.

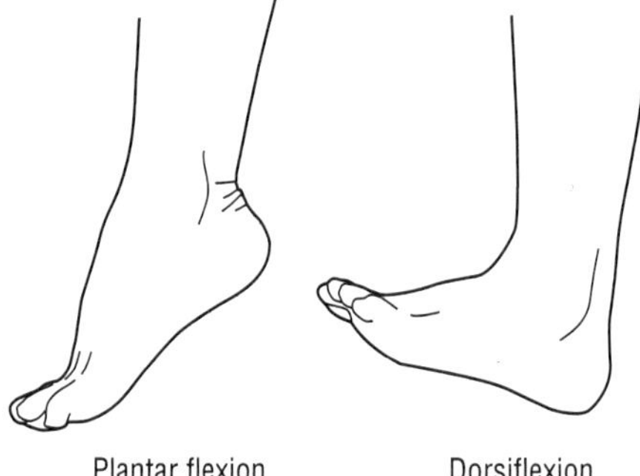

Figure 1-16 Plantar flexion and dorsiflexion of the ankle.

perspectives, depending on which bone is moving. Movement of the distal segment of bone about a relatively fixed proximal segment is often referred to as an **open-chain motion.** Conversely, movement of the proximal segment of bone about a relatively fixed, or stationary, distal segment is referred to as a **closed-chain motion.**

Figure 1-18 illustrates these two different movement perspectives for knee flexion. Figure 1-18, *A*, illustrates tibial-on-femoral flexion of the knee, indicating the tibia (distal segment) is moving on a relatively fixed femur; this is considered open-chain knee flexion. Figure 1-18, *B*, also illustrates knee flexion, but in this case the femur (proximal segment) is moving on a relatively fixed tibia (distal segment). This motion is referred to as closed-chain or femoral-on-tibial flexion of the knee.

Although these two motions appear to be different, both motions result in equal amounts of knee flexion. The only differences are which bone is moving and which bone remains stationary.

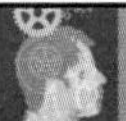

Consider this...

Open-Chain and Closed-Chain Motion

The terms *open-chain* and *closed-chain* are often used clinically to describe which bone is moving during a joint motion. *Open-chain motion* describes motion in which the distal segment of bone is moving about a relatively fixed proximal segment (Figure 1-18, *A*). *Closed-chain motion,* on the other hand, indicates movement of the proximal segment on a relatively fixed distal segment of bone (Figure 1-18, *B*).

Closed-chain exercises are widely used by physical therapists and physical therapist assistants. These types of exercises tend to be more functional in nature and capitalize on the benefits of weight bearing and the natural biomechanical advantages that closed-chain positions often provide. Open-chain motions, although not nearly as functional, are widely used therapeutically. Open-chain exercises offer an increased ability to target specific muscle groups and are easily employable through the use of weights, elastic bands, or tubing.

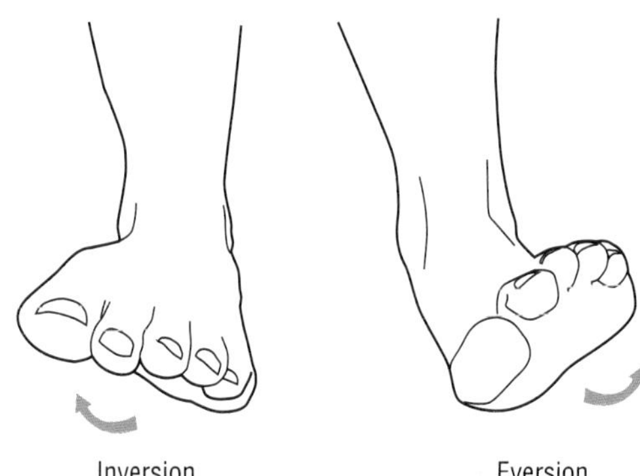

Figure 1-17 Inversion and eversion of the ankle and foot.

Arthrokinematics

Arthrokinematics describes the motion that occurs between the articular surfaces of joints. This concept differs from osteokinematics, which describes only the path of the moving bones. Consider the analogy of a bone and joint to a door and hinge. A door swings open in the horizontal plane (osteokinematics) about the spinning of a hinge (arthrokinematics).

Generally, the articular surfaces of joints are curved, with one surface being relatively concave and the other relatively convex (Figure 1-19). This concave-convex relationship of joints improves joint **congruency** (fit) and stability, thereby helping to guide motion between the bones. The motion that occurs between the articular surfaces follows specific rules depending on whether a concave articular surface is moving on a fixed convex surface or vice versa (see later discussion).

FUNDAMENTAL MOVEMENTS BETWEEN JOINT SURFACES

Three fundamental movements exist between joint surfaces: roll, slide, and spin, as follows:

1. *Roll:* Multiple points along one rotating articular surface contact multiple points on another articular surface (Figures 1-20, A, and 1-21, A). *Analogy:* A tire rotating across a stretch of pavement.
2. *Slide:* A single point on one articular surface contacts multiple points on another articular surface

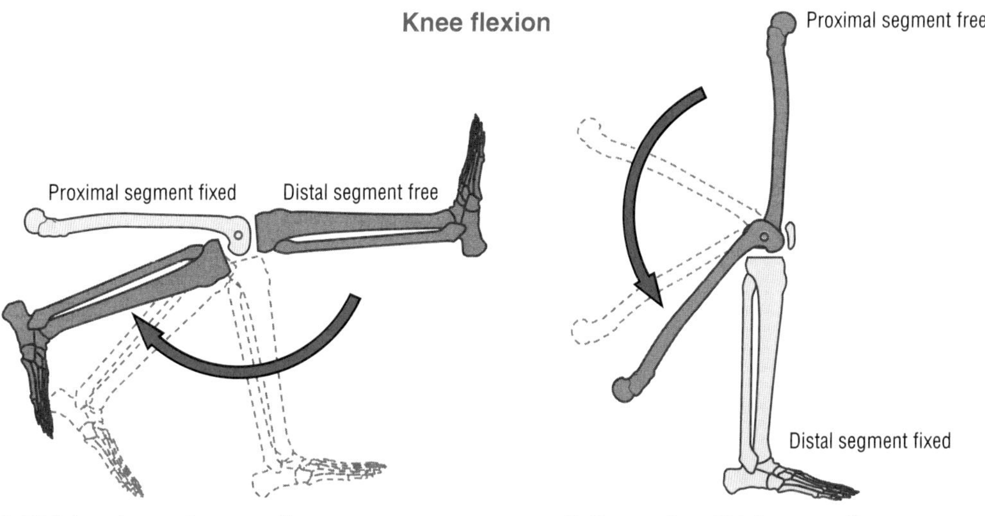

Figure 1-18 Two different ways to flex the knee. **A**, Open-chain or tibial-on-femoral flexion of the knee, **B**, Closed-chain or femoral-on-tibial flexion of the knee. (From Neumann DA: *Kinesiology of the musculoskeletal system: foundations for physical rehabilitation*, St Louis, 2002, Mosby, Figure 1-6.)

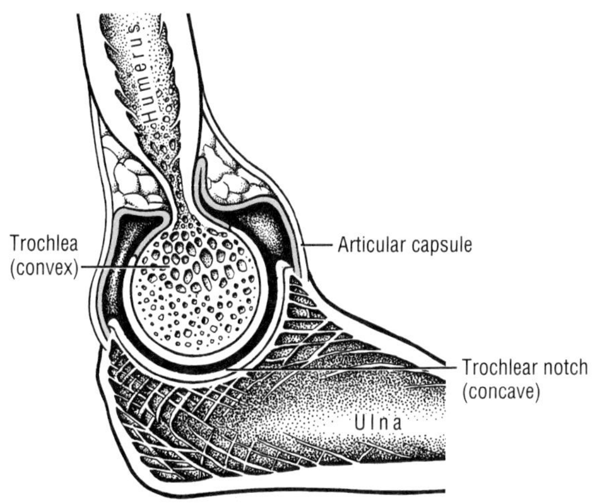

Figure 1-19 The humeroulnar (elbow) joint displaying the concave-convex relationship between articular surfaces. (From Neumann DA: *Kinesiology of the musculoskeletal system: foundations for physical rehabilitation*, St Louis, 2002, Mosby, Figure 1-7.)

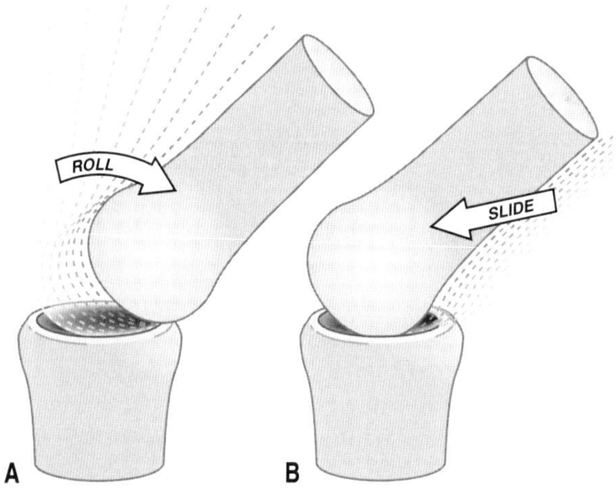

Figure 1-20 Convex-on-concave arthrokinematics. The arthrokinematic roll **(A)** and arthrokinematic slide **(B)** occur in opposite directions. (From Neumann DA: *Kinesiology of the musculoskeletal system: foundations for physical rehabilitation*, St Louis, 2002, Mosby, Figure 1-8.)

(Figures 1-20, *B*, and 1-21, *B*). *Analogy*: A stationary tire skidding across a stretch of icy pavement.

3. *Spin*: A single point on one articular surface rotates on a single point on another articular surface (Figure 1-22). *Analogy*: A rotating toy top spinning on one spot on the floor.

Roll-and-Slide Mechanics

The arthrokinematic motions that occur between articular surfaces follow specific rules. These movements, although subtle, are a necessary and healthy component of normal joint function.

> **Rule #1 Convex-on-Concave**
>
> When a convex joint surface moves on a concave joint surface, the roll and slide occur in *opposite* directions.

Figure 1-20, A, illustrates a convex joint surface rolling atop a fixed concave joint surface. Of note, however, is that the bone has literally rolled out of the joint. Figure 1-20, *B*, illustrates the opposite direction slide that would normally accompany the arthrokinematic roll. The combination of the roll and *opposite* direction slide maintains the articular stability of the joint surfaces.

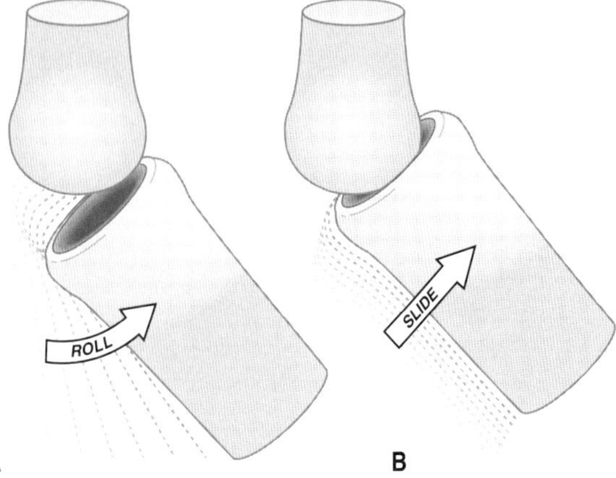

Figure 1-21 Concave-on-convex arthrokinematics. The arthrokinematic roll **(A)** and arthrokinematic slide **(B)** occur in the same direction. (From Neumann DA: *Kinesiology of the musculoskeletal system: foundations for physical rehabilitation*, St Louis, 2002, Mosby, Figure 1-8.)

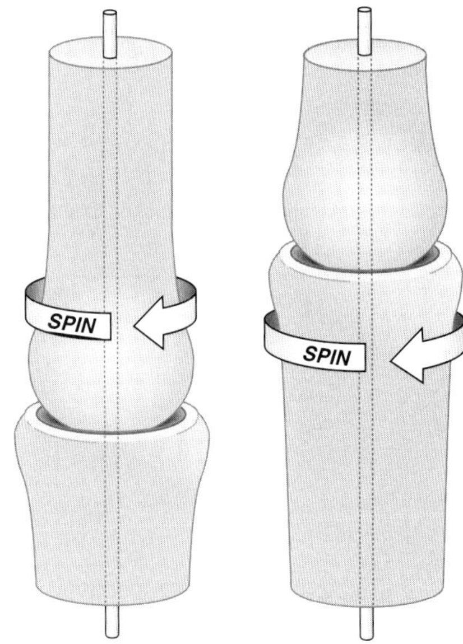

Figure 1-22 An illustration of an arthrokinematic spin. (From Neumann DA: *Kinesiology of the musculoskeletal system: foundations for physical rehabilitation*, St Louis, 2002, Mosby, Figure 1-8.)

Rule #2 Concave-on-Convex

When a concave joint surface moves about a stationary convex joint surface, the roll and slide occur in the *same* direction.

Figure 1-21, A, illustrates a concave joint surface rolling under a relatively fixed convex joint surface without an arthrokinematic slide; again this results in joint dislocation. To maintain firm contact between the articular surfaces, this motion must be accompanied by a slide in the *same* direction. As illustrated in Figure 1-21, B, this maintains proper joint alignment and congruency.

Spin Mechanics

An arthrokinematic spin occurs about a central longitudinal axis of rotation, regardless of whether a concave joint surface is spinning about its paired convex member or vice versa (see Figure 1-22). An example of an arthrokinematic spin occurs at the proximal humeroradial joint. During pronation and supination the radial head spins about its own longitudinal axis of rotation.

FUNCTIONAL CONSIDERATIONS

Normally, the arthrokinematic roll and slide between joint surfaces occurs naturally, without conscious effort, and is

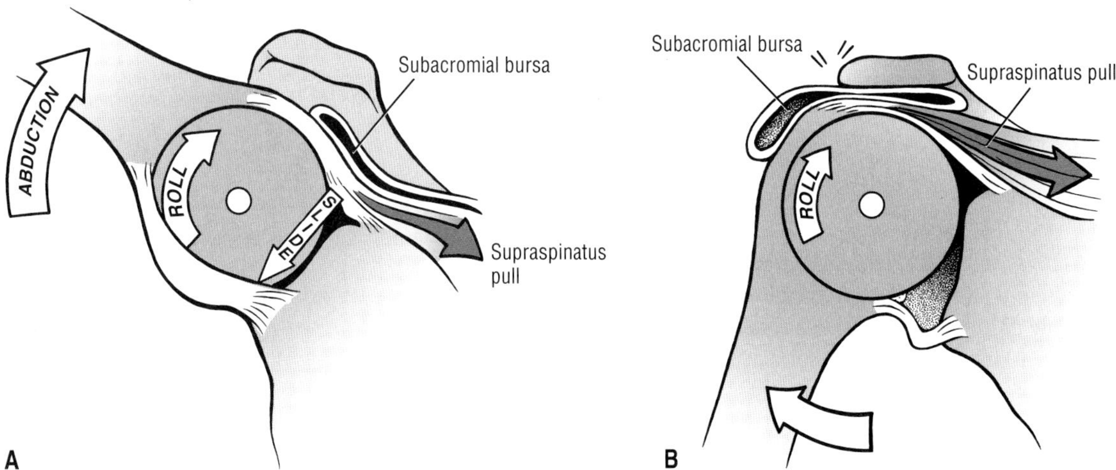

Figure 1-23 Arthrokinematics of the glenohumeral joint during shoulder abduction. **A**, Proper convex-on-concave arthrokinematic motion. The superior roll of the humeral head is offset by an inferior slide. **B**, Consequences of a superior roll occurring without an offsetting inferior slide. (From Neumann DA: *Kinesiology of the musculoskeletal system: foundations for physical rehabilitation*, St Louis, 2002, Mosby, Figure 1-9.)

integral to the proper functioning of a joint. However, for any number of reasons, the normal arthrokinematic motion of a joint may become dysfunctional. The classic example of the necessity for proper roll-and-slide arthrokinematics is the abducting shoulder (glenohumeral joint). Figure 1-23 contrasts normal versus abnormal arthrokinematic motions during glenohumeral abduction. During proper glenohumeral abduction (see Figure 1-23, *A*), the superior roll of the convex humeral head is accompanied by an inferior slide. These two opposite motions maintain the humeral head soundly within the concavity of the glenoid fossa. Figure 1-23, *B*, illustrates the consequences of a superior roll *without* an inferior slide. Without the offsetting inferior slide, the humeral head translates (rolls) upward, impinging the delicate structures within the subacromial space. This relatively common phenomenon is known as impingement syndrome and often leads to tendonitis or bursitis of the shoulder.

> **Clinical INSIGHT**
>
> **Joint Mobilization and Arthrokinematics**
>
> Clinicians often encounter patients who lack full range of motion of a joint. Although there may be many reasons for this, improper arthrokinematics may be a contributing factor. Joint mobilization is a treatment technique used by many therapists as a way to help restore normal joint motion.
>
> Figure 1-24 illustrates a physical therapist performing a joint mobilization technique to an individual who lacks full shoulder abduction. The pressure from the therapist's hands is directed inferiorly, near the proximal humerus, even though the goal of the treatment is to increase shoulder abduction. The downward pressure through the shoulder is an attempt to manually provide the inferior slide that would normally accompany the superior roll of an abducting humerus.
>
> 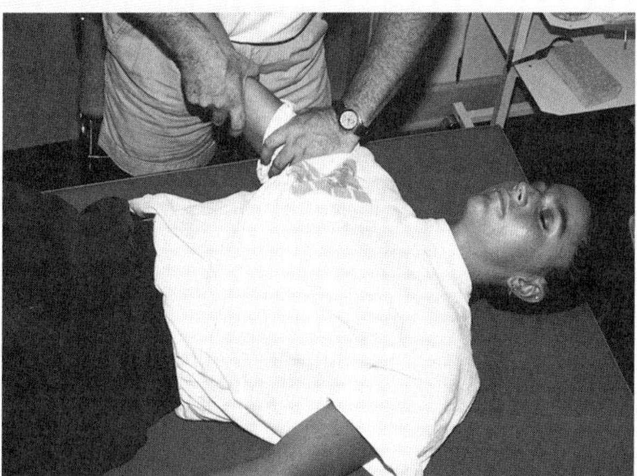
>
> **Figure 1-24** A therapist performing a joint mobilization technique to help improve shoulder abduction. Manual pressure provides the inferior slide that should normally accompany the superior roll of the humeral head. (From Shankman G: *Fundamental orthopedic management for the physical therapy assistant,* ed 2, St Louis, 2004, Mosby, Figure 22-38.)

Kinetics

Kinetics is a branch of mechanics that describes the effect of forces on the body. From a kinesiologic perspective, a **force** can be considered a push or pull that can produce, modify, or halt a movement. Forces therefore provide the ultimate impetus for movement and stabilization of the body.

In regard to body movement, forces can be classified as either internal or external (Figure 1-25). **Internal forces** are forces generated from within the body. Generally, these are active forces generated by muscular contraction, but many times passive internal forces such as tension generated from ligamentous or muscular elongation must be considered as well. **External forces** are forces originating from outside the body. Examples of this include gravity, an external load such as a suitcase or a barbell, or a therapist applying resistance to a movement.

Torque

Torque can be considered the rotational equivalent of force. Because nearly all joint motions occur about an axis of rotation, the internal and external forces acting at a joint are expressed as a torque. The amount of torque generated across a joint depends on two things: (1) the amount of force exerted and (2) the distance between the force and the axis of rotation. This distance, called the moment arm, is the length between the axis of rotation and the perpendicular intersection of the force. The product of a force and its moment arm is equal to the torque (or rotational force) generated about an axis of rotation.

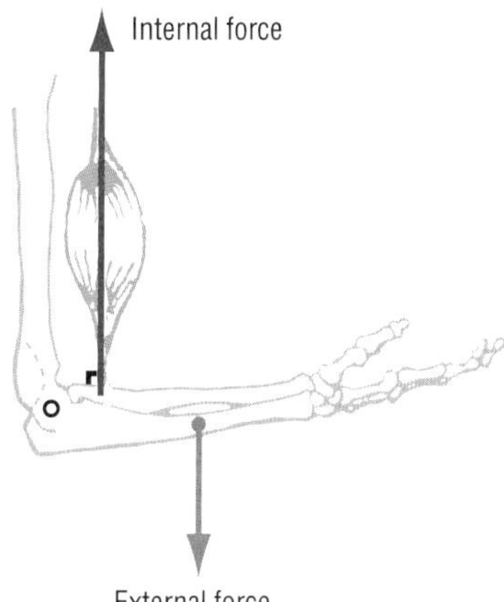

Figure 1-25 A sagittal plane view of the upper extremity illustrating the internal force provided by the biceps and the external force provided by gravity. (From Neumann DA: *Kinesiology of the musculoskeletal system: foundations for physical rehabilitation,* St Louis, 2002, Mosby, Figure 1-16, *A*.)

Force × Moment arm = Torque
Muscular force × Internal moment arm = Internal torque
External force × External moment arm = External torque

Torques generated from internal forces such as muscle are called **internal torques**, whereas torques generated from external forces such as gravity are called **external torques** (Figure 1-26). Movement of the body or a body segment is the result of the competition between the internal and external torques about a joint.

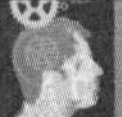

Consider this...

Strength

Measuring a person's strength really measures an individual's torque production. Torque considers not only muscular force, but also the length of the moment arm used by a particular muscle or muscle group. Both factors are equally important in determining an individual's functional strength.

Clinicians often perform manual muscle tests to objectify an individual's strength. Because force production and the corresponding internal moment arm of a muscle are highly dependent on muscular length and joint angle, standard-specific-positions (joint angles) are used in order to obtain more reliable measurements.

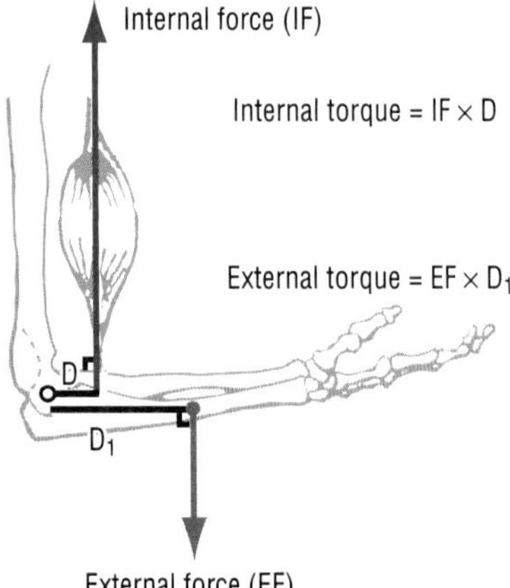

Figure 1-26 The internal and external torques produced about the medial-lateral axis of rotation of the elbow. The internal torque is the product of the internal force (provided by the biceps) multiplied by the internal moment arm (*D*). The external torque is the product of the external force (gravity) multiplied by the external moment arm (D_1). (Modified from Neumann DA: *Kinesiology of the musculoskeletal system: foundations for physical rehabilitation,* St Louis, 2002, Mosby, Figure 1-17.)

Biomechanical Levers

The interaction of internal and external forces ultimately controls our movement and posture. As described earlier, internal forces usually arise from muscular activation, whereas external forces arise from gravity or other external sources. These competing forces interact through a system of bony levers, with the pivot point, or fulcrum, located at the axis of rotation of our joints. Through these systems of levers, the internal and external forces are converted to internal and external torques, ultimately causing movement—or rotation—of the joints.

THREE CLASSES OF LEVERS

Three classes of levers exist: first, second, and third. Although the concept of a lever was originally defined for the design of tools, this concept applies to the musculoskeletal system as well. Figure 1-27 shows examples of the three types of lever systems used in the body.

First-Class Levers

The first-class lever is similar to a see-saw, with its axis of rotation (or fulcrum) located between the internal and external force, as exemplified by the neck extensor muscle acting to support the weight of the head (see Figure 1-27, *A*). Note that the muscular forces act about an **internal moment arm** (IMA); gravity (acting at the center of mass of the head), in contrast, acts with an **external moment arm** (EMA). These moment arms convert the forces into rotary torques.

Second-Class Levers

Second-class levers have an axis of rotation located at one end of the bony lever and always have an IMA that is *longer* than the EMA. This lever system is often said to provide "good **leverage**" because a relatively small force is able to lift a much larger external load. Figure 1-27, *B*, compares the plantar flexors to a wheelbarrow as an example of a second-class lever system. Because of the good leverage provided by the second-class lever, the weight of the body is more easily elevated by a relatively small force produced by the plantar flexor muscles.

Third-Class Levers

Third-class levers also have an axis of rotation located at one end of the bony lever. However, they always have an IMA that is *smaller* than the EMA (see Figure 1-27, C). In third-class biomechanical lever systems, gravity has more leverage than muscle. In other words, a relatively large muscular force is required to lift a relatively small external load.

BIOMECHANICAL LEVERS: DESIGNED FOR FORCE, OR SPEED AND RANGE OF MOTION?

Musculoskeletal lever systems that have larger IMAs than EMAs (e.g., second-class levers) are said to provide good leverage—or favor force—because small muscular (internal) forces are able to move larger external loads. In contrast, levers that have smaller IMAs than EMAs (e.g., third-class levers) favor speed and distance, meaning that the distal end of the bone (like the hand relative to the elbow) moves at a greater distance and speed than the contracting muscle. Any lever system that favors speed and distance does so at the expense of demanding increased muscle force. Conversely, any lever system that favors force does so at the expense of decreased distance and speed of the distal end of the lever. (Realize that first-class levers can function similar to a second- or third-class lever, depending on the precise location of the fulcrum.) Table 1-2 compares the biomechanical advantages and disadvantages of first-, second-, and third-class lever systems.

Depending on mechanical need, certain joint systems of the body are designed as first-, second-, or third-class levers. Muscle and joint systems that require great speed and displacement of the distal end of the bone are usually designed as third-class levers (see Figure 1-27, *C*). In contrast, muscle and joint systems that may benefit from a force advantage (as opposed to a speed and distance advantage) are usually designed as second-class levers (see Figure 1-27, *B*).

The overwhelming majority of bony lever systems in the body are designed as third-class levers. This is necessary because it is usually essential that the distal ends of our limbs move faster than our muscles can physiologically contract. For example, the biceps may be able to contract at a speed of only 4 inches per second, but the hand would be vertically displaced at speeds greater than 2 feet per second. (The reverse situation is not only impractical but physiologically impossible.) Great speed and distance of the hand and foot are necessary to impart large power or thrust against objects, as well as for rapid advancement of the foot during walking and running.

As stated, because most biomechanical lever systems in the body are third-class levers, most of the time a muscle must exert a force greater than the load being lifted. The muscle is usually willing to pay a high "force tax" in order to favor speed and distance of the distal point of the lever. The joint, however, must be able to tolerate the high force tax by being able to disperse large muscular forces that are transferred through the articular and bony surfaces. This explains why most joints are lined with relatively thick articular cartilage, have bursae, and contain synovial fluid. Without these elements, the high forces produced by most muscles would likely lead to excessive wear and tear of the ligaments, tendons, and bones composing a joint—possibly leading to joint degeneration or osteoarthritis.

Line of Pull

A muscle's **line of pull**, sometimes called the line of force, describes the direction of muscular force, typically represented as a vector. The relationship between a muscle's line of pull and the axis of rotation of a joint determines

First-class lever

IMA EMA

MF

HW

A

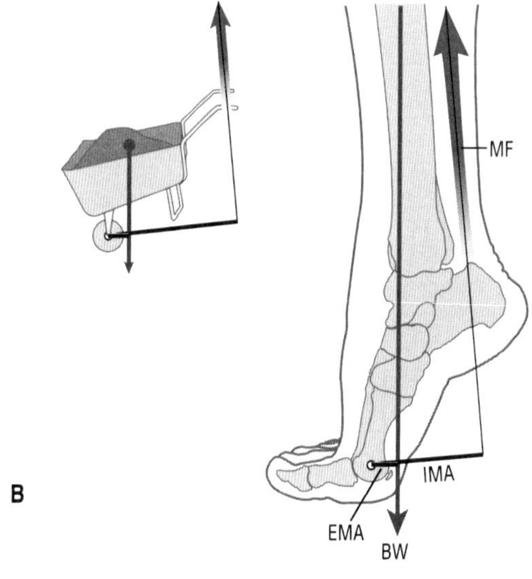

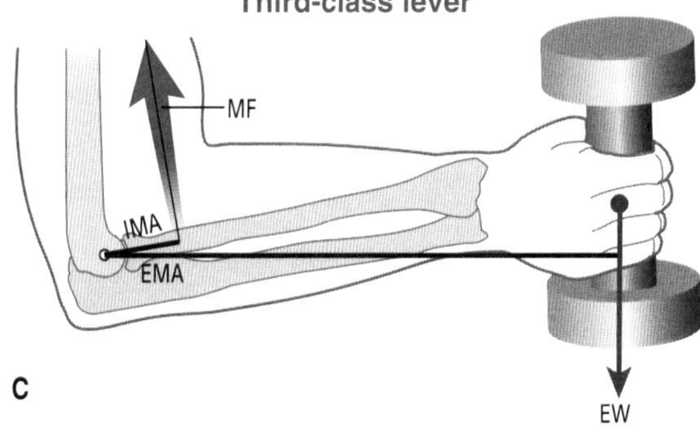

Figure 1-27 Anatomic examples are shown displaying first-class **(A)**, second-class **(B)**, and third-class **(C)** lever systems. Note that the small open circles represent the axis of rotation at each joint. *BW,* Body weight; *EMA,* external moment arm; *EW,* external weight; *HW,* head weight; *IMA,* internal moment arm; *MF,* muscle force. (From Neumann DA: *Kinesiology of the musculoskeletal system: Foundations for physical rehabilitation,* St Louis, 2002, Mosby, Figure 1-22.)

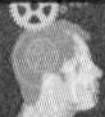

Consider this...

Selecting the Best Muscle for the Job: Biceps versus Brachioradialis

Even though most musculoskeletal lever systems in the body function as third-class levers, the muscles that operate these levers are uniquely different and therefore possess different sizes of internal moment arms (IMAs). A certain muscle therefore may be slightly better designed to favor force or speed and distance, even though both are third-class levers.

Figure 1-28 illustrates this concept by comparing two different elbow flexors: the biceps and the brachioradialis. Both muscles are shown supporting a 10-lb weight held 15 inches away from the axis of the elbow. In order to support the weight, each muscle must produce an internal torque of 150 inch-lbs. Because the IMA of the biceps is only 1 inch, the biceps must produce 150 lb of force to support the weight (see Figure 1-28, *A*). The larger 3-inch IMA of the brachioradialis, however, has a more favorable force advantage—requiring only 50 lb of force to support the same weight (see Figure 1-28, *B*).

Figure 1-29 further compares these two muscles in regard to speed and distance. As illustrated, a 1-inch contraction of the biceps results in a 15-inch lift of the hand (see Figure 1-29, *A*), whereas the brachioradialis (also contracting 1 inch) lifts the hand just 5 inches—one third the distance (see Figure 1-29, *B*). If both muscles were contracting at the same speed, the biceps would be elevating the hand (and weight) three times faster than the brachioradialis. Clearly, the biceps muscle has the advantage in regard to displacement and speed of the held object, and the brachioradialis has the advantage in terms of requiring less force.

Interestingly, the nervous system can determine and activate the most efficient muscle for the job, depending on whether force or speed and range of motion is most needed for the task at hand.

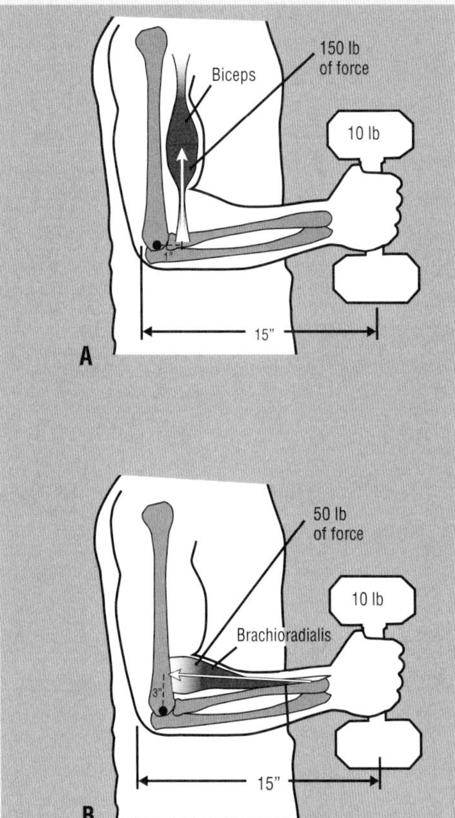

Figure 1-28 An illustration of two different elbow flexor muscles functioning as third-class levers but possessing different-length internal moment arms (IMAs). The small IMA of the biceps **(A)** requires three times the amount of muscular force as the brachioradialis **(B)** to lift the same external weight. The threefold force advantage of the brachioradialis is based on its threefold greater length in IMA.

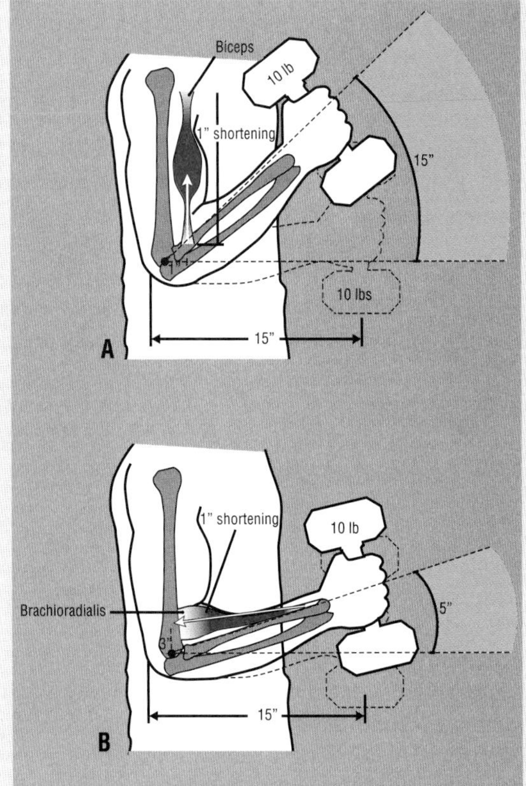

Figure 1-29 This illustration highlights the difference in speed and distance of the distal end of the forearm resulting from the same amount of shortening from two muscles with different moment arm lengths. The 1 inch of muscular shortening (contraction) of the biceps results in lifting the external weight 15 inches upward, **A**. In contrast, 1 inch of shortening of the brachioradialis results in only a 5-inch lift of the external weight **(B)**.

TABLE 1-2 BIOMECHANICAL ADVANTAGES AND DISADVANTAGES OF LEVER SYSTEMS

Lever Class	Advantages	Disadvantages	Examples
First	Mixed: depends on placement of axis	Mixed: depends on placement of axis	Upper trapezius muscle extending the head Seesaw
Second	Allows functions to be carried out with relatively small amounts of muscle force	Distal end of lever moves slower than the muscle shortens (contracts)	Gastrocnemius plantar flexing the ankle (standing on tiptoes) Wheelbarrow
Third	Favors greater displacement (range of motion) and speed of the distal end of the lever	Requires proportionally greater muscle force	Biceps flexing the elbow Quadriceps extending the knee

the action or actions that a particular muscle can produce. The beauty of analyzing a muscle's line of pull is that it allows the student or clinician to figure out the various actions of any muscle in the body, instead of relying solely on memorization. Consider the following examples that highlight muscles of the shoulder.

LINE OF PULL ABOUT A MEDIAL-LATERAL AXIS OF ROTATION

Muscles with a line of pull anterior to the medial-lateral axis of rotation of a joint will produce flexion in the sagittal plane. Consider, for example, the anterior deltoid, depicted in red in Figure 1-30, *A*. Conversely, a line of pull that courses posterior to the medial-lateral axis of rotation, such as the posterior deltoid, produces extension in the sagittal plane (Figure 1-30, *B*).

LINE OF PULL ABOUT AN ANTERIOR-POSTERIOR AXIS OF ROTATION

Muscles with a line of pull passing superior or lateral to the anterior-posterior axis of rotation at a joint will produce abduction in the frontal plane. Consider, for example, the middle deltoid, depicted in red in Figure 1-31, *A*. In contrast, a muscle such as the teres major, depicted in red in Figure 1-31, *B*, has a line of pull that courses inferior and medially relative to the anterior-posterior axis of rotation. This line of pull produces adduction in the frontal plane.

LINE OF PULL ABOUT A VERTICAL AXIS OF ROTATION

Muscles often wrap around bones, making it difficult to cite a specific direction to their line of pull. This is especially evident when referring to muscles that function about a vertical axis of rotation. However, once you know the line of pull of a muscle relative to a vertical axis of rotation, its function is relatively easy to predict. Consider, for example, the anterior deltoid, depicted in red in Figure 1-32, *A*. This muscle produces internal rotation about a vertical axis. In contrast, the posterior deltoid, depicted in red in Figure 1-32, *B*, has a line of pull that produces external rotation of the shoulder.

Vectors

Vectors are used in kinesiology to represent the magnitude and direction of a force. The magnitude of the force is indicated by the relative length of the vector line, and the direction is indicated by the orientation of the arrowhead. Figure 1-33 illustrates two different force vectors in red that represent two different muscles pulling on the same bone. The combined force of these two muscular vectors produces the **resultant force** (indicated by the black arrow). The resultant force can literally be viewed as the result of combining the individual force vectors. Because in this example each vector is equal, the resultant vector is directed exactly between the middle of the two composite vectors, similar to two people with equal strength pulling an object with ropes (see Figure 1-33, *B*). In the study of kinesiology, however, muscles that produce an action are often not equally matched, both in terms of strength and their line of pull. In the case of an unequal pair of muscular forces, the resultant force (and subsequent movement) will be distorted and pulled toward the stronger muscle (Figure 1-34, *A*). Similar to the analogy in Figure 1-34, *B*, the object will be pulled toward the side with two people because there is twice as much force.

In kinesiology, vectors are often used to study the effect of several muscles pulling in multiple directions. For example, the anterior and posterior deltoids have opposite directed lines of pull (vectors) but nearly equal force potential. Clinically it is not uncommon to see such a balanced

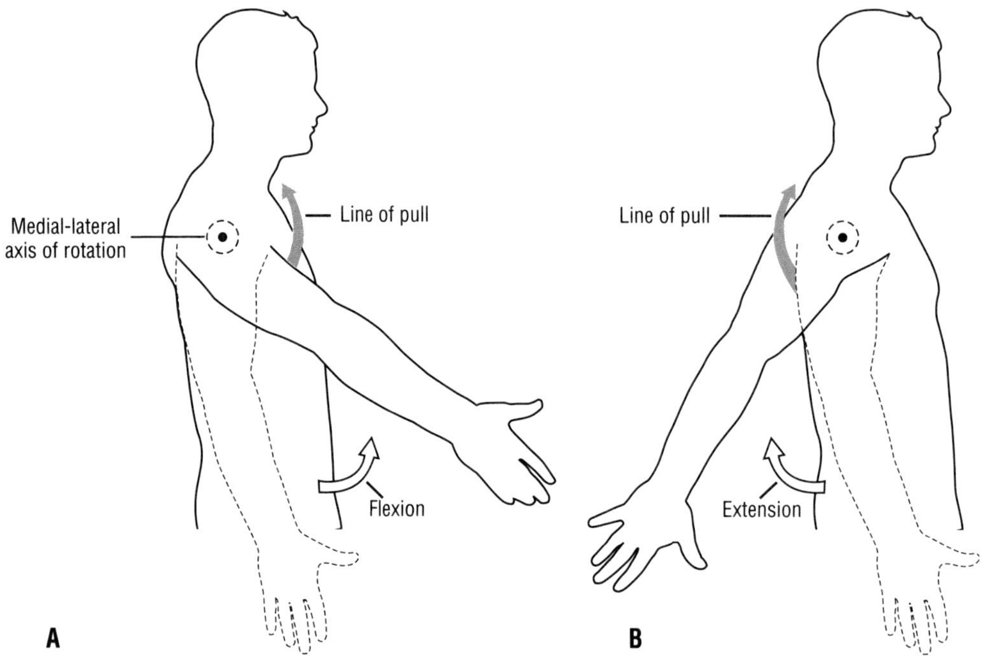

Figure 1-30 Lines of pull about a medial-lateral axis of rotation producing the sagittal plane motions of **(A)** flexion and **(B)** extension.

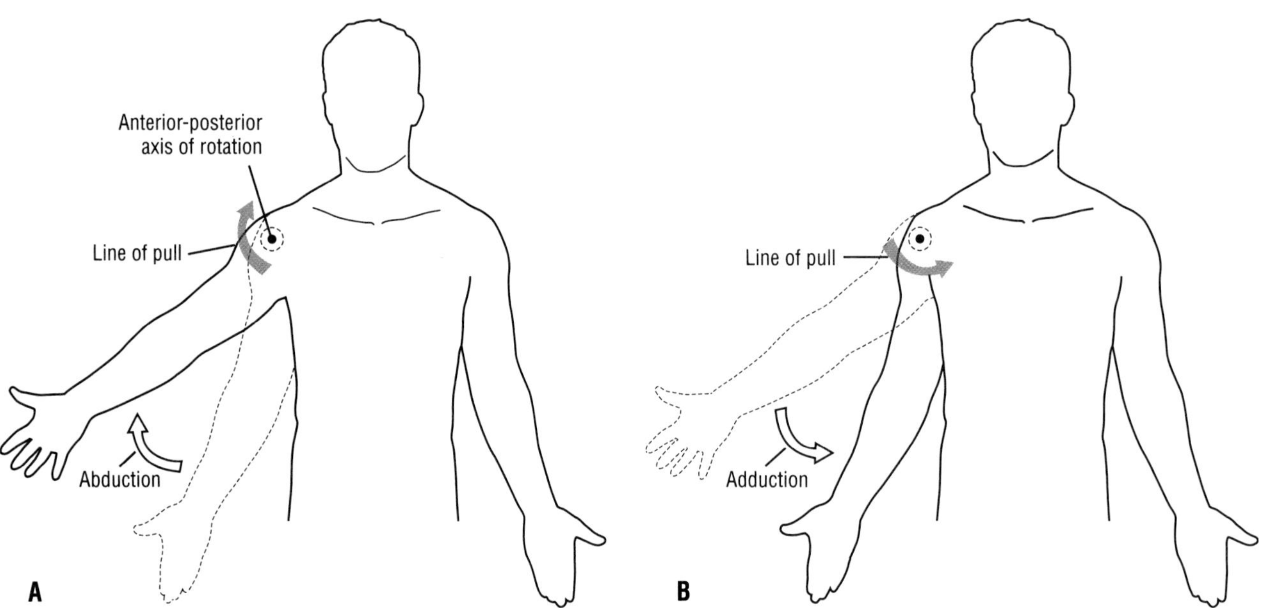

Figure 1-31 Lines of pull about an anterior-posterior axis of rotation producing the frontal plane motions of **(A)** abduction and **(B)** adduction.

muscular system such as this become upset. For example, if the posterior deltoid is weakened from injury or disease, the anterior deltoid muscle takes on a much more dominant role in the forces produced during shoulder movement. As a consequence, shoulder motion would be pulled toward the stronger muscle; in this case, the anterior deltoid. Clinicians must carefully observe movements of their patients in order to detect potential asymmetry in muscle forces. Over time, an individual's posture may become biased toward the stronger muscle group, which can lead to a painful and dysfunctional disruption in the kinesiology throughout the entire region.

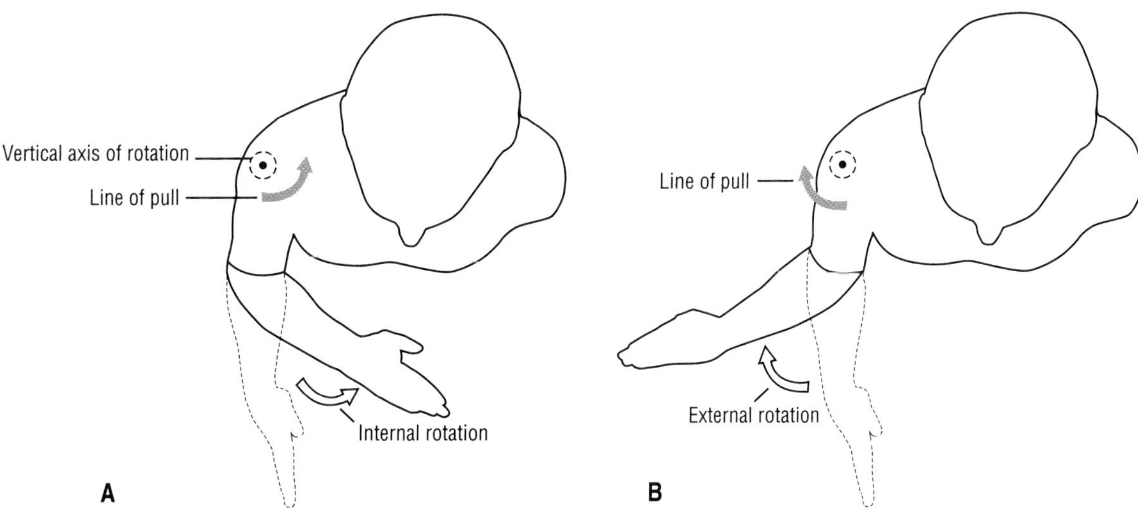

Figure 1-32 Lines of pull about a vertical axis of rotation producing the horizontal plane motions of **(A)** internal rotation and **(B)** external rotation.

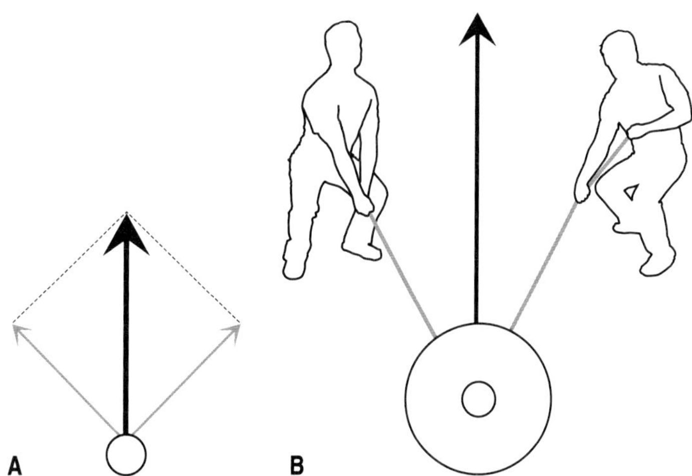

Figure 1-33 **A,** Two equal force vectors *(red)* producing a resultant *(black)*. **B,** An analogy of two equal force vectors resulting in motion of a load exactly between the two vectors.

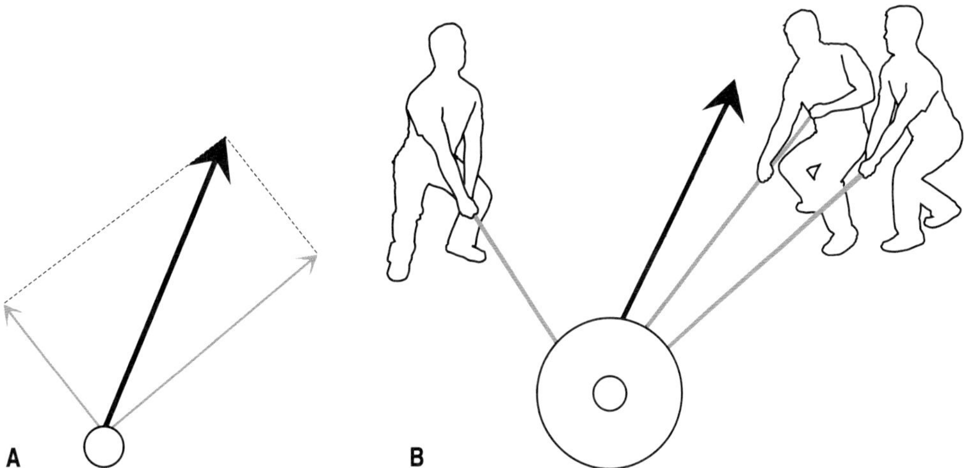

Figure 1-34 **A,** Two unequal force vectors *(red)* with the resultant *(black)* biased toward the stronger vector quantity. **B,** An analogy that shows the resultant force being pulled to the strong side.

Summary

In kinesiology the body may be viewed as a biologic machine that rotates bony levers, powered by muscules. Some of these musculoskeletal levers are designed to produce large torques, whereas others are designed for producing high speeds or covering large distances.

Although the body, or a body segment, rarely moves in a straight plane, movements are described relative to the three cardinal planes. The active motions of the body—powered by muscle—are determined by the muscle's line of pull relative to the axis of rotation of a joint. A large portion of this text will focus on the various functions of muscle, based on an understanding of this concept.

The motion that occurs at a joint follows specific (arthrokinematic) rules that help guide bony movement and stabilize the joint as the distal segment of the joint moves through various planes of motion. Other factors such as bony conformation and ligamentous support determine the available motion (degrees of freedom) of the limb or body segment.

Although this text will discuss the kinesiology of individual joints and regions of the body, our study of kinesiology focuses on the application of the form and function of the musculoskeletal system. Very rarely does a single muscle act in isolation, and rarely does movement at one joint occur without affecting another. The principles discussed in this first chapter should become increasingly meaningful as they are applied to the various joints and regions of the body.

Study Questions

1. Which of the following motions occurs around a medial-lateral axis of rotation?
   a. Shoulder abduction
   b. Knee flexion
   c. Shoulder extension
   d. A and B
   e. B and C
2. Which of the following lever systems is most commonly used by the musculoskeletal system?
   a. First class
   b. Second class
   c. Third class
3. When a convex member of a joint is moving over a relatively stationary concave member, the arthrokinematic roll and slide occur:
   a. In the same direction
   b. In opposite directions
4. Which of the following terms describes the proximal attachment of a muscle?
   a. Caudal
   b. Insertion
   c. Cephalad
   d. Origin
   e. A and B
5. Which of the following lever systems *always* provides good leverage, allowing an external load to be lifted with comparatively less muscular force?
   a. First class
   b. Second class
   c. Third class
6. The torque generated by a muscle is calculated by:
   a. Dividing the muscular force by the internal moment arm
   b. Multiplying the muscular force by the external moment arm
   c. Dividing the muscular force by the external moment arm
   d. Multiplying the muscular force by the internal moment arm
7. A closed-chain motion:
   a. Always provides larger ranges of motion than an open-chain motion
   b. Occurs when the distal segment of the joint moves relative to a stationary proximal segment
   c. Occurs when the proximal segment of a joint moves relative to a fixed distal segment
   d. Is typically not used when treating a patient
8. The shoulder is __________ to the elbow.
   a. Caudal
   b. Proximal
   c. Distal
   d. Deep
   e. A and B
9. Internal rotation of the shoulder occurs about a(n) __________ axis of rotation.
   a. Anterior-posterior
   b. Medial-lateral
   c. Longitudinal (or vertical)
   d. Reciprocal
10. The term *osteokinematics* describes the:
    a. Motion between joint surfaces
    b. Motion of bones relative to the three cardinal planes
    c. Forces transferred from muscles through joints
    d. Force of a muscle contraction acting on an internal moment arm
11. Which of the following statements is true?
    a. The proximal attachment of a muscle is known as the insertion.
    b. A vector is a representation of a force's magnitude and direction.
    c. Flexion of the hip occurs in the frontal plane.
    d. A *closed-chain motion* refers to the distal segment of a joint moving on a relatively fixed proximal segment.
12. Second-class lever systems favor range of motion and speed.
    a. True
    b. False

CONTENTS

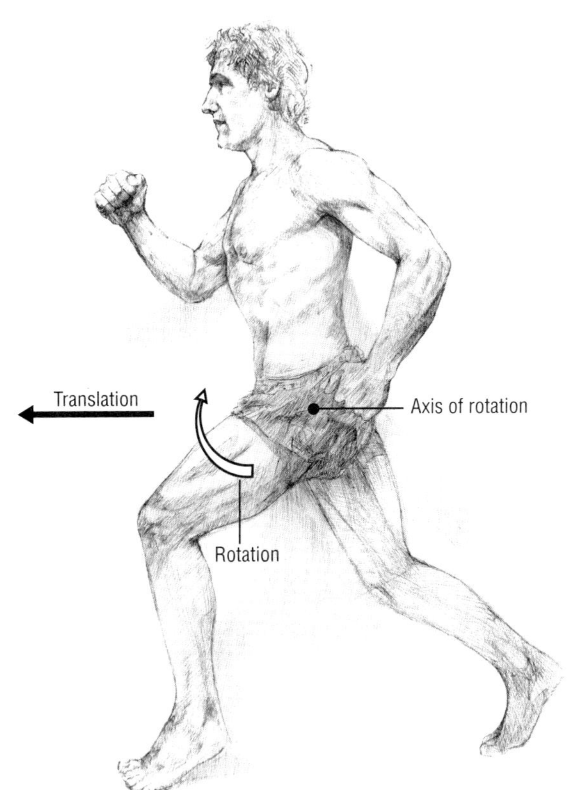

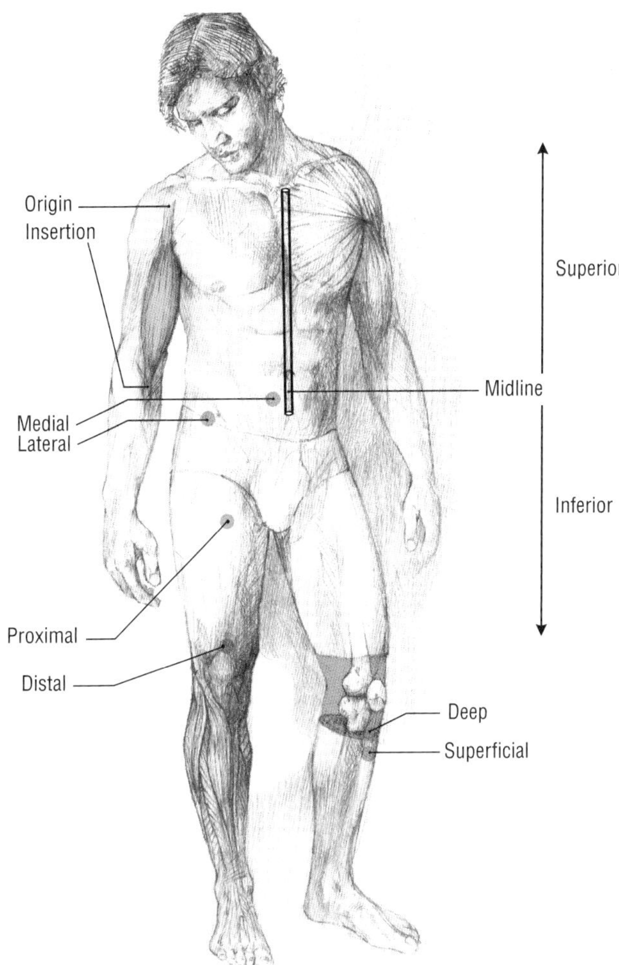

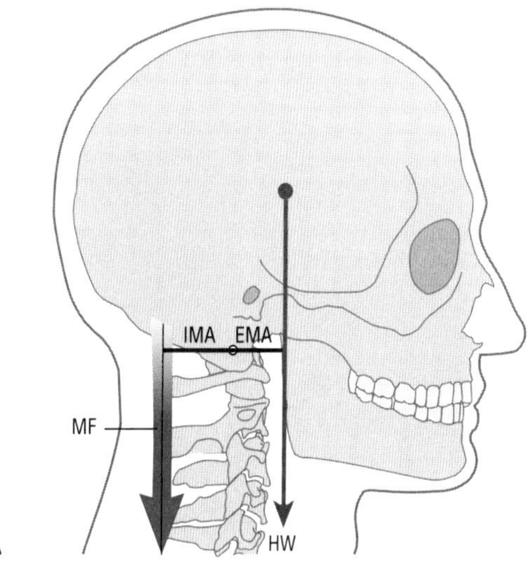

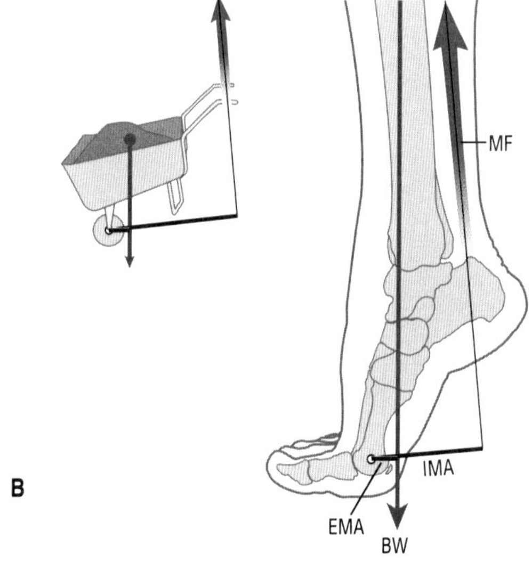

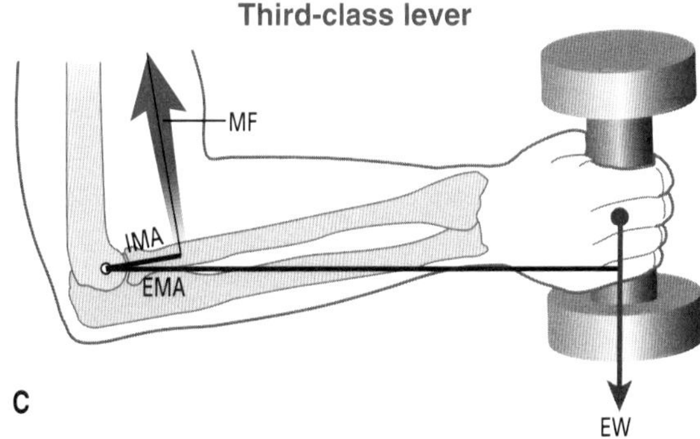

13. Which of the following movements occur in the frontal plane?
    a. Shoulder adduction
    b. Hip flexion
    c. Pronation of the forearm
    d. A and C
    e. B and C
14. Which of the following movements occur about a longitudinal or vertical axis of rotation?
    a. Internal rotation of the shoulder
    b. Extension of the shoulder
    c. Flexion of the hip
    d. Abduction of the hip
15. Which of the following movements occur in the sagittal plane?
    a. Extension of the hip
    b. Flexion of the shoulder
    c. Internal rotation of the shoulder
    d. A and B
    e. All of the above
16. Which of the following movements occur about an anterior-posterior axis of rotation?
    a. Extension of the hip
    b. Supination of the forearm
    c. Abduction of the hip
    d. Internal rotation of the shoulder
17. Based on a front view of the shoulder, which motion will occur by a muscular line of pull that courses lateral and superior to the anterior-posterior axis of rotation?
    a. Shoulder abduction
    b. Shoulder flexion
    c. Shoulder internal rotation
    d. Plantar flexion
18. Which of the following motions occurs about a vertical axis of rotation?
    a. Internal rotation of the shoulder
    b. External rotation of the shoulder
    c. Rotation of the head and neck
    d. A and B
    e. All of the above
19. Which of the above motions would be produced by a muscular line of pull that courses anterior to the medial-lateral axis of rotation?
    a. Hip flexion
    b. Shoulder extension
    c. Plantar flexion
    d. Shoulder adduction
20. The shoulder adductor muscles are antagonists to
    a. Shoulder abductors
    b. Shoulder flexors
    c. Shoulder extensors
    d. Shoulder internal rotators
21. Third-class levers favor range of motion and speed over force.
    a. True
    b. False
22. A muscle that courses anterior to a medial-lateral axis of rotation will produce motion in the sagittal plane.
    a. True
    b. False
23. The term *strength* refers solely to the force that a muscle can produce, not its torque production.
    a. True
    b. False
24. A *resultant force* refers to the amount of force that is lost because of tissue elasticity.
    a. True
    b. False
25. A first-class lever *always* favors force over range of motion.
    a. True
    b. False
26. *Passive movements* refer to forces that produce body movement other than that caused by muscular activation.
    a. True
    b. False
27. A joint that allows 2 degrees of freedom is likely to permit volitional motion in all three planes.
    a. True
    b. False
28. A joint must allow motion in at least two planes in order for it to circumduct.
    a. True
    b. False
29. A motion such as flexing and extending the elbow with the hand free is an example of a closed-chain motion.
    a. True
    b. False
30. When a convex joint surface moves about a stationary concave joint surface, the arthrokinematic roll and slide occur in the same direction.
    a. True
    b. False

ADDITIONAL READINGS

Greene D, Roberts S: *Kinesiology: movement in the context of activity*, ed 2, St Louis, 2005, Mosby.

Mosby's medical dictionary, ed 7, Philadelphia, 2005, Mosby.

Neumann D: *Kinesiology of the musculoskeletal system: foundations for physical rehabilitation*, St Louis, 2002, Mosby.

Rasch P: *Kinesiology and applied anatomy*, Philadelphia, 1989, Lea & Febiger.

Smith LK, Weiss EL, Lehmkuhl LD: *Brunnstrom's clinical kinesiology*, Philadelphia, 1983, FA Davis.

Wirhed R: *Athletic ability and the anatomy of motion*, ed 3, St Louis, 2007, Mosby.

CHAPTER 2

Structure and Function of Joints

CHAPTER OUTLINE

OBJECTIVES

- Describe the components of the axial versus appendicular skeleton.
- Define the primary components found in bone.
- Describe the five types of bones found in the human skeleton.
- Describe the three primary classifications of joints and give an anatomic example of each.
- Identify the components of a synovial joint.
- Describe the seven different classifications of synovial joints in terms of mobility (degrees of freedom) and stability.
- Provide an anatomic example of each of the seven different classifications of synovial joints.
- Describe the three primary materials found in connective tissue.
- Explain how tendons and ligaments support the structure of a joint.
- Explain how muscles help to stabilize a joint.
- Describe the effects of immobilization on the connective tissues of a joint.

KEY TERMS

amphiarthrosis
appendicular skeleton
articular cartilage
axial skeleton
cancellous bone
cortical (compact) bone
diaphysis
endosteum
epiphyses
medullary canal
periosteum
synarthrosis

A joint is the articulation, or junction, between two or more bones that acts as a pivot point for bony movement. Motion of the entire body or a particular body segment generally occurs through the rotation of bones about individual joints. The specific anatomic features of a joint play a large role in determining its range of motion, degrees of freedom, and overall functional potential. This chapter is intended to provide an overview of the basic structure and function of joints as a foundation for understanding the motion of individual body segments and the body as a whole.

Axial versus Appendicular Skeleton

The bones of the skeletal system can be grouped into two categories: the appendicular skeleton and the axial skeleton. The **axial skeleton** consists of the skull, hyoid bone, sternum, ribs, and vertebral column, including the

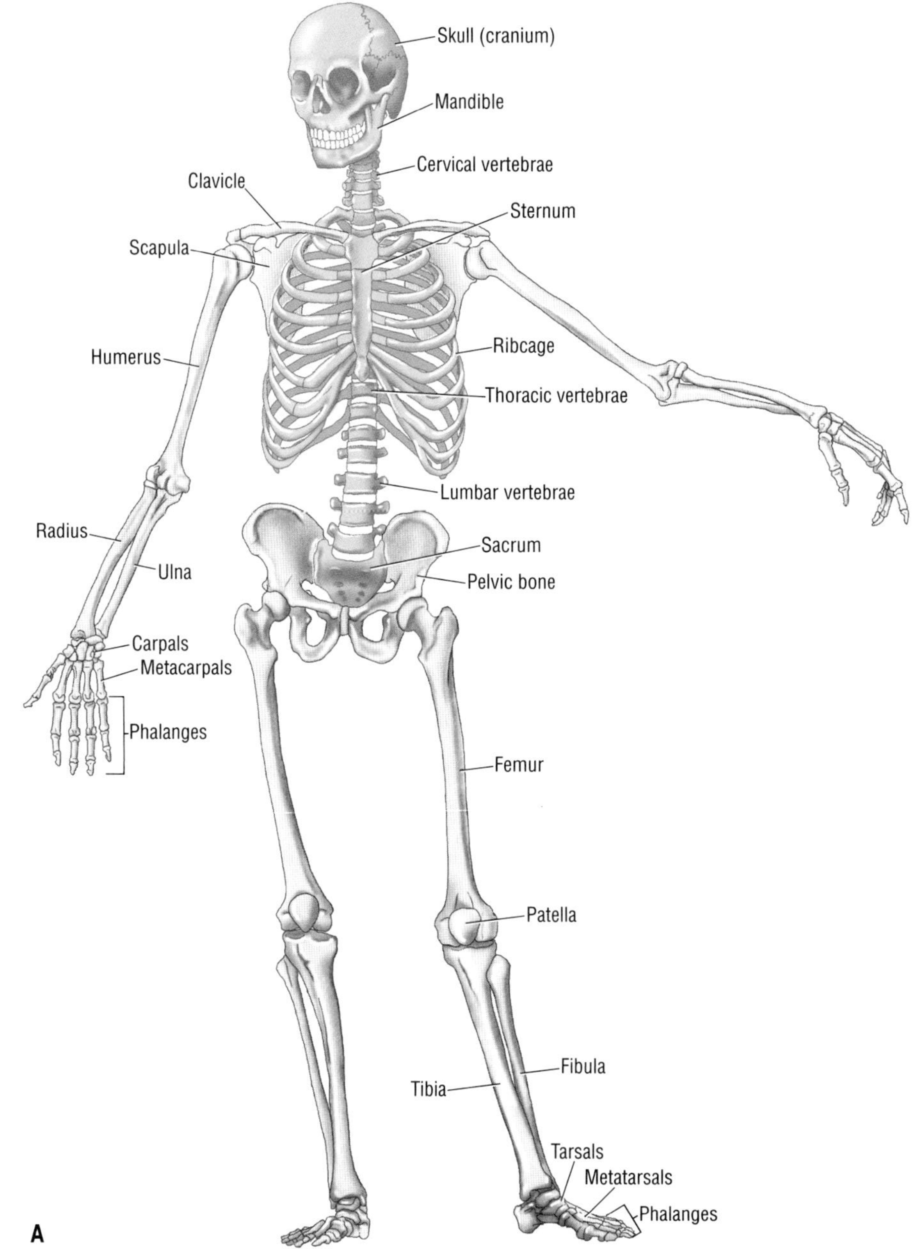

Figure 2-1 An illustration of the human skeleton highlighting the axial skeleton *(red)* and appendicular skeleton *(white)*. **A**, Anterior view. (From Muscolino JE: *Kinesiology: the skeletal system and muscle function,* St Louis, 2006, Mosby, Figure 4-2.)

sacrum and coccyx, forming the central, bony axis of the body. The **appendicular skeleton** is composed of the bones of the appendages, or extremities. All bones of the upper extremity, including the scapula and clavicle, and all bones in the lower extremity, including the pelvis, are part of the appendicular skeleton. Figure 2-1 differentiates the axial and appendicular skeleton and labels the major bones of the body.

Bone: Anatomy and Function

Bone provides the rigid framework of the body and equips muscles with a system of levers. This text describes bone as having two primary types of tissue: cortical (compact) bone and cancellous bone (Figure 2-2).

Cortical (compact) bone is relatively dense and typically lines the outermost portions of bones. This type of bone is extremely strong, especially in regard to absorbing compressive forces through a bone's longitudinal axis.

Cancellous bone is porous and typically composes the inner portions of a bone. The porous, web-like structure of cancellous bone not only lightens bones but, similar to a series of mechanical struts, redirects forces toward weight-bearing surfaces covered by articular cartilage.

Most bones have common structural features important to maintaining their health and integrity.

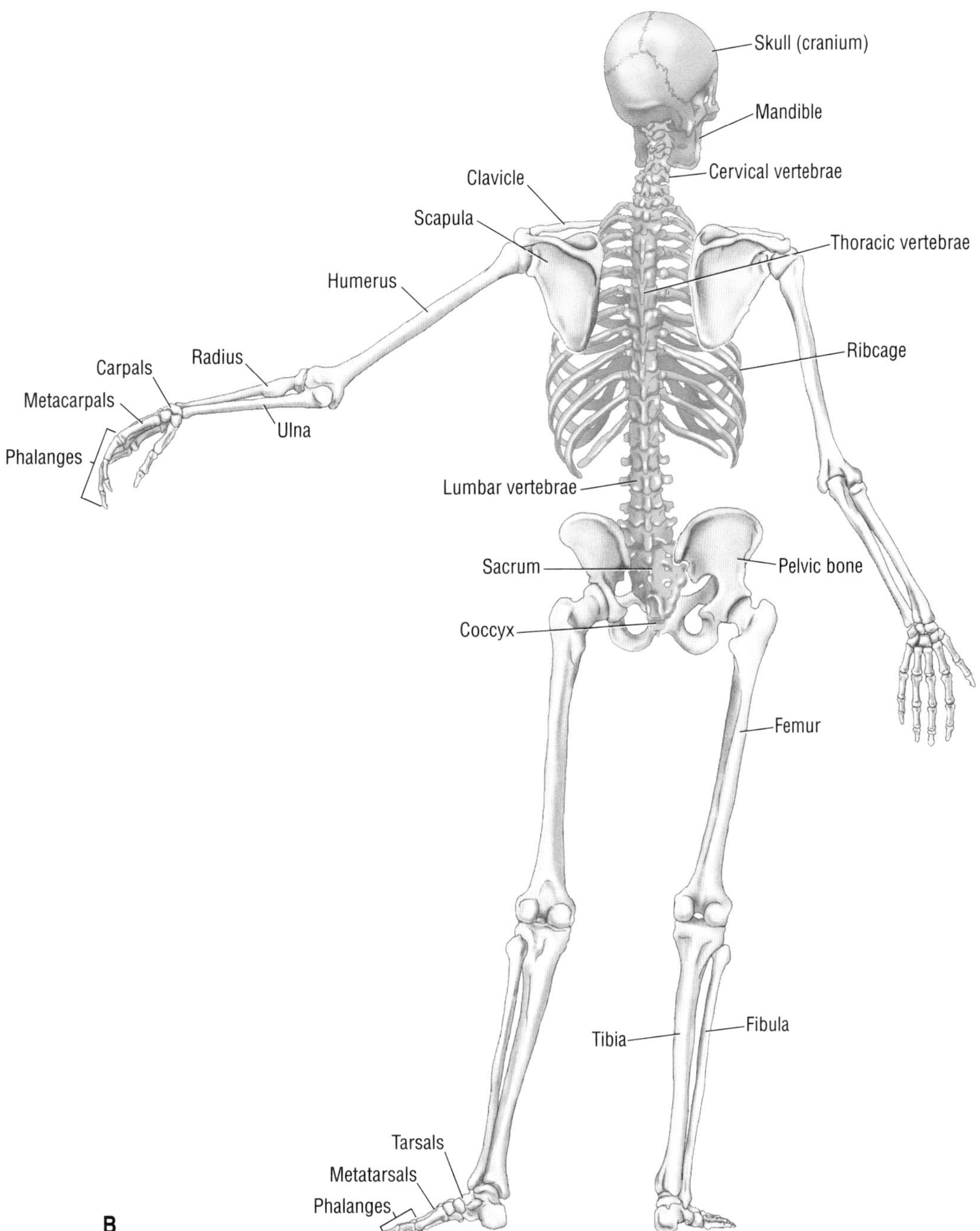

Figure 2-1, cont'd B, Posterior view. (From Muscolino JE: *Kinesiology: the skeletal system and muscle function,* St Louis, 2006, Mosby, Figure 4-2.)

Figure 2-3 illustrates the primary components found in a bone.

The **diaphysis** is the central shaft of the bone. It is similar to a thick, hollow tube and is composed mostly of cortical bone to withstand the large compressive forces from weight bearing. The **epiphyses** are the expanded portions of bone that arise from the diaphysis (shaft); each long bone has a proximal and a distal epiphysis. Primarily composed of cancellous (spongy) bone, each epiphysis typically articulates with another bone, forming a joint, and helps transmit weight-bearing forces across regions of the body. **Articular cartilage** lines the articular surface of each epiphysis, acting as a shock absorber between joints.

Each long bone is covered by a thin, tough membrane called the **periosteum.** This highly vascular and innervated membrane helps secure the attachments of muscles and ligaments to bone. The **medullary canal** (cavity) is the central hollow tube within the diaphysis of a long bone. This region is important for storing bone marrow and provides a passageway for nutrient-carrying arteries.

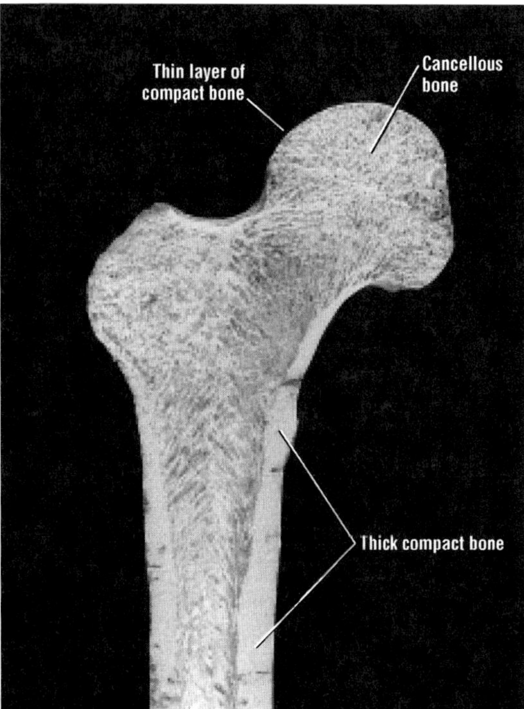

Figure 2-2 A cross section showing the internal architecture of the proximal femur. Note the thicker areas of compact bone around the shaft and the lattice-like cancellous bone occupying most of the inner regions. (From Neumann DA: *An arthritis home study course. The synovial joint: anatomy, function, and dysfunction,* Lacrosse, Wis, 1998, The Orthopedic Section of the American Physical Therapy Association.)

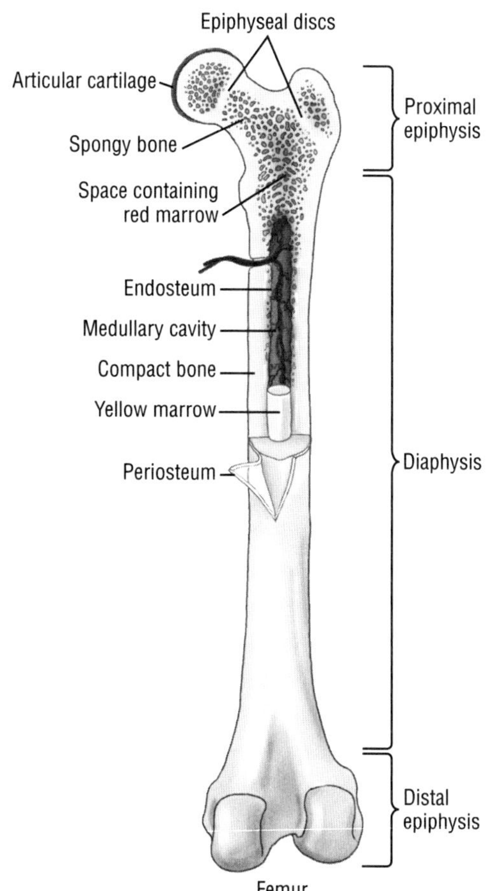

Figure 2-3 The primary components of a bone. (From Muscolino JE: *Kinesiology: the skeletal system and muscle function,* St Louis, 2006, Mosby, Figure 3-2.)

The **endosteum** is a membrane that lines the surface of the medullary canal. Many of the cells important for forming and repairing bone are housed within the endosteum.

Bone is a dynamic tissue that is constantly being remodeled in response to internal and external forces. Clinically this is an important fact because bones will become stronger from forces caused by weight-bearing activities and muscular contraction or significantly weaker after joint immobilization, periods of restricted weight bearing, or extended inactivity such as those who have been on bed rest.

Types of Bones

Bones can be classified into five basic categories based on their structure, or shape: long, short, flat, irregular, and sesamoid (Figure 2-4).

Long bones comprise the majority of the appendicular skeleton. As the name implies, they are long, containing obvious longitudinal axes or shafts. Generally, long bones contain an expanded portion of bone at each end of the shaft that articulates with another bone, forming a joint. The femur, humerus, metacarpals, and the radius are just some of the numerous examples of long bones found in the body.

Short bones are short, meaning their length, width, and heights are typically equal. The carpal bones of the hand provide a good example of short bones.

Flat bones such as the scapula or sternum are typically flat or slightly curved. Often the broad surface of these bones provides a wide base for expansive muscular attachments.

Irregular bones, as the name implies, come in a wide variety of shapes and sizes. Examples of irregular bones include vertebrae, most of the bones of the face and skull, and sesamoid bones.

Sesamoid bones are a subcategory of irregular bones, named so because their small, rounded appearance is similar to that of a sesame seed. These bones are encased within the tendon of a muscle, serving to protect the tendon and increase the muscle's leverage. For example, the patella (knee cap)—the largest sesamoid bone in the body—is embedded within the tendon of the quadriceps muscle. The patella increases the distance (internal moment arm) between the line of force of the quadriceps and the axis of rotation; as a result the patella augments the torque production of the quadriceps. Also, the patella protects the quadriceps tendon by absorbing some of the compressive and shear forces that occur during flexion and extension of the knee.

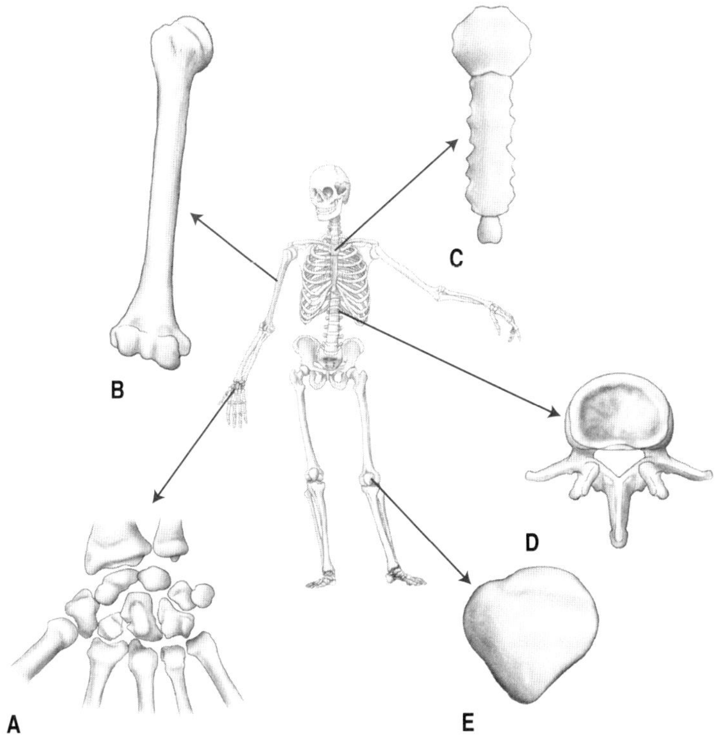

Figure 2-4 A figure highlighting the primary types of bones: short **(A)**, long **(B)**, flat **(C)**, irregular **(D)**, and sesamoid **(E).** (From Muscolino JM: Kinesiology: the skeletal system and muscle function, St Louis, 2006, Mosby, Figure 3-1.)

Classification of Joints

Joints are commonly classified by their anatomic structure and subsequent movement potential. On the basis of this system, there are three classifications of joints in the body: synarthrosis, amphiarthrosis, and diarthrosis.

Synarthrosis

A **synarthrosis** is a junction between bones that allows little to no movement. Examples include the sutures of the skull and the distal tibiofibular joint. The primary function of this type of joint is to firmly bind bones together and transmit forces from one bone to another (Figure 2-5).

Amphiarthrosis

An **amphiarthrosis** is a type of joint that is formed primarily by fibrocartilage and hyaline cartilage. Although these joints allow limited amounts of motion, they play an important role in shock absorption. For example, the intervertebral body joints of the spine allow relatively little motion, but the thick layers of fibrocartilage that form the intervertebral discs absorb and disperse the large compressive forces often transmitted through this region (Figure 2-6).

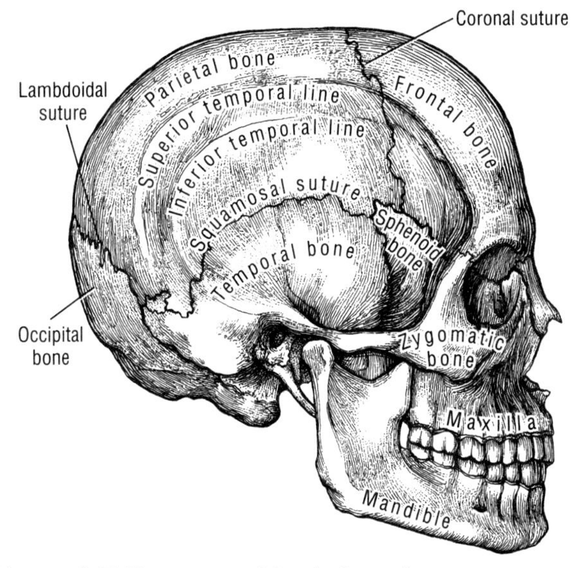

Figure 2-5 The sutures of the skull are shown as an example of a synarthrosis. (From Neumann DA: *Kinesiology of the musculoskeletal system: foundations for physical rehabilitation,* St Louis, 2002, Mosby, Figure 9-2.)

Diarthrosis: The Synovial Joint

A diarthrosis is an articulation that contains a fluid-filled joint cavity between two or more bones. Because of the presence of a synovial membrane, diarthrodial joints are frequently referred to as synovial joints. Seven different categories of diarthrodial (synovial) joints exist, each with unique functional abilities; however, all synovial joints contain the seven common elements listed below (Figure 2-7):

- *Synovial fluid:* provides joint lubrication and nutrition
- *Articular cartilage:* dissipates and absorbs compressive forces

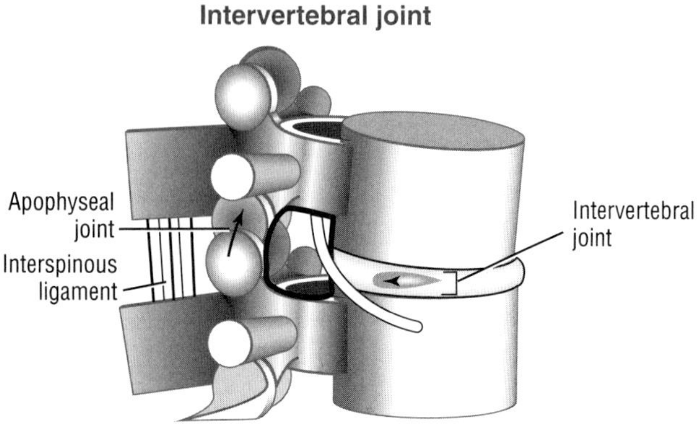

Intervertebral joint

Figure 2-6 An illustration of a lumbar intervertebral joint is shown as an example of an amphiarthrodial joint. (From Neumann DA: *Kinesiology of the musculoskeletal system: foundations for physical rehabilitation*, St Louis, 2002, Mosby, Figure 9-68, *D*.)

- *Articular capsule:* connective tissue that surrounds and binds the joint together
- *Synovial membrane:* produces synovial fluid
- *Capsular ligaments:* thickened regions of connective tissue that limit excessive joint motion
- *Blood vessels:* provide nutrients to the joint
- *Sensory nerves:* transmit signals regarding pain and proprioception

CLASSIFICATION OF SYNOVIAL JOINTS

Anatomists classify synovial joints into categories on the basis of their unique structural features. The unique structure of each joint determines its functional potential. The following analogies may be helpful in understanding the structure and function of most joints within the body.

Hinge Joint

Similar to the hinge of a door, the hinge joint (Figure 2-8) allows motion in only one plane about a single axis of rotation. Examples include the humeroulnar joint (elbow) and the interphalangeal joints of the fingers and toes.

Elements ALWAYS associated with diarthrodial (synovial) joints:
- Synovial fluid
- Articular cartilage
- Articular capsule
- Synovial membrane
- Capsular ligaments
- Blood vessels
- Sensory nerves

Elements SOMETIMES associated with diarthrodial (synovial) joints:
- Intraarticular discs or menisci
- Peripheral labrum
- Fat pads
- Synovial plicae

Figure 2-7 Elements associated with a typical diarthrodial (synovial) joint. (From Neumann DA: *Kinesiology of the musculoskeletal system: foundations for physical rehabilitation*, St Louis, 2002, Mosby, Figure 2-1.)

Pivot Joint

The pivot joint (Figure 2-9) allows rotation about a single longitudinal axis of rotation, similar to the rotation of a doorknob. Examples include the proximal radioulnar joint and the atlantoaxial joint between the first and second cervical vertebrae.

Ellipsoid Joint

An ellipsoid joint (Figure 2-10) has one partner with a convex elongated surface in one dimension mated with a matching concave surface on its partner. The structure of this type of joint allows motion to occur in two planes. The radiocarpal (wrist) joint provides a good example of an ellipsoid joint.

Ball-and-Socket Joint

The ball-and-socket joint (Figure 2-11) is composed of the articulation between a spherical convex surface and a matching cup-like socket. The glenohumeral (shoulder) joint and the hip joint are both ball-and-socket joints, allowing wide ranges of motion in all three planes.

Plane Joint

The plane joint (Figure 2-12) is composed of the articulation between two relatively flat bony surfaces. Plane joints typically allow limited amounts of motion, but the lack of bony restriction often allows these joints to slide and rotate in many directions. The intercarpal joints of the hand, many of which are plane joints, provide a good example of how minimal amounts of motion in several joints can be "added up" to provide a significant amount of mobility to a particular region.

Saddle Joint

Saddle joints (Figure 2-13) typically allow extensive motion, primarily in two planes. Each partner of a saddle joint has two surfaces: one concave, and one convex—similar to a horseback rider sitting on a saddle (see Figure 2-13, *A*). These reciprocally curved surfaces

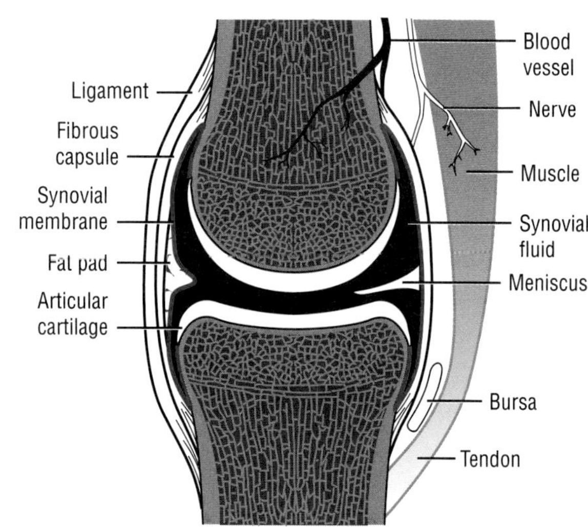

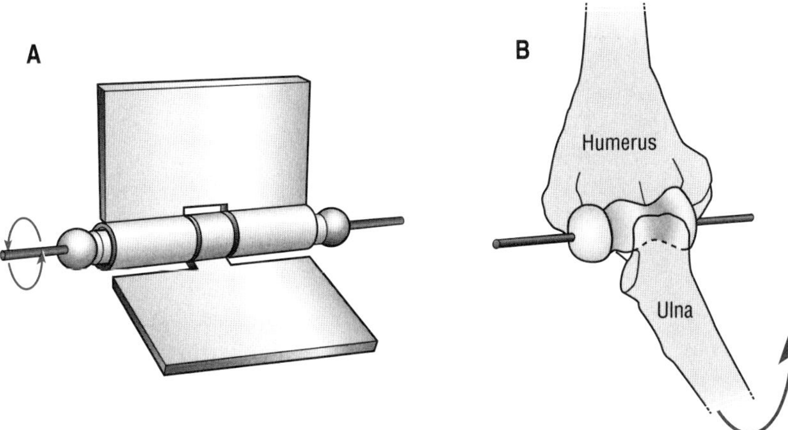

Figure 2-8 **A**, A hinge joint is illustrated as analogous to the humeroulnar joint **(B).** The axis of rotation is represented by the pin. (From Neumann DA: *Kinesiology of the musculoskeletal system: foundations for physical rehabilitation*, St Louis, 2002, Mosby, Figure 2-2.)

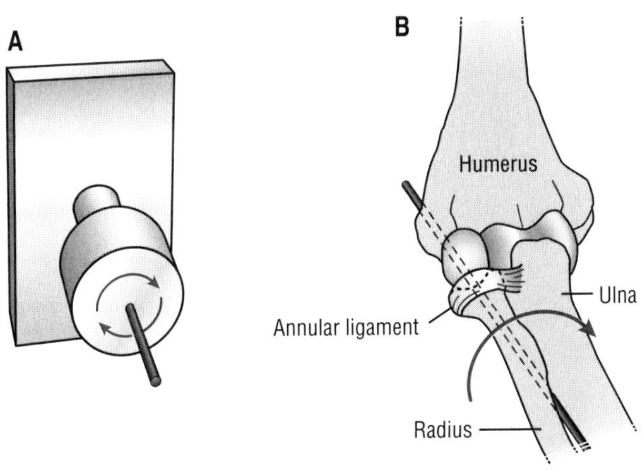

Figure 2-9 **A**, A pivot joint is shown as analogous to the proximal radioulnar joint **(B).** The axis of rotation is represented by the pin. (From Neumann DA: *Kinesiology of the musculoskeletal system: foundations for physical rehabilitation*, St Louis, 2002, Mosby, Figure 2-3.)

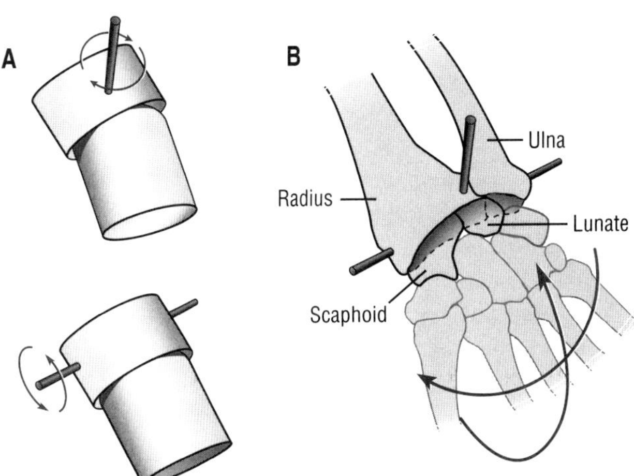

Figure 2-10 An ellipsoid joint **(A)** is shown as analogous to the radiocarpal joint (wrist) **(B).** The two axes of rotation are shown by the intersecting pins. (From Neumann DA: *Kinesiology of the musculoskeletal system: foundations for physical rehabilitation*, St Louis, 2002, Mosby, Figure 2-4.)

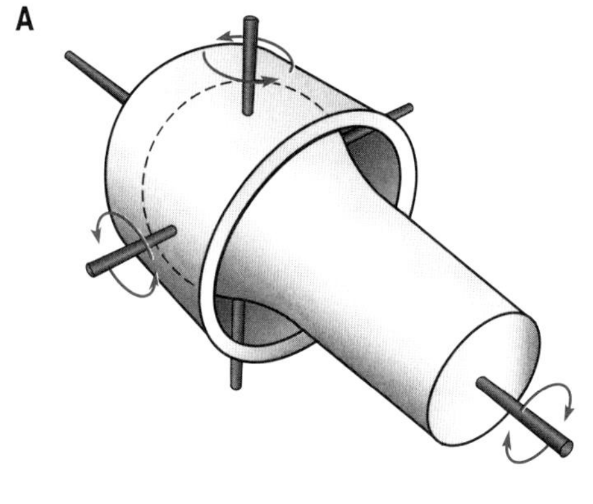

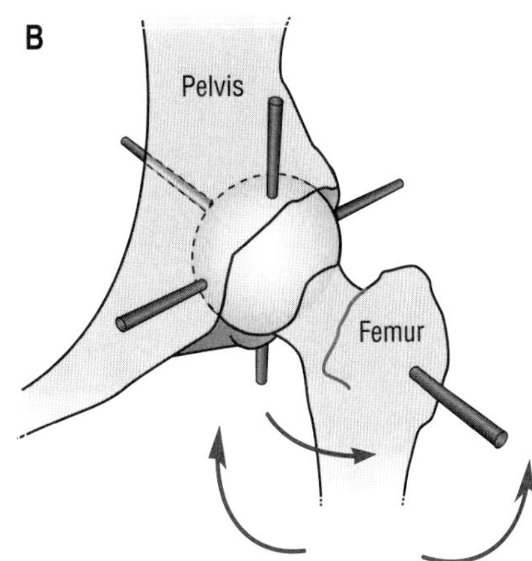

Figure 2-11 **A**, A ball-and-socket joint is shown as analogous to the hip joint, **B**. The three axes of rotation are represented by the three intersecting pins. (From Neumann DA: *Kinesiology of the musculoskeletal system: foundations for physical rehabilitation*, St Louis, 2002, Mosby, Figure 2-5.)

are oriented approximately at right angles to one another, producing a high degree of stability as the joint surfaces interlock. Examples include the sternoclavicular joint and the carpometacarpal joint of the thumb.

Condyloid Joint

Condyloid joints such as the tibiofemoral (knee) or metacarpophalangeal joints of the fingers (Figure 2-14) are composed of the articulation between a large, rounded, convex member and a relatively shallow concave member. Most often these joints allow 2 degrees of freedom; ligaments as well as the bony structure of the joint typically prevent motion from occurring in a third plane.

See Table 2-1 for a summary of the types of synovial joints.

Connective Tissue

Composition of Connective Tissue

All of the connective tissues that support the joints of the body are composed of only three types of biologic materials: fibers, ground substance, and cells. These biologic materials are blended in various proportions on the basis of the mechanical demands of the joint.

FIBERS

Three main fiber types comprise the connective tissues of joints: type I collagen, type II collagen, and elastin.

- Type I collagen fibers are thick and rugged, designed to resist elongation. These fibers primarily compose ligaments, tendons, and fibrous capsules.
- Type II collagen fibers are thinner and less stiff than type I fibers. This type of fiber provides a flexible woven framework for maintaining the general shape and consistency of structures such as hyaline cartilage.
- Elastin fibers, like the name implies, are elastic in nature. These fibers resist stretching (tensile) forces but have more "give" when elongated. Therefore they can be useful in preventing injury because they allow the tissue to bend a great deal before breaking.

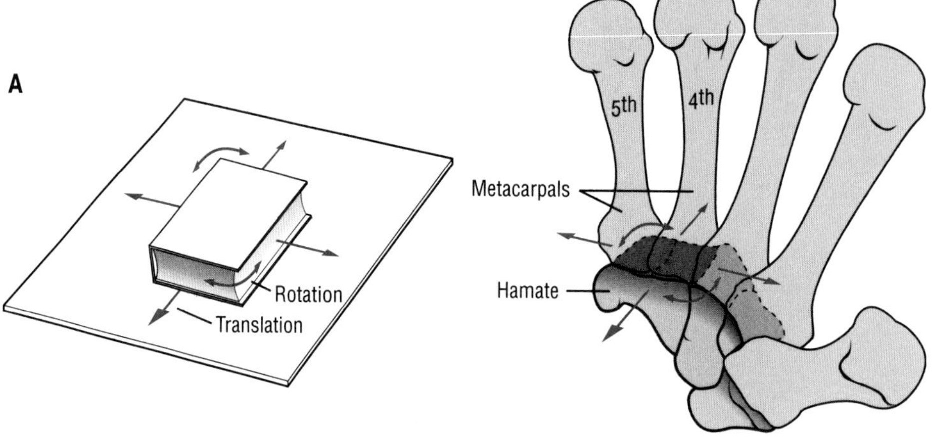

Figure 2-12 A plane joint is formed by the articulation of two flat surfaces. **A**, The book moving across the table is depicted as analogous to the combined slide and spin at the fourth and fifth carpometacarpal joints, **B**. (From Neumann DA: *Kinesiology of the musculoskeletal system: foundations for physical rehabilitation*, St Louis, 2002, Mosby, Figure 2-6.)

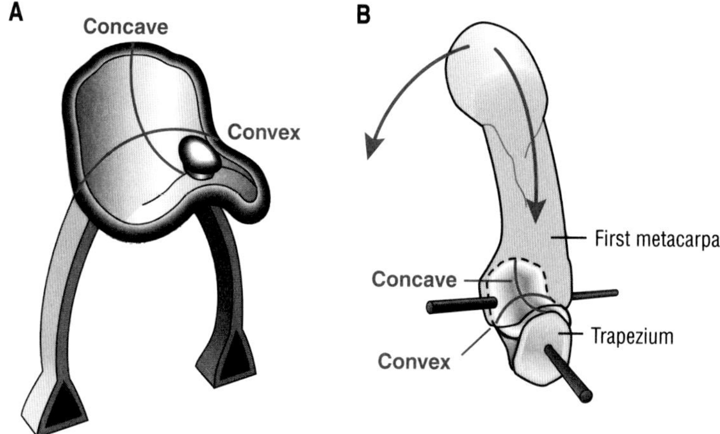

Figure 2-13 **A**, A saddle joint is illustrated as analogous to the carpometacarpal joint of the thumb. The two axes of rotation are represented by the pins in **B**. (From Neumann DA: *Kinesiology of the musculoskeletal system: foundations for physical rehabilitation*, St Louis, 2002, Mosby, Figure 2-7.)

GROUND SUBSTANCE

Collagen and elastin fibers are embedded within a water-saturated matrix known as *ground substance*. Ground substance (Figure 2-15) is composed primarily of glycosaminoglycans, water, and solutes. The combination of these materials allows many fibers of the body to exist in a fluid-filled environment that disperses millions of repetitive forces affecting a joint throughout a lifetime.

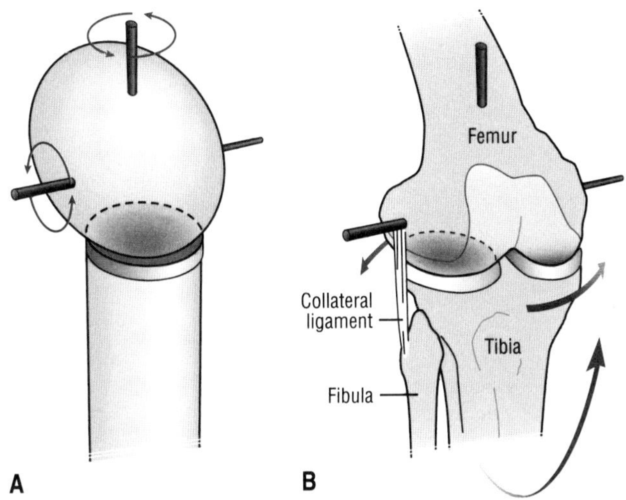

Figure 2-14 A, A condyloid joint is shown as analogous to the tibiofemoral (knee) joint **(B).** The two axes of rotation are represented by the pins. (From Neumann DA: *Kinesiology of the musculoskeletal system: foundations for physical rehabilitation,* St Louis, 2002, Mosby, Figure 2-8.)

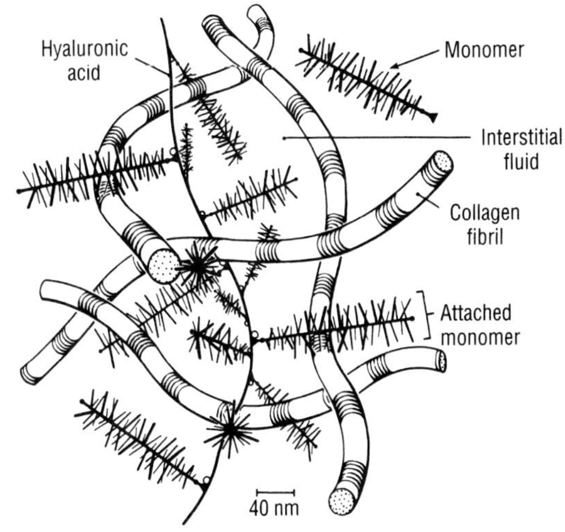

Figure 2-15 Schematic drawing of the molecular organization of cartilage. A glycosaminoglycan molecule is formed by a hyaluronic acid center thread to which proteoglycan monomers are attached, forming a bottle-brush configuration. Interlacing collagen fibrils and water fill much of the space within this matrix. (From Nordin M, Frankel VH: *Basic biomechanics of the musculoskeletal system,* ed 2, Philadelphia, 1989, Williams & Wilkins.)

TABLE 2-1 TYPES OF SYNOVIAL JOINTS

Joint	Degrees of Freedom	Primary Motions	Mechanical Analogy	Anatomic Examples
Hinge	1	Flexion and extension	Door hinge	Humeroulnar joint Interphalangeal joint
Pivot	1	Spinning of one member about a single axis of rotation	Door knob	Proximal radioulnar joint Atlantoaxial joint
Ellipsoid	2	Flexion-extension and abduction-adduction	Flattened convex ellipsoid paired with a concave trough	Radiocarpal joint
Ball-and-socket	3	Flexion-extension, abduction-adduction, internal and external rotation	Spherical convex surface paired with a concave cup	Glenohumeral (shoulder) joint Hip joint
Plane	Variable	Typical motions include a slide or rotation, or both	Book sliding or spinning on a table	Intercarpal joints Intertarsal joints
Saddle	2	Biplanar motion; generally excluding a spin	Horseback rider on a saddle	Carpometacarpal joint of the thumb Sternoclavicular joint
Condyloid	2	Biplanar motion	Spherical convex surface paired with a shallow concave cup	Tibiofemoral (knee) joint Metacarpophalangeal joint

Modified from Neumann DA: *Kinesiology of the musculoskeletal system: foundations for physical rehabilitation*, St Louis, 2002, Mosby, Table 2-2.

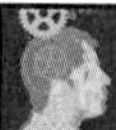

Consider this...

How to Protect the Joints of Our Patients

Surprisingly large forces cross the joints of the human body. During normal walking, forces at the hip, for example, routinely reach three times a person's body weight. How could this be? A person does not actually weigh three times his or her own body weight. Most of this joint force arises from the forces of muscle contraction; these are commonly referred to as *joint reaction forces*. The muscular forces that move and stabilize our limbs must be transferred across the surfaces of our joints. In healthy persons, these forces are usually well tolerated because they are dampened by a thick and moist articular cartilage, plus a slight "give" in the structure of the spongy component of bone and other tissues around the joint.

In addition to dampening or absorbing forces, healthy articular cartilage also increases the surface area at the joints. Increasing surface area reduces the actual stress on the cartilage. Disease, trauma, or simple overuse may wear out the cartilage, reducing its ability to tolerate even relatively small pressures. Excessive and repetitive stress on unprotected bone and nearby soft tissues often leads to inflammation and pain of the entire joint—or arthritis (from the Greek word *arthros* meaning "joint" and *itis* meaning "inflammation"). Severe arthritis can eventually reduce the range of motion and weaken all the soft tissues that normally help stabilize a joint. Over time, joints may actually dislocate (separate) or sublux (become overly loose). When increased pain and decreased function reach a critical level, the joint may need to be replaced by an arthroplasty, or artificial joint (Figure 2-16).

Many times, physical therapists and physical therapist assistants teach patients how to protect their joints from unnecessarily large and damaging muscle contractions. Joint protection principles for arthritis at the hip, for example, usually involve teaching the patients to move slower, use good body mechanics, avoid lifting large objects, and stretch to remain relatively flexible. These principles may help reduce stress and further wear and tear at the joint.

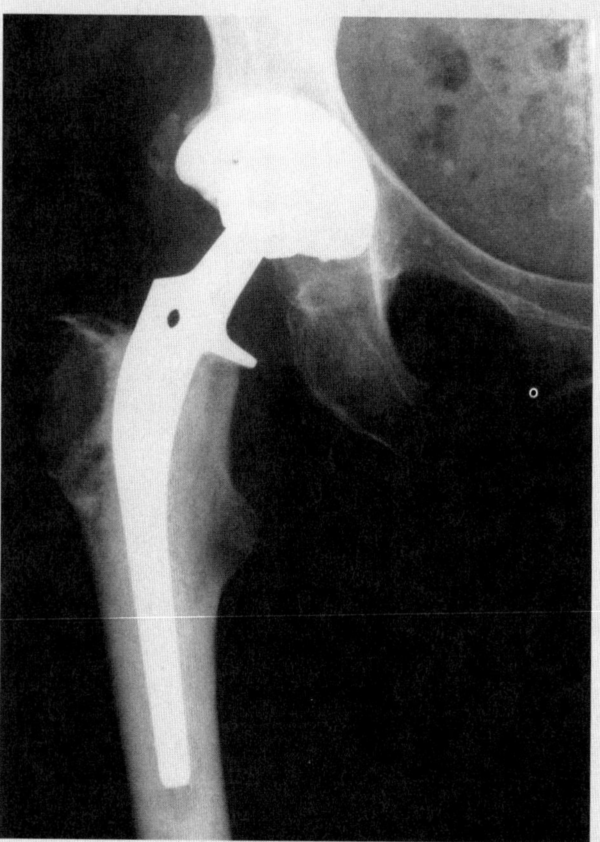

Figure 2-16 A radiograph of a total hip arthroplasty. (From Neumann DA: *Kinesiology of the musculoskeletal system: foundations for physical rehabilitation*, St Louis, 2002, Mosby, Figure 12-52. Courtesy Michael Anderson, MD, Blount Orthopedic Clinic, Milwaukee, Wis.)

CELLS

The cells within connective tissues of joints are primarily responsible for the maintenance and repair of tissues that constitute joints. The types of cells within a particular type of tissue help determine the properties of that tissue.

Types of Connective Tissue

In general, there are four basic types of connective tissue that form the structure of joints: dense irregular connective tissue, articular cartilage, fibrocartilage, and bone. A summary of the basic structure and function of these tissues is provided in Table 2-2.

Functional Considerations

TENDONS AND LIGAMENTS: SUPPORTING JOINT STRUCTURE

The fibrous composition of tendons and ligaments is quite similar; however, the arrangement of the fibers within ligaments is different than that of tendons. The unique fibrous architecture of these two different tissues helps to explain the primary function of each tissue.

Tendons, which connect muscle to bone, help convert muscular force into bony motion. These tissues are composed primarily of collagen fibers that are aligned parallel to one another (Figure 2-17, A). This parallel arrangement allows muscular force to be efficiently transmitted to the

TABLE 2-2 TYPES OF CONNECTIVE TISSUE THAT FORM THE STRUCTURE OF JOINTS

	Mechanical Specialization	Anatomic Location	Fiber Types	Clinical Correlation
Dense irregular connective tissue	Binds bones together and restrains unwanted movement of joints	Composes ligaments and the tough external layer of joint capsules	Primarily type I collagen fibers; low elastin fiber content	Rupture of the lateral collateral ligaments of the ankle can lead to medial-lateral instability of the talocrural joint
Articular cartilage	Resists and distributes compressive and shear forces transferred through articular surfaces	Covers the ends of articulating bones in synovial joints	High type II collagen fiber content; fibers help anchor the cartilage to bone	Wear and tear of articular cartilage often decreases its effectiveness in dispersing joint compression forces, often leading to osteoarthritis and joint pain
Fibrocartilage	Provides support and stabilization to joints; primarily functions to provide shock absorption by resisting and dispersing compressive and shear forces	Composes the intervertebral discs of the spine, and the menisci of the knee	Multidirectional bundles of type I collagen	Tearing of the intervertebral disc within the vertebral column can allow the central nucleus pulposus (gel) to escape and press on a spinal nerve or nerve root
Bone	Forms the primary supporting structure of the body and provides a rigid lever to transmit muscle force to move and stabilize the body	Forms the internal levers of the musculoskeletal system	Specialized arrangement of type I collagen that provides a framework for hard mineral salts	Osteoporosis of the spine results in loss of mineral and bone content; may result in fractures of the vertebral body

Modified from Neumann DA: *Kinesiology of the musculoskeletal system: foundations for physical rehabilitation*, St Louis, 2002, Mosby, Table 2-3.

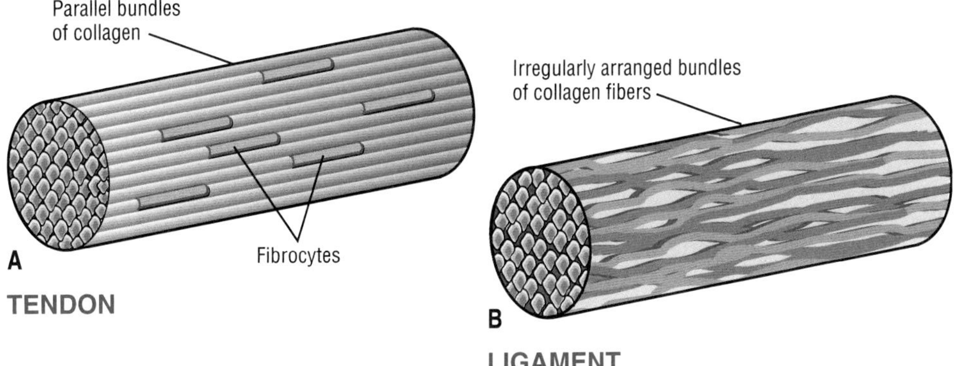

Figure 2-17 The fibrous organization of tendons versus ligaments. **A**, The bundles of collagen in a tendon are parallel to one another for efficient transmission of muscular forces. **B**, The collagen bundles of a ligament are in a criss-cross pattern to accept tensile forces from numerous directions. (From Neumann DA: *Kinesiology of the musculoskeletal system: foundations for physical rehabilitation*, St Louis, 2002, Mosby, Figure 2-12.)

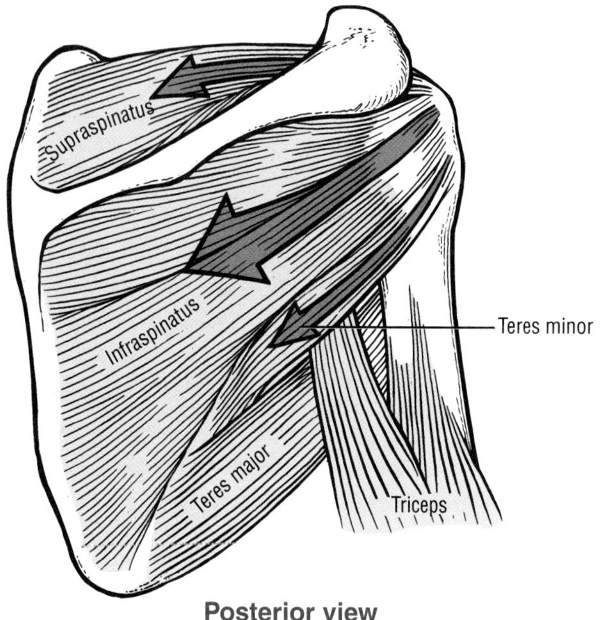

Figure 2-18 A posterior view of the right shoulder showing the supraspinatus, infraspinatus, and teres minor as active dynamic stabilizers of the glenohumeral joint. (From Neumann DA: *Kinesiology of the musculoskeletal system: foundations for physical rehabilitation*, St Louis, 2002, Mosby, Figure 5-53.)

bone with minimal loss of muscular energy as it is transferred into joint motion.

Ligaments, on the other hand, connect bone to bone and function primarily to maintain a joint's structure by resisting internal and external forces. The collagen fibers of a ligament are aligned in irregular crossing patterns (Figure 2-17, *B*). This fiber arrangement allows the ligament to accept tensile forces from several different directions while maintaining the integrity of the joint.

ACTIVE STABILIZATION OF JOINTS

Bony conformation and ligamentous networks often provide the majority of static stability to a joint. However, many times additional stability is required, especially as a body segment is moving; this additional dynamic stability is most often acquired by enlisting muscles, which function as active stabilizers of a joint (Figure 2-18).

Many rehabilitation programs are designed to strengthen the supporting musculature in an effort to stabilize a joint in which the passive stabilizing structures such as ligaments are insufficient. Although a muscle cannot respond as quickly as ligaments to a potentially damaging external force, muscles do allow a graded and more controlled response. Chapter 3 covers this in greater detail.

EFFECTS OF IMMOBILIZATION ON THE CONNECTIVE TISSUES OF A JOINT

Connective tissues protect, support, and maintain the integrity of a joint. Through normal physical activity, connective tissues accept and resist the natural range of forces imposed on the musculoskeletal system. However, if a joint is immobilized such as during bed rest or following a casting, there may be a significant increase in

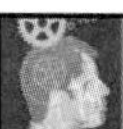

Consider this...

Long-Term Immobilization and Advanced Age: Different Populations, Comparable Results

The physiologic effects of long-term immobilization and the physiologic effects of advanced age are remarkably similar, especially in regard to connective tissues.

Persons with advanced age and those with long-term immobilization of their joints display three common changes in the connective tissue surrounding joints. These three interrelated changes, if severe, may give rise to a similar set of impairments in each of these two populations:

- **Tissue Weakness**
  As the tissue weakens, tears and microtrauma accumulate and significantly reduce a joint's ability to resist outside forces. This may result in abnormal posture because individuals begin to hold atypical postures in order to stabilize a particular joint, region, or body segment.
- **Tissue Dehydration**
  Tissue dehydration can cause tissue weakness, tissue stiffness, or both. It is primarily the water within the ground substance that allows the connective tissues to absorb and disperse the forces across a joint. If connective tissues become dehydrated, the fibrous (non-water) components of the joint will more likely become injured.
  Both hyaline and articular cartilage normally have a large water content. Dehydration of these tissues may significantly reduce joint space and the ability to disperse joint compression forces. Significant dehydration may therefore lead to bone-on-bone compression, eventually resulting in arthritis, bone spurs, or even fracture.
- **Tissue Stiffness**
  Tissue stiffness may be considered a primary factor in the reduced joint range of motion observed in these two different populations. This is clinically significant because decreased range of motion can lead to joint contractures and abnormal posture. These impairments therefore can begin a vicious cycle of postural adaptation and tissue shortening, which may result in functional limitations or even disablement.
  Clinicians attempt to prevent these cycles from beginning by promoting an early return to weight-bearing activities, active and passive range of motion, functional exercise, and patient education.

the overall stiffness of the joint's connective tissue and a decrease in the ability of these tissues to withstand forces.

Immobilization of a joint for a period of time may be necessary to promote healing following an injury such as a fracture of a bone; however, this may make the involved joints more susceptible to injury or instability. Rehabilitation programs, involving a relatively quick return to weight bearing, and specific strengthening exercises may be indicated to help restore connective tissue strength and joint stability.

Summary

Numerous types of joints exist throughout the body, each having specific functional capabilities. The available range of motion and relative stability of a joint depends not only on its bony structure but also on the surrounding muscles and connective tissues.

Upon studying the structure and function of joints, it becomes clear that there is a tradeoff between the stability and the mobility of a joint. For example, the elbow (humeroulnar) joint is highly stable. Its bony conformation and ligamentous network provides ample support to the joint. The inherent stability of the elbow, however, comes at the cost of mobility—the elbow (humeroulnar) joint is limited to motion in only one plane.

In contrast, consider the glenohumeral (shoulder) joint. The ball-and-socket structure and relatively loose ligamentous network of this joint allows extensive ranges of motion in all three planes. Because of this design, the glenohumeral joint is one of the most unstable joints of the body and therefore prone to injury. To combat the inherent instability at the glenohumeral joint, the body incorporates muscular force to help actively stabilize the joint throughout the wide ranges of motion.

As this text progresses, keep in mind that every joint in the body must find the balance between mobility and stability to properly function. The joint-specific chapters that follow provide insight into the various ways in which this is accomplished.

Study Questions

1. Which of the following types of joints allows the least amount of motion?
   a. Diarthrosis
   b. Synarthrosis
   c. Condyloid
   d. Amphiarthrosis
2. Which of the following joints allows only 1 degree of freedom?
   a. Ellipsoid
   b. Ball-and-socket
   c. Hinge
   d. Saddle
   e. B and C
3. Which of the following connective tissues are designed to "give" when stretched, thereby resisting injury?
   a. Type I collagen fibers
   b. Type II collagen fibers
   c. Elastin
   d. Glycosaminoglycans
4. The intervertebral discs of the spine are primarily composed of which type of connective tissue?
   a. Dense, irregular connective tissue
   b. Articular cartilage
   c. Fibrocartilage
   d. Bone
5. Which of the following structures connect bone to bone and function primarily to resist internal and external forces?
   a. Tendons
   b. Ligaments
   c. Articular cartilage
   d. Bursae
6. The glenohumeral joint of the shoulder is an example of which type of joint?
   a. Saddle
   b. Ball-and-socket
   c. Ellipsoid
   d. Pivot
7. Which of the following is an example of a condyloid joint?
   a. Sternoclavicular
   b. Acromioclavicular
   c. Tibiofemoral (knee)
   d. Metacarpophalangeal
   e. C and D
8. Which of the following statements is true?
   a. Pivot joints typically allow 3 degrees of freedom.
   b. Cancellous bone is porous and typically lines the inner portions of a bone.
   c. Ground substance typically has almost no water content.
   d. Tendons connect bone to bone.
9. Immobilization of a joint generally leads to greater stiffness of the surrounding connective tissues.
   a. True
   b. False
10. The sutures of the skull are a good example of an amphiarthrodial joint.
    a. True
    b. False
11. Cortical bone is dense and strong, typically lining the outermost portions of a bone.
    a. True
    b. False
12. The humerus and the tibia are both bones considered to be part of the axial skeleton.
    a. True
    b. False

13. Bone is considered a non-dynamic tissue with limited ability to remodel itself.
    a. True
    b. False
14. Saddle joints, condyloid joints, and ellipsoid joints all permit motion in at least two planes.
    a. True
    b. False

Use the following images to answer Questions 15 through 20:

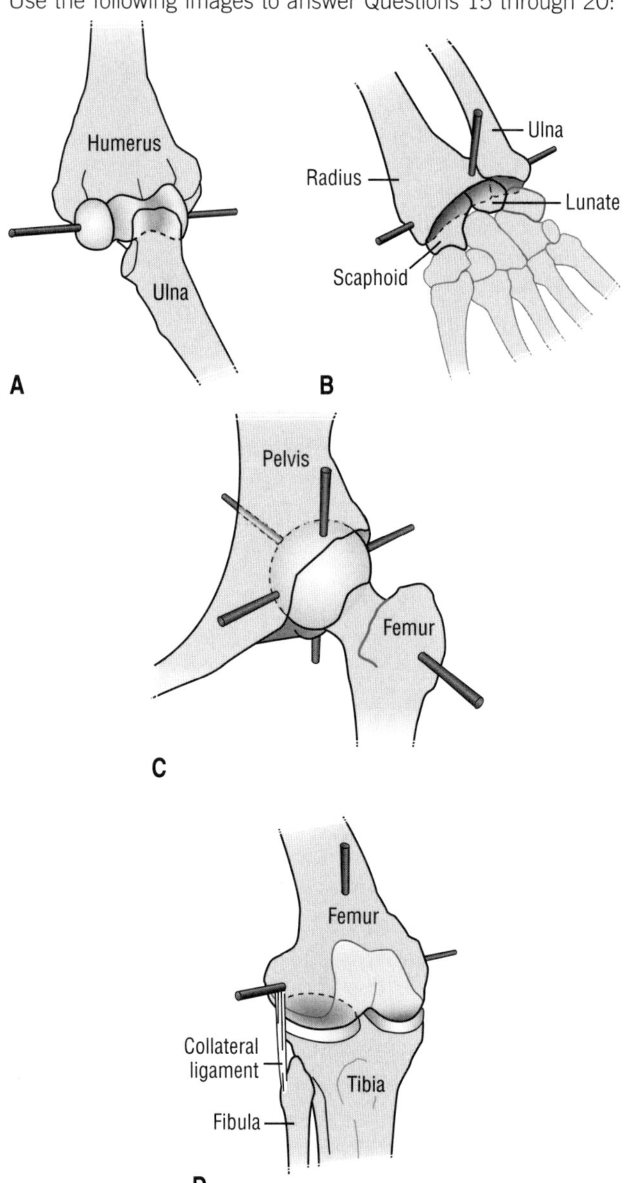

(Modified from Neumann DA: *Kinesiology of the musculoskeletal system: foundations for physical rehabilitation,* St Louis, 2002, Mosby. **A,** Figure 2-2, *B*; **B,** Figure 2-4, *B*; **C,** Figure 2-5, *B*; **D,** Figure 2-8, *B*.)

15. Which of the above joints allows motion to occur in only two planes?
    a. A
    b. B and C
    c. C and D
    d. B and D
16. Which of the above joints is considered the most mobile?
    a. A
    b. B
    c. C
    d. D
17. Which of the above joints allows flexion and extension?
    a. A and B
    b. B and C
    c. C and D
    d. All of the above
18. Which of the above joints allows motion in just one plane?
    a. A
    b. A and C
    c. B
    d. D
19. Which of the above joints does (do) not allow motion to occur in the frontal plane?
    a. D
    b. A and D
    c. A and C
    d. B and C
20. Which of the above joints allow(s) motion to occur about all three axes of rotation?
    a. A
    b. B
    c. C
    d. D
    e. B and C

ADDITIONAL READINGS

Abrahams P, Logan B, Hutchings R, et al: *McMinn's the human skeleton*, ed 2, St Louis, 2007, Mosby.

Gunn C: *Bones and joints: a guide for students*, ed 5, Edinburgh, 2007, Churchill Livingstone.

MacConaill M, Basmajian J: *Muscles and movements: a basis for human kinesiology*, Baltimore, 1969, Williams & Wilkins.

Neumann D: *Kinesiology of the musculoskeletal system: foundations for physical rehabilitation*, St Louis, 2002, Mosby.

Whiten S: *The flesh and bones of anatomy*, Philadelphia, 2007, Mosby.

CHAPTER 3

Structure and Function of Skeletal Muscle

CHAPTER OUTLINE

OBJECTIVES

- Describe concentric, eccentric, and isometric activation of muscle.
- Identify the anatomic components that comprise a whole muscle.
- Describe the sliding filament theory.
- Describe how cross-sectional area, line of pull, and shape help determine the functional potential of a muscle.
- Describe the active length-tension relationship of muscle.
- Describe the passive length-tension relationship of muscle.
- Explain why the force production of a multi-articular muscle is particularly affected by its operational length.
- Describe the principles of stretching muscular tissue.
- Describe the basic principles of strengthening muscular tissue.

KEY TERMS

actin-myosin cross bridge
active insufficiency
agonist
antagonist
co-contraction
concentric activation
contracture
cross-sectional area
distal attachment
eccentric activation
endomysium
epimysium
excursion
fasciculus
force-couple
hypertrophy
insertion
isometric activation
muscle belly
muscle fiber
myofibril
origin
passive insufficiency
perimysium
proximal attachment
sarcomere
sliding filament theory
stabilizer
synergist
vector

Nearly all physical rehabilitation programs involve stretching, strengthening, or the retraining of muscles. As the sole producer of active force in the body, muscle is ultimately responsible for all active motions and therefore plays a fundamental role in kinesiology. Muscles also control and stabilize our posture by their action at joints. Clinicians therefore often advocate strengthening muscles to stabilize the underlying joints, especially when structures such as ligaments have been weakened by disease or trauma. This chapter provides a basic overview of the structure and function of skeletal muscle and reviews the important features of muscle as it relates to our study of kinesiology.

Fundamental Nature of Muscle

Muscles develop active force after receiving input from the nervous system. Once stimulated, a muscle produces a contractile, or pulling, force. By pulling on bones, muscles create movement. Although not always obvious, it is important to understand that muscles act by *pulling*, not pushing, regardless of whether the muscle is shortening, lengthening, or remaining a constant length.

A fundamental principle of kinesiology states that when a muscle contracts, the freest (or less constrained) segment moves. This principle applies whether a muscle is pulling its distal attachment toward its proximal attachment or vice versa (Figure 3-1).

Types of Muscular Activation

An active muscle develops a force in only one of the following three ways:

1. Shortening (or contracting)
2. Attempting to resist elongation
3. Remaining at a constant length

These muscle activations are referred to as concentric, eccentric, and isometric, respectively.

CONCENTRIC

Concentric activation occurs as a muscle produces an active force and simultaneously shortens; as a result, the muscle decreases the distance between its proximal and distal attachments. During a concentric contraction, the internal torque produced by the muscle is greater than the external torque produced by an outside force (Figure 3-2, A).

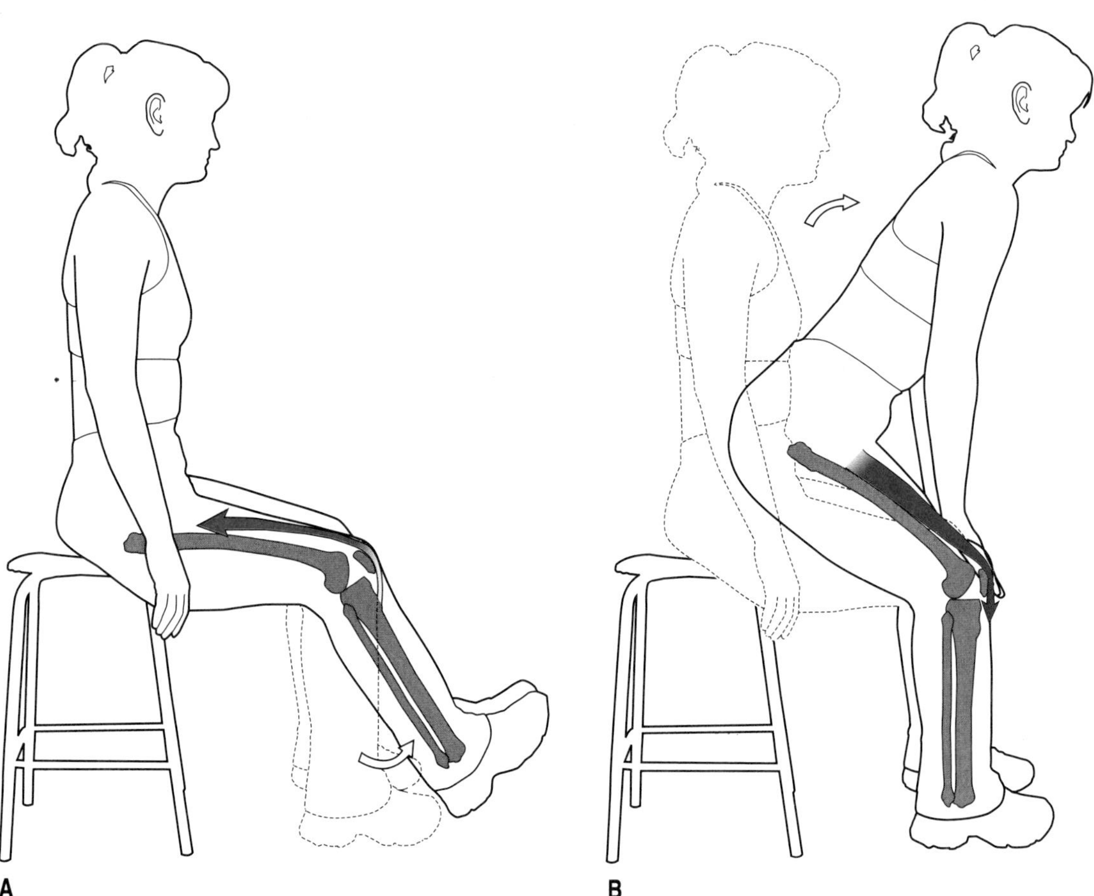

Figure 3-1 When a muscle contracts, the freest kinematic segment moves. This figure illustrates the knee extensor muscles contracting in an open and closed chain. **A**, The tibia (distal segment) is most free to move. **B**, The femur (proximal segment) is most free to move.

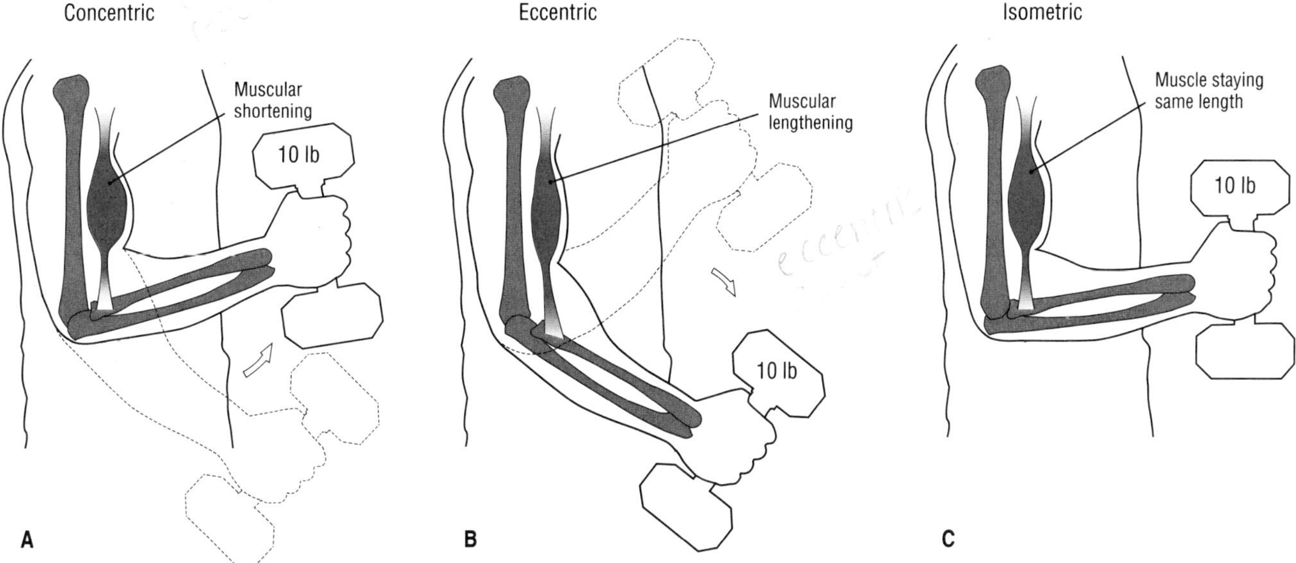

Figure 3-2 The three types of muscular activation: concentric **(A)**, eccentric **(B)**, and isometric **(C)**.

ECCENTRIC

Eccentric activation occurs as a muscle produces an active force—attempts to contract—but is simultaneously pulled to a longer length by a more dominant external force. During eccentric muscular activation, the external torque, often generated by gravity, exceeds the internal torque produced by muscle. Most often, gravity or a held weight is allowed to "win," effectively lengthening the muscle in a controlled manner. For example, slowly lowering a barbell involves eccentric activation of the elbow flexors. As a consequence, the proximal and distal attachments of the muscle become farther apart (Figure 3-2, *B*).

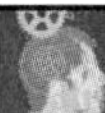

Consider this...

Eccentric Activation—the Lowering Force of Muscle

Eccentric activation occurs when a muscle is active but lengthening. Almost invariably, eccentric activation of a muscle is used to control the rate of descent, effectively lowering or decelerating the body or body segment in the direction of gravity. Lowering one's self from standing to sitting, lowering an arm to one's side, or lowering a weight to one's chest such as during the lowering phase of a bench press all require eccentric muscular activation.

If an action is described as "lowering," it is almost 100% certain that the muscles controlling the action are eccentrically activated. During an eccentric activation, gravity usually powers the movement; the eccentric activation of muscle is used to decelerate the rate of descent of the body.

ISOMETRIC

Isometric activation occurs when a muscle generates an active force while remaining at a constant length (Figure 3-2, *C*). This results when the muscle generates an internal torque equal to the external torque; as a consequence, there is no motion or change in joint angle.

Muscle Terminology

Specific terminology is commonly used when describing muscle or the actions of muscles, and the following paragraphs outline some of these terms and their definitions.

The terms *proximal attachment* and *distal attachment* are used throughout this text to describe the relative points of attachment of muscle to bone. The **proximal attachment**, or **origin**, of a muscle refers to the point of attachment that is closest to the midline, or core of the body, when in the anatomic position. The **distal attachment**, or **insertion**, refers to the muscle's point of attachment that is farthest from the midline, or core, of the body.

An **agonist** is a muscle or muscle group that is most directly related to performing a specific movement. For example, the quadriceps (knee extensors) are the agonists for knee extension. An **antagonist**, on the contrary, is the muscle or muscle group that can oppose the action or actions of the agonist. Usually, the antagonist muscle passively elongates as the agonist actively contracts. For example, when performing elbow flexion, the biceps are considered the agonists as they perform elbow flexion. The triceps (elbow extensors), which are the antagonists of this action, passively elongate as the elbow is flexed. Therefore an overly stiff antagonist muscle that fails to elongate can significantly limit the action of an agonist muscle.

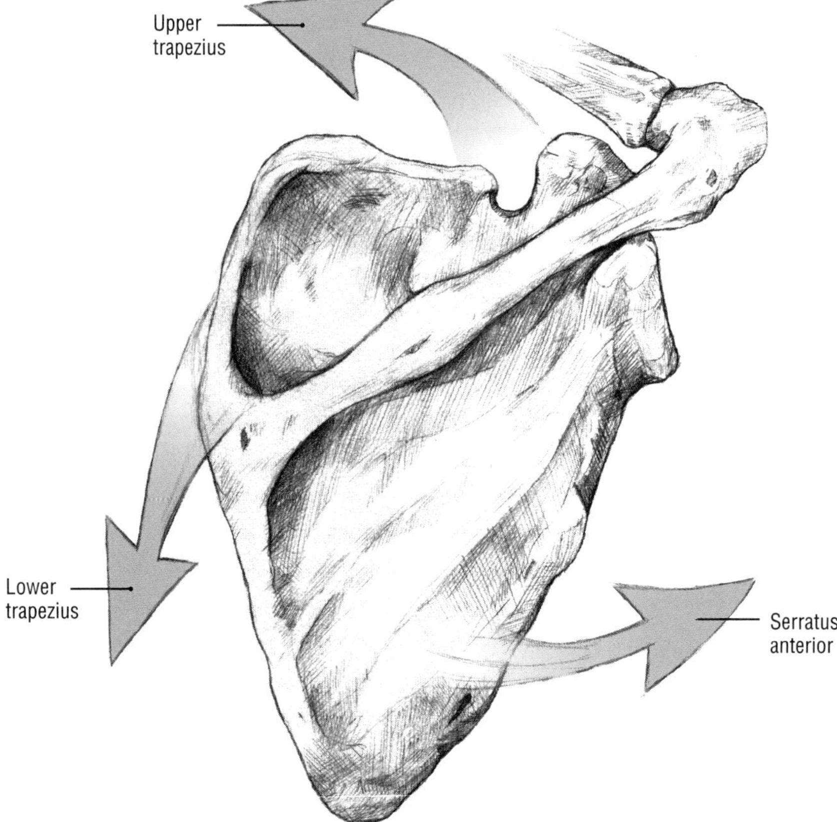

Figure 3-3 A muscular force-couple producing upward rotation of the scapula. All three muscles have different lines of pull, but all assist in rotating the scapula the same direction.

A **co-contraction** occurs when agonist and antagonist muscles are simultaneously activated in a pure or near isometric fashion. Co-contractions of muscle often stabilize and therefore protect a joint. Similarly, a muscle that fixes or holds a body segment relatively stationary so that another muscle can more effectively perform an action is referred to as a **stabilizer**.

Muscles that work together to perform a particular action are known as **synergists;** furthermore, most meaningful movements of the body involve the synergistic action of muscles. A **force-couple** is a type of synergistic action that occurs when two or more muscles produce force in different linear directions but produce torque in the same rotary direction. Figure 3-3 illustrates the force-couple generated by three different shoulder muscles to upwardly rotate the scapula.

Muscles are elastic in nature and are therefore constantly being lengthened or shortened. This change in length of a muscle is known as its **excursion**. Typically, a muscle can only shorten or elongate about half of its resting length. For example, a muscle 8 inches long at its resting length could contract to roughly 4 inches or elongate to about 12 inches in length.

Muscular Anatomy

Figure 3-4 illustrates the primary functional components that constitute skeletal muscle, whereas Box 3-1 describes each of these components. A whole muscle consists of three main components, each surrounded by a particular type of connective tissue that supports its function.

The Sarcomere: The Basic Contractile Unit of Muscle

A **sarcomere** is the basic contractile unit of muscle fiber. Each sarcomere is composed of two main protein filaments—actin and myosin—which are the active structures responsible for muscular contraction. The most popular model that describes muscular contraction is called the **sliding filament theory.** In this theory, active force is generated as actin filaments slide past the myosin filaments, resulting in contraction of an individual sarcomere.

Figure 3-5 illustrates a sarcomere and emphasizes the physical orientation of the actin and myosin filaments. The thick myosin filament contains numerous heads, which when attached to the thinner actin filaments create **actin-myosin cross bridges**. In essence a myosin head is similar to a cocked spring, which on binding with an actin filament flexes and produces a *power stroke*. The power stroke slides the actin filament past the myosin, resulting in force generation and shortening of an individual sarcomere (Figure 3-6). Because sarcomeres are joined

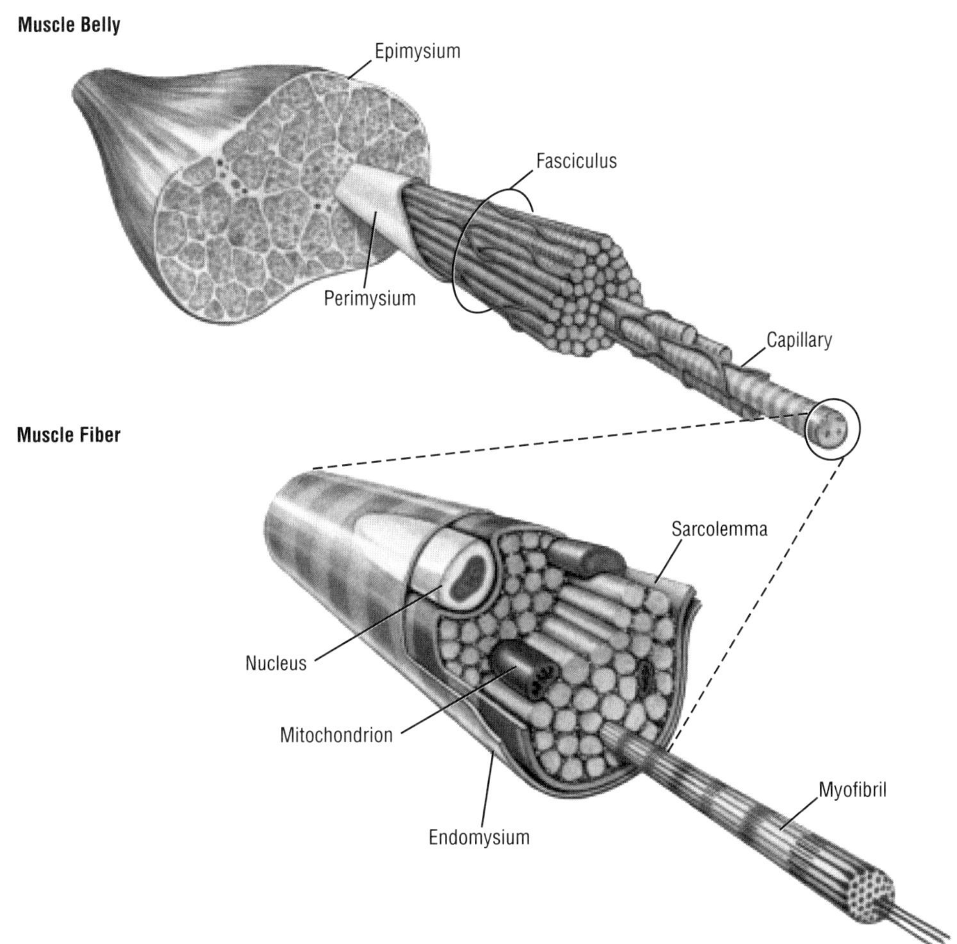

Figure 3-4 The structures and connective tissue that comprise a skeletal muscle. (Modified from Williams PL: *Gray's anatomy: the anatomical basis of medicine and surgery*, ed 38, New York, 1995, Churchill Livingstone.)

end to end throughout an entire muscle fiber, their simultaneous contraction shortens the entire muscle.

Each myosin filament has numerous heads, and each actin filament has numerous binding sites. This is important because in order for a sarcomere to maximally contract, numerous power strokes must occur. In fact, the force of a muscular contraction is determined largely by the number of actin-myosin cross bridges that are formed. This concept is addressed later in the section on the importance of muscular length.

Form and Function of Muscle

The three following factors help determine the functional potential of a muscle: cross-sectional area, shape, and line of pull.

Cross-Sectional Area

The physiologic **cross-sectional area** of a muscle describes its thickness—an indirect and relative measure of the amount of contractile elements available to generate force. The larger a muscle's cross-sectional area, the greater its force potential. This simple concept explains why a

> **BOX 3-1**
>
> **Functional Components of Skeletal Muscle**
>
> - **Muscle belly:** The muscle belly is the bulk, or body, of the muscle and is composed of numerous fasciculi.
>   Surrounding connective tissue: The **epimysium** surrounds the outer layer, or belly, of the muscle and helps to hold the shape of a muscle.
> - **Fasciculus:** Each fasciculus consists of a bundle of muscle fibers.
>   Surrounding connective tissue: The **perimysium** surrounds individual fasciculi. It functions to support the fasciculi and serves as a vehicle to support the nerves and blood vessels.
> - **Muscle fiber:** A muscle fiber is actually an individual cell with multiple nuclei. The fiber contains all the contractile elements within muscle.
>   Surrounding connective tissue: The **endomysium** surrounds each muscle fiber. It is composed of a relatively dense meshwork of collagen fibrils that help to transfer contractile force to the tendon.
> - **Myofibril:** Each muscle fiber is composed of several myofibrils. Myofibrils contain contractile proteins, packaged within each sarcomere.

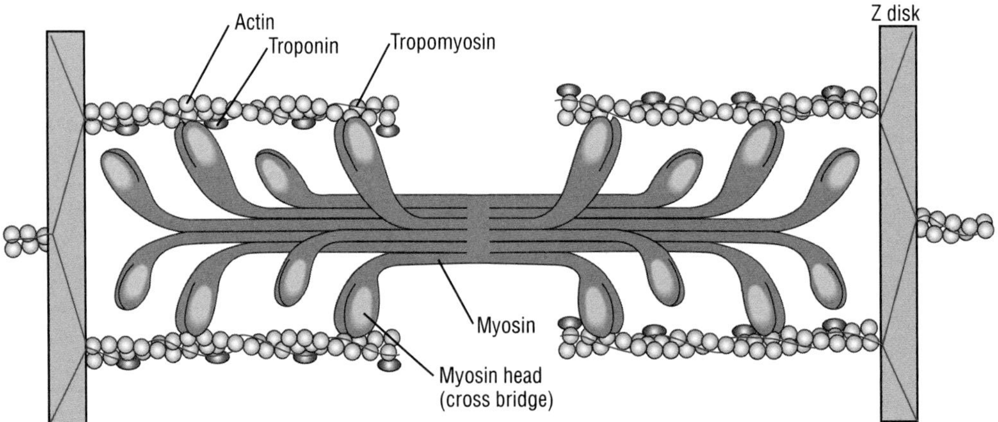

Figure 3-5 An illustration of a single sarcomere showing the cross-bridge structure created by the myosin heads and their attachment to the actin filaments. The proteins troponin and tropomyosin are also shown. Troponin is responsible for exposing the actin filament to the myosin head, thereby allowing cross-bridge formation. (Modified from Berne RM, Levy MN: *Principles of physiology,* ed 2, St Louis, 1996, Mosby.)

person with larger muscles can usually generate larger muscular forces.

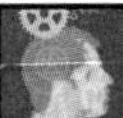

Consider this...

Cross-Sectional Area of the Quadriceps: From Force to Torque

In general a maximally activated muscle produces approximately 50 lb of force for every square inch of muscular tissue; this varies surprisingly little among different people or different muscles.

The quadriceps muscle has an average cross-sectional area of about 25 square inches. If each square inch of muscle produces approximately 50 lb of force, then a maximal effort contraction of the quadriceps would theoretically produce 1250 lb of force (25 inches^2 × 50 lb/inches^2 = 1250 lb): almost enough force to lift a Volkswagen bug! When considering the internal moment arm provided by the patella (≈1.5 inches), the average knee extension torque provided by the quadriceps reaches 1875 inch-lbs (1.5 inches × 1250 lb). Typically described in foot-pounds, this magnitude of torque (≈155 foot-lbs) can be expected from a healthy, strong, young male.

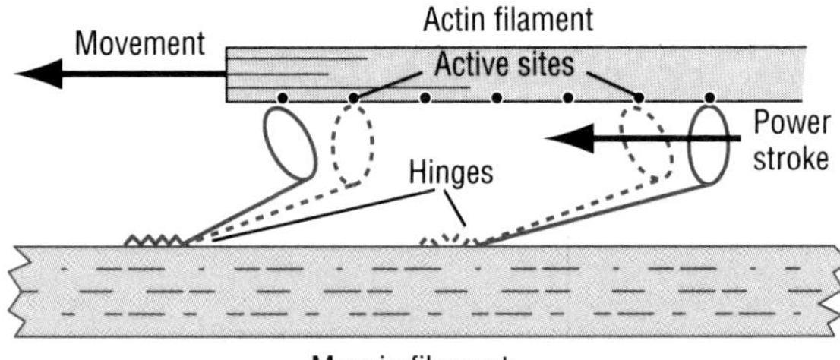

Figure 3-6 The sliding filament action that occurs as myosin heads attach and then release from the actin filament. Contractile force is generated during the power stroke of the cycle. (From Guyton AC, Hall JE: *Textbook of medical physiology,* ed 10, Philadelphia, 2000, Saunders.)

Shape

A muscle's shape is one important indicator of its specific action. For example, long, strap-like muscles typically provide large ranges of motion, whereas thick, short muscles typically provide large forces. Most muscles appear as one of four basic shapes: fusiform, triangular, rhomboidal, and pennate (Figure 3-7).

Fusiform muscles such as the brachioradialis have fibers that run parallel to one another (see Figure 3-7, A). Typically, these muscles are built to provide large ranges of motion.

Triangular muscles such as the gluteus medius have expansive proximal attachments that converge to a small distal attachment (see Figure 3-7, B). The large proximal attachments provide a well-stabilized base for generating force.

Rhomboidal muscles such as the rhomboids or gluteus maximus have expansive proximal and distal attachments (see Figure 3-7, C). As the name implies, these muscles are generally shaped like large rhomboids or offset squares. The expansive attachments make them well suited to either stabilize a joint or provide large forces, depending on the cross-sectional area of the muscle.

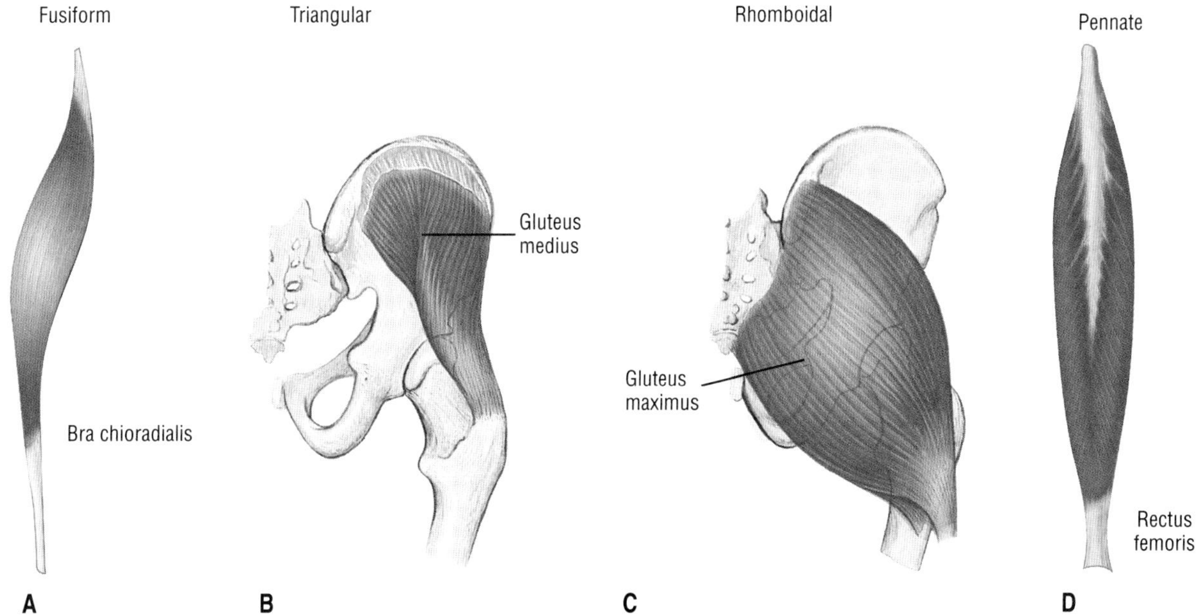

Figure 3-7 Four common shapes of skeletal muscle: fusiform **(A)**, triangular **(B)**, rhomboidal **(C)**, and pennate **(D)**. (From Thibodeau GA, Patton KT: *Anatomy & physiology*, ed 6, St Louis, 2006, Mosby, Figures 10-2, *CD*, and 10-29, *AC*.)

Pennate muscles resemble the shape of a feather, with muscle fibers approaching a central tendon at an oblique angle (see Figure 3-7, *D*). The diagonal orientation of the fibers maximizes the muscle's force potential. Many more muscle fibers fit into the muscle compared with a similar-sized fusiform muscle. However, because the muscle fibers are oriented obliquely, the actual range of motion, or excursion, of the muscle is limited. Pennate structure is found in muscles such as the rectus femoris and gastrocnemius—muscles that are often required to produce large forces to support or propel the weight of the body.

Pennate muscles may be further classified as uni-pennate, bi-pennate, or multi-pennate depending on the number of similarly angled sets of fibers that attach to the central tendon.

Line of Pull

Muscle forces can be described as a **vector** because they possess both a direction and a magnitude. The direction of a muscle's force is referred to as the muscle's line of pull (or line of force). Assumed to act in a straight line, a muscle's line of pull relative to the axis of rotation of a joint dictates the muscle's action. For example, a muscle's line of pull that crosses anterior to the medial-lateral axis of rotation of the shoulder performs flexion. Conversely, if a muscle's line of pull courses posterior to the medial-lateral axis of rotation at the shoulder, it will perform extension (Figure 3-8). This concept is discussed in Chapter 1.

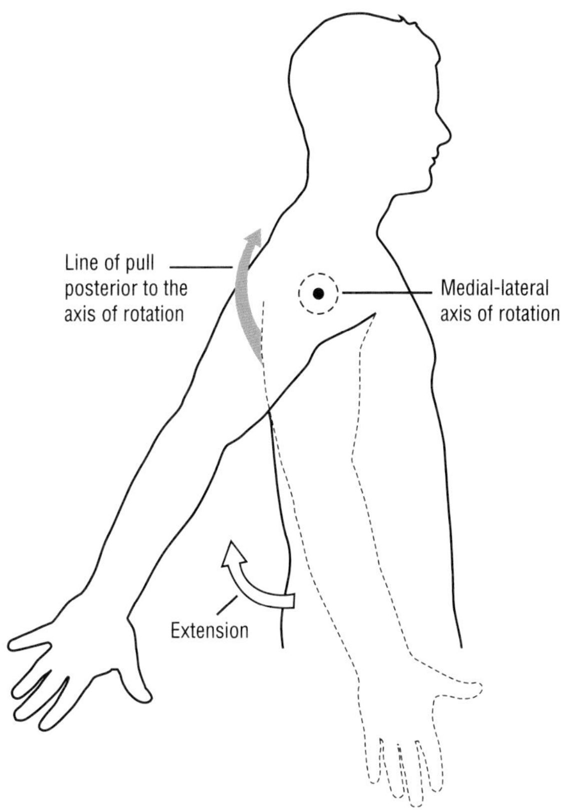

Figure 3-8 The line of pull of a shoulder muscle is shown traveling posterior to the medial-lateral axis of rotation. Activation of this muscle results in extension of the shoulder.

Clinical **INSIGHT**

Surgically Altering a Muscle's Line of Pull

The triceps muscle courses posterior to the medial-lateral axis of rotation at the elbow and is therefore an extensor of this joint. By surgically altering the insertion of one of the three heads of the muscle, the line of pull can be shifted anterior to the medial-lateral axis of the elbow. This part of the muscle is therefore converted to an elbow flexor (Figure 3-9).

This type of procedure, known as a tendon transfer, may be performed on individuals who have paralysis of key muscles such as those that flex the elbow or oppose the thumb. To be successful, however, there must be a relatively strong and healthy muscle in a nearby location suitable for transfer. Therapists must help retrain the patient on how to perform the new action of the transferred muscle.

This procedure is an excellent example of how medicine uses principles of kinesiology: In this case the principle that a muscle's ultimate action is determined by its line of pull relative to the axis of rotation.

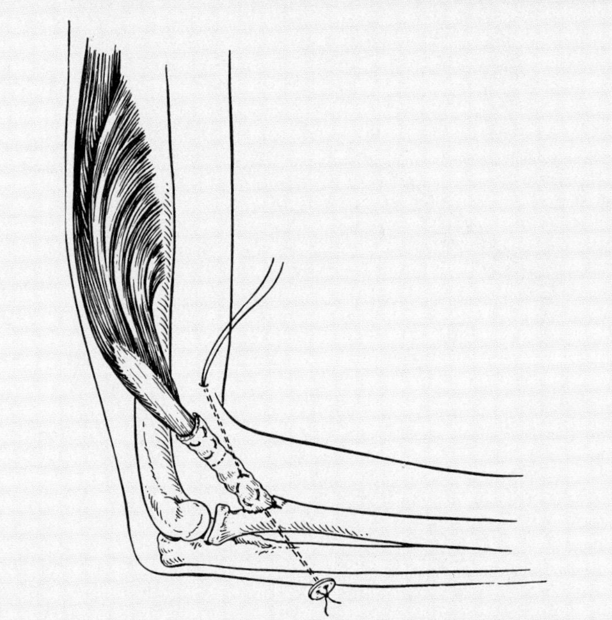

Figure 3-9 An anterior transfer of the triceps muscle changing the function of this muscle from elbow extension to elbow flexion. (From Bunnell S: Restoring flexion to the paralytic elbow, *J Bone Joint Surg Am* 33-A(3):566-571, 1951.)

Length-Tension Relationship of Muscle

The operational length of a muscle describes the degree to which it is either stretched or shortened at the time of its activation. This factor, known as the length-tension relationship, has a significant impact on the force output of muscle. The concept that muscle length strongly influences muscle force is interwoven into many clinical activities, including the testing and strengthening of muscles and the use of splints or braces to immobilize or control joints. Specific examples are provided throughout this chapter and textbook.

Active Length-Tension Relationship

As described previously, a muscle produces a force by a sliding of thin actin filaments relative to the thicker myosin filaments. The amount of force generated by such a process is highly dependent on the relative length of the sarcomere (Figure 3-10). Length is critical because it determines the number of effective actin-myosin cross bridges that exist at any given time. Similar to the number of men pulling a carriage, more cross bridges yield a greater contraction force (Figure 3-11).

The length-tension relationship of a single sarcomere helps explain how the relative length (or degree of stretch) of a whole muscle affects its force production. Consider, for example, the change in maximal strength of the elbow flexor muscles in different amounts of elbow flexion. Similar to the length-tension relationship at the sarcomere level, the strength of the elbow flexor muscles is characterized by a bell-shaped curve (Figure 3-12). Elbow

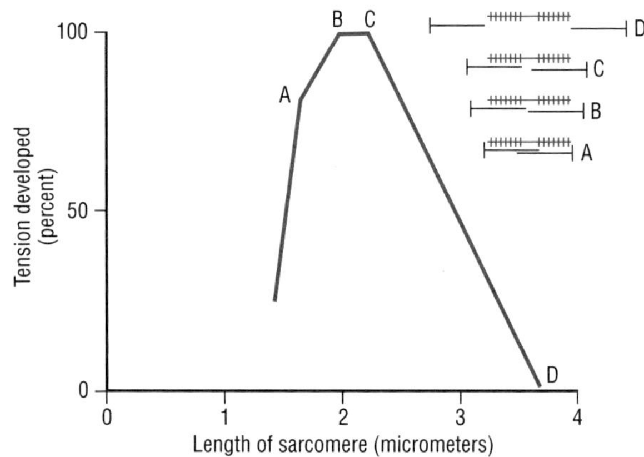

Figure 3-10 The active length-tension curve of a sarcomere for four specified sarcomere lengths (*upper right, A-D*). *A*, Actin filaments overlap, so the number of cross-bridge formations is reduced. *B* and *C*, Actin and myosin filaments are positioned to allow an optimal number of cross bridges to be formed. *D*, Actin filaments are positioned out of the range of the myosin heads, so cross-bridge formation is limited. (From Guyton AC, Hall JC: *Textbook of medical physiology,* ed 10, Philadelphia, 2000, Saunders.)

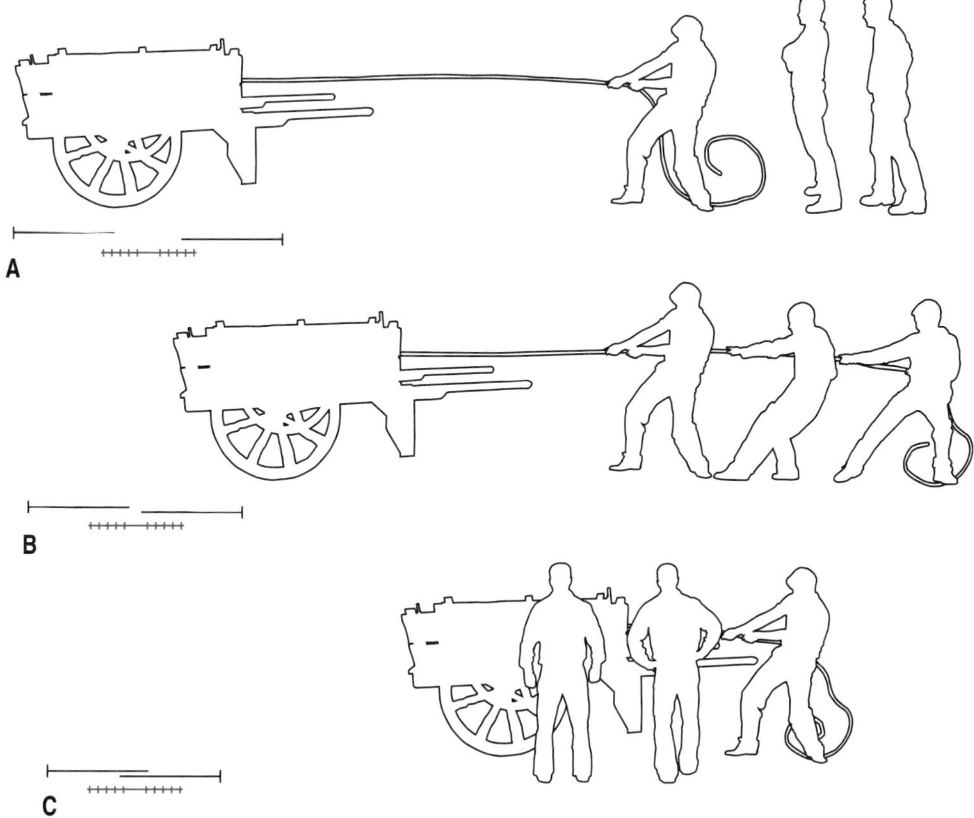

Figure 3-11 Men pulling a cart as an analogy for force production relative to sarcomere length. The black and red notched lines represent actin and myosin filaments in an **A,** elongated position; **B,** optimal length; and **C,** shortened position. At either very long **(A)** or very short **(B)** sarcomere lengths, the ability to produce contractile force is reduced.

flexion strength is least in full elbow flexion (where the muscles are short) and again in full elbow extension (where the muscles are relatively elongated). Elbow flexion strength is greatest at midrange of elbow flexion, a joint angle that is associated with maximal overlap of the cross bridges within the muscles. Because strength of the elbow flexors (as with any muscle group) is expressed clinically as a torque, both muscle force and internal moment arm need to be considered. Regardless, the important concept is that a muscle's active force is generally greatest at its midlength and least at both extremes.

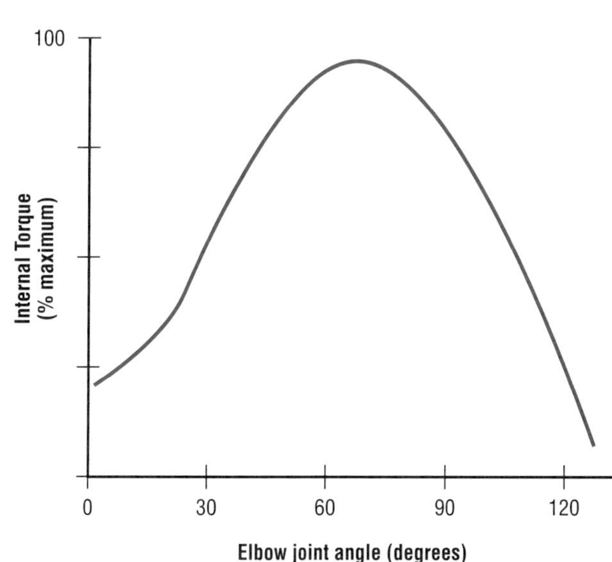

Figure 3-12 A curve showing the internal torque produced by the elbow flexors relative to elbow joint angle. The highest amount of internal torque is produced with the elbow flexed to 70 to 80 degrees, a joint angle that provides maximal actin-myosin cross-bridge formation, as well as a large internal moment arm. (From Neumann DA: *Kinesiology of the musculoskeletal system: foundations for physical rehabilitation,* St Louis, 2002, Mosby, Figure 3-12, *A.*)

Passive Length-Tension Relationship

Although muscles are most often discussed as the active force producers in the body, because of their elastic nature, they also produce force passively. In this way, a muscle is similar to a rubber band. Like a rubber band, a muscle generates greater internal elastic force when stretched. This elastic behavior is demonstrated by a muscle's passive length-tension curve (Figure 3-13).

Length-Tension Relationship Applied to Multi-Articular Muscles

Mono-articular muscles cross only one joint. Multi-articular (or poly-articular) muscles, on the other hand, cross multiple joints. As expected, a multi-articular muscle can be stretched or elongated to a much greater amount than a mono-articular muscle. For this reason, the range in force output of a multi-articular muscle can vary to large degrees—much more so than a mono-articular muscle. This can have important clinical implications when addressing the activation of multi-articular muscles.

Consider, for example, the multi-articular biceps brachii, which crosses the shoulder and the elbow. Furthermore, consider this muscle during an unnatural movement that rapidly combines elbow flexion with full shoulder flexion. Such an active motion requires that the biceps simultaneously contracts at both ends. As a result, the muscle becomes shortened in a short period of time. This type of movement significantly reduces the force-producing potential of the muscle, as fewer and fewer actin-myosin cross bridges can be formed.

In contrast to the previously mentioned movement, consider the biceps muscle during a more natural and effective movement that combines simultaneous and rapid elbow flexion with shoulder extension, such as pulling an object toward you. As the biceps contracts to perform elbow flexion, it is simultaneously elongated or stretched across the extending shoulder. Such an activity helps maintain a near constant (and optimal) overall length of biceps during the activity. In this way the biceps produces a more constant force throughout the range of motion. This strategy is important to consider when designing functional exercises or teaching functional activities that involve the activation of multi-articular muscles.

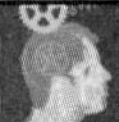

Consider this...

Quick-Stretch for Maximal Muscle Power

Many high-powered activities use the elasticity of muscle to a functional advantage. Consider, for example, a jumping motion. Typically, jumping involves a loading motion, which flexes the hips, knees, and ankles before "exploding" upward. The quick-bend provides a quick stretch to the hip extensors, knee extensors, and plantar flexors, all of which contribute to the jumping force.

A quick-stretch, similar to quickly stretching a rubber band, spring loads the muscle, allowing the stored energy to be released during the desired action—in this case, the jumping motion.

Clinicians often use a quick-stretch to engage or improve the performance of a particular muscle group. Plyometrics, as another example, are a specific group of exercises often used by athletes to improve training and performance. These exercises incorporate a quick-stretch of a muscle group immediately before its action to enhance force production.

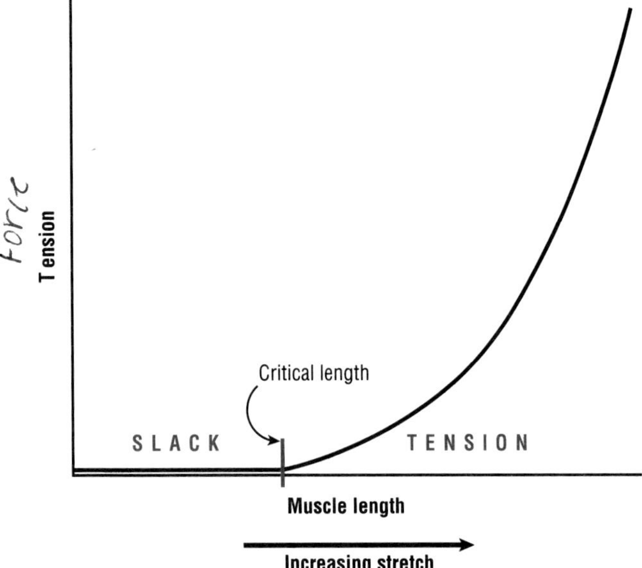

Figure 3-13 A generalized passive length-tension curve is shown. As a muscle is progressively stretched, the tissue is slack during its initial shortened lengths until it reaches a critical length where it begins to generate tension. Beyond this critical length, the tension builds exponentially. (From Neumann DA: *Kinesiology of the musculoskeletal system: foundations for physical rehabilitation,* St Louis, 2002, Mosby, Figure 3-5.)

Force-Velocity Relationship of Muscle: Speed Matters

The velocity of a muscular contraction (activation) can have a significant impact on its force production. During a concentric contraction, a muscle produces *less* force as the speed of contraction increases. This concept should be self-evident and can be verified by comparing the greatest speed at which you can repeatedly lift a heavy versus a light object. At higher speeds of contraction, the actin-myosin cross bridges do not have sufficient time to form (pull) and re-form. Therefore the muscle's ability to produce force is decreased.

Isometric activation of a muscle creates greater force than any speed concentric contraction. Because the velocity of an isometric contraction is zero, nearly all the available actin-myosin cross bridges are formed, and all are given enough time to reach their maximal force-producing potential.

The force-velocity relationship of muscle also applies to eccentric activation. During an eccentric activation, force production *increases* slightly as the speed of the elongation increases. This is explained, in part, by the elasticity of the connective tissues within a muscle. Similar to quickly stretching a rubber band, the muscle's resistance to elongation increases with increased speed of elongation. At a

Clinical INSIGHT

Active versus Passive Insufficiency

Because multi-articular muscles can experience extreme shortening or elongation across multiple joints, such muscles are often associated with functional weakness, regardless of effort. Two terms help describe the reason for this weakness: active insufficiency and passive insufficiency.

Passive insufficiency occurs when a particular action is weakened because the antagonist muscle of the action is over-stretched across two or more joints, preventing the full range of motion of the intended action. Verify this phenomenon on yourself by trying the following activity: Hold the wrist in a fully flexed position and then attempt to make a fist without letting the wrist extend. The reason a full fist cannot be effectively made is largely because of passive insufficiency, or excessive tightness within the over-stretched long finger extensor muscles. Because the long finger extensors are over-stretched across the flexed wrist, they prevent the finger flexor muscles from making an effective fist.

Active insufficiency occurs when a particular action is weakened because the multi-articular agonist muscle performing the action is too short to produce a useful or effective force. The weakness in making the fist, for example, is also caused by the long finger flexor muscles being too short (slackened) over the flexed wrist and flexed fingers. Note that the weakness in making the fist is caused by two factors acting simultaneously: (1) active insufficiency of the agonist and (2) passive insufficiency of the antagonist.

Clinicians should be aware of active and passive insufficiency issues when they design exercise programs or immobilize joints.

Clinical INSIGHT

Isolating One-Joint versus Two-Joint Muscles for a Manual Muscle Test

Many times the principles of active insufficiency are used therapeutically to isolate certain muscles (e.g., when isolating the gluteus maximus from the rest of the hip extensor muscles during a manual muscle test).

Figure 3-14, *A*, illustrates a therapist performing a manual muscle test to determine the maximal strength of the hip extensor muscles. By testing hip extensor strength with the knee in a fully extended position, the hamstrings and the gluteus maximus are at favorable lengths to produce near-maximal forces. Thus a good measure of overall hip extensor strength can be ascertained. However, it may become necessary to determine the relative strength of just the gluteus maximus muscle. By placing the knee in a flexed position (Figure 3-14, *B*), the hamstrings become shortened across the hip and the knee, thereby making them actively insufficient and thus significantly reducing their ability to contribute to hip extension force. Because the hamstrings are effectively taken out of the equation, the gluteus maximus is said to be isolated, as it becomes responsible for the majority of the hip extension torque produced.

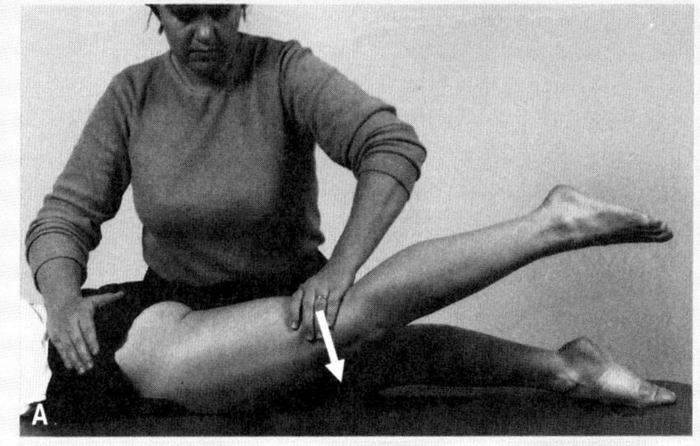

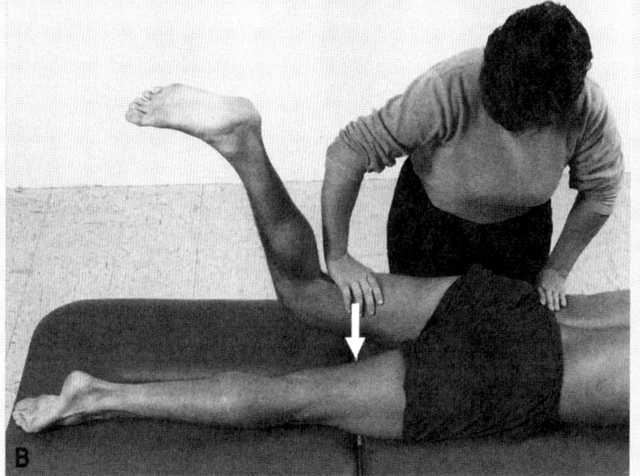

Figure 3-14 A clinician is shown performing a manual muscle test to all the hip extensor muscles **(A)** and to the gluteus maximus **(B)**. By placing the knee in a flexed position, the hamstrings are put "on slack," and therefore the gluteus maximus is said to be isolated. (From Reese NB: *Muscle and sensory testing,* ed 2, Philadelphia, 2005, Saunders.)

high enough speed or force output, the connective tissue elements within muscle may become strained. This explains why persons often feel greater muscle soreness following high-velocity eccentric activities.

Table 3-1 highlights the force-velocity relationships for concentric, eccentric, and isometric muscular activations.

Important Clinical Considerations: Taking the Principles to the Patient

Many patients receiving physical therapy services display some form of muscular weakness or tightness, which often compromises overall mobility and joint stability. Many interventions to treat these impairments are based on the principles described in this chapter. These principles are reinforced in the following sections, which highlight clinical examples and definitions of common clinical terminology.

TABLE 3-1 FORCE-VELOCITY RELATIONSHIP OF MUSCLE

Type of Muscle Activation	Force-Velocity Relationship	Reasoning
Concentric	Slower-speed contraction produces greater force	Maximal time for actin-myosin cross-bridge formation
Eccentric	Higher-speed elongation produces greater force	Stretching of passive elements of muscle
Isometric	Force from isometric activation is greater than any speed concentric contraction	Velocity of isometric contraction is zero, allowing more time for maximal cross-bridge formation

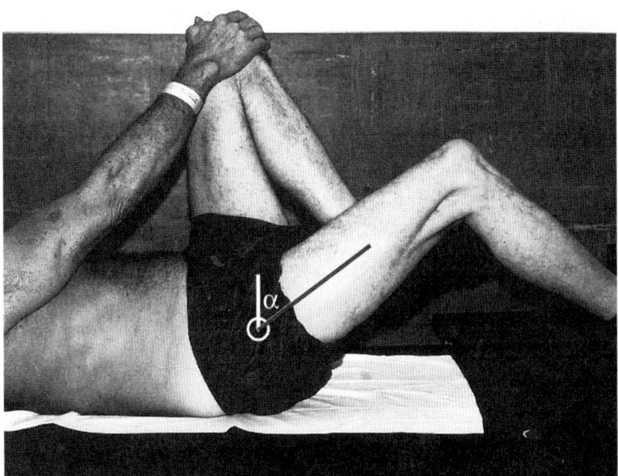

Figure 3-15 An individual performing a Thomas test showing a significant contracture (shortening) of the hip flexor muscles in the right lower extremity. The left hip is held flexed to stabilize the pelvis. (From Neumann DA: *Kinesiology of the musculoskeletal system: foundations for physical rehabilitation,* St Louis, 2002, Mosby, Figure 9-69, *A.*)

Muscular Tightness

Muscles are highly adaptable and often adapt to the length in which they are most often held. Simply stated, a muscle held in a shortened position over time will shorten; a muscle held in an elongated position, over time, will lengthen.

Disease, immobility, or simply poor posture often results in some degree of adaptive shortening in muscle. Muscles that become shorter often become stiffer and experience an increased resistance to elongation, or stretch. This phenomenon is referred to clinically as being "tight." The degree and functional consequence of muscular tightness varies considerably. Many people have some tightness in their hamstring muscles, for example, but suffer little, if any, loss in function or quality of life. A muscle so tight that it severely restricts joint movement, however, is pathologic; it is referred to as a **contracture** (Figure 3-15).

A muscle contracture can significantly alter posture and reduce functional mobility of the entire body. Muscle stretching for muscle tightness or contracture is an important component of many exercise programs.

Stretching Muscular Tissue

An overly tight muscle causes the associated joints to assume a posture that mimics the muscle's primary actions. For example, a tightened hamstring muscle caused by severe spasticity causes a posture of hip extension and knee flexion—two primary actions of this muscle. To stretch the muscle, therefore, the limb must be held in some tolerable amount of hip flexion and knee extension. Note that as a general principle, optimal

BOX 3-2

Guidelines for Stretching

Proper Stretching

- Stretch the muscle by attempting to position the joint (or joints) in a manner that is opposite to all of the tightened muscles normal actions.
- Hold the stretch at least 20 to 30 seconds.
- Perform stretches frequently.
- When feasible, encourage positions throughout the day that maintain some stretch on the muscle.
- When feasible, strengthen the muscles that are antagonist to the tightened muscle.
- Do not over-stretch the muscle; this may cause injury.

Preventing Tightness

- Avoid extended periods of time in the same position.
- Embrace an active lifestyle.
- Maintain ideal posture as much as possible.

Clinical INSIGHT

Muscular Atrophy: Use It or Lose It

Muscular atrophy refers to muscle wasting or a decrease in muscle mass (Figure 3-16). This is clinically relevant because reduced muscle mass is directly proportional to the loss in muscle strength. Loss in muscle strength, or weakness, can significantly impair an individual's functional mobility and independence. Atrophy of muscle is often measured indirectly by making girth measurements of limbs. For example, decreased circumference of the calf or thigh indicates atrophy of the plantar flexor or knee extensor muscles, respectively.

Muscles begin to atrophy surprisingly quickly after immobilization. Often the role of a physical therapist or physical therapist assistant is to prevent atrophy by having patients begin exercise protocols as soon as possible following a period of immobilization.

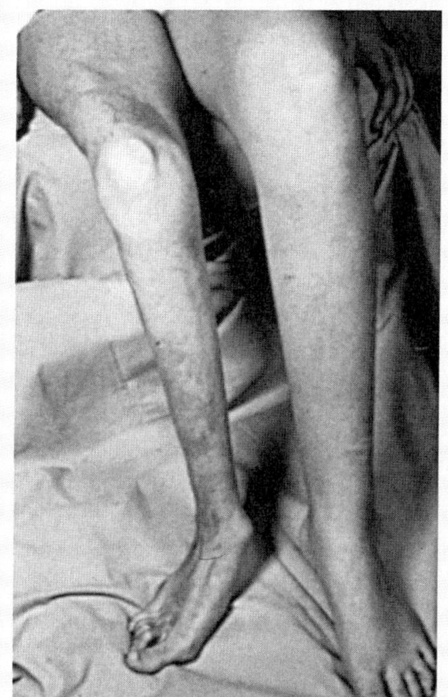

Figure 3-16 Atrophy of the right lower extremity. (From Harris ED, Budd RC, Firestein GS, et al: *Kelly's textbook of rheumatology,* ed 7, Philadelphia, 2005, Saunders, Figure 97-11.)

stretching of a muscle requires the therapist to hold a limb in a position that is opposite to all of the muscle's actions. Although research on the most effective method to stretch muscle is variable, Box 3-2 provides some helpful clinical tips for stretching and preventing muscular tightness.

Strengthening

Muscular weakness can result from injury, disease, or simply lack of use. Regardless of the cause, muscular weakness can significantly impair the ability to perform normal functional activities and may result in postural abnormalities and injury to joints.

Many times, therapists are called on to devise exercise programs to increase a patient's muscular strength. Many strengthening exercises employ the principles of overload and training specificity. The *overload* principle states that a muscle must receive sufficient level of resistance to stimulate hypertrophy. Without a critical amount of resistance (or overload), muscle strengthening will not occur. Therapists must make clinical judgments on how to apply the appropriate amount of resistance to stimulate hypertrophy but not cause injury.

The principle of *training specificity* implies that a muscle will adapt to the way in which it is challenged. Clinicians often use this principle by designing exercises that closely match the natural demands placed on the muscle. Specific examples of these exercises are given throughout this text.

Clinical INSIGHT

Muscular Hypertrophy

Muscular **hypertrophy** refers to muscular growth or enlargement. In healthy muscle, hypertrophy indicates an increase in strength. This occurs over time as a muscle is appropriately resisted or overloaded. Interestingly, muscle hypertrophy is not a result of more muscle fibers, but mostly from an increase in the size of individual muscle fibers. The increased size is caused by a synthesis of more proteins that are involved with muscle force (actin and myosin). As a result, more actin and myosin cross bridges can be formed, thereby resulting in greater maximal force.

Muscle as an Active Stabilizer

Although ligaments and capsules can stabilize joints, only muscle can adapt to the immediate and long-term external forces that can destabilize the body. Muscle tissue is ideally suited to stabilize a joint, because it is coupled to the external environment and to the internal control mechanisms offered by the nervous system.

Many types of injuries, such as ligamentous rupture, can significantly destabilize a joint. Often this can lead to postural compensations or further injury to the joint. Physical therapists and physical therapist assistants often improve stability of a joint by strengthening the surrounding muscles. By targeting the stabilizing musculature, specific exercises can be employed to support an injured, or unstable, joint. For example, most post-surgical anterior cruciate ligament rehabilitation programs begin by strengthening the musculature that can support and protect the new graft.

Summary

The force generated by muscle is the primary means by which an individual controls the intricate balance between stable posture and active movement. Throughout the remainder of this text, much of the discussion involves the multiple roles of muscle in controlling the postures and movements that are used in common functional tasks.

Injuries or disease often impair normal muscular function, resulting in tightness, weakness, or postural instability. On the basis of clinical signs and functional limitations, a clinician often must decide on—and pursue—a particular course of therapeutic intervention. A fundamental understanding of the nature of muscle can be extremely helpful in determining and properly advancing a particular course of treatment.

Study Questions

1. Which of the following statements describes a concentric contraction?
   a. The proximal and distal attachments of the muscle become farther apart.
   b. The proximal and distal attachments of the muscle become closer together.
   c. The internal torque produced by the muscle is greater than the external torque produced by an outside force.
   d. A and C
   e. B and C
2. Which of the following types of muscular activation results in elongation of the muscle?
   a. Concentric
   b. Eccentric
   c. Isometric
3. Which of the following statements best describes an antagonist?
   a. A muscle that fixes or holds a body segment stationary so that another muscle can more effectively perform an action
   b. A muscle that always shortens when it is active
   c. A muscle or muscle group that opposes the action of an agonist
   d. The muscle or muscle group most directly responsible for performing a particular action
4. Which of the following statements best describes a muscular force-couple?
   a. Two or more muscles actively lengthening throughout an entire action
   b. Combined agonist and antagonist activity resulting in no or minimal joint movement
   c. When two or more muscles produce force in different linear directions but produce rotary torque in the same linear direction
   d. When an overly stiff or tight antagonist limits the action of the agonist muscle
5. Which of the following statements is true?
   a. The larger a muscle's cross-sectional area, the greater its force-producing potential.
   b. In pennate muscles, nearly all the muscle fibers run parallel to one another.
   c. A muscle is able to produce the most force as it nears a maximally shortened position.
   d. A and B
   e. A and C
6. A muscle with a line of pull anterior to the medial-lateral axis of rotation of the shoulder will perform:
   a. Abduction
   b. Flexion
   c. Adduction
   d. Extension
7. The primary reason a muscle can produce the most force near its midrange is:
   a. Elastic properties of muscle help add to the active force of a muscle in its midrange.
   b. Minimal actin-myosin cross-bridge formation is available in a muscle's midrange.
   c. Passive elements of muscular tissue are put "on slack."
   d. The number of actin-myosin cross bridges that can be formed is near maximal.
8. Which of the following statements is (are) true?
   a. The passive length-tension curve indicates that muscle produces more passive force when it is stretched, rather than slackened.
   b. The force a muscle produces during a concentric contraction increases as the velocity of the contraction increases.
   c. The force produced by a muscle activated isometrically is greater than any speed of concentric contraction.
   d. A and C
   e. B and C
9. The term *active insufficiency* describes:
   a. A muscle's inability to perform an action because of the tightness of its antagonist
   b. Decreased ability of a two-joint (multi-articular) muscle to produce significant force to complete an action because it has become too short

c. The inability of an action to be completed because the antagonist is stretched over multiple joints
d. When two or more muscles combine forces but fail to complete an action

10. If a muscle that performs both hip flexion and knee extension becomes tight, which of the following combination of actions will likely be limited?
    a. Hip flexion and knee extension
    b. Hip extension and knee flexion
    c. Hip flexion and knee flexion
    d. Hip extension and knee extension
11. During a concentric contraction, the muscle is active and shortening.
    a. True
    b. False
12. According to the sliding filament theory, contraction of a sarcomere is the result of actin filaments sliding past myosin filaments.
    a. True
    b. False
13. Isometric activation of muscle results in the proximal and distal attachments of a muscle becoming farther apart.
    a. True
    b. False
14. Regardless of whether a muscle is lengthening or shortening, a muscle can produce only a contractile, or pulling, force.
    a. True
    b. False
15. A muscle's *excursion* refers to the maximal force that the muscle can produce.
    a. True
    b. False
16. A *multi-articular* muscle refers to a muscle that crosses two or more joints.
    a. True
    b. False
17. Fusiform muscles can typically produce more force than similar-sized pennate muscles.
    a. True
    b. False
18. The overload principle states that a muscle must receive a sufficient amount of resistance to stimulate hypertrophy.
    a. True
    b. False
19. *Atrophy* refers to muscular enlargement or an increase in muscle mass.
    a. True
    b. False
20. In order to stretch or maximally elongate a muscle, the muscle must be placed in a position opposite that of all its actions.
    a. True
    b. False

ADDITIONAL READINGS

Hoppenfield S: *Physical examination of the spine and extremities*, New York, 1976, Appleton-Century-Crofts.

Mosby's anatomy coloring book, St Louis, 2004, Mosby.

Muscolino JM: *The muscular system manual: the skeletal muscles of the human body*, St Louis, 2005, Mosby.

Patton KT: *Survival guide for anatomy & physiology*, St Louis, 2005, Mosby.

Standring S: *Gray's anatomy: the anatomical basis of clinical practice*, ed 39, Edinburgh, 2005, Churchill Livingstone.

Thibodeau GA, Patton KT: *Anatomy & physiology*, ed 6, St Louis, 2005, Mosby.

Whyte G, Spurway N, MacLaren D: *The physiology of training*, Edinburgh, 2006, Churchill Livingstone.

CHAPTER 4

Structure and Function of the Shoulder Complex

CHAPTER OUTLINE

OBJECTIVES

- Identify the bones and primary bony features relevant to the shoulder complex.
- Describe the location and primary function of the ligaments that support the joints of the shoulder complex.
- Cite the normal ranges of motion for shoulder flexion and extension, abduction and adduction, and internal and external rotation.
- Describe the planes of motion and axes of rotation for the primary motions of the shoulder.
- Cite the proximal and distal attachments, actions, and innervation of the muscles of the shoulder complex.
- Describe the muscular interactions involved with active shoulder abduction.
- Describe the scapulohumeral rhythm.
- Explain the force-couple that occurs to produce upward rotation of the scapula.
- Identify the primary muscles involved with dynamic stabilization of the glenohumeral joint.
- Explain how the shoulder depressor muscles can be used to elevate the thorax.
- Describe the interaction between the internal and external rotators of the shoulder during a throwing motion.

KEY TERMS

downward rotation
dynamic stabilization
force-couple
impingement
muscular substitution
reverse action
scapulohumeral rhythm
static stability
subluxation
upward rotation
winging

Our study of the upper limb begins with the shoulder complex, a set of four articulations involving the sternum, clavicle, ribs, scapula, and humerus (Figure 4-1). This series of joints works together to provide large ranges of motion to the upper extremity in all three planes. Rarely does a single muscle act in isolation at the shoulder complex. Rather, muscles work in teams to produce highly coordinated movements that are expressed over multiple joints. The cooperative nature of the shoulder musculature increases the versatility, control, and range of active

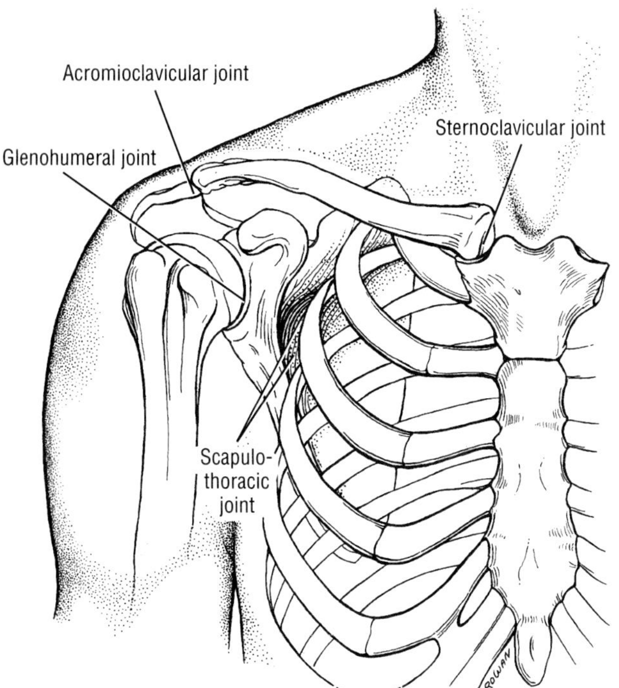

Figure 4-1 The joints of the right shoulder complex. (From Neumann DA: *Kinesiology of the musculoskeletal system: foundations for physical rehabilitation,* St Louis, 2002, Mosby, Figure 5-1.)

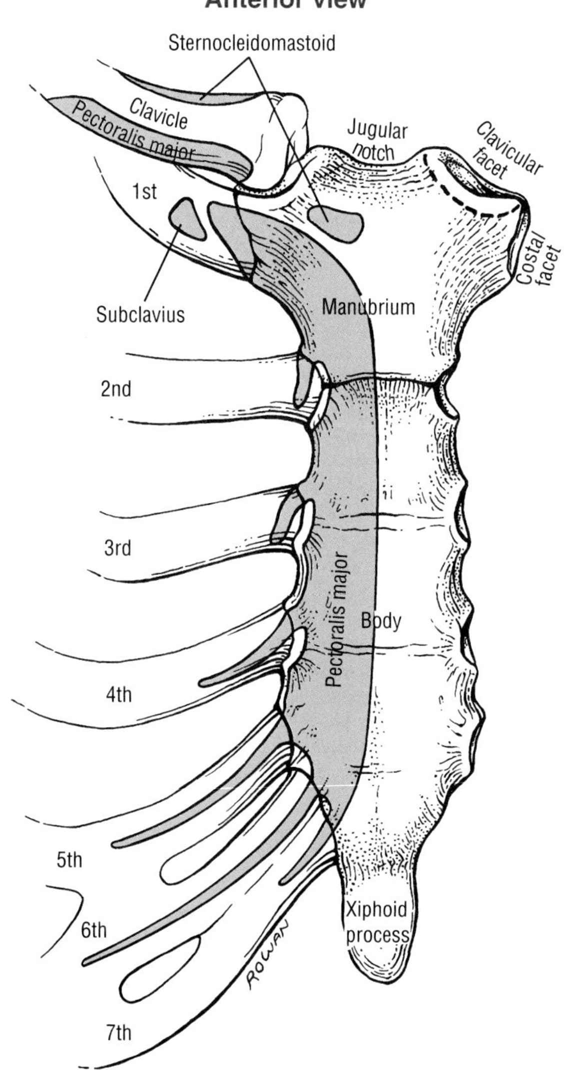

Figure 4-2 An anterior view of the sternum with the left clavicle and ribs removed. The proximal attachments of surrounding muscles are shown in red. (From Neumann DA: *Kinesiology of the musculoskeletal system: foundations for physical rehabilitation,* St Louis, 2002, Mosby, Figure 5-2.)

movements available to the upper extremity. Because of the nature of this functional relationship among the shoulder muscles, paralysis, weakness, or tightness of any single muscle can disrupt the natural kinematic sequencing of the entire shoulder complex. This chapter provides an overview of the kinesiology of the four joints of the shoulder complex and the important muscular synergies that support proper function of the shoulder (Figure 4-1).

Osteology

Sternum

The sternum, often called the breast bone, is located at the midpoint of the anterior thorax; composed of the manubrium, body, and xiphoid process (Figure 4-2). The *manubrium* is the most superior portion of the sternum that articulates with the clavicle—forming the *sternoclavicular joint.* The *body* or middle portion of the sternum serves as the anterior attachment for ribs 2 through 7. The inferior tip of the sternum is called the *xiphoid process,* meaning "sword shaped."

Clavicle

The clavicle, commonly called the collar bone, is an S-shaped bone that acts like a mechanical rod that links the scapula to the sternum (Figure 4-3). The flattened lateral portion—called the *acromial end*—articulates with the acromion of the scapula, forming the *acromioclavicular joint.* The medial or *sternal end* of the clavicle articulates with the manubrium of the sternum, forming the *sternoclavicular joint.*

Scapula

Commonly called the shoulder blade, the scapula is a highly mobile, triangular-shaped bone that rests on the posterior side of the thorax (Figure 4-4). The slightly concave anterior aspect of the bone is called the *subscapular fossa,* which allows the scapula to glide smoothly along the convex posterior rib cage. The *glenoid fossa* is the slightly concave, oval-shaped surface that accepts the head of the humerus, composing the *glenohumeral joint.* The *superior*

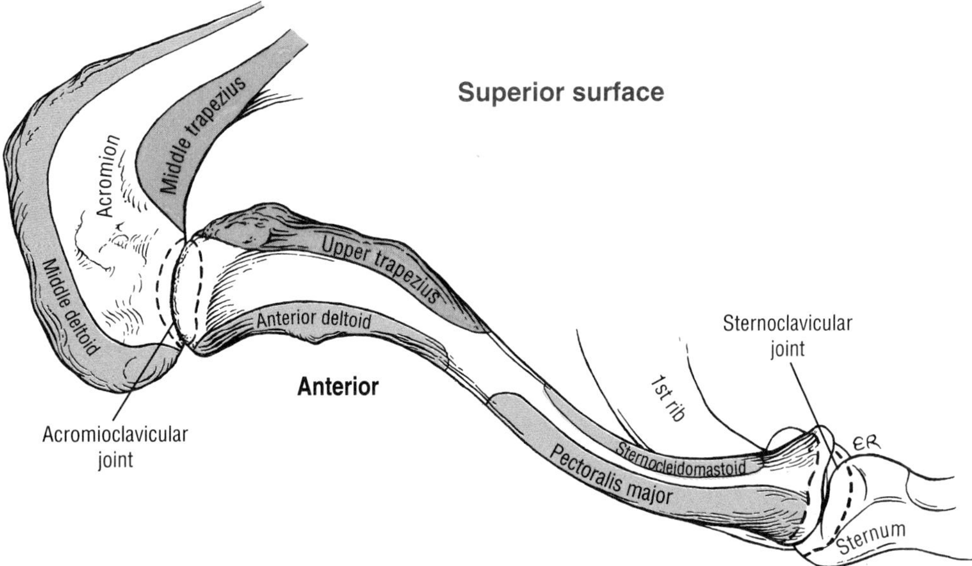

Figure 4-3 A superior view of the right clavicle articulating with the sternum and acromion. Proximal attachments of muscles are shown in red, distal attachments in gray. (From Neumann DA: *Kinesiology of the musculoskeletal system: foundations for physical rehabilitation,* St Louis, 2002, Mosby, Figure 5-3.)

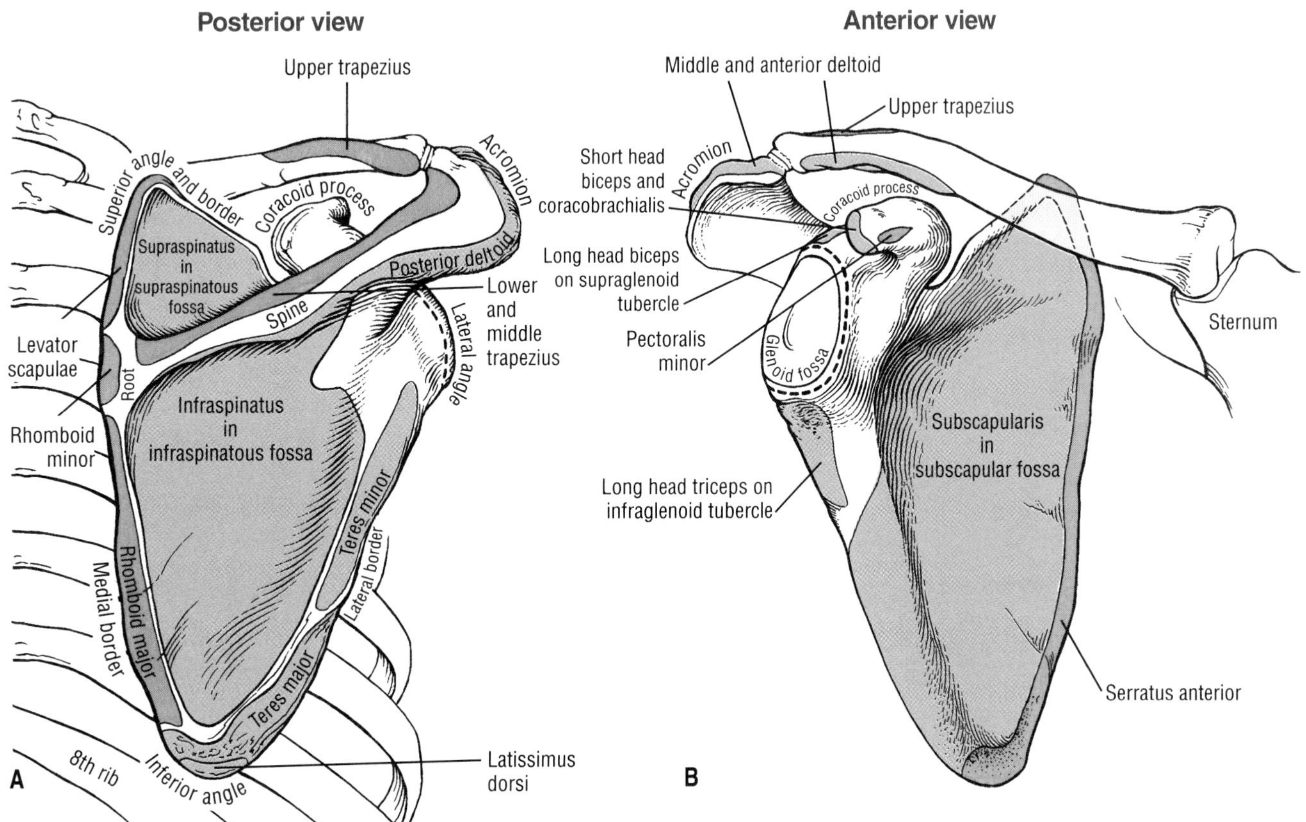

Figure 4-4 Posterior **(A)** and anterior **(B)** surfaces of the right scapula. Proximal attachments of muscles are shown in red, distal attachments in gray. (From Neumann DA: *Kinesiology of the musculoskeletal system: foundations for physical rehabilitation,* St Louis, 2002, Mosby, Figure 5-5.)

and *inferior glenoid tubercles* border the superior and inferior aspects of the glenoid fossa and serve as proximal attachments for the long head of the biceps and long head of the triceps, respectively. The *scapular spine* divides the posterior aspect of the scapula into the *supraspinatous fossa* (above) and *infraspinatous fossa* (below). The *acromion process* is a wide, flattened projection of bone from the most superior-lateral aspect of the scapula. The acromion forms a functional "roof" over the humeral head to help protect the delicate structures within that area. The *coracoid process*

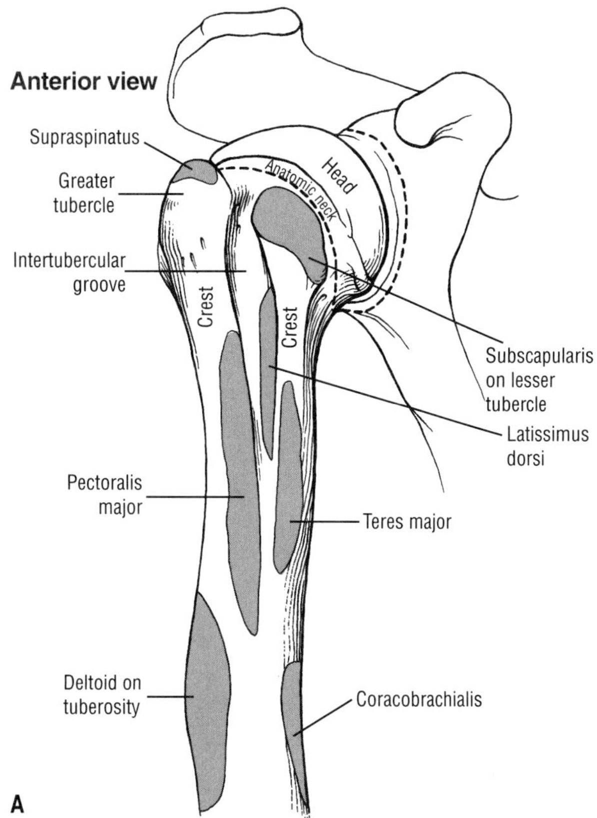

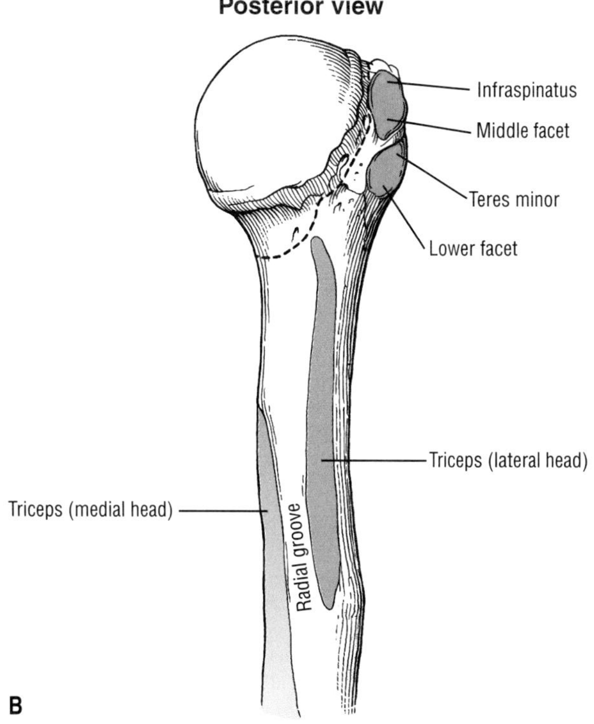

Figure 4-5 Anterior **(A)** and posterior **(B)** views of the right humerus. Proximal attachments of muscles are shown in red, distal attachments in gray. (From Neumann DA: *Kinesiology of the musculoskeletal system: foundations for physical rehabilitation*, St Louis, 2002, Mosby, Figures 5-8, *A*, and 5-10.)

is the finger-like projection of bone from the anterior surface of the scapula, palpable about 1 inch below the most concave portion of the distal clavicle. The coracoid process is the site of attachment for several muscles and ligaments of the shoulder complex. The *medial* and *lateral borders* of the scapula meet at the *inferior angle*, or tip, of the scapula. Clinically, the inferior angle is important in helping track scapular motion.

Proximal-to-Mid Humerus

The proximal humerus (Figure 4-5) is the point of attachment for a multitude of ligaments and muscles. The distal humerus is discussed in the next chapter.

The *humeral head* is nearly one half of a full sphere that articulates with the glenoid fossa forming the *glenohumeral joint*. The *lesser tubercle* is a sharp, anterior projection of bone just below the humeral head. The larger, more rounded lateral projection of bone is the *greater tubercle*. The greater and lesser tubercles are divided by the *intertubercular groove*, often called the *bicipital groove* because it houses the tendon of the long head of the biceps. More distally, on the lateral aspect of the upper one third of the shaft of the humerus is the *deltoid tuberosity*—the distal insertion of all three heads of the deltoid muscle. The *radial (spiral) groove* runs obliquely across the posterior surface of the humerus. The radial nerve follows this groove and helps define the proximal attachment for the lateral and medial heads of the triceps.

Arthrology

The shoulder complex functions through the interactions of four joints: the (1) sternoclavicular, (2) scapulothoracic, (3) acromioclavicular, and (4) glenohumeral joints. To fully understand how the shoulder functions as a whole, we must first examine the structure and kinematics of each individual joint.

Joints of the Shoulder Complex

- Sternoclavicular
- Scapulothoracic
- Acromioclavicular
- Glenohumeral

Sternoclavicular Joint

GENERAL FEATURES

The sternoclavicular (SC) joint is created by the articulation of the medial aspect of the clavicle with the

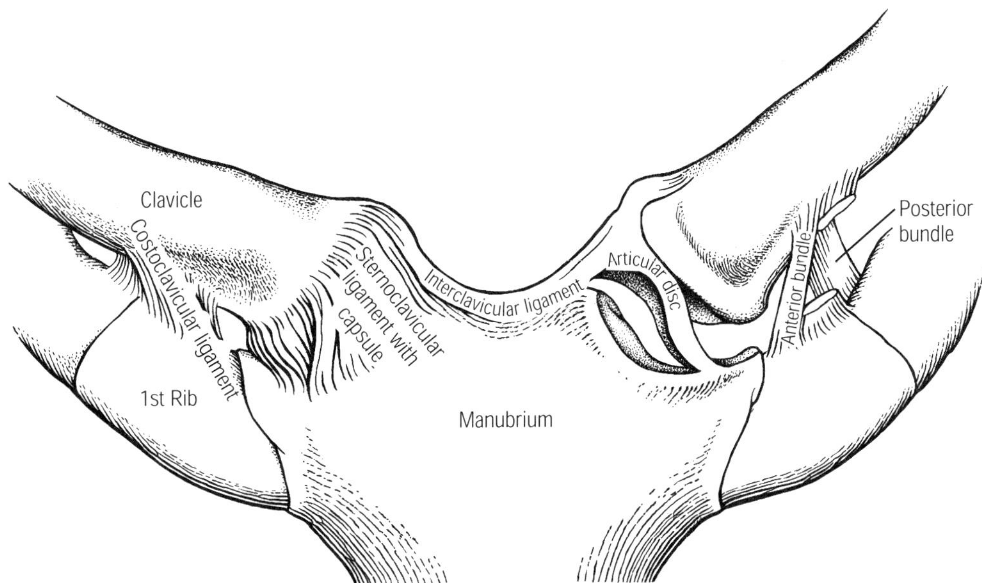

Figure 4-6 An anterior view of the sternoclavicular joints with the capsule and some of the ligaments removed on the left side. (From Neumann DA: *Kinesiology of the musculoskeletal system: foundations for physical rehabilitation,* St Louis, 2002, Mosby, Figure 5-12.)

sternum (Figure 4-6). This joint provides the only direct bony attachment of the upper extremity to the axial skeleton—accordingly, the joint must be stable while also allowing extensive mobility.

The SC joint allows motion in all three cardinal planes, and it is supported by a thick network of ligaments, an articular disc, and a joint capsule. The high degree of stability provided by this thick ligamentous network explains, in part, why fractures of the clavicle occur more frequently than dislocations of the SC joint.

SUPPORTING STRUCTURES OF THE STERNOCLAVICULAR JOINT

Figure 4-6 illustrates the supporting structures of the SC joint.

- *Sternoclavicular Ligament:* Contains anterior and posterior fibers that firmly join the clavicle to the manubrium
- *Joint Capsule:* Surrounds the entire SC joint; reinforced by the anterior and posterior SC joint ligaments
- *Interclavicular Ligament:* Spans the jugular notch, connecting the superior medial aspects of the clavicles
- *Costoclavicular Ligament:* Firmly attaches the clavicle to the costal cartilage of the first rib and limits the extremes of all clavicular motion except depression
- *Articular Disc:* Acts as a shock absorber between the clavicle and the sternum; helps improve joint congruency

KINEMATICS

The SC joint structure is a saddle joint with concave and convex surfaces on each of the joint's articular surfaces (Figure 4-7). This conformation allows the clavicle to move in all three planes. Motions include elevation and depression, protraction and retraction, and axial rotation (Figure 4-8).

In essence, all movements of the shoulder girdle (i.e., the scapula and clavicle) originate at the SC joint. A fused SC joint would therefore significantly limit movement of the clavicle and scapula and hence limit movement of the entire shoulder.

Elevation and Depression

Elevation and depression of the SC joint is a near-frontal plane movement about a near–anterior-posterior axis of rotation, allowing roughly 45 degrees of clavicular elevation and 10 degrees of depression.

Protraction and Retraction

Protraction and retraction of the SC joint occur in the horizontal plane about a vertical axis of rotation, allowing about 15 to 30 degrees of clavicular motion in either direction.

Axial Rotation

During abduction or flexion of the shoulder, the clavicle rotates posteriorly about its longitudinal axis. As the shoulder is abducted, the coracoclavicular ligament becomes taut and spins the clavicle posteriorly. The clavicle rotates anteriorly, back to its rest position, as the shoulder is extended or adducted.

Scapulothoracic Joint

GENERAL FEATURES

The scapulothoracic joint is not a "true" joint in the traditional sense. It refers to the junction created by the anterior aspect of the scapula on the posterior thorax. Scapulothoracic joint motion typically describes the motion of the scapula relative to the posterior rib cage.

Normal movement and posture of the scapulothoracic joint are essential to the normal function of the shoulder. Clinicians therefore focus a great deal on evaluating

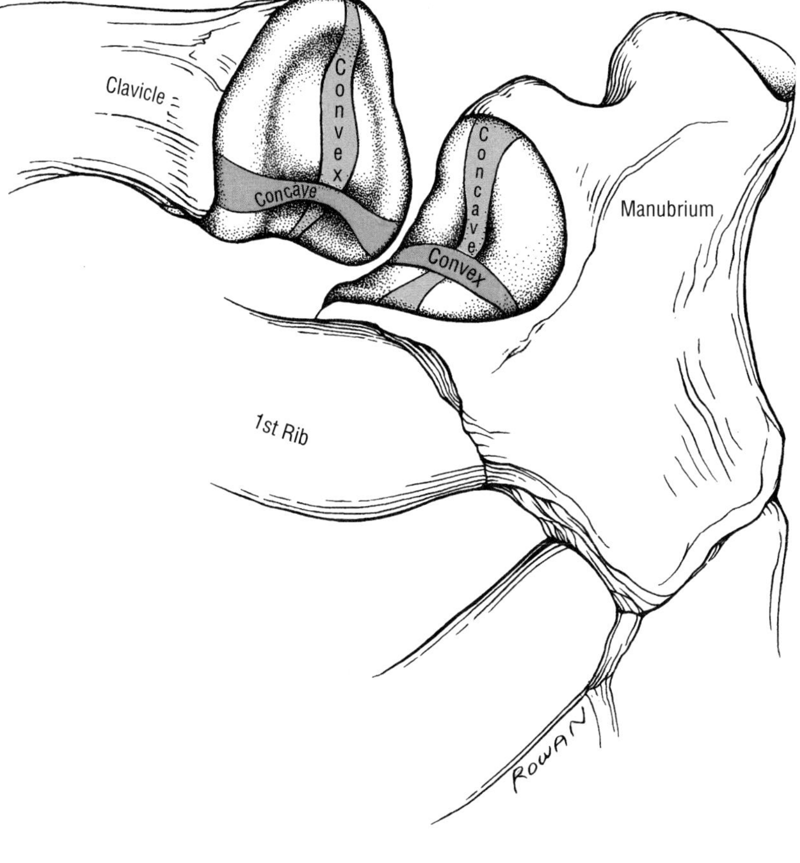

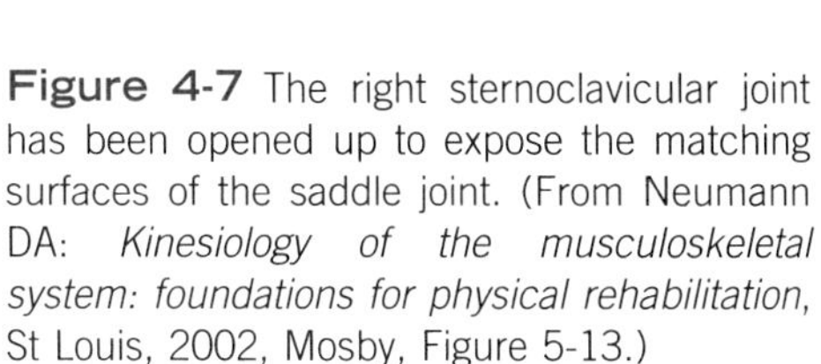

Figure 4-7 The right sternoclavicular joint has been opened up to expose the matching surfaces of the saddle joint. (From Neumann DA: *Kinesiology of the musculoskeletal system: foundations for physical rehabilitation*, St Louis, 2002, Mosby, Figure 5-13.)

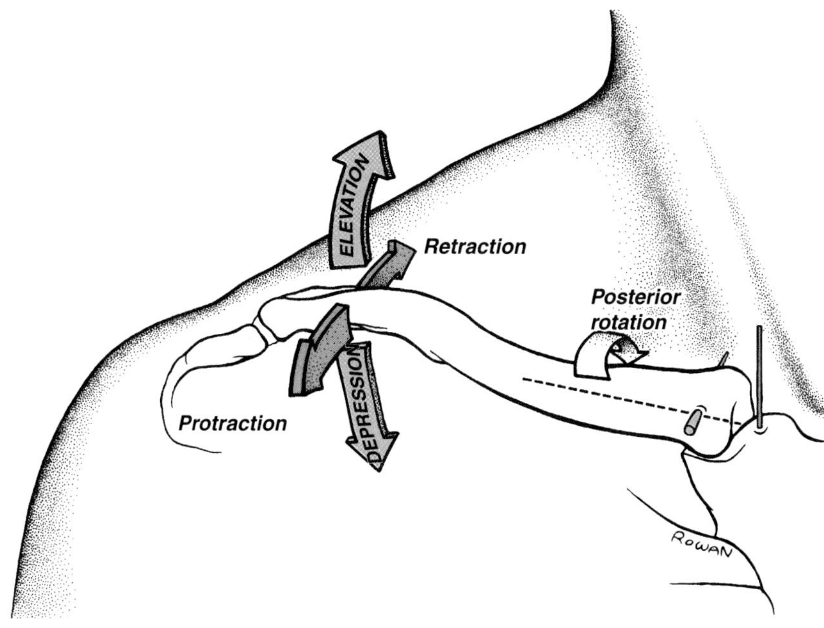

Figure 4-8 The right sternoclavicular joint showing the osteokinematic motions of the clavicle. The axes of rotation are color coded with the associated planes of motion. (From Neumann DA: *Kinesiology of the musculoskeletal system: foundations for physical rehabilitation*, St Louis, 2002, Mosby, Figure 5-14.)

and treating the quality and amount of motion between the scapula and the thorax.

KINEMATICS

Motions at the scapulothoracic joint include elevation and depression, retraction and protraction, and upward and downward rotation (Figure 4-9). All motions are functionally linked to the motions that occur at the other three joints of the shoulder complex; these functional relationships are discussed in depth later.

Elevation and Depression

Scapular elevation involves the scapula sliding superiorly on the thorax (e.g., shrugging the shoulders). Depression occurs when the scapula slides inferiorly on the thorax (see Figure 4-9, *A*; e.g., returning shrugged shoulders to a resting position, or depressing entire shoulder, such as occurs when pushing up from a sitting position).

Protraction and Retraction

Protraction describes the motion of the scapula sliding laterally on the thorax, away from midline, whereas *retraction* describes movement of the scapula toward the midline (see Figure 4-9, *B*).

Upward and Downward Rotation

Upward rotation occurs as the glenoid fossa of the scapula rotates upwardly; this occurs as a natural component of raising the arm overhead (see Figure 4-9, *C*). **Downward rotation** occurs as the scapula returns from an upwardly rotated position to its resting position. This motion naturally occurs as an elevated upper extremity is lowered to one's side.

Acromioclavicular Joint

GENERAL FEATURES

The acromioclavicular (AC) joint is considered a gliding or plane joint, created by the articulation between the lateral aspect of the clavicle and the acromion process of the scapula (Figure 4-10). In essence, this joint links the motion of the scapula (and attached humerus) to the lateral end of the clavicle. Because strong forces are frequently transferred across the AC joint, several important stabilizing structures are required to maintain its structural integrity.

SUPPORTING STRUCTURES OF THE ACROMIOCLAVICULAR JOINT

Figure 4-10 illustrates the supporting structures of the AC joint.

- *Acromioclavicular Ligament:* Joins the clavicle to the acromion; helps to prevent dislocations of the scapula and links motion of the scapula to the clavicle
- *Coracoclavicular Ligament:* Composed of the conoid and trapezoid ligaments. Together, these ligaments help suspend the scapula from the clavicle and prevent dislocation.
- *Coracoacromial Ligament:* Attaches the coracoid process to the acromion process. One of the few ligaments of the body that attaches proximally and distally to the same bone. Along with the acromion, the coracoacromial ligament completes the coracoacromial arch—a functional "roof" that protects the head of the humerus.

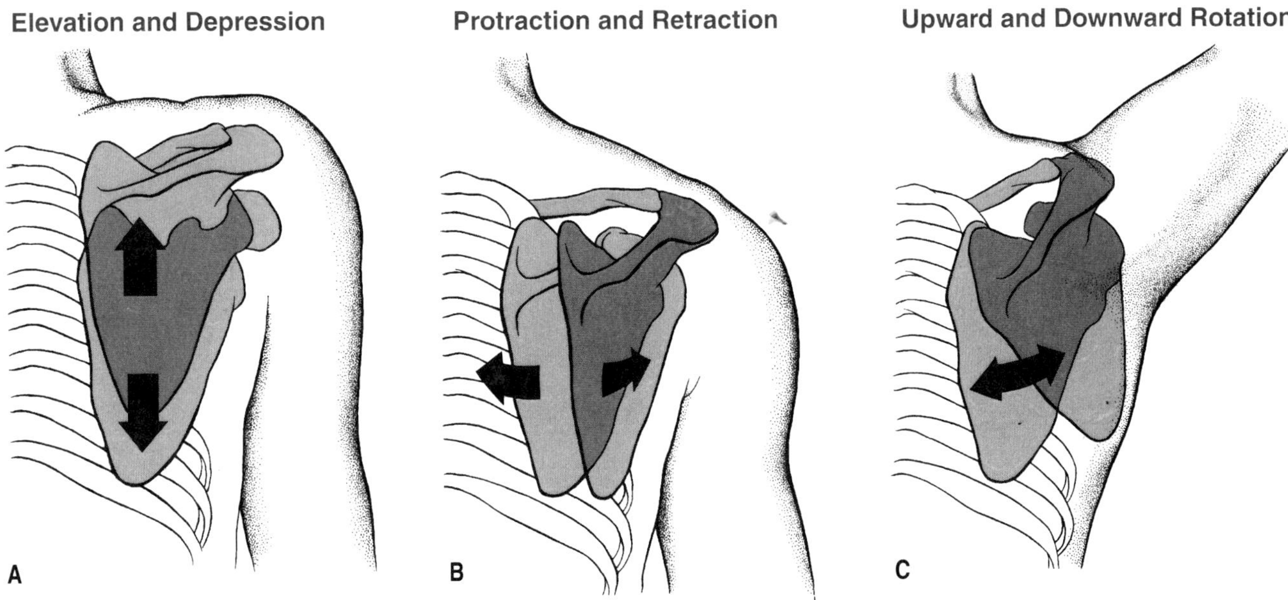

Figure 4-9 Motions of the right scapula against the posterior-lateral thorax. **A**, Elevation and depression. **B**, Protraction and retraction. **C**, Upward and downward rotation. (From Neumann DA: *Kinesiology of the musculoskeletal system: foundations for physical rehabilitation*, St Louis, 2002, Mosby, Figure 5-11.)

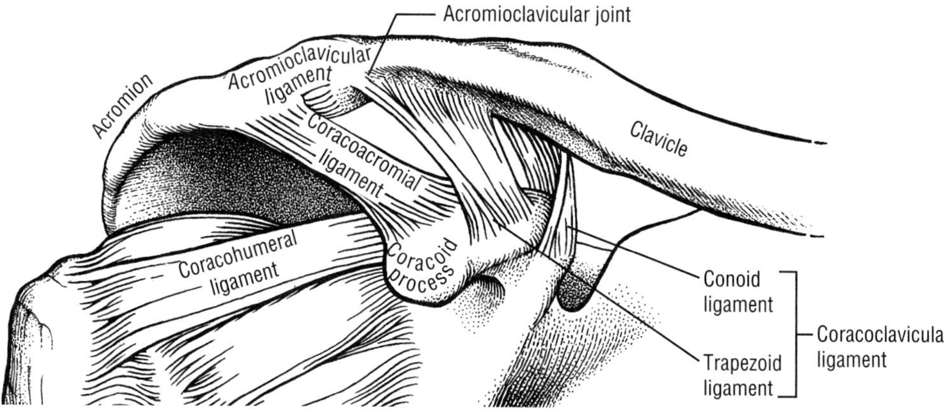

Figure 4-10 An anterior view of the right acromioclavicular joint including many of the surrounding ligaments. (From Neumann DA: *Kinesiology of the musculoskeletal system: foundations for physical rehabilitation*, St Louis, 2002, Mosby, Figure 5-18.)

KINEMATICS

The AC joint allows motion in all three planes: upward and downward rotation, rotation in the horizontal plane, and rotation in the sagittal plane (Figure 4-11). These relatively slight but important adjustment motions help to fine-tune the movements between the scapula and humerus. Equally important, these motions allow the scapula to maintain firm contact with the posterior thorax.

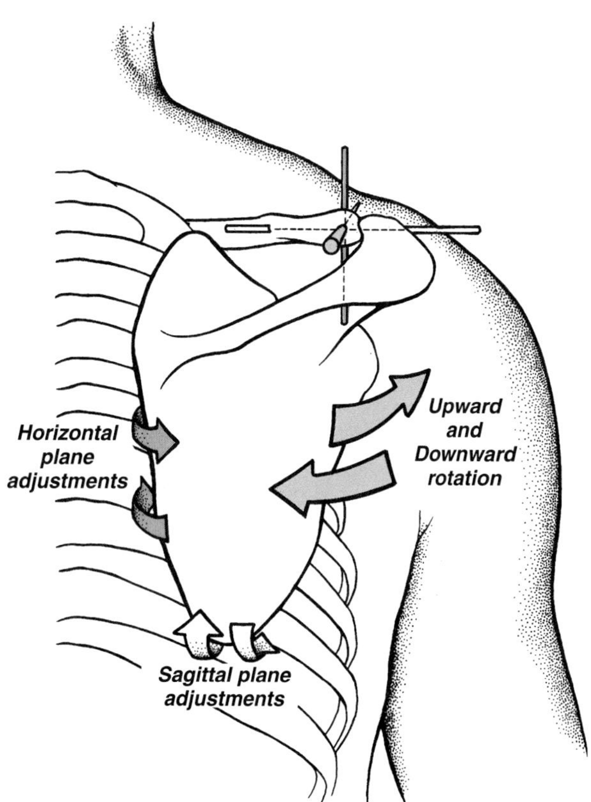

Figure 4-11 The osteokinematics of the right acromioclavicular joint. The axes of rotation are color coded with the associated planes of motion. (From Neumann DA: *Kinesiology of the musculoskeletal system: foundations for physical rehabilitation*, St Louis, 2002, Mosby, Figure 5-20, *A*.)

Glenohumeral Joint

GENERAL FEATURES

The glenohumeral (GH) joint is created by the articulation of the humeral head with the glenoid fossa of the scapula (Figure 4-12). Recall that the head of the humerus is a large, rounded hemisphere, and the glenoid fossa is relatively flat. This bony conformation, in conjunction with the highly mobile scapula, allows for abundant motion in all three planes but does not promote a high degree of stability. Interestingly, the ligaments and capsule of the GH joint are relatively thin and provide only secondary stability to the joint. The primary stabilizing force of this joint is garnered from the surrounding musculature, particularly the rotator cuff muscles.

SUPPORTING STRUCTURES OF THE GLENOHUMERAL JOINT

- *Rotator Cuff:* A group of four muscles including the supraspinatus, infraspinatus, subscapularis, and teres minor. These muscles surround the humeral head and actively hold the humeral head against the glenoid fossa. These muscles are discussed at length in a subsequent section.
- *Capsular Ligaments:* A thin fibrous capsule that includes the superior, middle, and inferior glenohumeral ligaments. This relatively loose capsule attaches between the rim of the glenoid fossa and the anatomic neck of the humerus (see Figure 4-12).
- *Coracohumeral Ligament:* Attaches between the coracoid process and the anterior side of the greater tubercle. It helps limit the extremes of external rotation, flexion, and extension, as well as inferior displacement of the humeral head (see Figure 4-12).
- *Glenoid Labrum:* A fibrocartilaginous ring that encircles the rim of the glenoid fossa. The labrum serves to deepen the socket of the GH joint, nearly doubling the functional depth of the glenoid fossa. The labrum also helps seal the joint, thereby contributing to stability by maintaining a suction effect between the humerus and glenoid fossa.

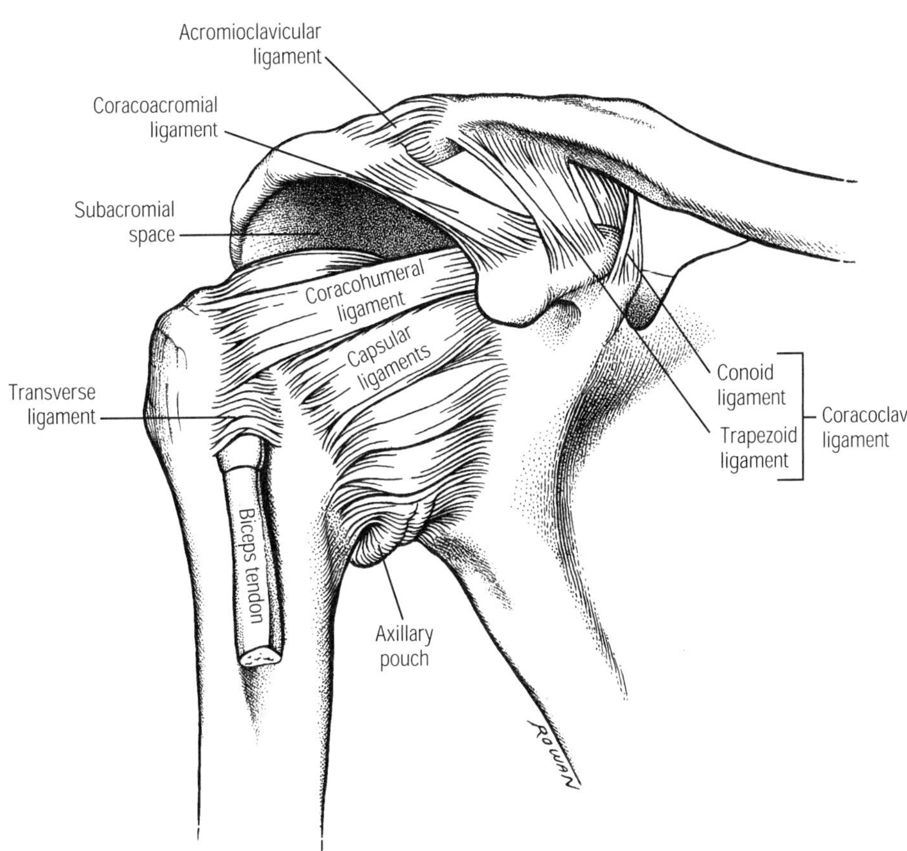

Figure 4-12 An anterior view of the right glenohumeral joint showing many of the surrounding ligaments. (From Neumann DA: *Kinesiology of the musculoskeletal system: foundations for physical rehabilitation,* St Louis, 2002, Mosby, Figure 5-26.)

- *Long Head of the Biceps:* The proximal portion of the tendon wraps around the superior aspect of the humeral head, attaching to the superior glenoid tubercle. This tendon helps provide anterior stability because it acts as a partial extension of the glenoid labrum.

KINEMATICS

The GH joint is a ball-in-socket joint that allows 3 degrees of freedom. The primary motions of this joint are abduction and adduction, flexion and extension, and internal and external rotation (Figure 4-13). Horizontal abduction and horizontal adduction are commonly used terms to describe special motions of the shoulder and are described below.

Abduction and Adduction

Abduction and adduction of the GH joint occur in the frontal plane about an anterior-posterior axis of rotation, which courses through the humeral head. Normally, the GH joint allows approximately 120 degrees of abduction; the full 180 degrees of shoulder abduction normally occurs by combining 60 degrees of scapular upward rotation with the abduction of the GH joint. This important concept is discussed further in a subsequent section.

The arthrokinematics of abduction involve the convex head of the humerus rolling superiorly while simultaneously sliding inferiorly (Figure 4-14, *A*). Without an inferior slide, the upward roll of the humerus will result in the humeral head jamming into the acromion. This is known as **impingement** and often results in damage to the supraspinatus muscle or the subacromial bursa, which become pinched between these two bony structures (Figure 4-14, *B*). The arthrokinematics of GH joint adduction are the same as that of shoulder abduction but in the reverse direction.

Flexion and Extension

Flexion and extension of the GH joint occur in the sagittal plane about a medial-lateral axis of rotation. During these actions the humeral head spins on the glenoid fossa about a relatively fixed axis—an arthrokinematic roll and slide is not necessary.

Approximately 120 degrees of flexion and 45 degrees of extension are available to the GH joint. Similar to abduction, the full 180 degrees of shoulder flexion is obtained by incorporating approximately 60 degrees of scapular upward rotation.

Internal and External Rotation

Internal and external rotation of the GH joint occurs in the horizontal plane about a vertical (longitudinal) axis of rotation (see Figure 4-13). Internal rotation results in the anterior surface of the humerus rotating medially, toward the midline, whereas external rotation results in the anterior surface of the humerus rotating laterally, away from the midline.

Horizontal Adduction and Abduction

With the shoulder in roughly 90 degrees of abduction, movement of the humerus toward the midline in the

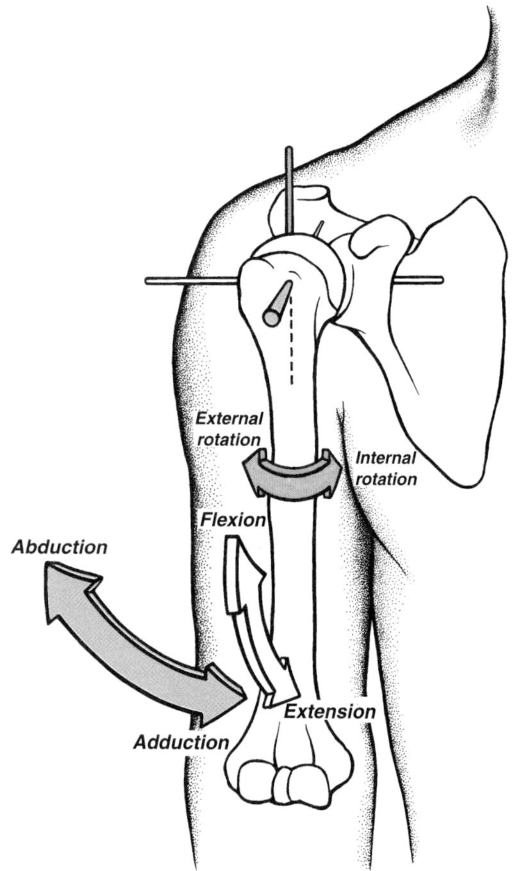

Figure 4-13 The right glenohumeral joint showing the conventional osteokinematic motions of the humerus. The axes of rotation are color coded with the associated planes of motion. (From Neumann DA: *Kinesiology of the musculoskeletal system: foundations for physical rehabilitation*, St Louis, 2002, Mosby, Figure 5-30.)

horizontal plane is considered horizontal adduction. Movement away from the midline in the horizontal plane is considered horizontal abduction. Examples of these actions include a rowing motion or a push-up.

Interaction among the Joints of the Shoulder Complex

Up to this point, we have discussed the arthrology and kinematics of each joint of the shoulder complex. It must be understood, however, that movement of the entire shoulder is the result of movement in each of its four joints. All four joints must properly interact for normal shoulder motion to occur. An excellent example of this interaction is the **scapulohumeral rhythm**.

SCAPULOHUMERAL RHYTHM

During normal shoulder abduction (or flexion), a natural 2:1 ratio or rhythm exists between the GH joint and the scapulothoracic joint. This means that for every 2 degrees of GH abduction, the scapula must simultaneously upwardly rotate roughly 1 degree. For example, if the shoulder is abducted to 90 degrees, only about 60 degrees of that motion occurs from GH abduction; the additional 30 degrees or so is achieved through upward rotation of the scapula. The full 180 degrees of abduction normally attained at the shoulder is the summation of 120 degrees of GH joint abduction and 60 degrees of scapular upward rotation (Figure 4-15).

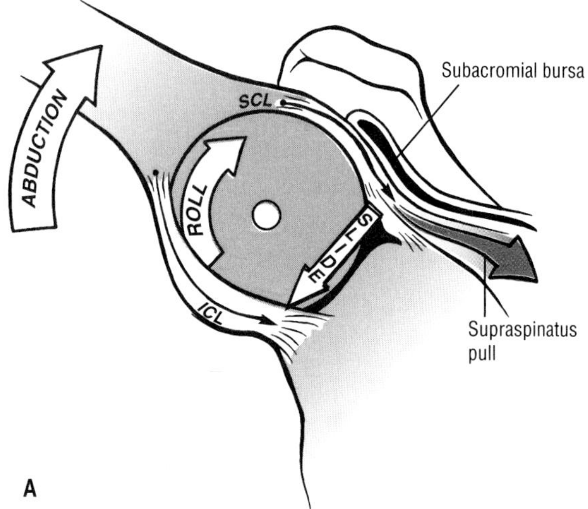

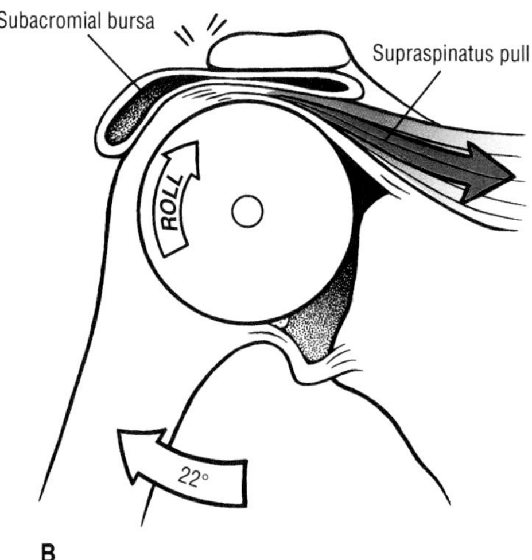

Figure 4-14 **A**, Proper arthrokinematics of the glenohumeral (GH) joint during abduction involving a superior roll and inferior slide of the humeral head. **B**, A superior roll without an inferior slide resulting in impingement of the subacromial bursa and supraspinatus. *ICL*, Inferior capsular ligament; *SCL*, superior capsular ligament. (From Neumann DA: *Kinesiology of the musculoskeletal system: foundations for physical rehabilitation*, St Louis, 2002, Mosby, Figures 5-31 and 5-32, *B*.)

120 degrees of glenohumeral joint abduction
+60 degrees of scapulothoracic joint upward rotation
= 180 degrees of shoulder abduction

Acromioclavicular and Sternoclavicular Joint Interaction within the Scapulohumeral Rhythm

Scapulothoracic motion is an integral part of nearly every shoulder movement. Furthermore, motion at the scapulothoracic joint is dependent on the combined movements of the AC and SC joints. The full 60 degrees of scapulothoracic upward rotation is achieved by combining about 30 degrees of clavicular elevation with 30 degrees of AC joint upward rotation (see Figure 4-15).

30 degrees of sternoclavicular joint elevation
+30 degrees of acromioclavicular joint upward rotation
= 60 degrees scapulothoracic joint upward rotation

In the treatment of a patient with a shoulder dysfunction, it is important to remember the integrated relationship of the joints within the shoulder complex because a problem in one joint will likely affect the other three.

Box 4-1 summarizes the interactions among the joints during common shoulder motions.

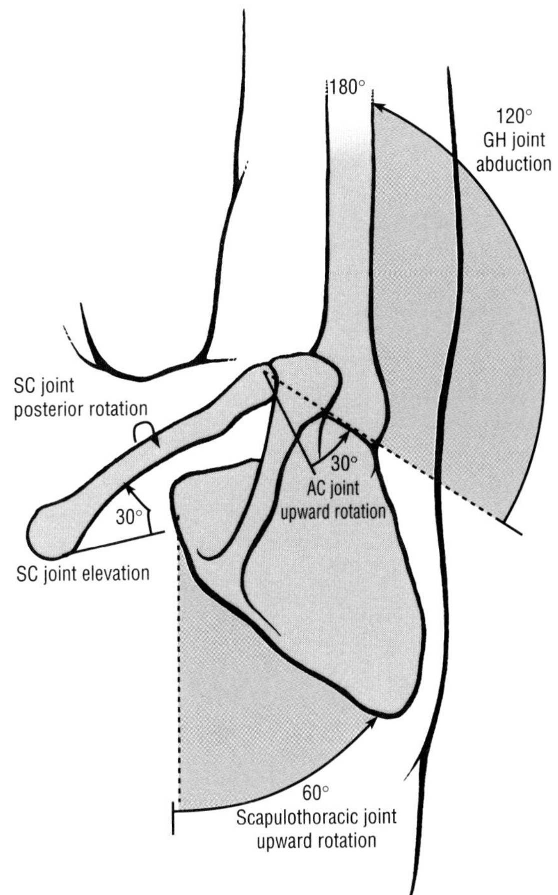

Figure 4-15 A posterior view of the right shoulder complex after the arm has abducted 180 degrees. The 60 degrees of scapular upward rotation and 120 degrees of glenohumeral *(GH)* joint abduction are shaded in red. The scapular upward rotation is depicted as a summation of 30 degrees of elevation at the sternoclavicular *(SC)* joint and 30 degrees of upward rotation at the acromioclavicular *(AC)* joint. (From Neumann DA: *Kinesiology of the musculoskeletal system: foundations for physical rehabilitation*, St Louis, 2002, Mosby, Figure 5-37.)

BOX 4-1

Summary of Bony Movements during Common Shoulder Motions

The following provides a summary of the normal kinematic interactions among the humerus, scapula, and clavicle during common shoulder motions.

Horizontal Abduction
- Horizontal abduction of the humerus
- Retraction of the scapula
- Retraction of the clavicle

Horizontal Adduction
- Horizontal adduction of the humerus
- Protraction of the scapula
- Protraction of the clavicle

Shoulder Flexion
This motion involves the typical scapulohumeral rhythm: a 2:1 ratio of glenohumeral flexion and scapulothoracic upward rotation.
- Flexion of the humerus
- Upward rotation of the scapula
- Elevation and posterior rotation of the clavicle

Shoulder Extension
The exact kinematics of this joint vary depending on the range of motion through which the shoulder is being extended. The following movements occur during a pulling motion, beginning at 90 degrees of shoulder flexion and moving to 10 degrees of extension.
- Extension of the humerus
- Downward rotation and retraction of the scapula
- Depression and retraction of the clavicle

Shoulder Abduction
Abduction involves the 2:1 ratio of glenohumeral abduction to scapular upward rotation—the scapulohumeral rhythm.
- Abduction of the humerus
- Upward rotation of the scapula
- Clavicular elevation and posterior rotation

Clinical INSIGHT

Two Ways to Help Prevent Shoulder Impingement

To achieve full range of motion during abduction, the prominent greater tuberosity must be positioned to clear the undersurface of acromion; this can be accomplished by externally rotating the shoulder or performing abduction in the scapular plane.

To illustrate this, first try to perform frontal plane abduction with your arm in full internal rotation (thumb pointing down), in a neutral position (palm facing down), and finally in full external rotation (thumb pointing up). The limited range of motion experienced in a neutral or internally rotated position is caused by the greater tuberosity impinging against the acromion process. However, if the shoulder is externally rotated, the greater tuberosity is positioned posterior to the coracoacromial arch, thereby avoiding full impact with the acromion.

Even with the humerus in full external rotation, complete abduction of the shoulder may still result in impingement if performed in the *true* frontal plane (Figure 4-16, *A*). Therapists often request that their patients perform shoulder exercises in the scapular plane as a way to prevent recurring impingement. The *scapular plane* is about 35 degrees anterior to the frontal plane (Figure 4-16, *B*). Shoulder abduction in the scapular plane, often referred to as scaption, positions the greater tuberosity of the humerus under the highest point of the acromion and helps to prevent bony impingement, regardless of the amount of rotation of the glenohumeral joint. This can be verified by performing abduction in the scapular plane, with the upper extremity positioned in internal rotation, neutral, and external rotation.

Scapular plane abduction is more natural than abduction in the pure frontal plane. The humeral head fits better against the glenoid fossa, and the ligaments and muscles (in particular, the supraspinatus) are more optimally aligned to promote proper shoulder mechanics.

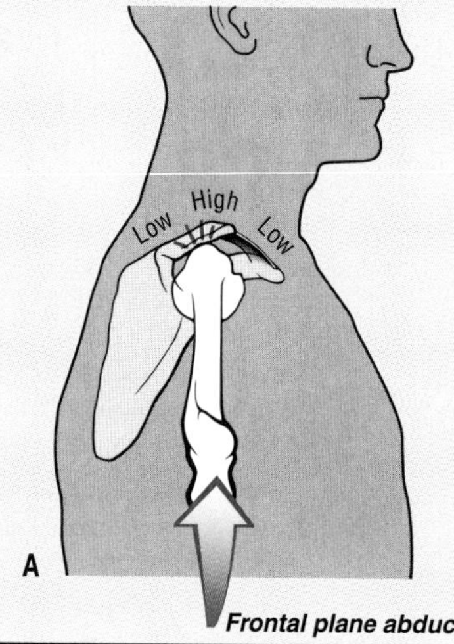

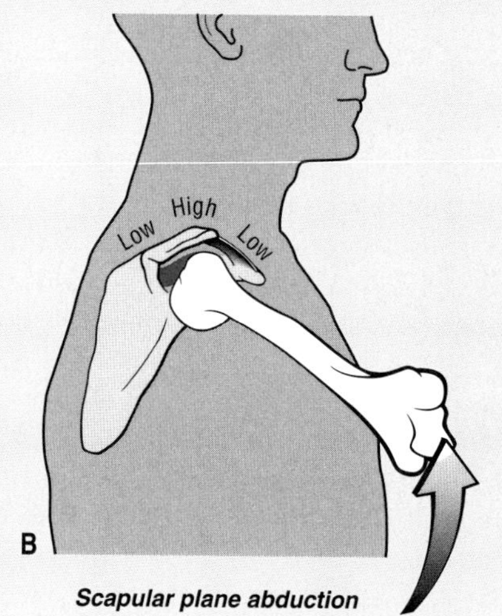

Figure 4-16 A side view of the right glenohumeral joint comparing abduction of the humerus in the **(A)** true frontal plane and **(B)** scapular plane. (From Neumann DA: *Kinesiology of the musculoskeletal system: foundations for physical rehabilitation*, St Louis, 2002, Mosby, Figure 5-34.)

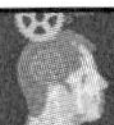

Consider this...

Static Passive Locking Mechanism of the Glenohumeral Joint

When the arm is at rest, near the side of the body, the head of the humerus is held flush against the glenoid fossa, in part, by the static locking mechanism of the glenohumeral (GH) joint. Interestingly, with optimal posture of the scapula, little GH joint muscle activity is required for stability at rest. Recall that the glenoid fossa is relatively flat and shallow, whereas the humeral head is large and round, making the anatomy of this joint more like a golf ball sitting on a quarter than a ball-and-socket joint. The static locking mechanism helps provide stability to this loose-fitting joint.

Ideal posture of the scapula positions the glenoid fossa so that it is tilted about 5 degrees upward (Figure 4-17, *A*). This position not only improves the contact of the articulation but allows the surrounding soft tissues to help support this joint. The superior capsular ligaments provide an upward force vector to counteract the downward force of gravity. When these forces are combined, the resultant vector is a compressive force directed through the middle of the glenoid fossa, enhancing the static stability of the GH joint.

As illustrated in Figure 4-17, *B*, when the scapula becomes downwardly rotated, such as commonly occurs following a stroke involving weakness or paralysis of the trapezius muscles, the static locking mechanism becomes ineffective. Not only does the humeral head lose its ledge to rest on, but the direction of the upward forces created by the superior capsular ligaments are changed, reducing the overall potential of these structures to produce a passive compression force (*CF*).

The relatively large amount of GH joint instability produced by relatively small alterations in the posture of the scapula is good evidence that proper posture of the scapula contributes significantly to the stability of the GH joint.

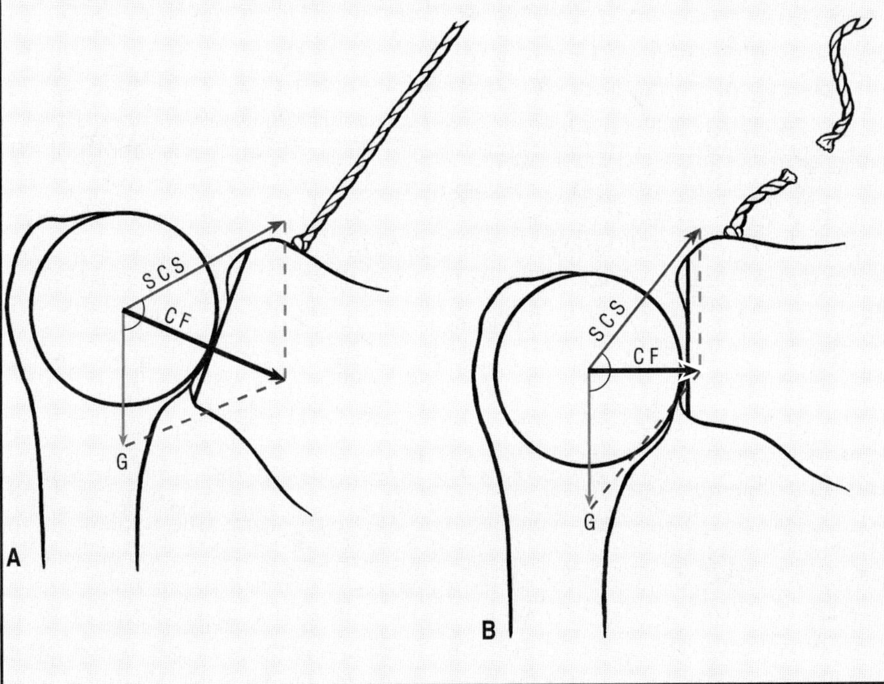

Figure 4-17 The static locking mechanism of the glenohumeral joint. **A**, The rope indicates a muscular force that holds the glenoid fossa slightly upward. **B**, Loss of the upward force—indicated by the cut rope—allows the glenoid fossa to downwardly rotate with a resultant inferior slide of the humerus. *CF*, Compression force; *G*, gravity; *SCS*, superior capsular structure. (From Neumann DA: *Kinesiology of the musculoskeletal system: foundations for physical rehabilitation*, St Louis, 2002, Mosby, Figure 5-28.)

Muscle and Joint Interaction

As discussed, all four joints of the shoulder must cooperate to produce normal shoulder motion. The muscles of the shoulder complex, therefore, must work in a highly coordinated fashion. For organizational purposes this text divides these muscles into two categories: (1) muscles of the shoulder girdle and (2) muscles of the GH joint. A brief summary of the innervation scheme of the entire upper extremity is provided in the following section.

Innervation of the Shoulder Complex

The entire upper extremity receives innervation primarily through the brachial plexus (Figure 4-18). The brachial plexus is formed by a network of nerve roots from the spinal nerves C5-T1. Nerve roots C5 and C6 form the upper trunk, C7 forms the middle trunk, and C8 and T1 form the lower trunk. The trunks travel a short distance before forming the anterior or posterior divisions. The divisions then reorganize into the lateral, medial, and posterior cords, named by their position relative to the axillary artery.

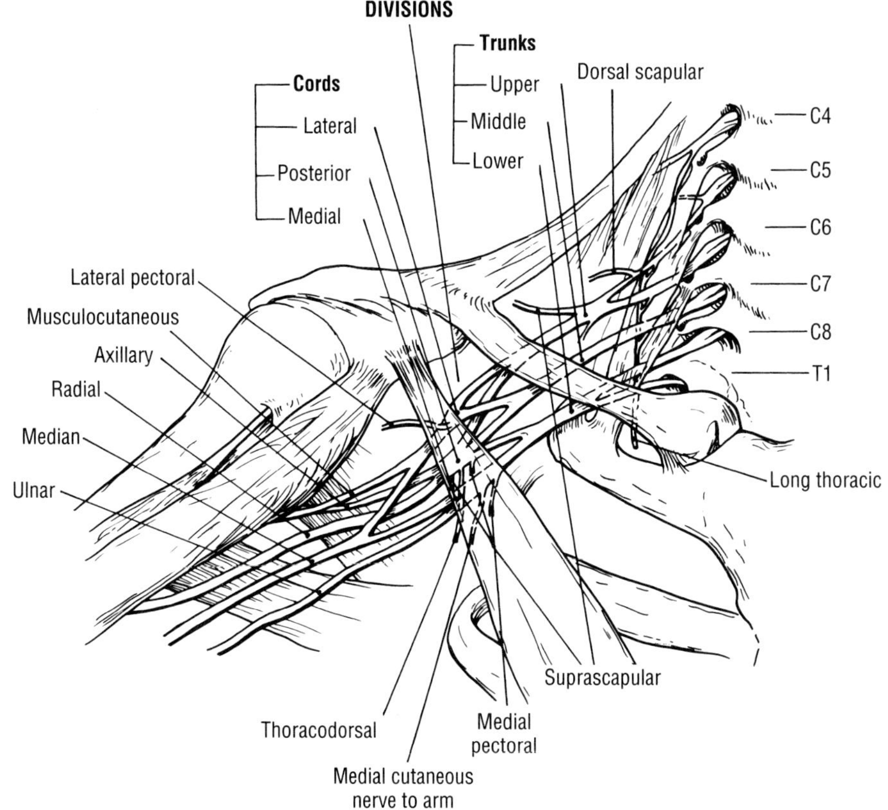

Figure 4-18 The brachial plexus. (From Jobe MT, Wright PE: Peripheral nerve injuries. In Canale ST, editor: *Campbell's operative orthopaedics*, ed 9, vol 4, St Louis, 1998, Mosby.)

The cords eventually branch into nerves that primarily innervate muscles of the upper extremity.

The majority of muscles of the shoulder complex receive their innervation from two regions of the brachial plexus: (1) nerves that branch from the posterior cord such as the axillary, subscapular, and thoracodorsal nerves and (2) nerves that branch from the more proximal segments of the plexus such as the dorsal scapular, long thoracic, pectoral, and suprascapular nerves. An exception to this innervation scheme is the trapezius muscle, which is innervated primarily by cranial nerve XI (spinal accessory nerve).

Muscles of the Shoulder Girdle

The shoulder girdle can be considered the combination of the scapula and clavicle. The scapulothoracic muscles control the shoulder girdle—each attaching proximally on the axial skeleton and distally to the scapula or clavicle. In general the primary function of these muscles is to position or stabilize the scapula to augment the function of the shoulder as a whole.

The following section provides an atlas style format of the individual scapulothoracic muscles. The discussion of the interaction of these muscles will resume on p. 69.

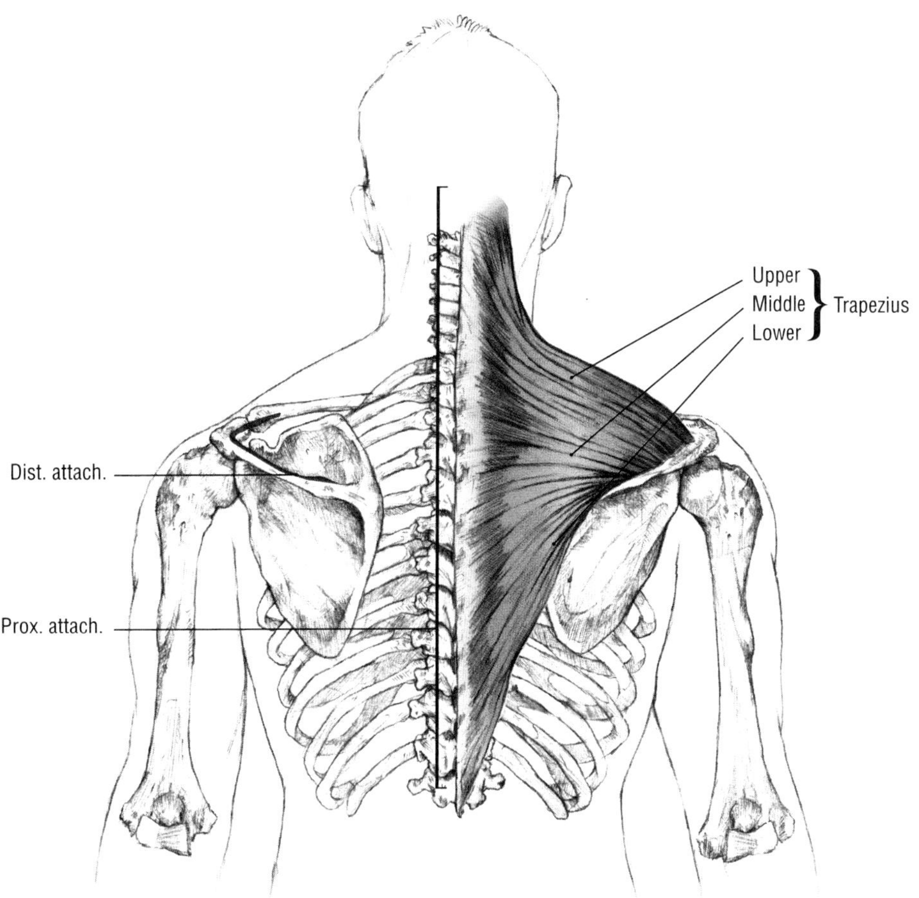

Upper Trapezius

Proximal Attachment: External occipital protuberance, ligamentum nuchae (on cervical vertebrae), and medial portion of the superior nuchal line

Distal Attachment: Posterior-superior aspect of the lateral one third of the clavicle

Innervation: Spinal accessory nerve (cranial nerve XI)

Actions:

- Elevation of the scapula
- Upward rotation of the scapula (with serratus anterior and lower trapezius)

Comments: One primary motion of the upper trapezius is scapular elevation; however, it also plays an important role in the force-couple that produces scapular upward rotation. In addition, with the scapula and clavicle fixed, the upper trapezius can perform lateral flexion and contralateral rotation of the cervical spine.

Middle Trapezius

Proximal Attachment: Ligamentum nuchae and spinous processes of C7-T5

Distal Attachment: Medial aspect of the acromion

Innervation: Spinal accessory nerve (cranial nerve XI)

Action: Retraction of the scapula

Comments: The middle trapezius has a favorable line of pull to perform scapular retraction and often plays an essential role in stabilizing the scapula against strong forces produced by other scapulothoracic muscles such as the serratus anterior—a powerful protractor.

Lower Trapezius

Proximal Attachment: Spinous processes of the middle and lower thoracic vertebrae (T6-T12)

Distal Attachment: Upper lip of the spine of the scapula near the medial border

Innervation: Spinal accessory nerve (cranial nerve XI)

Actions:

- Depression of the scapula
- Upward rotation of the scapula (with serratus anterior and upper trapezius)
- Retraction of the scapula

Comments: The lower trapezius is the largest of the three trapezius muscles. Along with being a prime mover of scapular depression, the lower trapezius is integral to performing both scapular upward rotation and scapular retraction.

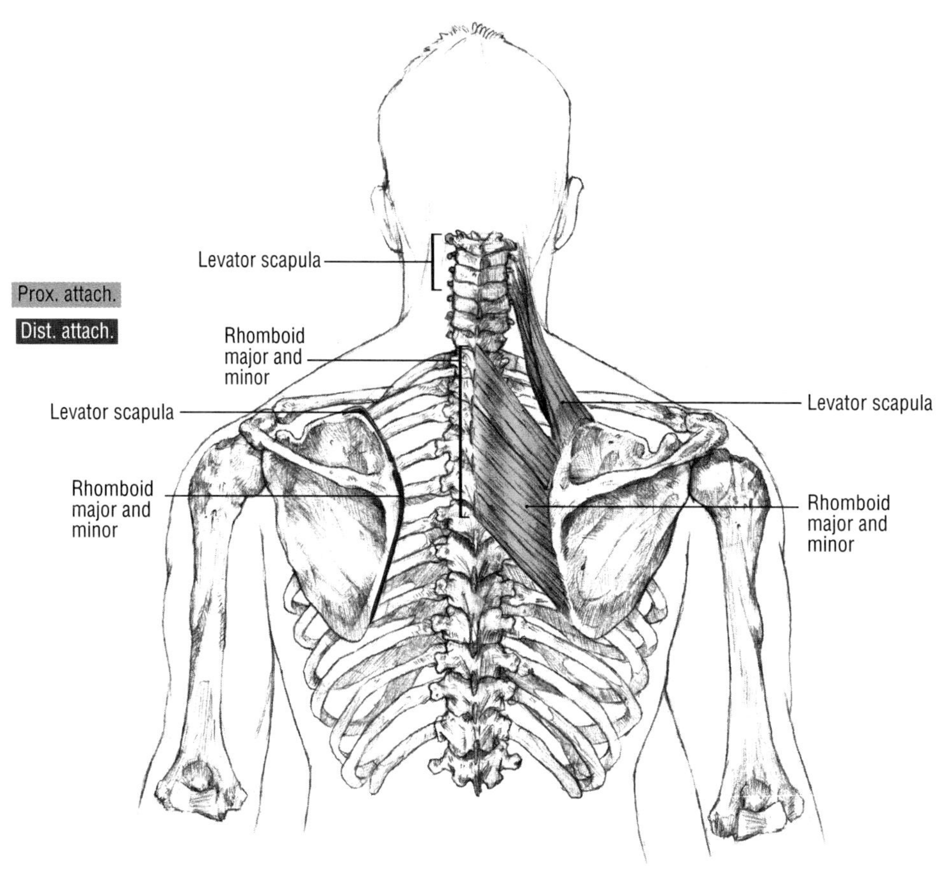

Levator Scapulae

Proximal Attachment: Transverse processes of C1-C4

Distal Attachment: Medial border of the scapula between the superior angle and the root of the scapular spine

Innervation: Dorsal scapular nerve (spinal nerves C3-C5)

Actions:
- Elevation of the scapula
- Downward rotation of the scapula

Comments: The levator scapula is palpable just superior and medial to the superior angle of the scapula. Painful trigger points often develop within this muscle, typically as a result of strain from poor, slouched posture.

Rhomboids

The rhomboid major and minor are usually grouped together as one muscle group.

Proximal Attachment: Ligamentum nuchae and spinous processes of C7-T5

Distal Attachment: Medial border of the scapula from the root of the scapular spine to the inferior angle of the scapula

Innervation: Dorsal scapular nerve

Actions:
- Retraction of the scapula
- Elevation of the scapula
- Downward rotation of the scapula

Comments: The wide, flat shape of this muscle group provides firm control of the entire medial border of the scapula. The rhomboids act with the middle trapezius as scapular retractors and stabilizers, helping to prevent unwanted scapular motions. The rhomboids are active during nearly any pulling activity of the upper extremity.

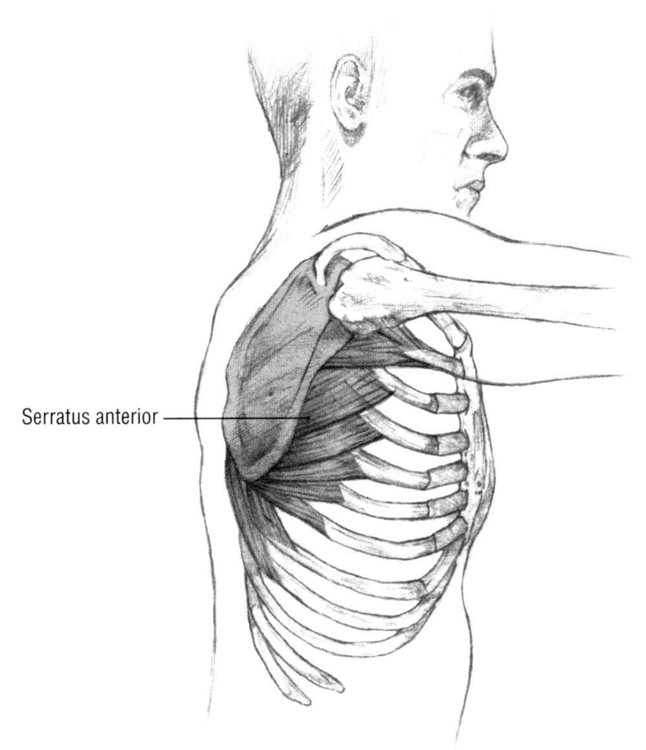

Serratus Anterior

Proximal Attachment: External surface of the lateral region of the first nine ribs

Distal Attachment: Entire medial border of the scapula with a concentration of fibers near the inferior angle

Innervation: Long thoracic nerve

Actions:
- Protraction of the scapula
- Upward rotation of the scapula
- Holds the scapula firmly against the posterior thorax

Comments: The serratus anterior courses between the anterior surface of the scapula and the outer surface of the rib cage. The extensive attachments and line of pull of this muscle make it the most powerful upward rotator and protractor of the scapula.

Weakness of the serratus anterior can significantly decrease the effectiveness of pushing activities. Also, because the serratus anterior is the primary upward rotator of the scapula, weakness of this muscle severely compromises motions involving active flexion or abduction of the shoulder.

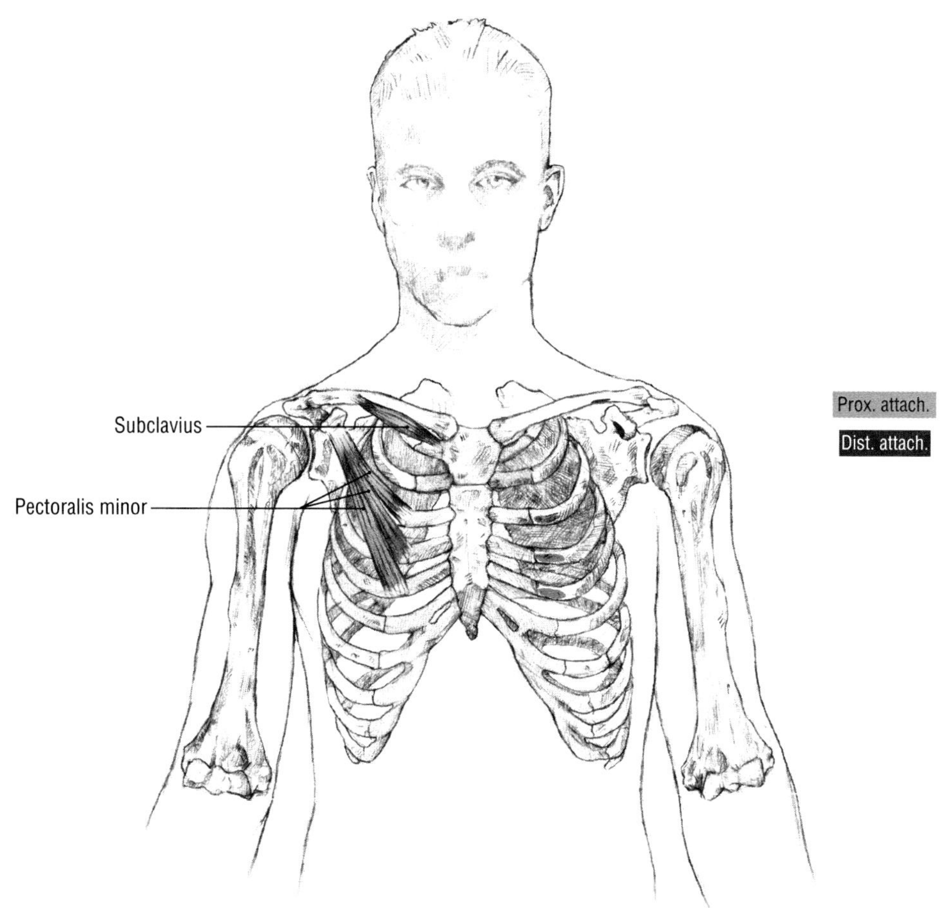

Pectoralis Minor

Proximal Attachment: Anterior surface of ribs 3 to 5
Distal Attachment: Coracoid process of the scapula
Innervation: Medial pectoral nerve
Actions:
- Depression of the scapula
- Downward rotation of the scapula
- Anterior tilt of the scapula (sagittal plane)

Comments: The pectoralis minor plays a significant role in stabilizing the scapula and neutralizing unwanted motions of the scapula produced by other muscles such as the lower trapezius. With the scapula fixed, the pectoralis minor may be used to assist with inspiration by elevating the ribs.

Subclavius

Proximal Attachment: Near the cartilage of the first rib
Distal Attachment: Inferior surface of the clavicle
Innervation: Branch from the upper trunk of the brachial plexus (C5-C6)
Action: Depression of the clavicle
Comments: The line of pull of the subclavius muscle is nearly parallel with the clavicle, indicating that it primarily functions as a clavicular stabilizer.

Clinical INSIGHT

Upper Trapezius and Rhomboids: Offsetting Scapular Rotators

The upper trapezius is an upward rotator of the scapula, whereas the rhomboids are downward rotators of the scapula; however, both of these muscles function as scapular elevators. How is this possible? During simultaneous activation of these muscles, the rotational component of each is offset or neutralized by the other muscle. The tendency of the upper trapezius to upwardly rotate the scapula is negated by the downward rotation pull of the rhomboids. Because the rotational component of each muscle is offset, the muscular energy of these muscles is combined and channeled into a single action—scapular elevation.

Putting It All Together

Now that the anatomy and function of the individual scapulothoracic muscles has been covered, we will begin discussion on how these muscles interact to produce functional movements of the entire shoulder complex.

ELEVATORS OF THE SCAPULOTHORACIC JOINT

The upper trapezius, levator scapulae, and, to a lesser extent, the rhomboids are responsible for elevating the scapula and supporting proper scapulothoracic posture. Optimal scapulothoracic posture is normally described as a slightly retracted and slightly elevated position of the scapula, resulting in the glenoid fossa facing slightly upward.

Primary Scapular Elevators

- Upper trapezius
- Levator scapula
- Rhomboids

Functional Consideration: Weakness of the Upper Trapezius

Weakness or paralysis of the upper trapezius, over time, will likely lead to a depressed and downwardly rotated scapula. A chronically depressed clavicle may eventually lead to a superior dislocation of the SC joint. With the lateral end of the clavicle excessively lowered, the medial end is forced upward because of the fulcrum action on the underlying first rib.

Perhaps more commonly, weakness of the upper trapezius will lead to **subluxation** of the GH joint. As described in Figure 4-17, the **static stability** of the GH joint is provided, in part, by the slightly naturally inclined position of the glenoid fossa. Long-term weakness of the upper trapezius may result in a downwardly rotated position of the glenoid fossa, allowing the humerus to slide inferiorly. The downward pull of gravity on an unsupported arm may strain the supporting musculature and the GH joint capsule, eventually leading to subluxation. This complication is commonly observed following flaccid hemiplegia.

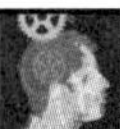

Consider this...

Levator Scapula—Fighting Poor Posture

Poor posture of the neck and shoulder region commonly involves forward, rounded shoulders combined with a forward head, a posture commonly attained while typing on a computer. Rounded shoulders are often accompanied by scapular protraction and slight upward rotation; a forward head involves a flexed mid to lower cervical spine. The combination of these two positions elongates the levator scapula. Over time, the levator scapula may become inflamed and begin to spasm or become knotted from resisting this scapulothoracic posture. Although tightness of this muscle is often attributed to mental stress, it is often the result of habitual poor posture while working, regardless of whether the job is stressful or not.

DEPRESSORS OF THE SCAPULOTHORACIC JOINT

Scapulothoracic depression is performed by the lower trapezius, latissimus dorsi, pectoralis minor, and subclavius. These muscles work together to depress the shoulder girdle and humerus, resulting in shoulder depression (Figure 4-19).

Primary Scapular Depressors

- Lower trapezius
- Latissimus dorsi
- Pectoralis minor
- Subclavius

Functional Consideration: "Reverse Action" of the Shoulder Depressors

The line of pull of the latissimus dorsi and lower trapezius is perfectly suited to produce depression of the shoulder complex. However, if the arm is physically blocked from being depressed, these muscles can be used to effectively elevate the trunk as illustrated in Figure 4-20. This **reverse action** of the shoulder depressors can be extremely useful clinically because elevation of the trunk is required for many functional rehabilitation activities such as crutch walking, pushing up from sitting to standing, ambulation with a walker, or performing a boost while transferring to a bed or wheelchair.

Numerous conditions significantly weaken or even paralyze the lower extremities but do not affect the upper extremities. Many times persons with this paralysis are able to ambulate with the help of assistive devices, orthotics, and creative **muscular substitution**. With the humerus firmly stabilized such as when weight bearing on a crutch, the latissimus dorsi can be substituted as a "hip hiker," effectively elevating the ipsilateral pelvis so that the lower extremity can be lifted and advanced.

UPWARD ROTATORS AND PROTRACTORS OF THE SCAPULA

Upward Rotators: The Classic Muscular Force-Couple

Upward rotation of the scapula is an extremely important component of flexion or abduction of the shoulder. Recall the scapulohumeral rhythm: 1 degree of scapular upward rotation for every 2 degrees of GH flexion or abduction. Upward rotation of the scapula is performed by an

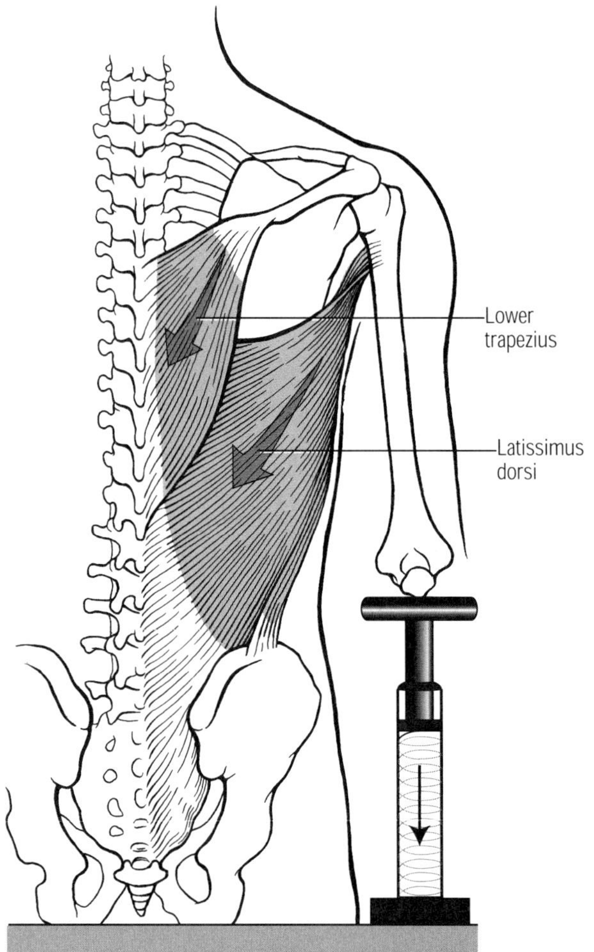

Figure 4-19 A posterior view of the lower trapezius and the latissimus dorsi depressing the scapulothoracic joint. (From Neumann DA: *Kinesiology of the musculoskeletal system: foundations for physical rehabilitation,* St Louis, 2002, Mosby, Figure 5-43, *A*.)

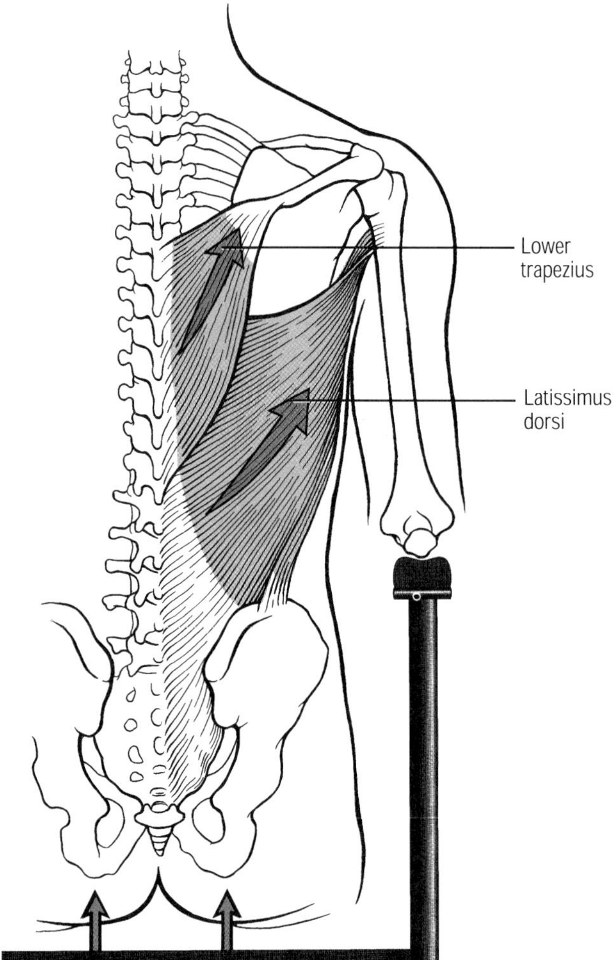

Figure 4-20 The lower trapezius and latissimus dorsi are shown working in reverse, elevating the ischial tuberosities from the seat of the wheelchair. The contraction of these muscles lifts the pelvic and trunk segment up toward the fixed scapula and arm segment. (From Neumann DA: *Kinesiology of the musculoskeletal system: foundations for physical rehabilitation,* St Louis, 2002, Mosby, Figure 5-44.)

important **force-couple** generated by the serratus anterior, upper trapezius, and lower trapezius (Figure 4-21, A). Even though all three muscles have different lines of pull, they all rotate the scapula in the same direction, resulting in upward rotation. As illustrated in Figure 4-21, *B*, the force-couple generated by these three muscles is similar to two hands turning a steering wheel. Even though each hand is moving in a different linear direction, both are producing force in the same rotary direction.

Primary Scapular Upward Rotators

- Serratus anterior
- Upper trapezius
- Lower trapezius

Serratus Anterior: The Sole Scapular Protractor

Scapulothoracic protraction describes the horizontal plane movement of the scapula away from the midline of the body; this action occurs primarily as a result of the force generated by the serratus anterior (Figure 4-22). Force produced by this muscle is transferred through the scapula to the humerus, ultimately used for forward reaching and pushing activities.

Functional Consideration: Winging of the Scapula. One of the most obvious signs of serratus anterior weakness is scapular "winging." **Winging** refers to the medial border of the scapula lifting away from the rib cage, giving the appearance of a bird's wing (Figure 4-23). Clinically this is observed during resisted shoulder abduction, as illustrated in Figure 4-23, or during a standard push-up. Rehabilitation programs designed to strengthen the serratus anterior incorporate what is often called a push-up-plus maneuver. This exercise exaggerates the final phase of a push-up, which involves additional protraction of the scapula at the end phase of the push-up, raising the chest farther from the floor.

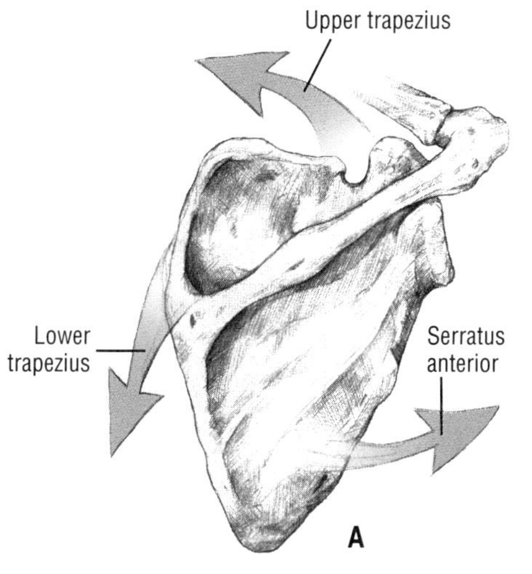

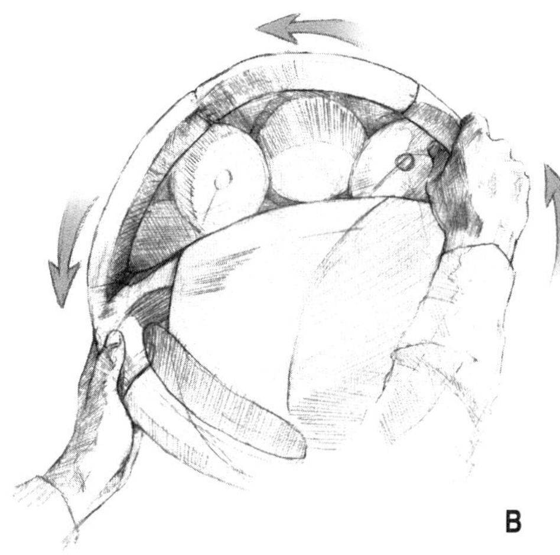

Figure 4-21 A, The force-couple to upward rotate the scapula, produced by the upper trapezius, lower trapezius, and serratus anterior. **B**, Two hands turning a steering wheel as an analogy to the upward rotation force-couple.

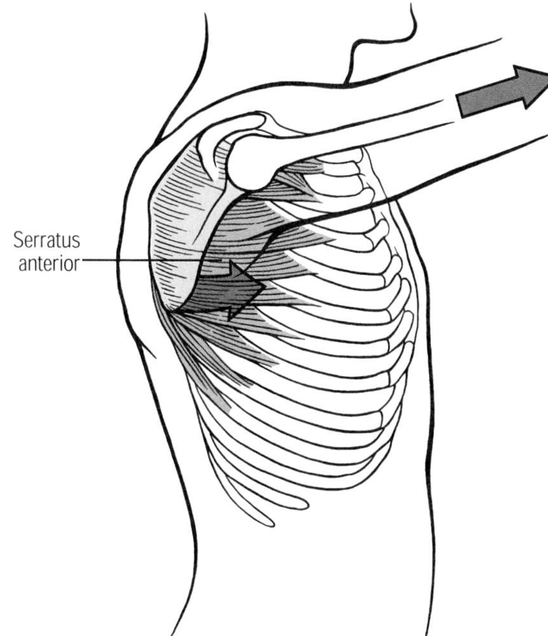

Figure 4-22 The right serratus anterior muscle. The muscle's line of pull is shown protracting the scapula and arm in a forward reaching or pushing motion. (From Neumann DA: *Kinesiology of the musculoskeletal system: foundations for physical rehabilitation*, St Louis, 2002, Mosby, Figure 5-45, *A*.)

DOWNWARD ROTATORS AND RETRACTORS OF THE SCAPULA

Downward Rotators

Downward rotation of the scapula is an important component of shoulder adduction and extension. The primary muscles involved with this action are the rhomboids and pectoralis minor. Because of its attachment on the inferior angle of the scapula, the latissimus dorsi can assist with downward rotation as well. Similar to the upward rotators of the scapula, the latissimus dorsi and the rhomboids have significantly different lines of pull but produce scapular motion in the same rotary direction.

Primary Scapular Downward Rotators

- Rhomboids
- Pectoralis minor

Clinical **INSIGHT**

Scapular Stability and Independent Transfers

Many individuals who suffer from quadriplegia (at the C6 level and below) demonstrate the ability to independently transfer themselves from a wheelchair to a bed. Persons with C5 quadriplegia (just one spinal segment higher), however, typically require maximal assistance to perform the same activity. One of the many reasons for the reduced function in the person with C5 quadriplegia is the severely weakened serratus anterior. Observation of an individual with C5 quadriplegia attempting a boost (elevating the trunk by pushing down on the bed or wheelchair) often reveals winging in both scapulae. The weakened serratus anterior is unable to stabilize the scapulae firmly against the thorax. Although the lower trapezius is typically innervated and therefore theoretically capable of acting in a reverse action to elevate the trunk, the severe winging interferes with the associated biomechanics. With a fully functional serratus anterior, the scapula is adequately stabilized and the trunk is able to be elevated by the lower trapezius, enabling the potential for an independent transfer.

Retractors

Retraction of the scapulae is often referred to as "pinching your shoulder blades together" and is linked to upper-extremity movements such as rowing or pulling. The primary scapular retractors are the rhomboids and the middle trapezius. However, all three of the trapezius muscles can assist with retraction. Figure 4-24 shows how the scapular elevation potential of the rhomboids is neutralized by the downward line of pull of the lower trapezius, resulting in pure retraction.

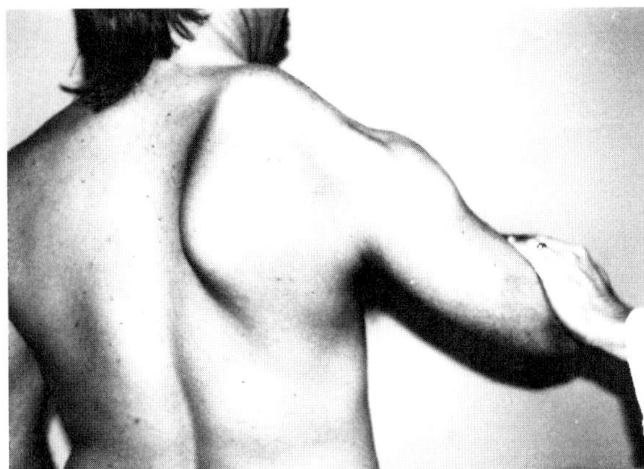

Figure 4-23 Winging of the right scapula. (From Neumann DA: *Kinesiology of the musculoskeletal system: foundations for physical rehabilitation,* St Louis, 2002, Mosby, Figure 5-52, *A.*)

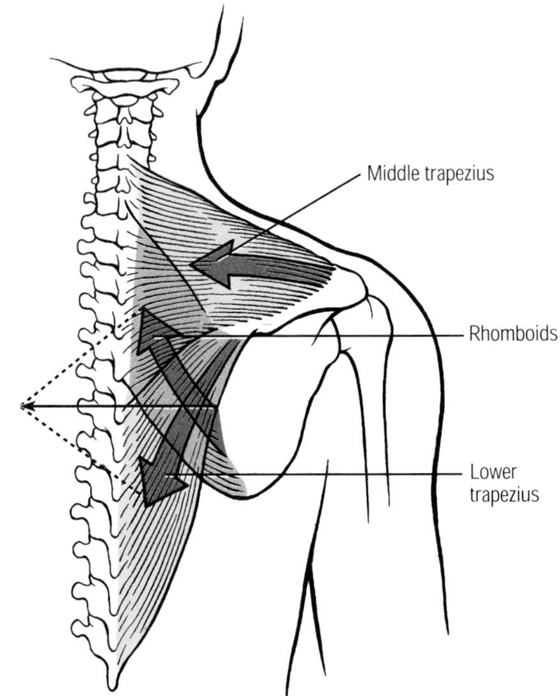

Figure 4-24 The lines of pull of the middle trapezius, lower trapezius, and rhomboids combining to retract the scapula. (From Neumann DA: *Kinesiology of the musculoskeletal system: foundations for physical rehabilitation,* St Louis, 2002, Mosby, Figure 5-46.)

Primary Scapular Retractors

- Rhomboids
- Middle trapezius

Functional Consideration: Controlling Scapular Motion. Resisted shoulder adduction requires optimal interaction between the GH joint adductors and the scapular downward rotators (Figure 4-25). Consider, for example, the teres major and latissimus dorsi. Without the stabilizing force of strong retractor and downward rotator muscles (such as the rhomboids), the strong unopposed contraction of these GH joint muscles would inevitably pull the scapula upward and outward toward the humerus. Such an abnormal movement of the scapula would quickly over-shorten the GH joint muscles, thereby significantly reducing their force-generating ability. In practice therefore the shoulder adductor and extensor muscles can be no stronger than the scapulothoracic retractor and downward rotator muscles.

Muscles of the Glenohumeral Joint

Often the terms *shoulder movement* and *GH joint movement* are used interchangeably. Technically, this is incorrect; shoulder movement is a combination of GH and scapulothoracic joint motions. Muscles that move the GH joint therefore control only a part of overall shoulder motion.

The motion of the scapula is of particular significance to the GH joint because the vast majority of GH joint muscles attach to the highly mobile scapula. The motion or stability of the scapula, or both, therefore plays a significant role in determining the lines of pull and functional potential of all GH joint muscles.

The following section provides an atlas style format of the individual muscles of the GH joint. The discussions regarding the interactions between these muscles will resume on p. 83.

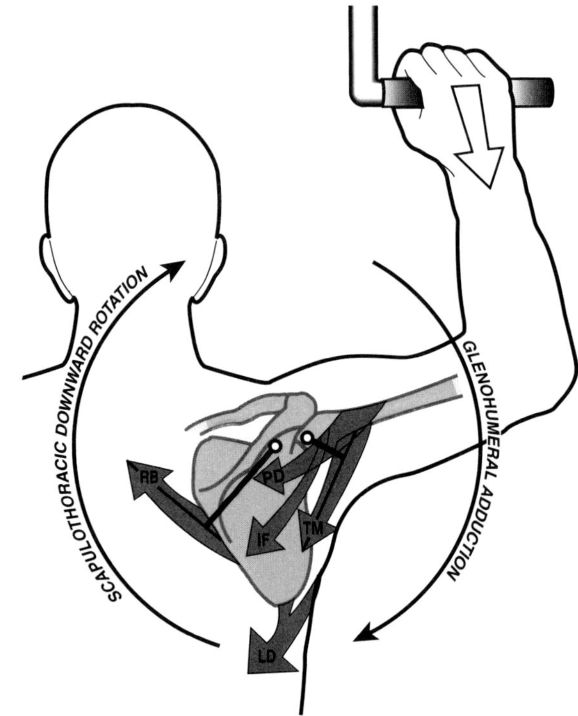

Figure 4-25 A posterior view of the right shoulder showing the muscular interactions between the scapulothoracic downward rotators and the glenohumeral adductors. *IF,* Infraspinatus; *LD,* latissimus dorsi; *PD,* posterior deltoid; *RB,* rhomboids; *TM,* teres major. (From Neumann DA: *Kinesiology of the musculoskeletal system: foundations for physical rehabilitation,* St Louis, 2002, Mosby, Figure 5-57.)

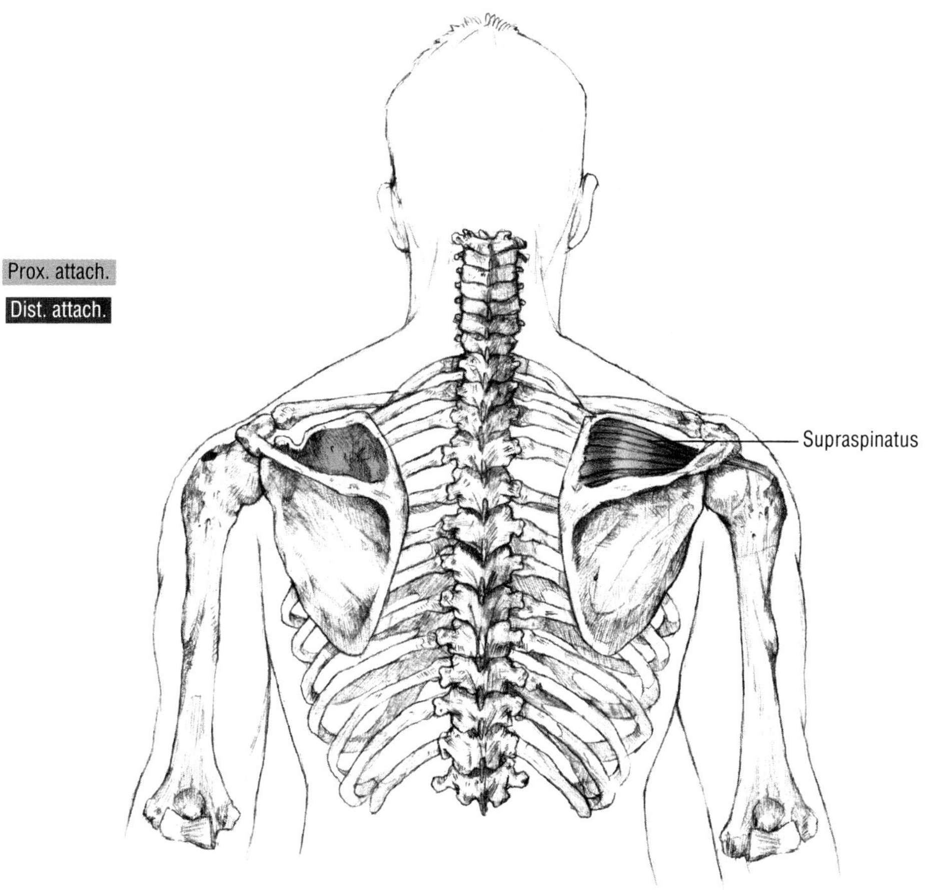

Supraspinatus

Proximal Attachment:	Supraspinatous fossa
Distal Attachment:	Greater tubercle of the humerus (superior facet)
Innervation:	Suprascapular nerve
Actions:	• Shoulder abduction • Stabilization of the GH joint
Comments:	The supraspinatus is one of the rotator cuff muscles; its position over the humeral head provides important superior stability to the GH joint. It is an important initiator of abduction because its horizontal line of pull is perfectly suited to begin the roll of the humeral head during GH abduction.

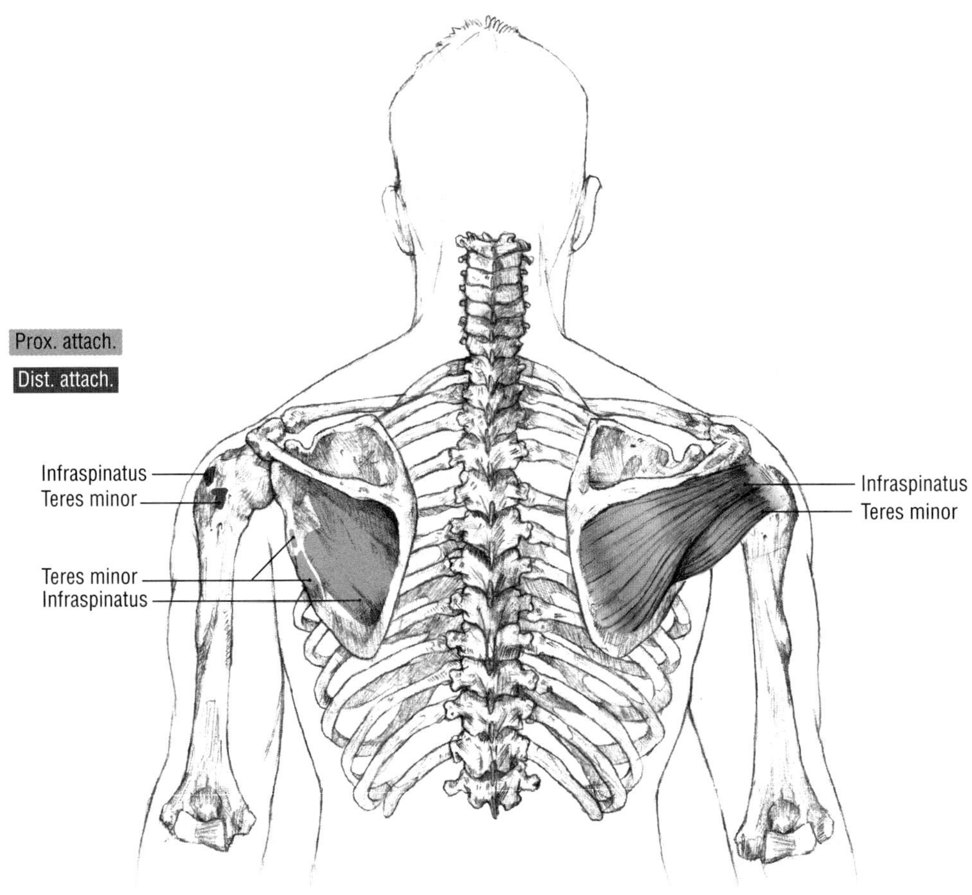

Infraspinatus

Proximal Attachment: Infraspinatous fossa

Distal Attachment: Greater tubercle of the humerus (middle facet)

Innervation: Suprascapular nerve

Actions:
- External rotation of the shoulder
- Stabilization of the GH joint

Comments: The infraspinatus and the teres minor are both external rotators of the shoulder. Throwing motions such as pitching a baseball or spiking a volleyball generate huge internal rotation torques that must be decelerated, primarily through eccentric activation of these two muscles. Often, one or both of these muscles may become injured or torn while trying to resist these large forces. This injury is often referred to as a rotator cuff tear.

Teres Minor

Proximal Attachment: Posterior surface of the lateral border of the scapula, near the inferior angle

Distal Attachment: Greater tubercle of the humerus (lower facet)

Innervation: Axillary nerve

Actions:
- External rotation of the shoulder
- Stabilization of the GH joint

Comments: The inferior-medially directed line of pull of the teres minor and infraspinatus plays an important role in the normal arthrokinematic motion of the GH joint. During flexion or abduction of the shoulder, these muscles actively direct the inferior slide of the humerus to avoid GH joint impingement. Also, the teres minor and infraspinatus play an important role in abduction by externally rotating the humerus to ensure that the greater tubercle can clear the acromion.

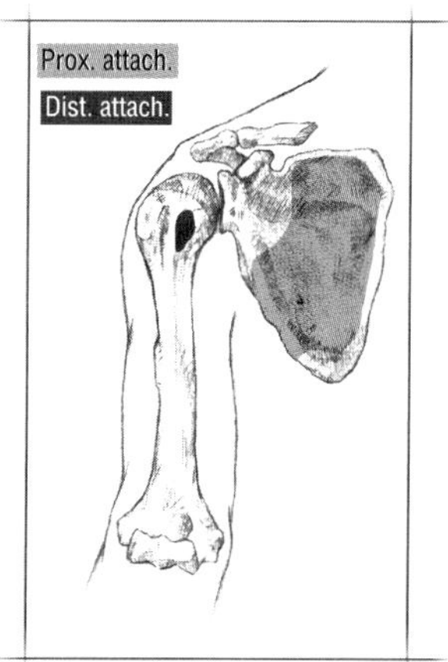

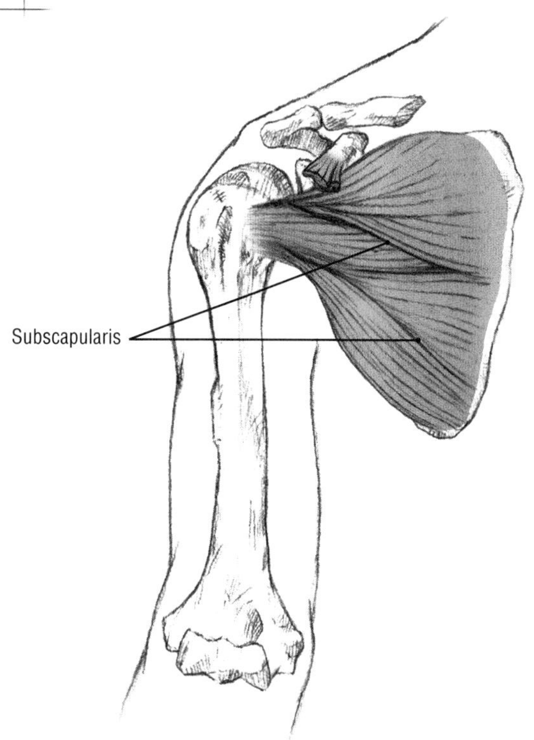

Subscapularis

Proximal Attachment: Subscapular fossa

Distal Attachment: Lesser tubercle of the humerus

Innervation: Upper and lower subscapular nerves

Actions:
- Internal rotation of the shoulder
- Stabilization of the GH joint

Comments: The subscapularis provides anterior stability to the GH joint while also balancing the external rotation pull of the other rotator cuff muscles, specifically the teres minor and infraspinatus. This synergistic action enables the rotator cuff as a whole to help hold the humeral head firmly on the glenoid fossa.

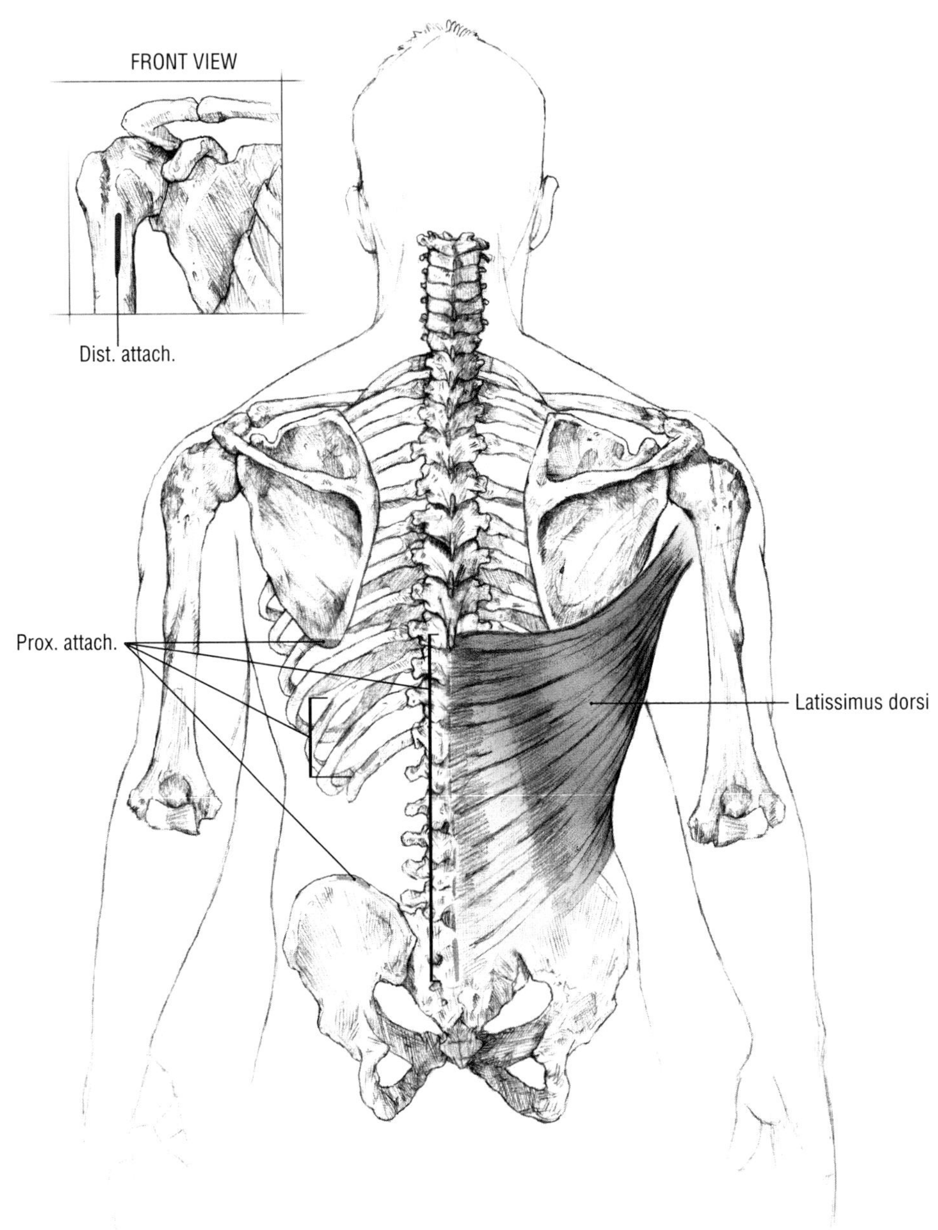

Latissimus Dorsi

Proximal Attachment: Thoracolumbar fascia, spinous processes of lower thoracic and all of the lumbar vertebrae, posterior crest of the ilium, the lower four ribs, and inferior angle of the scapula

Distal Attachment: Floor of the intertubercular groove of the humerus

Innervation: Thoracodorsal nerve (middle subscapular nerve)

Actions:
- Shoulder adduction
- Shoulder extension
- Shoulder internal rotation
- Scapular depression

Comments: The attachments of the latissimus dorsi to the humerus and the scapula allow this muscle to help coordinate the kinetics of shoulder adduction and extension. The ability to simultaneously adduct/extend the humerus and downwardly rotate the scapula make it an excellent choice for activities that incorporate pulling motions such as rowing or a wide-grip pull-up.

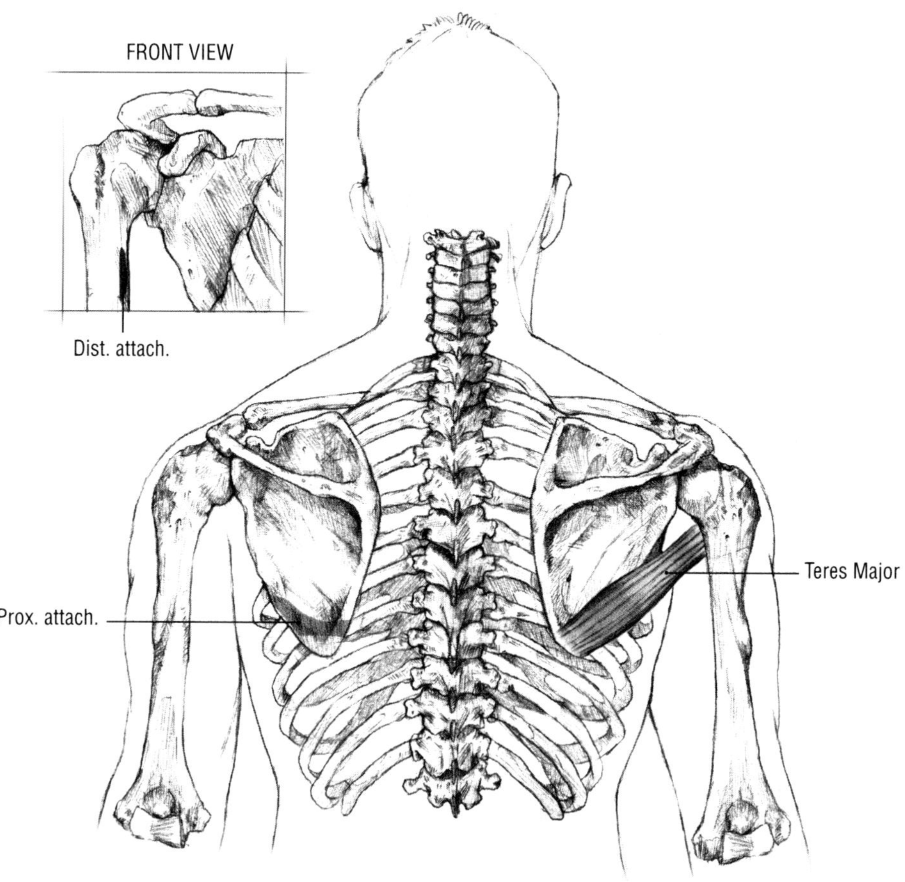

Teres Major

Proximal Attachment:	Inferior angle of the scapula
Distal Attachment:	Crest of the lesser tubercle of the humerus
Innervation:	Lower subscapular nerve
Actions:	• Shoulder adduction • Shoulder extension • Internal rotation of the shoulder
Comments:	The teres major has a good line of pull to perform GH joint adduction and extension. This muscle is sometimes referred to as "latissimus dorsi's little helper" because it performs all of the same actions as the latissimus dorsi, except scapular depression.

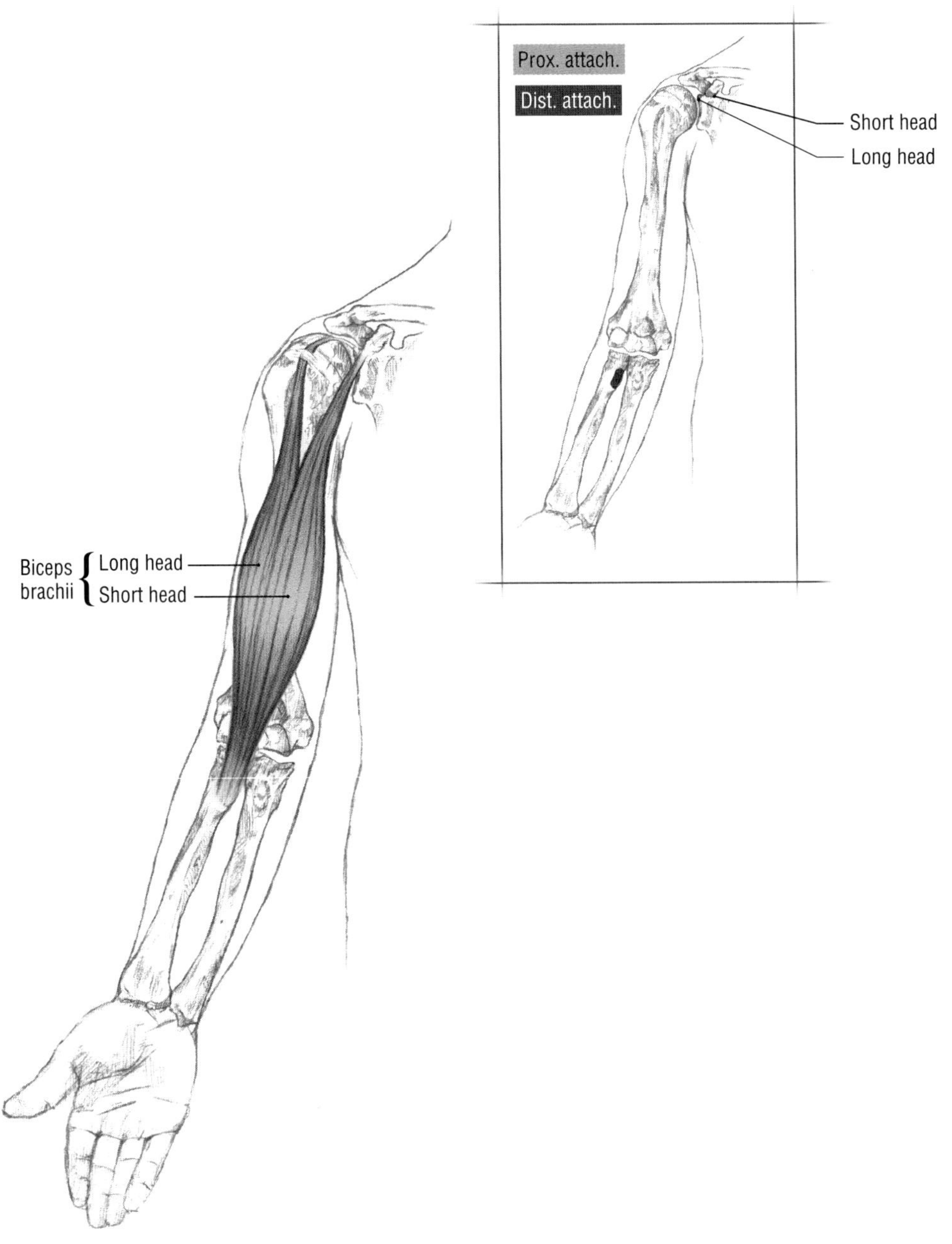

Biceps Brachii

Proximal Attachment:
- Long head: supraglenoid tubercle of the glenoid fossa
- Short head: coracoid process of the scapula

Distal Attachment: Via a common tendon to the bicipital tuberosity (radial tuberosity) of the radius

Innervation: Musculocutaneous nerve

Actions:
- Shoulder flexion
- Elbow flexion
- Supination of the forearm

Comments: The biceps brachii is a primary elbow flexor, but because both heads cross anterior to the medial-lateral axis of the shoulder, this muscle is also an effective shoulder flexor. The proximal tendon of the long head of the biceps brachii courses over the superior aspect of the humeral head, making it vulnerable to damage caused by shoulder impingement. Palpation of the tendon as it courses through the intertubercular (bicipital) groove of the humerus is often used to verify bicipital tendonitis.

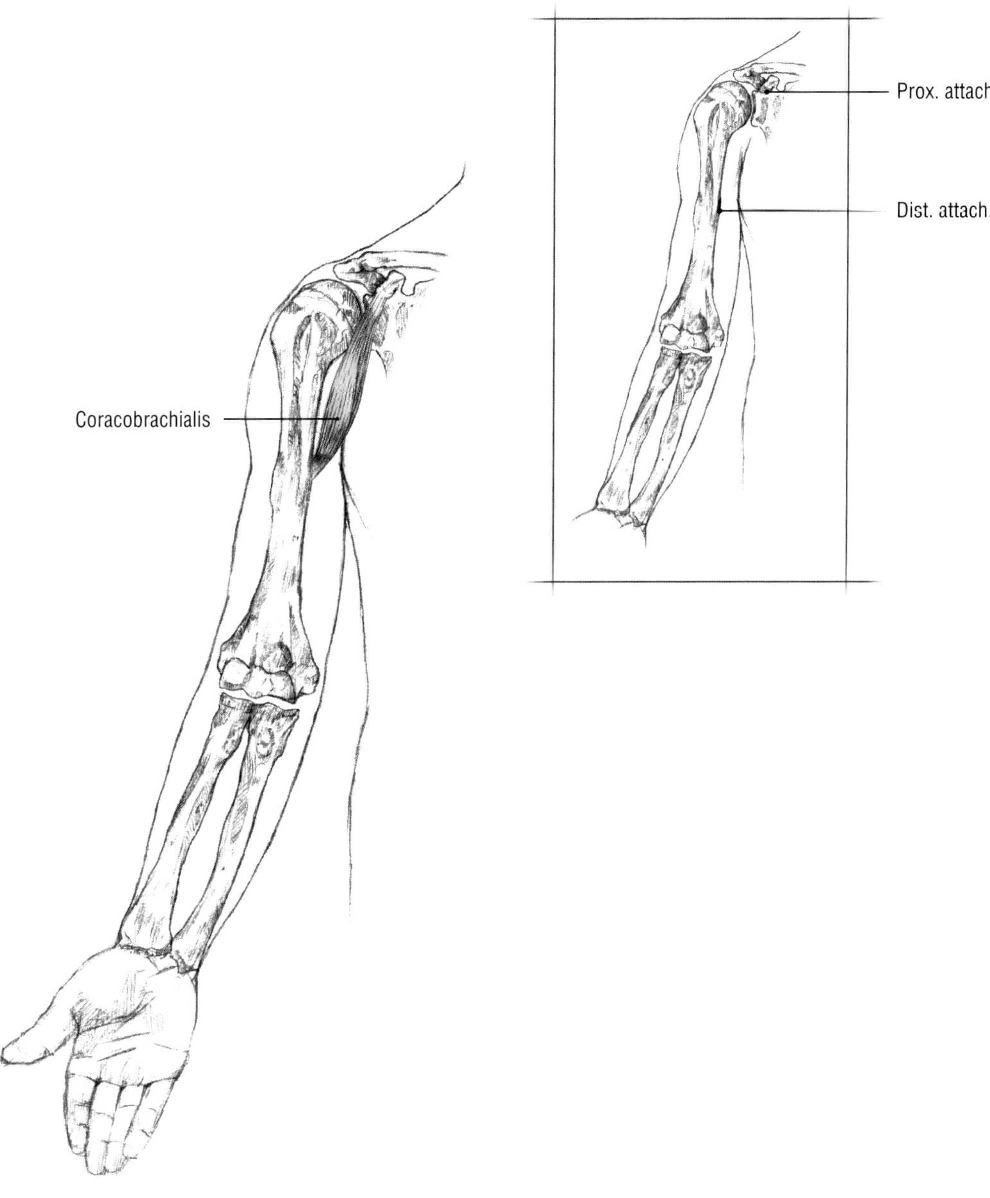

Coracobrachialis

Proximal Attachment:	Coracoid process of the scapula
Distal Attachment:	Medial aspect of the proximal shaft of the humerus
Innervation:	Musculocutaneous nerve
Action:	Shoulder flexion
Comments:	This muscle is a GH joint flexor, but because its line of pull is so close to the joint's axis of rotation, it is likely more useful as a stabilizer of the GH joint. Such an action may help fixate the head of the humerus on the glenoid fossa as the shoulder moves through various ranges of motion.

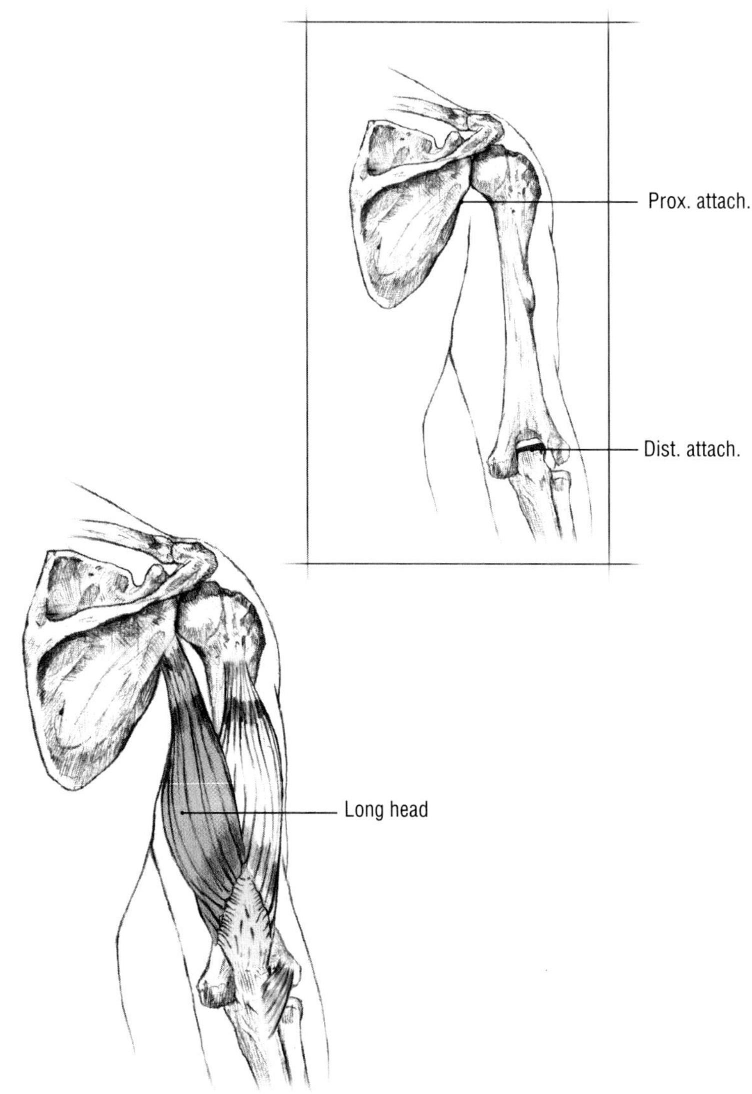

Long Head of the Triceps

Proximal Attachment:	Infraglenoid tubercle of the scapula
Distal Attachment:	Olecranon process of the ulna
Innervation:	Radial nerve
Actions:	• Shoulder extension • Elbow extension
Comments:	The two-joint long head of the triceps is often described as an elbow extensor. On the basis of the long head's proximal attachment, however, it is a strong shoulder extensor. This important muscle is discussed in greater detail in Chapter 5.

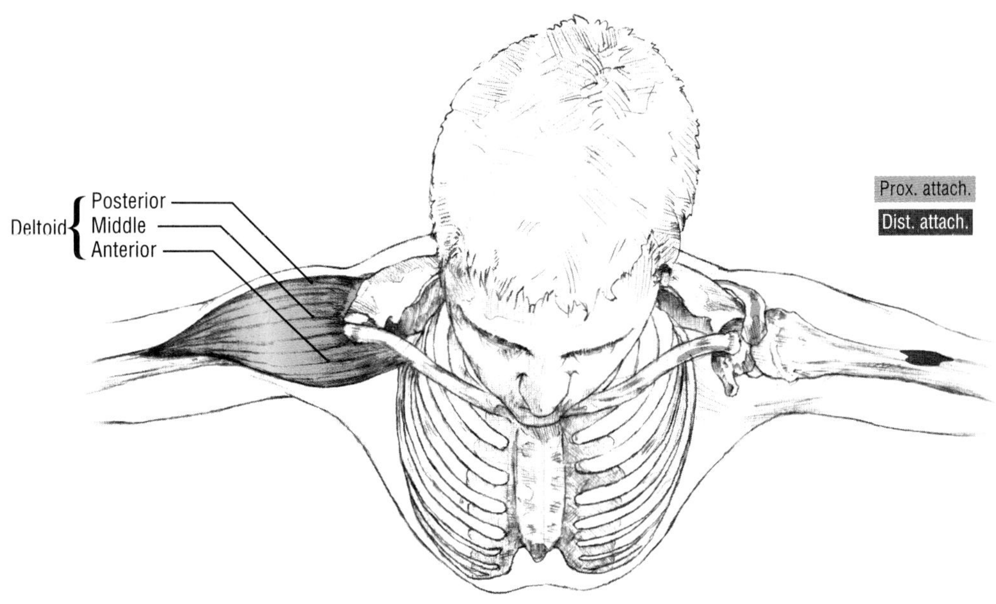

Deltoid

Proximal Attachment:
- Anterior deltoid: Anterior surface of the lateral aspect of the clavicle
- Middle deltoid: Superior-lateral surface of the acromion
- Posterior deltoid: Spine of the scapula

Distal Attachment: Deltoid tuberosity of the humerus

Innervation: Axillary nerve

Actions:

- *Anterior Deltoid:*
  - Flexion of the shoulder
  - Horizontal adduction of the shoulder
  - Internal rotation of the shoulder
  - Abduction of the shoulder
- *Middle Deltoid:*
  - Abduction of the shoulder
  - Flexion of the shoulder
- *Posterior Deltoid:*
  - Extension of the shoulder
  - Horizontal abduction of the shoulder
  - External rotation of the shoulder

Comments: The anterior deltoid assists with shoulder abduction. This muscle is also strongly activated during pushing activities, such as pushing open a heavy door.

The centralized position of the middle deltoid enables it to assist the other heads of the deltoid, depending on the relative position of the shoulder. If the shoulder is internally rotated, the line of pull of the middle deltoid is anterior to the medial-lateral axis of rotation, allowing it to assist the anterior deltoid with shoulder flexion. Conversely, with the shoulder in full external rotation, the line of pull is posterior to the medial-lateral axis of rotation, allowing it to assist the posterior deltoid with shoulder extension.

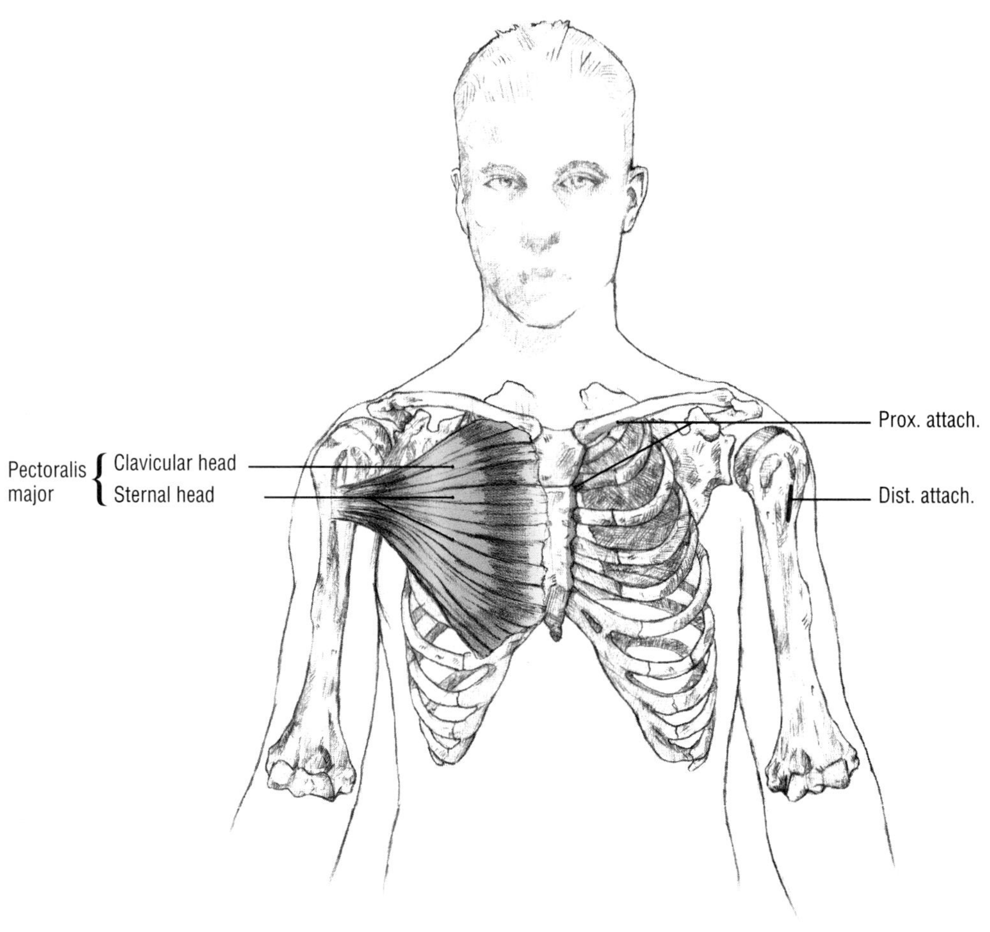

Pectoralis Major

Proximal Attachment:
- Clavicular head: anterior margin of the medial portion of the clavicle
- Sternal head: lateral margin of the manubrium and body of the sternum and cartilages of the first six to seven ribs

Distal Attachment: Crest of the greater tubercle of the humerus

Innervation:
- Clavicular head: lateral pectoral nerve
- Sternal head: lateral and medial pectoral nerves

Actions:

• *Clavicular Head:*
- Internal rotation of the shoulder
- Flexion of the shoulder
- Horizontal adduction of the shoulder

• *Sternal Head:*
- Horizontal Adduction
- Internal rotation of the shoulder
- Adduction and extension of the shoulder
- Depression of the shoulder (via its attachment to humerus)

Comments: The clavicular head of the pectoralis major has identical actions as the anterior deltoid: flexion, internal rotation, and horizontal adduction. The sternal head is important during pushing and pulling activities such as doing push-ups, performing a bench press, or pulling open a heavy door. The sternal head of the pectoralis major is the only GH joint muscle without an attachment to the scapula or clavicle.

Putting It All Together

Now that the anatomy and function of the individual GH joint muscles has been covered, we will begin discussion on how these muscles interact to produce functional movements of the entire shoulder complex.

ABDUCTORS AND FLEXORS

The abductors and flexors of the GH joint are grouped together because many of the muscles that perform abduction also perform flexion. The muscles that simultaneously upwardly rotate the scapula are also essential for normal shoulder abduction or flexion.

Abductors

The primary GH joint abductors are the supraspinatus, anterior deltoid, and middle deltoid (Figure 4-26).

Primary Glenohumeral Joint Abductors

- Supraspinatus
- Anterior deltoid
- Middle deltoid

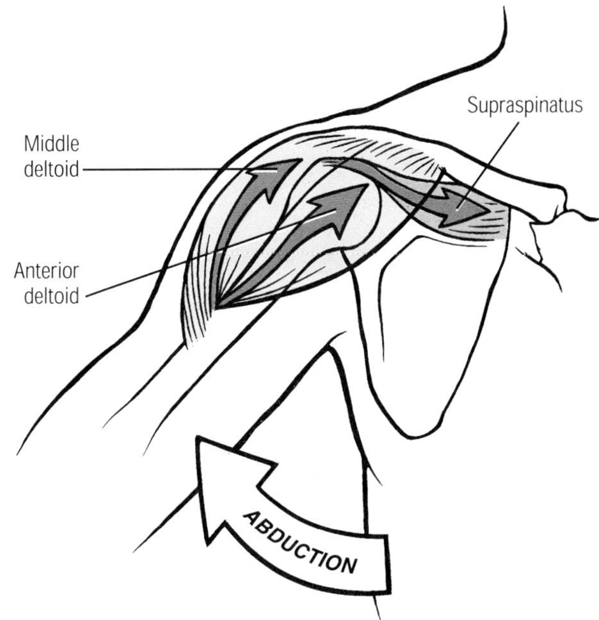

Figure 4-26 Anterior view showing the middle deltoid, anterior deltoid, and supraspinatus as abductors of the glenohumeral joint. (From Neumann DA: *Kinesiology of the musculoskeletal system: foundations for physical rehabilitation*, St Louis, 2002, Mosby, Figure 5-47.)

Flexors

The primary GH joint flexors are the anterior deltoid, clavicular head of the pectoralis major, coracobrachialis, and biceps brachii.

Primary Glenohumeral Joint Flexors

- Anterior deltoid
- Pectoralis major (clavicular head)
- Coracobrachialis
- Biceps brachii

Functional Consideration: Scapulohumeral Rhythm Revisited. Upward rotation of the scapula is an essential component of abduction or flexion of the shoulder. This important scapular motion is performed by the serratus anterior and upper and lower trapezius muscles (Figure 4-27). These muscles drive the scapula through upward rotation and, equally important, provide stable attachment sites for the muscles that produce GH joint motion. The middle trapezius is active to neutralize the strong protraction tendency of the serratus anterior.

Upward rotation of the scapula is important for several reasons. First, the motion augments the total range of motion of the shoulder. Recall that one third of the range of motion for shoulder abduction or flexion occurs from upward rotation of the scapula. Second, the upward rotation of the scapula helps maintain favorable length-tension relationship of the GH joint abductors and flexors throughout extensive ranges of motion. For example, if the scapula did *not* upwardly rotate, many of the GH joint

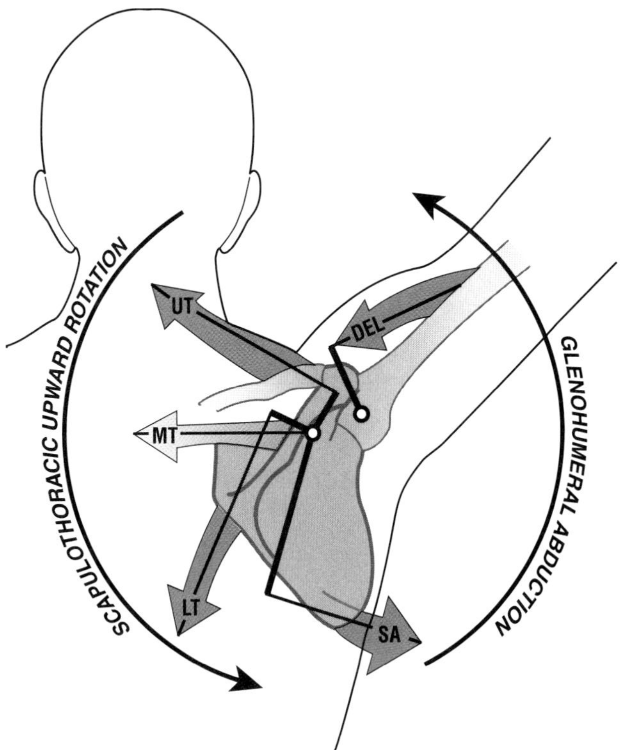

Figure 4-27 Posterior view of the right shoulder, showing the interaction between the scapulothoracic upward rotators and the glenohumeral abductors. *DEL*, Deltoid/supraspinatus; *LT*, lower trapezius; *MT*, middle trapezius; *SA*, serratus anterior; *UT*, upper trapezius. (From Neumann DA: *Kinesiology of the musculoskeletal system: foundations for physical rehabilitation*, St Louis, 2002, Mosby, Figure 5-49.)

Clinical INSIGHT

Impingement and Tendonitis of the Shoulder

The tendon of the supraspinatus and the long head of the biceps both reside between the acromion and humeral head. This vulnerable location places these structures at risk of injury. Excessive superior migration of the humeral head, for example, will likely impinge, or pinch, one or both of these structures (see Figure 4-14, *B*). Because these structures play a dominant role in the kinesiology of the shoulder, their injury often begins a vicious cycle of repeated injury, inflammation, and faulty mechanics. This helps explain the relatively high frequency of tendonitis that involves these muscles.

abductors or flexors would quickly become too short, too quickly, significantly reducing their ability to contribute to abduction or flexion torque.

ADDUCTORS AND EXTENSORS

Shoulder adduction and extension are powerful motions supported by strong muscles such as the latissimus dorsi and pectoralis major. The teres major, long head of the triceps, and posterior deltoid are also key players in these actions. Because the latter three muscles are attached proximally to the scapula, adequate stabilization forces are required from scapulothoracic muscles. Shoulder adduction and/or extension require simultaneous downward rotation of the scapula.

Adductors

The primary muscles that produce adduction of the GH joint are the teres major, latissimus dorsi, and pectoralis major. As illustrated in Figure 4-25, these muscles work closely with the scapular downward rotators to produce adduction of the shoulder as a whole.

Primary Glenohumeral Joint Adductors

- Teres major
- Latissimus dorsi
- Pectoralis major

Extensors

The primary muscles involved with GH joint extension are the latissimus dorsi, teres major, pectoralis major, posterior deltoid, and long head of the triceps. Note that these muscles are strong extensors, especially with the arm starting in a flexed position. However, once the arm becomes even with the midline of the thorax, only the posterior deltoid can continue to extend the arm well beyond the body.

Primary Glenohumeral Joint Extensors

- Latissimus dorsi
- Teres major
- Pectoralis major
- Posterior deltoid
- Long head of the triceps

Clinical Consideration: Horizontal Abduction and Adduction-Flexion and Extension Turned Sideways. A quick review of the musculature of the shoulder reveals an interesting phenomenon. The muscles that perform shoulder flexion also perform horizontal adduction, and muscles that perform shoulder extension also perform horizontal abduction. Examination of this phenomenon exposes the fact that, in regard to axes of rotation and lines of pull, these seemingly different actions are actually the same motions, just turned sideways.

Recall that shoulder flexion and extension occur about a medial-lateral axis of rotation: Muscles that course anterior to the medial-lateral axis perform flexion, whereas muscles with a line of pull posterior to the medial-lateral axis perform extension.

The motions of horizontal abduction and adduction, on the contrary, are typically described as occurring about a vertical axis of rotation. Muscles with a line of pull anterior to this vertical axis of rotation perform horizontal adduction, and muscles with a line of pull posterior to this axis of rotation perform horizontal abduction.

ROTATOR CUFF

The rotator cuff (Figure 4-28) is the common name that describes the supraspinatus, infraspinatus, teres minor, and subscapularis. This group of muscles shares an important function in driving the motions of internal and external rotation, as well as actively stabilizing the humeral head on the glenoid fossa.

Rotator Cuff Muscles

- Supraspinatus
- Infraspinatus
- Teres minor
- Subscapularis

The rotator cuff muscles surround the humeral head anteriorly, superiorly, and posteriorly, each providing a muscular force that pulls the humeral head toward the glenoid fossa. These muscles also play an important role in controlling GH joint arthrokinematics and function as **dynamic stabilizers;** giving stability to the loose-fitting

GH joint as the shoulder moves through a nearly infinite number of positions.

Functional Consideration: Rotator Cuff Function during Glenohumeral Motion

In the healthy shoulder, the rotator cuff controls much of the active arthrokinematics of an abducting GH joint (Figure 4-29). Contraction of the horizontally oriented supraspinatus produces a compression force directly into the glenoid fossa. This compression force stabilizes the humeral head against the fossa during its superior roll. In addition, the other three rotator cuff muscles provide an inferiorly directed force to counteract the tendency of the deltoids to pull the humerus superiorly. Without these stabilizing forces, the nearly vertical line of pull of the deltoid tends to jam or impinge the humeral head superiorly against the coracoacromial arch.

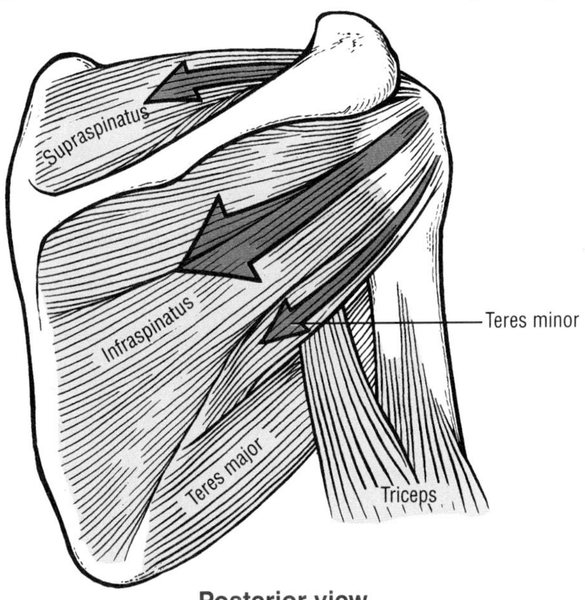

Figure 4-28 Posterior view of the right shoulder showing the supraspinatus, infraspinatus, and teres minor muscles. The subscapularis is not visible from this view; see p. 75. (From Neumann DA: *Kinesiology of the musculoskeletal system: foundations for physical rehabilitation*, St Louis, 2002, Mosby, Figure 5-53.)

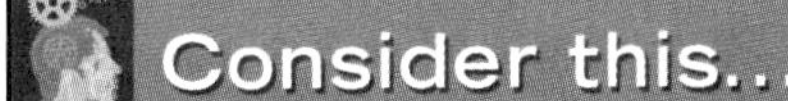

Consider this...

Rotator Cuff: The "SITS" Muscles

The rotator cuff muscles are often referred to as the SITS muscles. SITS is an acronym used to help individuals remember the four rotator cuff muscles, as follows:

S Supraspinatus
I Infraspinatus
T Teres minor
S Subscapularis

"The rotator cuff SITS in the center of the stable" is a mnemonic to help individuals not only remember the names of the four rotator cuff muscles but also their common function—centralizing and stabilizing the humeral head within the glenoid fossa.

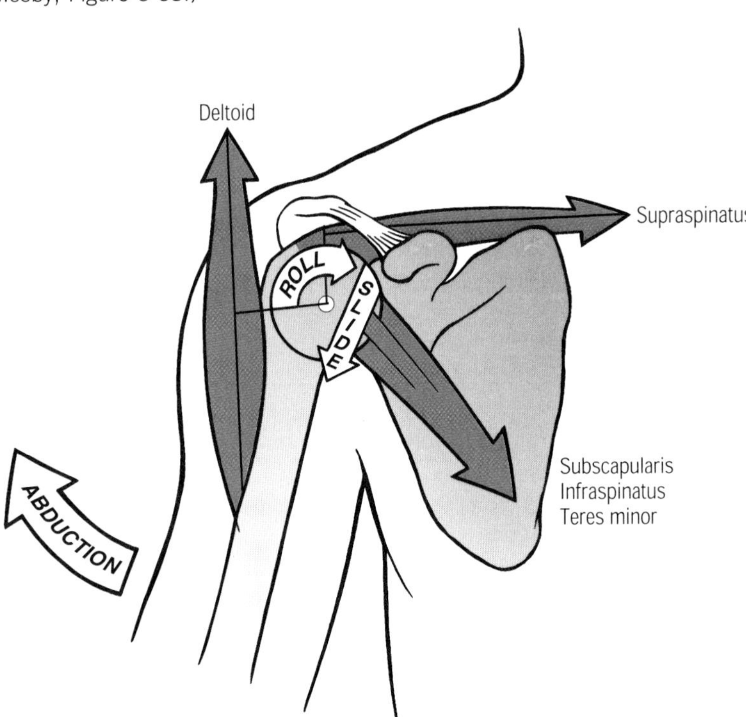

Figure 4-29 Anterior view of the right shoulder showing the force-couple between the deltoid and rotator cuff muscles during active shoulder abduction. (From Neumann DA: *Kinesiology of the musculoskeletal system: foundations for physical rehabilitation*, St Louis, 2002, Mosby, Figure 5-55.)

Functional Consideration: Summary of the Rotator Cuff in Controlling Glenohumeral Arthrokinematics

- *Supraspinatus:* Compresses the humeral head directly into the glenoid fossa
- *Subscapularis, infraspinatus,* and *teres minor:* Produce an inferiorly directed force on the humerus to counteract the superior-translation force of the deltoid
- *Infraspinatus* and *teres minor:* Externally rotate the humeral head, preventing an impingement between the greater tuberosity and the acromion

INTERNAL AND EXTERNAL ROTATORS

Internal Rotators

The primary muscles that internally rotate the GH joint are the teres major, pectoralis major, subscapularis, latissimus dorsi, and the anterior deltoid. Many of these muscles are also powerful shoulder extensors and adductors. Often, lifting activities incorporate all of these actions. Consider, for example, lifting a large box. The initial squeezing force to secure the box is typically an internal rotation force. Almost simultaneously, the shoulders will adduct and extend, further securing the box while bringing the box inward, toward the body's center of mass.

Primary Internal Rotators

- Teres major
- Pectoralis major
- Subscapularis
- Latissimus dorsi
- Anterior deltoid

The internal rotators are larger and more numerous than the external rotators. This fact explains why the internal rotators can produce about 1.75 times more isometric torque than the external rotators. This is generally advantageous because many more functional activities require strong forces into internal rotation than external rotation. However, this muscular imbalance can predispose an individual to poor posture—forward, rounded shoulders—and makes the weaker external rotator muscles more prone to injury.

External Rotators

The primary external rotators of the GH joint are the teres minor, infraspinatus, and posterior deltoid. These muscles contribute to a relatively small percentage of the total muscle mass of the shoulder. Accordingly, maximal effort external rotation produces the smallest torque of any muscle group at the shoulder. Regardless of the relatively low maximal torque potential, these muscles can still produce high-velocity concentric contractions such as when cocking the arm backward just before pitching a ball.

Primary External Rotators

- Teres minor
- Infraspinatus
- Posterior deltoid

Functional Consideration: Activation of the Rotators during a Throwing Motion. Activities such as pitching a baseball, spiking a volleyball, or serving a tennis ball all incorporate a similar type of motion. Typically, this motion occurs with the shoulder abducted to about 90 degrees. A quick concentric contraction of the external rotators cocks the shoulder and is followed by a concentric contraction of the internal rotators that generate huge amounts of internal rotation torque. The internal rotation velocity of the shoulder has been measured at nearly 7000 degrees/second during the release phase of pitching.

The large torques and high velocities produced during a vigorous throwing motion are good examples of how the elastic nature of muscle can be used for a functional advantage. Rotational torques such as those of the magnitude produced by major-league baseball pitchers cannot be generated solely by the activation of the internal rotator muscles. Instead, a portion of this force is generated indirectly by rotations of the lower extremities and trunk and eventually transmitted through the internal rotators of the shoulder to the baseball. The rotation of the legs and trunk stretch the internal rotators and, similar to stretching a rubber band, the shoulder harnesses part of this energy for the release phase of the pitch. Major league baseball pitchers take full advantage of this kinematic chain, enabling many of them to throw a ball in excess of 95 miles per hour. The great speed and internal rotation torque, however, often result in injury to the external rotators, which have the arduous task of decelerating the arm through eccentric activation.

Summary

The shoulder is one of the most complex musculoskeletal systems in the body. Almost any action that occurs at the shoulder complex involves the coordination of numerous muscles that can guide and support the shoulder through large ranges of motion. Muscles may be involved with stabilizing a proximal bone such as the scapula or clavicle, whereas others simultaneously produce motion of the humerus. All the while, ligaments and other soft tissues including muscle enable proper arthrokinematic motions at each of the four joints of the shoulder complex.

Because proper motion of the shoulder requires coordinated action of so many muscles across multiple joints, dysfunction of the shoulder is relatively common. However, the same factors that make this region of the body prone to dysfunction also make the shoulder complex highly adaptable. With careful consideration of the kinesiology of the shoulder complex, clinicians are typically able to rehabilitate a large majority of the impairments that affect this region.

Study Questions

1. Which of the following statements is true regarding upward rotation of the scapula?
   a. Occurs as a natural component of shoulder extension
   b. Occurs as a natural component of raising one's arm overhead
   c. Occurs primarily through activation of the teres major and teres minor muscles
   d. Results in the inferior tip of the scapula pointing medially
2. Which of the following statements is true regarding the glenohumeral joint?
   a. The glenohumeral joint has a ball-and-socket joint structure.
   b. The glenohumeral joint allows motion in all three planes.
   c. The glenohumeral joint is formed by the greater tubercle articulating with the distal clavicle.
   d. A and B
   e. All of the above
3. Which of the following joints is a saddle joint?
   a. Glenohumeral
   b. Sternoclavicular
   c. Acromioclavicular
   d. Scapulothoracic
4. Without upward rotation of the scapula, full shoulder abduction would be limited to approximately:
   a. 60 degrees
   b. 80 degrees
   c. 120 degrees
   d. 170 degrees
5. The acromion is a structure associated with which bone?
   a. Humerus
   b. Scapula
   c. Clavicle
   d. Sternum
6. A muscle that performs shoulder flexion:
   a. Must have a line of pull anterior to the medial-lateral axis of rotation of the shoulder
   b. Must course posterior to the medial-lateral axis of rotation of the shoulder
   c. Must also extend the elbow
   d. Is likely innervated by the radial nerve
7. Which of the following best describes the scapulohumeral rhythm?
   a. For every 3 degrees of scapular upward rotation, 1 degree of glenohumeral adduction must occur.
   b. For every 2 degrees of glenohumeral flexion or abduction, 1 degree of scapular upward rotation must occur.
   c. The scapulohumeral rhythm only occurs during passive flexion and extension motions of the shoulder.
   d. Protraction of the scapula must be accompanied by horizontal abduction of the humerus.
8. Which of the following muscles is *not* part of the force-couple that produces upward rotation of the scapula?
   a. Serratus anterior
   b. Upper trapezius
   c. Rhomboids
   d. Lower trapezius
9. Which of the following muscles does not attach to the humerus (proximally or distally)?
   a. Teres minor
   b. Anterior deltoid
   c. Serratus anterior
   d. Subscapularis
10. Which of the following muscles is *not* part of the rotator cuff?
    a. Supraspinatus
    b. Teres minor
    c. Infraspinatus
    d. Upper trapezius
11. Winging of the scapula is indicative of:
    a. Anterior deltoid weakness
    b. Posterior deltoid weakness
    c. Serratus anterior weakness
    d. Teres major and latissimus dorsi weakness
12. Which of the following statements is true regarding shoulder depression?
    a. Incorporates scapulothoracic depression and glenohumeral depression
    b. Can be used in a closed-chain to elevate the trunk
    c. Relies mostly on the combined action of the upper and middle trapezius muscles
    d. A and B
    e. B and C
13. Which of the following statements is true regarding the deltoid muscles?
    a. The anterior deltoid performs shoulder flexion.
    b. The posterior deltoid performs shoulder extension.
    c. All heads of the deltoid are innervated by the axillary nerve.
    d. A and C
    e. All of the above

14. What is the common similarity among the latissimus dorsi, posterior deltoid, and long head of the triceps?
    a. All three of these muscles attach to the humerus.
    b. All three of these muscles are strong internal rotators of the shoulder.
    c. All three of these muscles are innervated by the radial nerve.
    d. All three of these muscles can extend the shoulder.
15. Which of the following describes the common function of the rotator cuff muscles?
    a. All four muscles perform internal rotation of the shoulder.
    b. All four muscles help to stabilize the humeral head within the glenoid fossa.
    c. All four muscles produce a force-couple that upwardly rotates the scapula.
    d. All four muscles prevent excessive external rotation of the glenohumeral joint.
16. If the shoulder is abducted to 150 degrees, according to the scapulohumeral rhythm, how much upward rotation of the scapula has occurred?
    a. 50 degrees
    b. 100 degrees
    c. 120 degrees
    d. 25 to 30 degrees
17. Impingement can best be described as:
    a. Reduced activation of the internal rotators of the shoulder
    b. A superior migration of the humerus resulting in the humeral head colliding with the acromion
    c. The combined actions of scapular depression and glenohumeral protraction
    d. Complete rupture of the acromioclavicular and coracoclavicular ligaments
18. Performing abduction in the scapular plane helps avoid impingement because:
    a. The teres minor and teres major are put on slack.
    b. The greater tuberosity is positioned under the highest point of the acromion.
    c. The scapula becomes fixed to the medial aspect of the posterior thorax.
    d. The subscapularis becomes an external rotator of the shoulder in this position.
19. Which of the following muscles is *not* an internal rotator of the shoulder?
    a. Pectoralis major
    b. Latissimus dorsi
    c. Infraspinatus
    d. Teres major
20. Which of the following statements is true regarding external rotation of the shoulder?
    a. Occurs in frontal plane
    b. Occurs about a longitudinal axis of rotation
    c. Performed by two of the four rotator cuff muscles
    d. A and C
    e. B and C
21. The serratus anterior is a primary upward rotator of the scapula.
    a. True
    b. False
22. A muscle that performs glenohumeral abduction must have a line of pull superior to the anterior-posterior axis of rotation.
    a. True
    b. False
23. The shoulder complex is equipped with more external rotators than internal rotator muscles.
    a. True
    b. False
24. During abduction of the shoulder, the arthrokinematic roll and slide occur in the same direction.
    a. True
    b. False
25. The latissimus dorsi and lower trapezius often work together to depress the entire shoulder.
    a. True
    b. False
26. Horizontal abduction of the humerus is generally accompanied by retraction of the scapula.
    a. True
    b. False
27. The supraspinatus and the middle deltoid are both innervated by the same nerve.
    a. True
    b. False
28. The rhomboids and pectoralis minor are primary downward rotators of the scapula.
    a. True
    b. False
29. A pulling motion such as a "wide grip pull-up" will involve strong activation of the latissimus dorsi.
    a. True
    b. False
30. Shoulder impingement is likely to occur if the scapula does not upwardly rotate as the shoulder is actively abducted.
    a. True
    b. False

ADDITIONAL READINGS

Bagg SD, Forrest WJ: Electromyographic study of the scapular rotators during arm abduction in the scapular plane, *Am J Phys Med* 65(3): 111-124, 1986.

Bagg SD, Forrest WJ: A biomechanical analysis of scapular rotation during arm abduction in the scapular plane, *Am J Phys Med Rehabil* 67(6):238-245, 1988.

Bigliani LU, Kelkar R, Flatow EL, et al: Glenohumeral stability. Biomechanical properties of passive and active stabilizers, *Clin Orthop* September(330):13-30, 1996.

Borsa PA, Dover GC, Wilk KE, et al: Glenohumeral range of motion and stiffness in professional baseball pitchers, *Med Sci Sports Exerc* 38(1):21-26, 2006.

Borstad JD, Ludewig PM: The effect of long versus short pectoralis minor resting length on scapular kinematics in healthy individuals, *J Orthop Sports Phys Ther* 35(4):227-238, 2005.

Brunnstrom S: Muscle testing around the shoulder girdle, *J Bone Joint Surg Am* 23A:263-272, 1941.

Ebaugh DD, McClure PW, Karduna AR: Three-dimensional scapulothoracic motion during active and passive arm elevation, *Clin Biomech (Bristol, Avon)* 20(7):700-709, 2005.

Ebaugh DD, McClure PW, Karduna AR: Effects of shoulder muscle fatigue caused by repetitive overhead activities on scapulothoracic and glenohumeral kinematics, *J Electromyogr Kinesiol* 16(3): 224-235, 2006.

Graichen H, Stammberger T, Bonel H, et al: Three-dimensional analysis of shoulder girdle and supraspinatus motion patterns in patients with impingement syndrome, *J Orthop Res* 19(6): 1192-1198, 2001.

Halder AM, Itoi E, An KN: Anatomy and biomechanics of the shoulder, *Orthop Clin North Am* 31(2):159-176, 2000.

Hayes K, Callanan M, Walton J, et al: Shoulder instability: management and rehabilitation, *J Orthop Sports Phys Ther* 32(10):497-509, 2002.

Itoi E, Hsu HC, An KN: Biomechanical investigation of the glenohumeral joint, *J Shoulder Elbow Surg* 5(5):407-424, 1996.

Ludewig PM, Behrens SA, Meyer SM, et al: Three-dimensional clavicular motion during arm elevation: reliability and descriptive data, *J Orthop Sports Phys Ther* 34(3):140-149, 2004.

Ludewig PM, Cook TM, Nawoczenski DA: Three-dimensional scapular orientation and muscle activity at selected positions of humeral elevation, *J Orthop Sports Phys Ther* 24(2):57-65, 1996.

Ludewig PM, Hoff MS, Osowski EE, et al: Relative balance of serratus anterior and upper trapezius muscle activity during push-up exercises, *Am J Sports Med* 32(2):484-493, 2004.

McClure PW, Michener LA, Sennett B, et al: Direct 3-dimensional measurement of scapular kinematics during dynamic movements in vivo, *J Shoulder Elbow Surg* 10(3):269-277, 2001.

Michener LA, McClure PW, Karduna AR: Anatomical and biomechanical mechanisms of subacromial impingement syndrome, *Clin Biomech (Bristol, Avon)* 18(5):369-379, 2003.

Murray MP, Gore DR, Gardner GM, et al: Shoulder motion and muscle strength of normal men and women in two age groups, *Clin Orthop* January-February(192):268-273, 1985.

Safran MR: Nerve injury about the shoulder in athletes, part 1: suprascapular nerve and axillary nerve, *Am J Sports Med* 32(3):803-819, 2004.

Safran MR: Nerve injury about the shoulder in athletes, part 2: long thoracic nerve, spinal accessory nerve, burners/stingers, thoracic outlet syndrome, *Am J Sports Med* 32(4):1063-1076, 2004.

CHAPTER 5

Structure and Function of the Elbow and Forearm Complex

CHAPTER OUTLINE

OBJECTIVES

- Identify the primary bones and bony features relevant to the elbow and forearm complex.
- Describe the supporting structures of the elbow and forearm complex.
- Describe the structure and function of the four main joints within the elbow and forearm complex.
- Cite the normal range of motion for elbow flexion and extension and forearm supination and pronation.
- Describe the planes of motion and axes of rotation for the joints of the elbow and forearm complex.
- Cite the proximal and distal attachments and innervation of the muscles of the elbow and forearm complex.
- Justify the primary actions of the muscles of the elbow and forearm complex.
- Cite innervation of the muscles of the elbow and forearm complex.
- Explain the primary muscular interactions involved in performing a pushing and pulling motion.
- Explain the primary muscular interactions involved in tightening a screw with a screwdriver.

KEY TERMS

actively efficient
actively insufficient
Colles' fracture
cubitus varus
end feel
excessive cubitus valgus
valgus
varus

The ability to actively flex and extend the elbow is essential for many important functions such as those involved with feeding, grooming, reaching, throwing, and pushing. The elbow itself actually consists of two separate articulations: the humeroulnar and the humeroradial joint (Figure 5-1). The forearm complex allows the movements of pronation and supination—motions that rotate the palm upward (supination) or downward (pronation). As in the elbow, the forearm consists of two articulations: the proximal and distal radioulnar joint

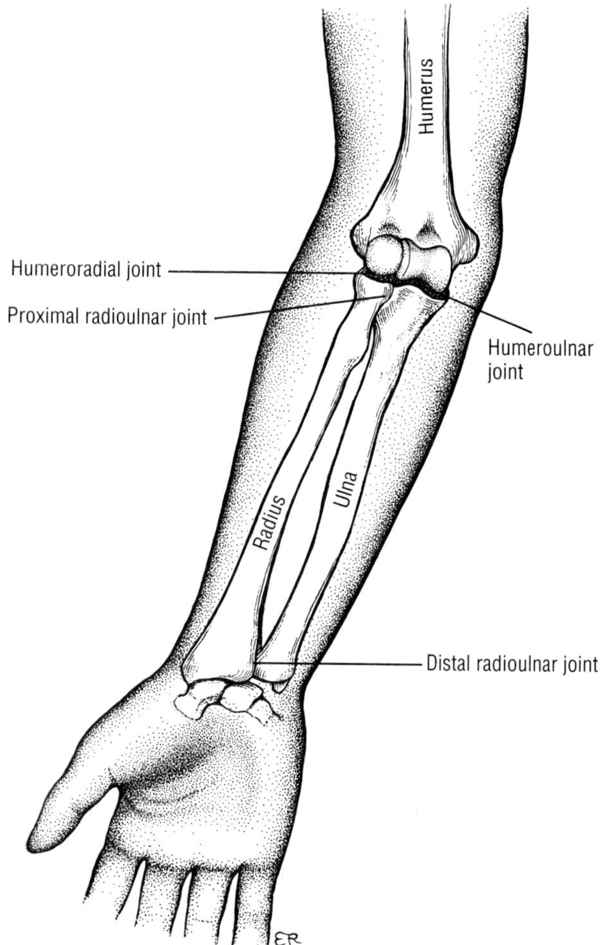

Figure 5-1 The articulations of the elbow and forearm complex. (From Neumann DA: *Kinesiology of the musculoskeletal system: foundations for physical rehabilitation,* St Louis, 2002, Mosby, Figure 6-1.)

(see Figure 5-1). The interaction among the four joints of the elbow and forearm enables the hand to be placed in a nearly infinite number of positions, greatly enhancing the functional potential of the entire upper extremity.

Joints of the Elbow and Forearm Complex

- Humeroulnar joint
- Humeroradial joint
- Proximal radioulnar joint
- Distal radioulnar joint

Osteology

The four bones that relate to the function of the elbow and forearm complex include the (1) scapula, (2) distal humerus, (3) ulna, and (4) radius.

Scapula

The scapula (Figure 5-2) has three bony features that are important to the muscles of the elbow. The *coracoid process* serves as the proximal attachment for the short head of the biceps. The *supraglenoid tubercle* serves as the proximal attachment for the long head of the biceps. The *infraglenoid tubercle* marks the proximal attachment for the long head of the triceps.

Distal Humerus

The *trochlea* is a spool-shaped structure located on the medial side of the distal humerus (Figures 5-3 and 5-4) that articulates with the ulna to form the *humeroulnar joint.* The *coronoid fossa* is a small pit located just superior to the trochlea that accepts the coronoid process of the ulna when the elbow is fully flexed. Just lateral to the trochlea is the ball-shaped *capitulum*, which articulates with the head of the radius to form the *humeroradial joint.*

The *medial epicondyle* is the prominent projection of bone on the medial side of the distal humerus. This easily palpable prominence serves as the proximal attachment for most of the wrist flexor muscles, the pronator teres, and the medial collateral ligament of the elbow. The *lateral epicondyle* is less prominent; however, it is the proximal attachment for most of the wrist extensor muscles, the supinator muscle, and the lateral collateral ligament of the elbow. Immediately proximal to both epicondyles are the *medial* and *lateral supracondylar ridges.*

The *olecranon fossa* is the relatively deep, broad pit located on the posterior side of the distal humerus. With the elbow fully extended, a portion of the olecranon process projects into this fossa.

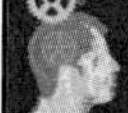

Consider this...

The "Funny Bone"

"Hitting your funny bone" technically means hitting your ulnar nerve. The ulnar nerve travels through a groove between the olecranon process and the medial epicondyle. When this area is bumped into a table edge, for example, the nerve is compressed between the table edge and its bony surroundings, sending tingling and numbness down the area of skin supplied by the nerve, specifically on the medial forearm and fourth and fifth digits (ring finger and small finger).

Ulna

The ulna (Figures 5-5 and 5-6) has a thick proximal end with distinct processes. The *olecranon process* is the large, blunt, proximal tip of the ulna commonly referred to as the elbow bone. The rough posterior surface of the olecranon process is the distal attachment for the triceps muscles.

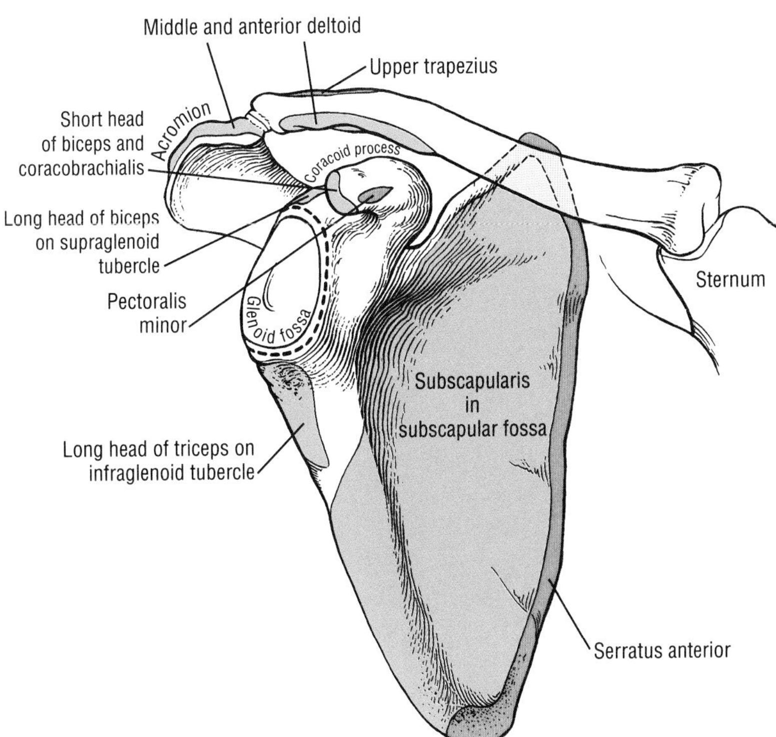

Figure 5-2 The anterior surface of the right scapula. Proximal attachments of muscles are shown in red, distal attachments in gray. (From Neumann DA: *Kinesiology of the musculoskeletal system: foundations for physical rehabilitation,* St Louis, 2002, Mosby, Figure 5-5, *B.*)

The *trochlear notch* is the large, jaw-like curvature of the proximal ulna that articulates with the trochlea (of the humerus) forming the humeroulnar joint (Figure 5-7). The inferior tip of the trochlear notch comes to a point, forming the coronoid process. The *coronoid process* strengthens the articulation of the humeroulnar joint by firmly grabbing the trochlea of the humerus. Slightly inferior and lateral to the trochlear notch is the *radial notch,* which articulates with the head of the radius to form the *proximal radioulnar joint.*

Located distally, the *styloid process* is a pointed projection of bone that arises from the *ulnar head.* Both of these structures can be palpated on the ulnar side of the dorsum of the wrist, with the forearm fully pronated.

Radius

In a fully supinated position, the radius lies parallel and lateral to the ulna (see Figures 5-5 and 5-6). The *radial head* is shaped like a wide disk on the proximal end of the radius. The superior surface of the radial head consists of a shallow cup-shaped depression called the *fovea* that articulates with the capitulum of the humerus, forming the *humeroradial joint.*

The *bicipital tuberosity,* sometimes called the *radial tuberosity,* is an enlarged ridge of bone located on the anterior-medial aspect of the proximal radius. The bicipital tuberosity is so named because it is the primary distal attachment for the biceps brachii.

The distal end of the radius is wide and flat with two notable structures, the styloid process and the ulnar notch. The *styloid process* is the pointed (and easily palpable) projection of bone off the distal lateral radius. The *ulnar notch* is a small depression on the medial side of the distal radius that articulates with the ulnar head, forming the *distal radioulnar joint.*

Arthrology of the Elbow

General Features

As mentioned in the previous section, the elbow joint is composed of two articulations, the humeroulnar joint and the humeroradial joint. The *humeroulnar joint* provides most of the structural stability to the elbow as a whole. This stability is provided primarily by the jaw-like trochlear notch of the ulna interlocking with the spool-shaped trochlea of the humerus (Figure 5-8). This hinge-like joint limits motion of the elbow to flexion and extension.

The *humeroradial joint* is formed by the ball-shaped capitulum of the humerus articulating with the bowl-shaped fovea of the radius (see Figure 5-8). This configuration permits continuous contact between the radial head and the capitulum during supination and pronation, as the radius spins about its own axis; and during flexion and extension, as the radial head rolls and slides over the rounded capitulum. Compared with the humeroulnar joint, the humeroradial joint provides only secondary stability to the elbow.

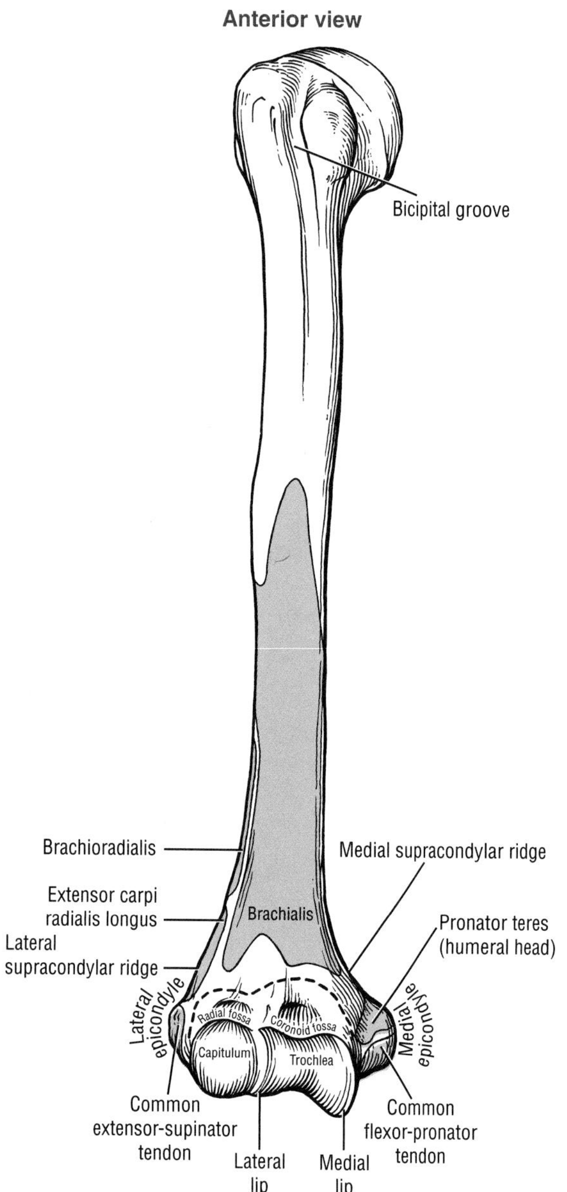

Figure 5-3 The anterior aspect of the right humerus. Proximal attachments of muscles are shown in red. The dotted line represents the capsular attachments of the elbow. (From Neumann DA: *Kinesiology of the musculoskeletal system: foundations for physical rehabilitation*, St Louis, 2002, Mosby, Figure 6-2.)

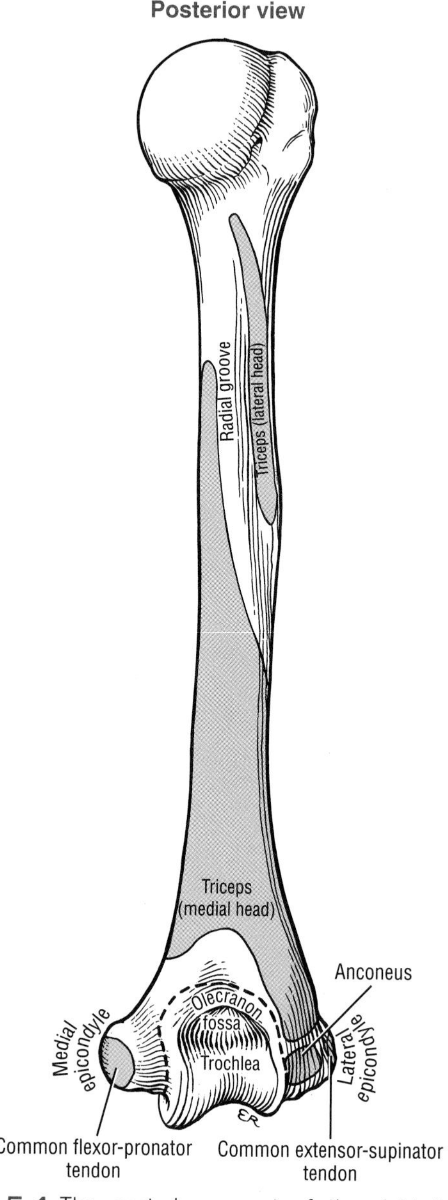

Figure 5-4 The posterior aspect of the right humerus. Proximal attachments of muscles are shown in red. The dotted line represents the capsular attachments of the elbow. (From Neumann DA: *Kinesiology of the musculoskeletal system: foundations for physical rehabilitation*, St Louis, 2002, Mosby, Figure 6-3.)

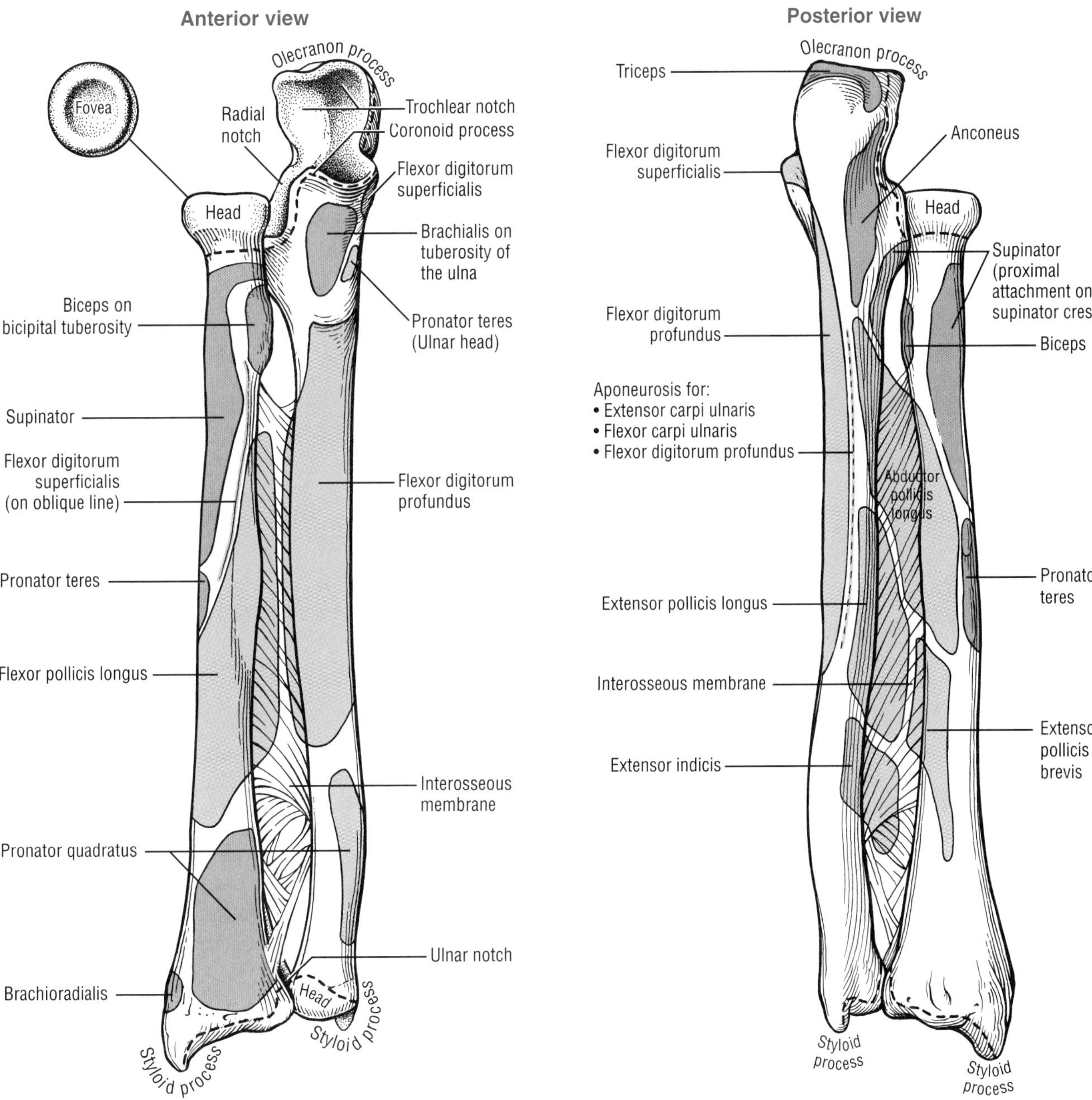

Figure 5-5 The anterior aspect of the right radius and ulna. The muscle's proximal attachments are shown in red and distal attachments in gray. The dotted lines represent the capsular attachments of the elbow and wrist. (From Neumann DA: *Kinesiology of the musculoskeletal system: foundations for physical rehabilitation*, St Louis, 2002, Mosby, Figure 6-5.)

Figure 5-6 The posterior aspect of the right radius and ulna. The muscle's proximal attachments are shown in red and distal attachments in gray. The dotted lines represent the capsular attachments of the elbow and wrist. (From Neumann DA: *Kinesiology of the musculoskeletal system: foundations for physical rehabilitation*, St Louis, 2002, Mosby, Figure 6-6.)

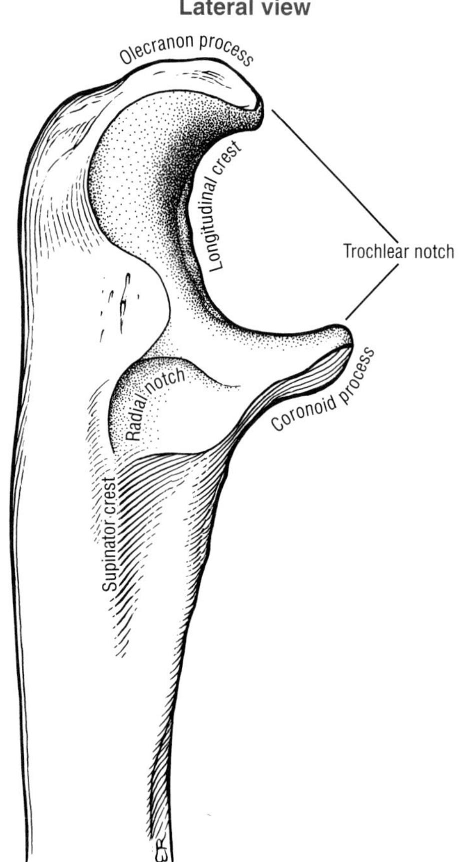

Figure 5-7 A lateral (radial) view of the right proximal ulna, with the radius removed. Note the jaw-like shape of the trochlear notch. (From Neumann DA: *Kinesiology of the musculoskeletal system: foundations for physical rehabilitation,* St Louis, 2002, Mosby, Figure 6-7.)

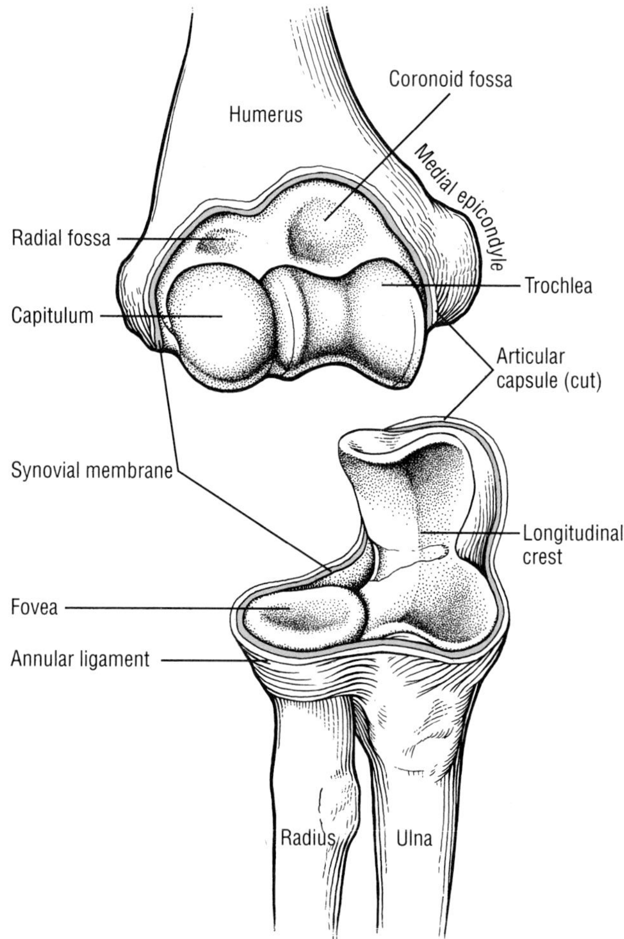

Figure 5-8 Anterior view of the right elbow disarticulated to expose the features of the humeroulnar and humeroradial joints. The synovial membrane lining the internal side of the capsule is shown in red. (From Neumann DA: *Kinesiology of the musculoskeletal system: foundations for physical rehabilitation,* St Louis, 2002, Mosby, Figure 6-11.)

Clinical INSIGHT

Position of Comfort—A Double-Edged Sword

Patients with a painful and inflamed elbow often hold their arm in about 70 to 90 degrees of elbow flexion. This so-called position of comfort reduces intra-capsular pressure and reduces pain on inflamed tissues. Although the flexed position improves comfort, extended periods of time in this flexed position significantly increase the chance of an elbow flexion contracture.

With the forearm supinated and elbow fully extended, it should be evident that the forearm projects laterally about 15 to 20 degrees relative to the humerus. This natural outward angulation of the forearm within the frontal plane is called *normal cubitus valgus* (Figure 5-9); **valgus** literally means to "bend outward." The natural cubitus valgus orientation is also called the *carrying angle* because of its apparent function of keeping a carried object away from the body. Trauma to the elbow can alter the normal valgus angle, resulting in either **excessive cubitus valgus** (see Figure 5-9, B) or **cubitus varus** (see Figure 5-9, C).

Supporting Structures of the Elbow Joint

The following structures are illustrated in Figure 5-10:

- *Articular Capsule*: A thin, expansive band of connective tissue that encloses three different articulations: the humeroulnar joint, the humeroradial joint, and the proximal radioulnar joint
- *Medial Collateral Ligament*: Contains fibers that attach proximally to the medial epicondyle and distally to the medial aspects of the coronoid and olecranon processes; provides stability by primarily resisting cubitus valgus–producing forces
- *Lateral Collateral Ligament*: Originates on the lateral epicondyle and ultimately attaches to the lateral aspect of the proximal forearm. These fibers provide stability to the elbow by resisting cubitus varus–producing forces.

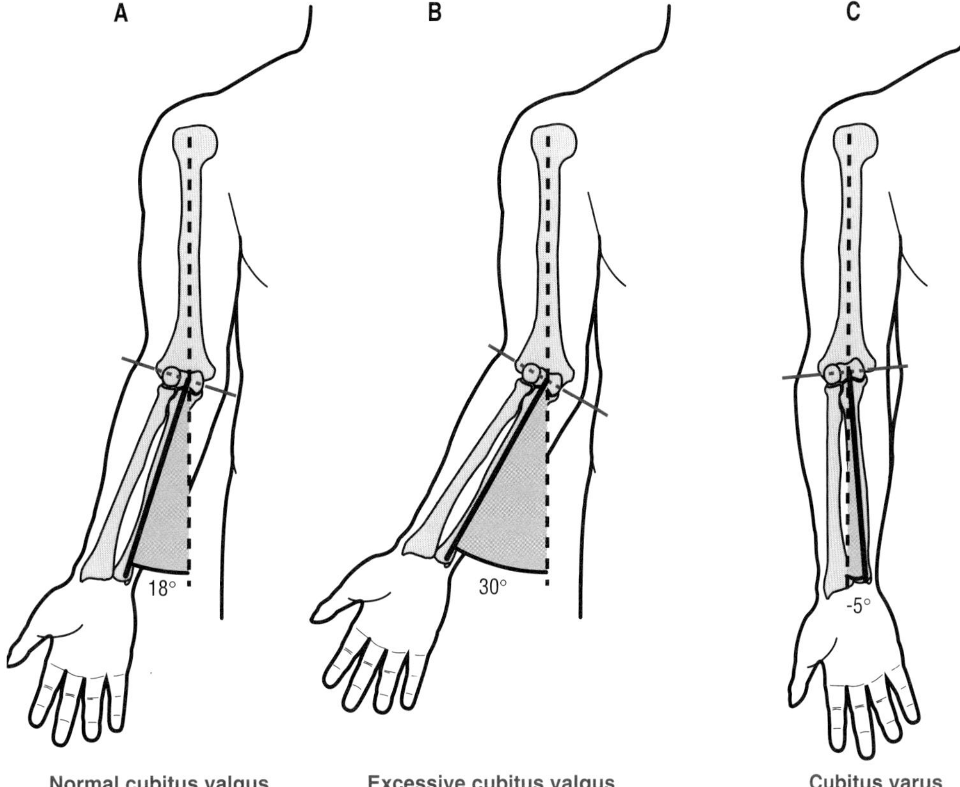

Figure 5-9 **A**, Normal cubitus valgus of the elbow. The radius and ulna deviate 18 degrees from the longitudinal axis of the humerus. The red line represents the medial-lateral axis of rotation of the elbow. **B**, Excessive cubitus valgus. **C**, Cubitus varus. (From Neumann DA: *Kinesiology of the musculoskeletal system: foundations for physical rehabilitation,* St Louis, 2002, Mosby, Figure 6-9.)

The primary function of the collateral ligaments is to limit excessive **varus** and valgus deformations of the elbow. The medial collateral ligament is most often injured during attempts to catch oneself from a fall (Figure 5-11). Because these ligaments also become taut at the extremes of flexion and extension, the extremes of these sagittal plane motions—if sufficiently forceful—can also damage the collateral ligaments.

Kinematics

From the anatomic position, elbow flexion and extension occur in the sagittal plane about a medial-lateral axis of rotation, which courses through both epicondyles. The range of motion at the elbow normally spans from 5 degrees beyond extension to 145 degrees of flexion (Figure 5-12). Most typical activities of daily living, however, use a more limited 100-degree arc of motion, between 30 and 130 degrees of flexion. Excessive extension is normally limited by the bony articulation between the olecranon and the olecranon fossa.

The elbow can be flexed and extended while the forearm is free, such as when performing a biceps curl, or fixed, such as performing a push-up. Although both open and closed chained functions are important, unless stated otherwise, this chapter describes open-chain motions. In either case, restricted mobility of the elbow can greatly decrease a person's functional abilities.

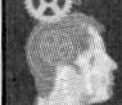

Consider this...

Assessing a Joint's End Feel

Clinicians must be able to describe the feel of a joint as it reaches its maximal range of motion. The term **end feel** has evolved for this purpose. Compare the end feel of full elbow extension versus full elbow flexion. Full extension results in an abrupt stop or bony end feel as the olecranon runs into the bony floor of the olecranon fossa. Full flexion, in contrast, results in a springy or soft end feel because of the soft tissue approximation of the forearm with the elbow flexor muscles and other soft tissues.

Clinicians with an awareness of the normal end feel of a joint can better determine the reason for the joint's lack of motion (or excessive motion) and can therefore implement more effective treatments to address the underlying problem.

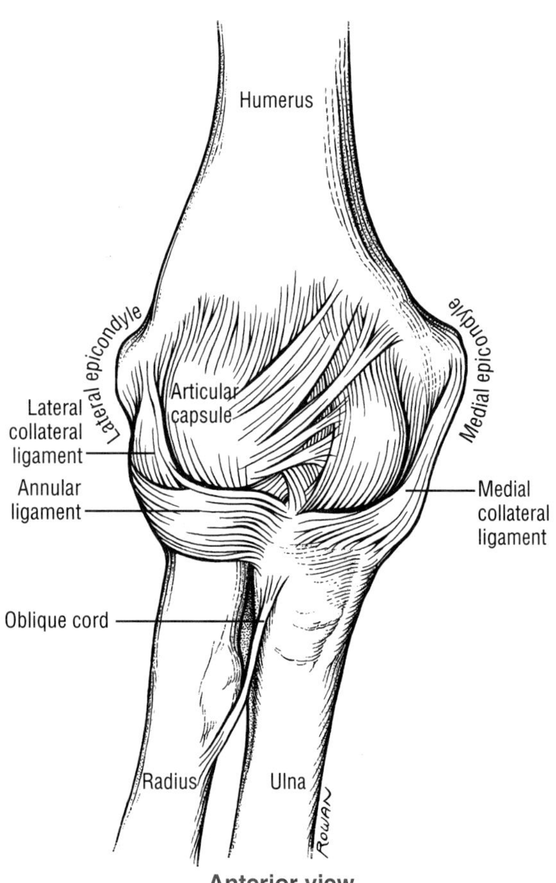

Figure 5-10 An anterior view of the right elbow showing the capsule and collateral ligaments. (From Neumann DA: *Kinesiology of the musculoskeletal system: foundations for physical rehabilitation*, St Louis, 2002, Mosby, Figure 6-10.)

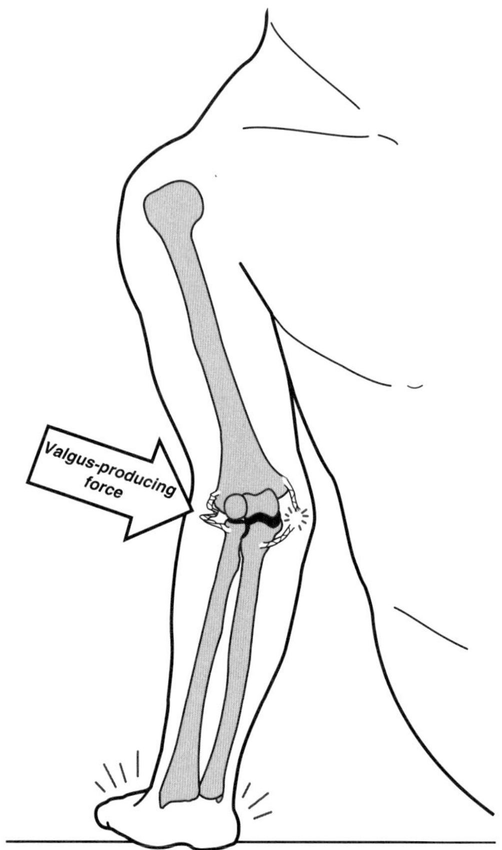

Figure 5-11 Attempts at catching oneself from a fall may induce a severe valgus-producing force that over-stretches or ruptures the medial collateral ligament. (From Neumann DA: *Kinesiology of the musculoskeletal system: foundations for physical rehabilitation*, St Louis, 2002, Mosby, Figure 6-22.)

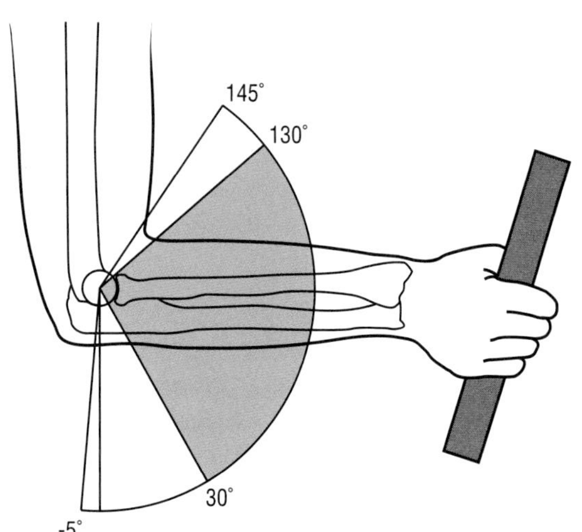

Figure 5-12 Normal range of motion at the elbow allows an arc of motion from 5 degrees of hyperextension to 145 degrees of flexion. The red area signifies the "functional arc" from 30 to 130 degrees of flexion. (Modified from Morrey BF, Bryan RS, Dobyns JH et al: Total elbow arthroplasty: a five-year experience at the Mayo Clinic, *J Bone Joint Surg Am* 63[7]:1050-1063, 1981.)

Arthrology of the Forearm

General Features

The forearm is composed of the proximal and distal radioulnar joints (see Figure 5-1). As the names imply, these joints are located at the proximal and distal ends of the forearm. Pronation and supination occur as a result of motion at each of these two joints. As shown in Figure 5-13, *A*, in full supination, the radius and ulna lie parallel to one another. However, in full pronation the radius crosses over the ulna (Figure 5-13, *B*). As emphasized in subsequent sections of this chapter, pronation and supination involve the radius rotating around a relatively fixed ulna. Although pronation and supination are typically used to describe motions or positions of the hand, these motions occur at the forearm. However, it is useful to observe this motion by noting the position of the hand relative to the humerus. The firm articulation between the distal radius and carpal bones (at the wrist) requires that the hand follows the rotation of the radius; the ulna typically remains relatively stationary because of its firm attachment at the humeroulnar joint.

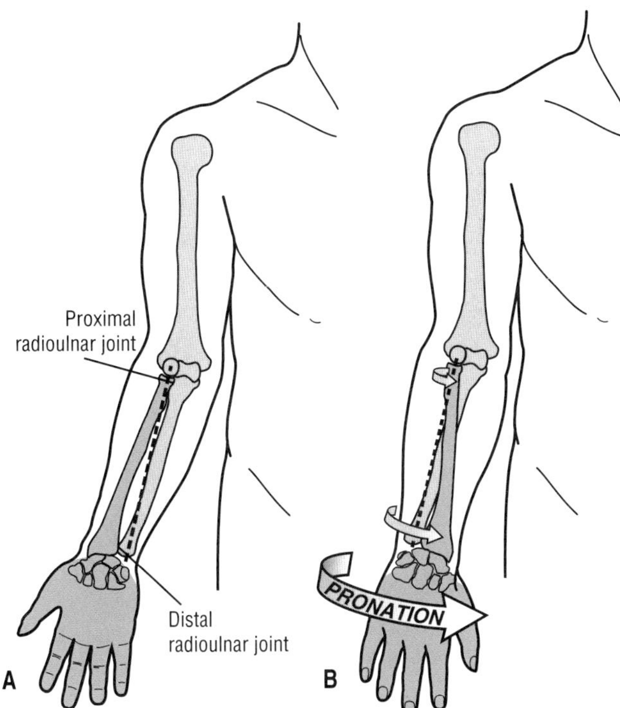

Figure 5-13 Anterior view of the right forearm. **A**, In full supination, the radius (*red*) and ulna (*gray*) are parallel. **B**, In full pronation, the radius is crossed over the ulna. The dotted line signifies the axis of rotation that extends from the radial head to the ulnar head. Note how the hand follows the radius. (From Neumann DA: *Kinesiology of the musculoskeletal system: foundations for physical rehabilitation*, St Louis, 2002, Mosby, Figure 6-24.)

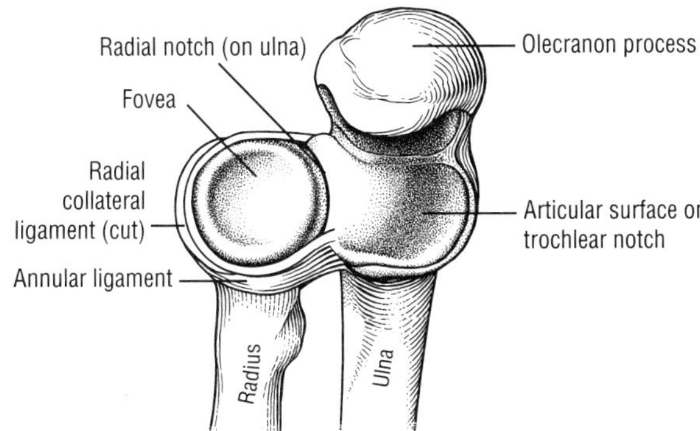

Figure 5-14 The right proximal radioulnar joint as viewed from above. Note how the radius is held against the radial notch of the ulna by the annular ligament. (From Neumann DA: *Kinesiology of the musculoskeletal system: foundations for physical rehabilitation*, St Louis, 2002, Mosby, Figure 6-25, *A*.)

Supporting Structures of the Proximal and Distal Radioulnar Joints

- *Annular Ligament*: A thick circular band of connective tissue that wraps around the radial head and attaches to either side of the radial notch of the ulna (Figures 5-10 and 5-14). This ring-like structure holds the radial head firmly against the ulna, allowing it to spin freely during supination and pronation.
- *Distal Radioulnar Joint Capsule*: Reinforced by palmar and dorsal capsular ligaments; this structure provides stability to the distal radioulnar joint
- *Interosseous Membrane* (see Figure 5-6): Helps bind the radius to the ulna; serves as a site for muscular attachments, and as a mechanism to transmit forces proximally through the forearm

Kinematics

Supination occurs in many functional activities that require the palm to be turned up, such as in feeding, washing your face, or holding a bowl of soup. Pronation, in contrast, is involved with activities such as grabbing an object from a table or pushing up from a chair, which require the palm to be turned down.

Supination and pronation occur as the radius rotates around an axis of rotation that travels from the radial head to the ulnar head (see Figure 5-13). The 0-degree or neutral position of the forearm is the thumb-up position (Figure 5-16). From this position, normally 85 degrees of supination and 75 degrees of pronation occur. People who lack full range of motion of these movements often compensate by internally or externally rotating the shoulder, so clinicians must be aware of this possible substitution when testing the range of motion of the forearm.

> **Consider this...**
>
> **Pronation and Supination—Don't Be Fooled!**
>
> Active internal and external rotation at the shoulder is functionally linked with active pronation and supination of the forearm. Shoulder internal rotation often occurs with pronation, whereas shoulder external rotation is linked with supination. Combining these shoulder and forearm rotations allows the hand to rotate nearly 360 degrees in space, rather than the 170 to 180 degrees by pronation and supination alone. When clinically testing range of motion, care must be taken not to be fooled by the extra motion that may have originated from the shoulder. To prevent these substitutions, pronation and supination can be tested with the elbow flexed to 90 degrees and with the medial side of the humerus pressed against the side of the body. In this position, any undesired motion at the shoulder is easily detected.

Supination and pronation occur as a result of simultaneous motion at the proximal and distal radioulnar joint; a restriction at one joint will therefore result in limited motion at the other. With the humerus fixed and forearm free to move, the arthrokinematics of supination and

Clinical INSIGHT

"Pulled" Elbow Syndrome

Pulled elbow syndrome is the common name given when the radial head is traumatically pulled out of its "home" within the annular ligament. This is generally caused by a sharp pull on a person's wrist or radius. This occurs most often to small children because of their ligamentous laxity, undeveloped musculature, and likelihood of others pulling on their arms (see Figure 5-15).

Common scenarios associated with a pulled arm syndrome include the following:

- Arm being pulled sharply distally during dressing
- Being forcefully pulled up steps by one arm
- Holding the leash of a dog that suddenly darts after an object

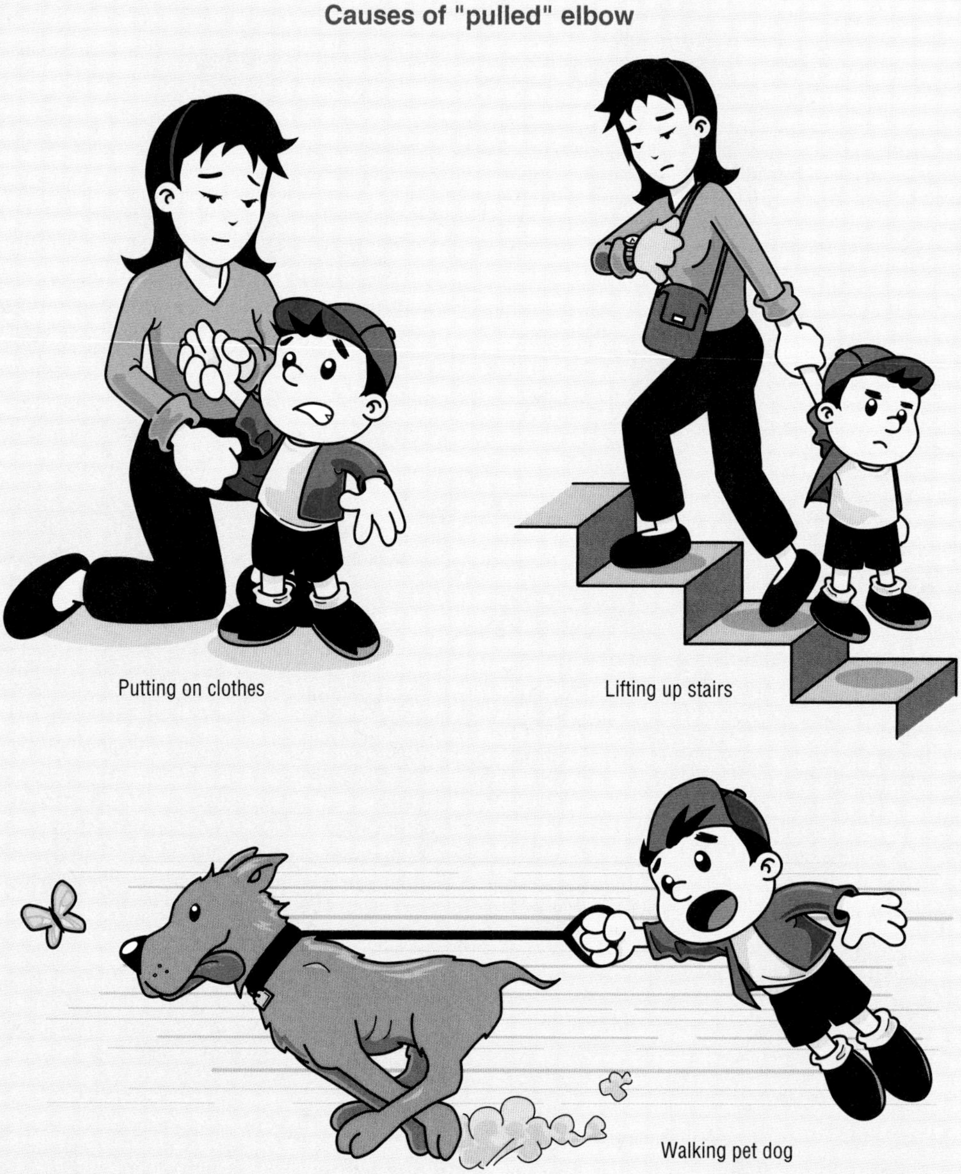

Figure 5-15 Three examples of causes of pulled elbow syndrome. (Redrawn from Letts RM: Dislocations of the child's elbow. In Morrey BF, editor: *The elbow and its disorders*, ed 3, Philadelphia, 2000, Saunders. With permission from the Mayo Foundation for Medical Education and Research.)

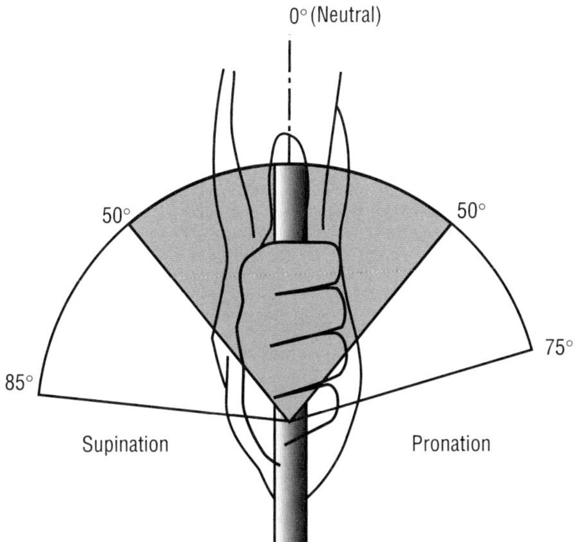

Figure 5-16 Ranges of motion for pronation and supination: 0 to 85 degrees of supination; 0 to 75 degrees of pronation. The 0-degree or neutral forearm position is shown with the thumb pointing up. The 100-degree functional arc is displayed in red. (Modified from Morrey BF, Bryan RS, Dobyns JH et al: Total elbow arthroplasty: a five-year experience at the Mayo Clinic, *J Bone Joint Surg Am* 63[7]:1050-1063, 1981.)

pronation are based on the following three premises (Figure 5-17):

1. Only the radius moves; the ulna stays essentially stationary.
2. The radial head spins in place, in the direction of the moving thumb.
3. The distal radius rolls and slides in the same direction relative to the ulnar head.

During supination, the radial head within the *proximal radioulnar joint* spins in the direction of the thumb within its "home" created by the annular ligament and the radial notch of the ulna (see Figure 5-17, *bottom right*). By necessity, the spinning head of the radius also makes contact with the capitulum of the humerus. At the *distal radioulnar joint*, the concave surface of the distal radius rolls and slides in the same direction across the stationary ulna (see Figure 5-17, *top right*).

The arthrokinematics of pronation are essentially the same as supination, except that they occur in reverse directions. In full pronation the shaft of the radius is rotated across the shaft of the ulna. This is a position of relative stability of the forearm region because the radius (and attached wrist) is braced against the ulna, which is firmly anchored to the humerus at the humero-ulnar joint.

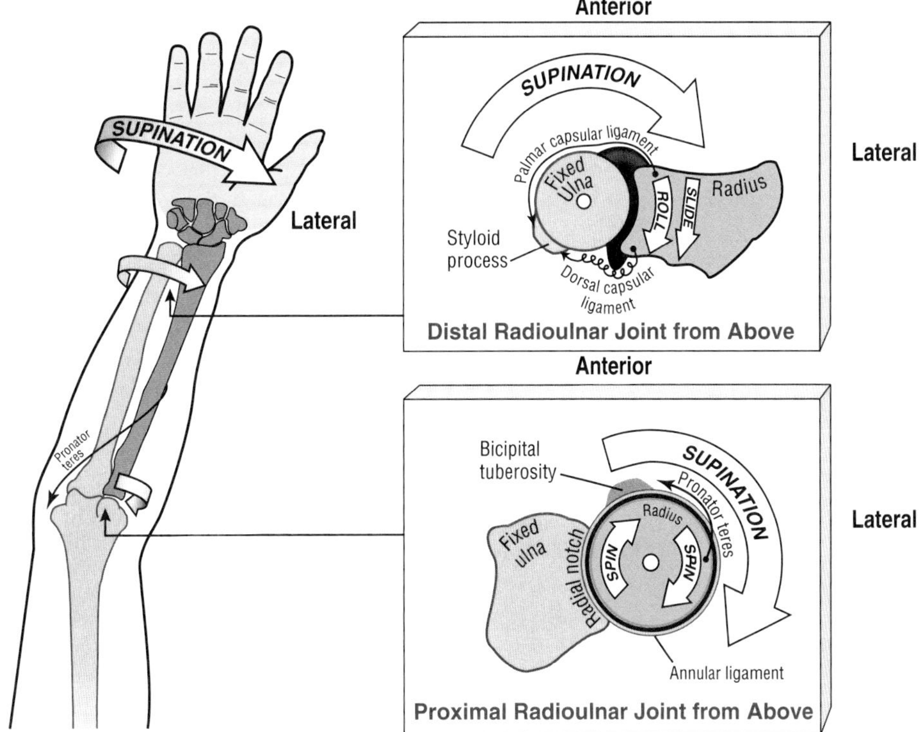

Figure 5-17 *Left,* Anterior aspect of the right forearm after completing full supination. Note the pronator teres muscle is pulled taut. *Top right,* Arthrokinematics of the distal radioulnar joint following full supination; note that the roll and slide occur in the same directions. *Bottom right,* Radial head spinning about its own axis as the forearm is fully supinated; this figure is a cross section, to be viewed as if looking down the forearm. *Wavy lines,* Slackened structures; *thin lines,* stretched (taut) structures. (From Neumann DA: *Kinesiology of the musculoskeletal system: foundations for physical rehabilitation,* St Louis, 2002, Mosby, Figure 6-29.)

TABLE 5-1 SUMMARY OF JOINTS OF ELBOW AND FOREARM

Joint	Motions Allowed	Normal Range of Motion	Axis of Rotation	Comments
Humeroulnar	Flexion and extension	5 degrees of hyperextension to 145 degrees of flexion	Medial-lateral through the trochlea	Primary hinge-like structure of the elbow
Humeroradial	Flexion and extension		Medial-lateral through the capitulum	The shared joint: functional link between the elbow and forearm
Proximal radioulnar	Pronation and supination	75 degrees of pronation to 85 degrees of supination	Radial head to the ulnar head	Radial head palpable during pronation and supination
Distal radioulnar	Pronation and supination		Radial head to the ulnar head	Full pronation exposes the ulnar head as a bump on the dorsal aspect of the distal forearm

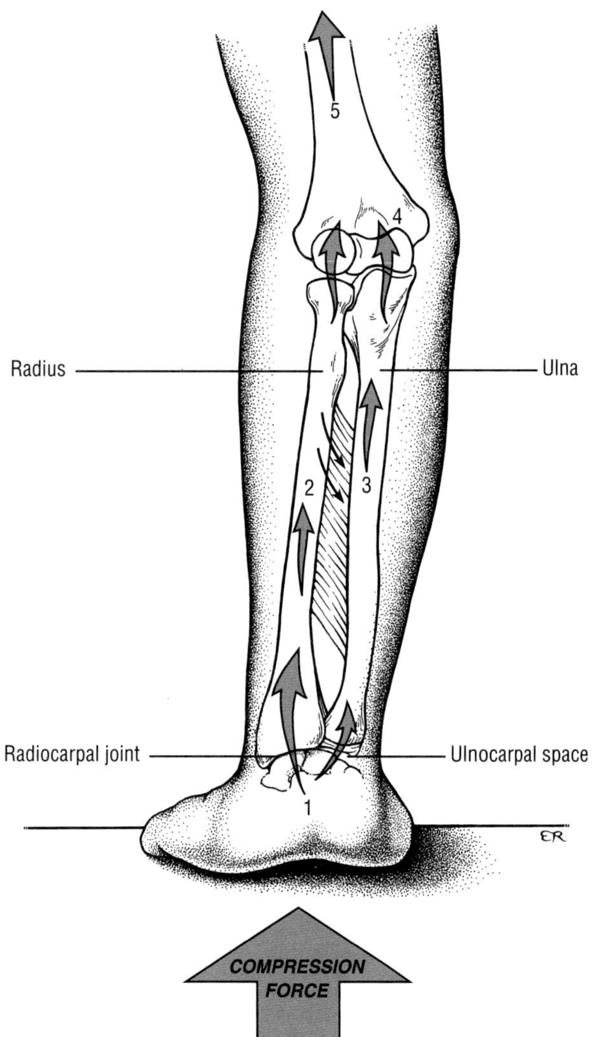

Figure 5-18 A compression force through the hand is transmitted through the wrist *(1)* at the radiocarpal joint and transmitted primarily through the radius *(2)*. This force stretches the interosseous membrane and transfers a part of the compression force to the ulna *(3)*. This allows the force to be shared more equally through the humeroulnar joint and the humeroradial joint *(4)*. The compression forces that cross the elbow are finally directed toward the shoulder *(5)*. (From Neumann DA: *Kinesiology of the musculoskeletal system: foundations for physical rehabilitation*, St Louis, 2002, Mosby, Figure 6-20.)

Table 5-1 summarizes the joints of the elbow and forearm.

Force Transmission through the Interosseous Membrane

The interosseous membrane of the forearm helps attach the radius with the ulna. Interestingly, most of the fibers of the interosseous membrane travel in an oblique fashion—distally and medially (ulnarly) from the radius (Figure 5-18). As explained, this unique fiber direction helps transmit compressive forces from the hand to the upper arm.

An action such as a push-up or pushing down on a walker, for example, creates a compressive force that first passes through the hand to the wrist, 80% of which is transmitted directly through the radius at the radiocarpal joint (see Figure 5-18, *1*). The proximal-directed force passes up the radius and, because of the specific angulation of the interosseous membrane, is transferred partly to the ulna (see Figure 5-18, *2*, *3*). As a result, the compressive force that enters the distal forearm at the wrist and radius exits the proximal forearm through both humeroulnar and humeroradial joints (see Figure 5-18, *4*) and is transferred up to the shoulder (see Figure 5-18, *5*).

The direction and alignment of the interosseous membrane helps distribute the compression force more evenly across both joints of the elbow. If the interosseous membrane were oriented 90 degrees to its actual orientation, a compressive force directed up through the radius would slacken (rather than tense) the membrane. A slackened or loose membrane—like a loose rope—cannot transmit a pull. This load distribution mechanism, based on the

Clinical **INSIGHT**

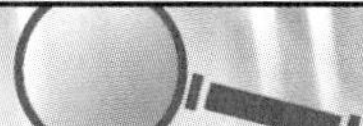

The Colles' Fracture

One of the most frequent fractures in the body involves the distal end of the radius. This injury, known as a **Colles' fracture** (named after orthopedic surgeon Abraham Colles in 1814) (Figure 5-19) often occurs while attempting to catch oneself from a fall with an outstretched hand. During the attempted catch, the weight of the body is transmitted through the hand and wrist. As mentioned earlier, most of this force is transmitted primarily *through the radius.* A fracture results when the force of the impact exceeds the strength of the distal radius. The fact that the radius is the primary force acceptor explains why the radius, and not the ulna, is fractured much more frequently during this type of accident.

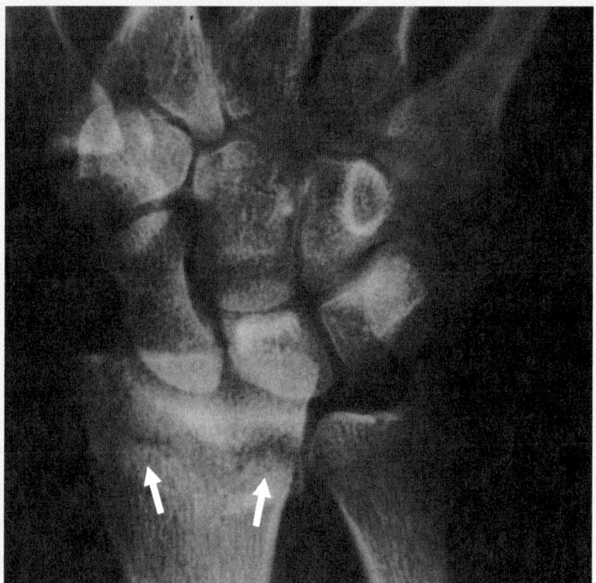

Figure 5-19 Posterior-anterior view of a Colles' fracture of the distal radius. (From Grainger R, Allison D, Dixon A: *Grainger & Allison's diagnostic radiology: a textbook of medical imaging,* ed 4, Edinburgh, 2002, Churchill Livingstone, Figure 78-49, *B.*)

actual fiber direction of the interosseous membrane, is certainly at work when pushing open a heavy door or as a patient bears weight through the upper extremities when using a walker.

Muscles of the Elbow and Forearm Complex

Innervation of Muscles

The following is the general theme of the innervation of the elbow and forearm muscles. The musculocutaneous nerve (Figure 5-20) supplies most of the elbow flexors, except the brachioradialis and pronator teres. The radial nerve (Figure 5-21) supplies all the muscles that extend the elbow, and the median nerve (Figure 5-22) supplies all the pronators of the forearm.

Interestingly, the elbow flexor muscles are innervated by three different nerves. This may reflect the importance of performing hand-to-mouth activities, especially feeding. Total paralysis of *all* elbow flexor muscles requires damage to all three nerves; fortunately a relatively unlikely event. In contrast, total paralysis of the elbow extensor muscles (the triceps) can occur by damage to the radial nerve only.

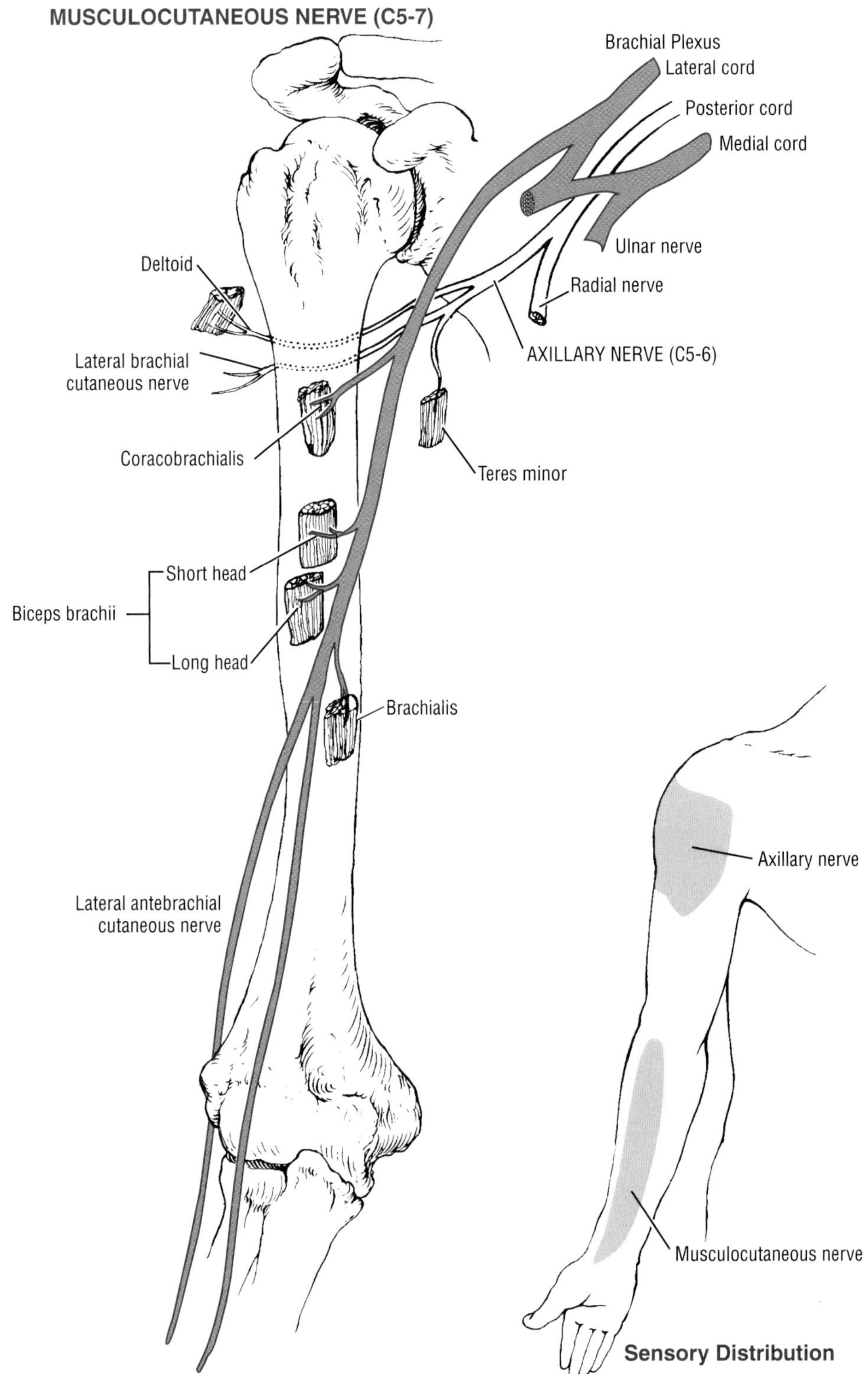

Figure 5-20 The path of the right musculocutaneous nerve innervating the coracobrachialis, biceps brachii, and brachialis. Sensory distribution is shown on the right. (Modified from Waxman S: *Correlative neuroanatomy*, ed 24, New York, 2000, Lange Medical Books/McGraw-Hill.)

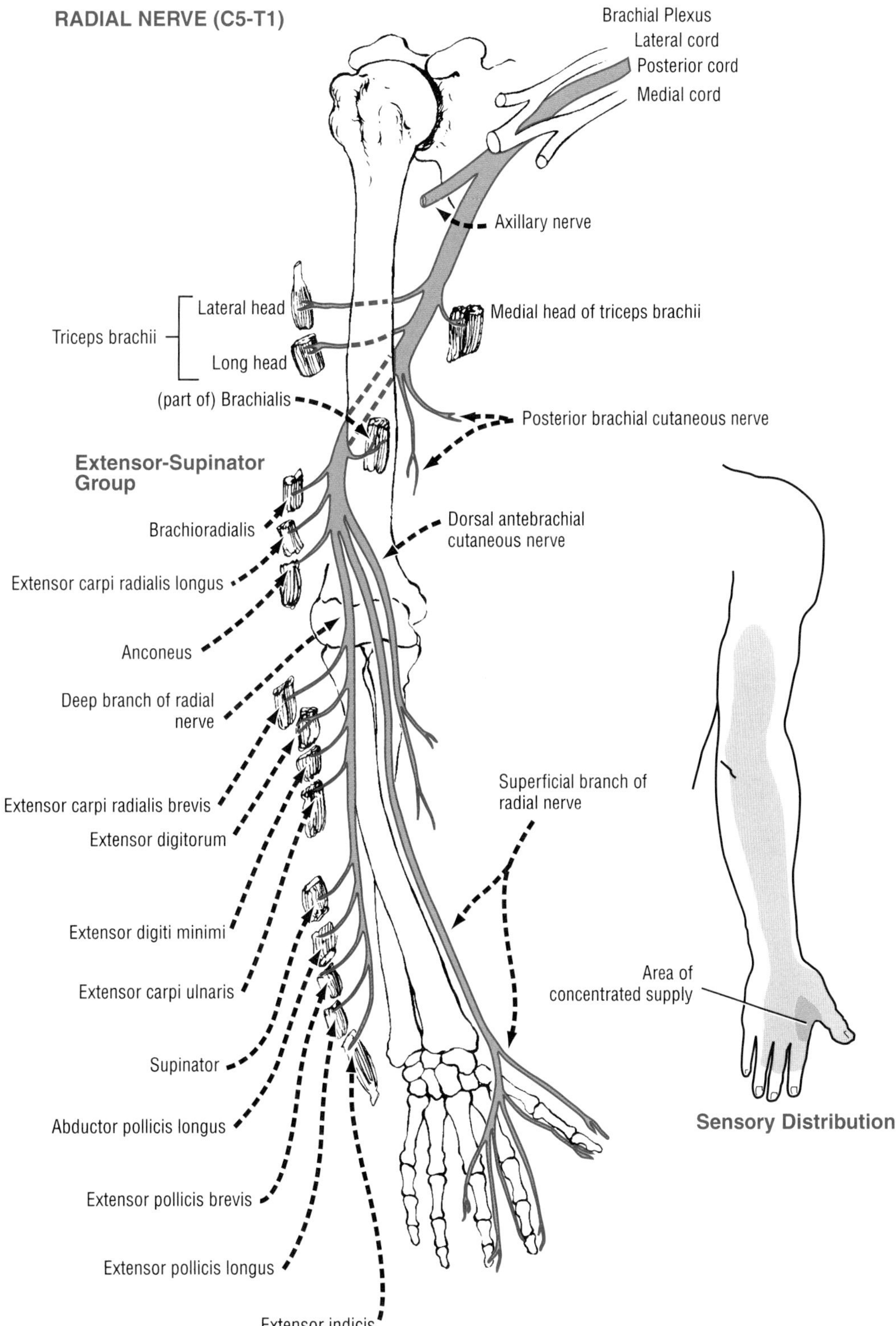

Figure 5-21 The path of the right radial nerve wraps around the posterior humerus to emerge on the lateral aspect of the forearm. The nerve innervates most of the extensors of the elbow, forearm, wrist, and digits. Sensory distribution is shown on the right. (Modified from Waxman S: *Correlative neuroanatomy*, ed 24, New York, 2000, Lange Medical Books/McGraw-Hill.)

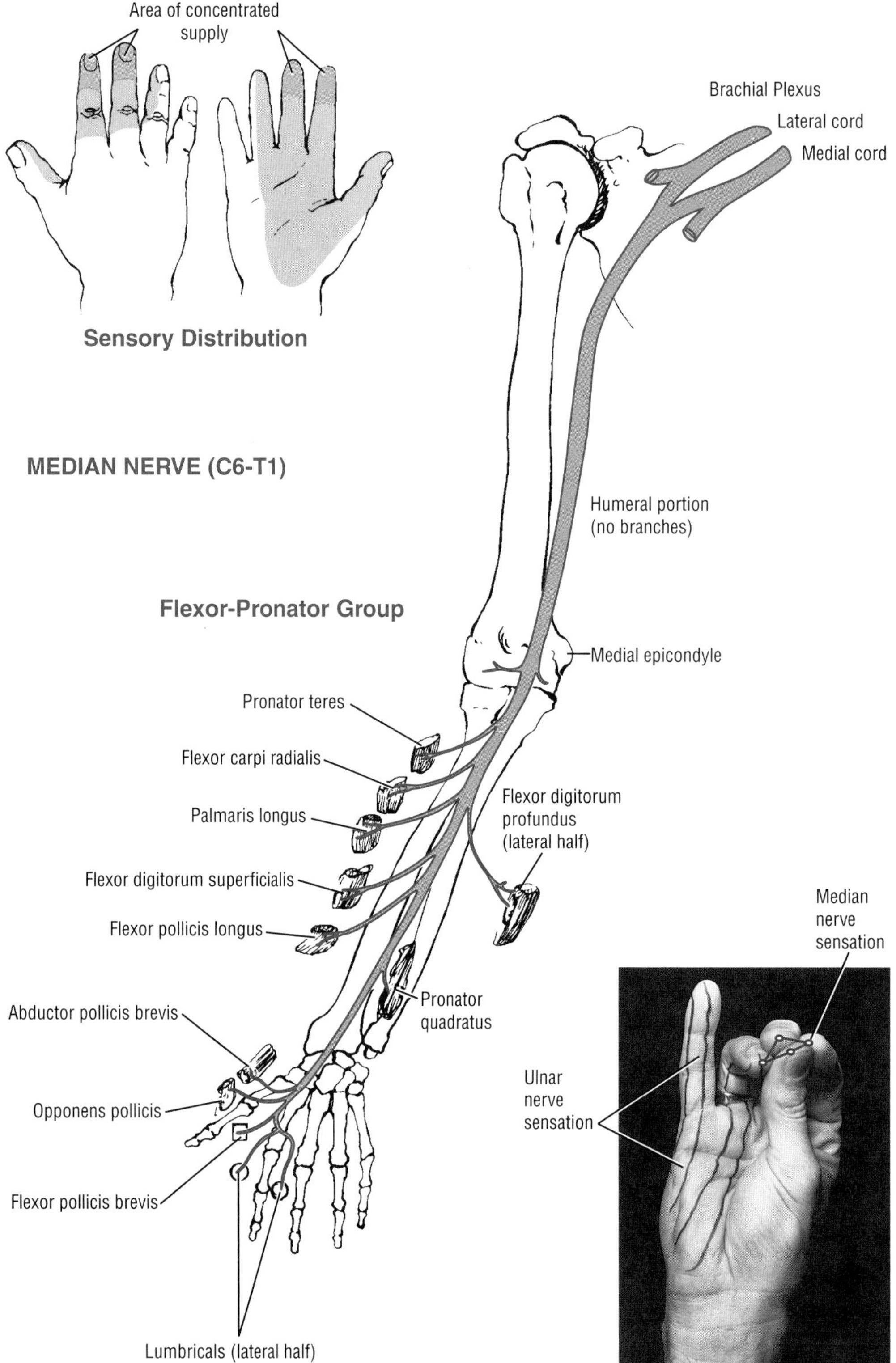

Figure 5-22 The path of the right median nerve innervating the pronators, most wrist flexors, long (extrinsic) flexors of the digits (except the flexor digitorum profundus to the ring and little finger), most of the intrinsic muscles of the thumb, and the two lateral lumbricals. The sensory distribution of the median nerve covers most of the palmar aspect of the thumb and digits 2 to 4; this figure illustrates the importance of the median nerve in "pinch sensation." (Modified from Waxman S: *Correlative neuroanatomy*, ed 24, New York, 2000, Lange Medical Books/McGraw-Hill.)

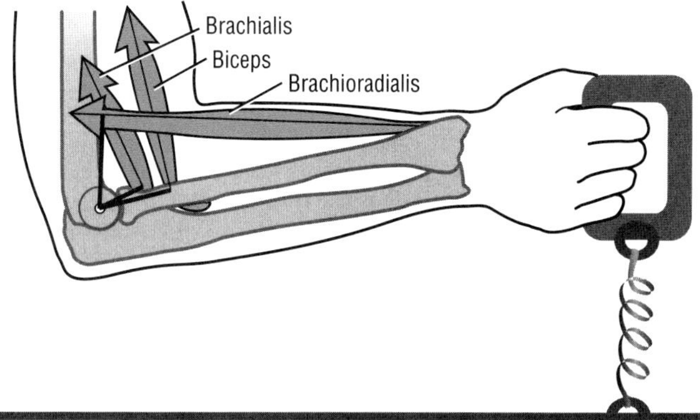

Figure 5-23 A lateral view of the right elbow showing the line of force of the three primary elbow flexors. The black lines represent the internal moment arm of each muscle. (From Neumann DA: *Kinesiology of the musculoskeletal system: foundations for physical rehabilitation*, St Louis, 2002, Mosby, Figure 6-37.)

Elbow Flexors

The prime movers of elbow flexion are the biceps brachii, the brachialis, and the brachioradialis. These muscles have a line of force that passes anterior to the elbow's axis of rotation (Figure 5-23). The pronator teres is considered a secondary elbow flexor. Three of the four flexors also have the potential to pronate *or* supinate the forearm. Note that any elbow flexor muscle that attaches distally to the radius (versus the ulna) will also pronate or supinate the forearm. These forearm functions bestow a unique action on each muscle—an important consideration when testing the strength or attempting to maximally stretch a specific elbow flexor muscle.

Primary Elbow Flexors

- Biceps brachii
- Brachialis
- Brachioradialis

Secondary Elbow Flexor

- Pronator teres

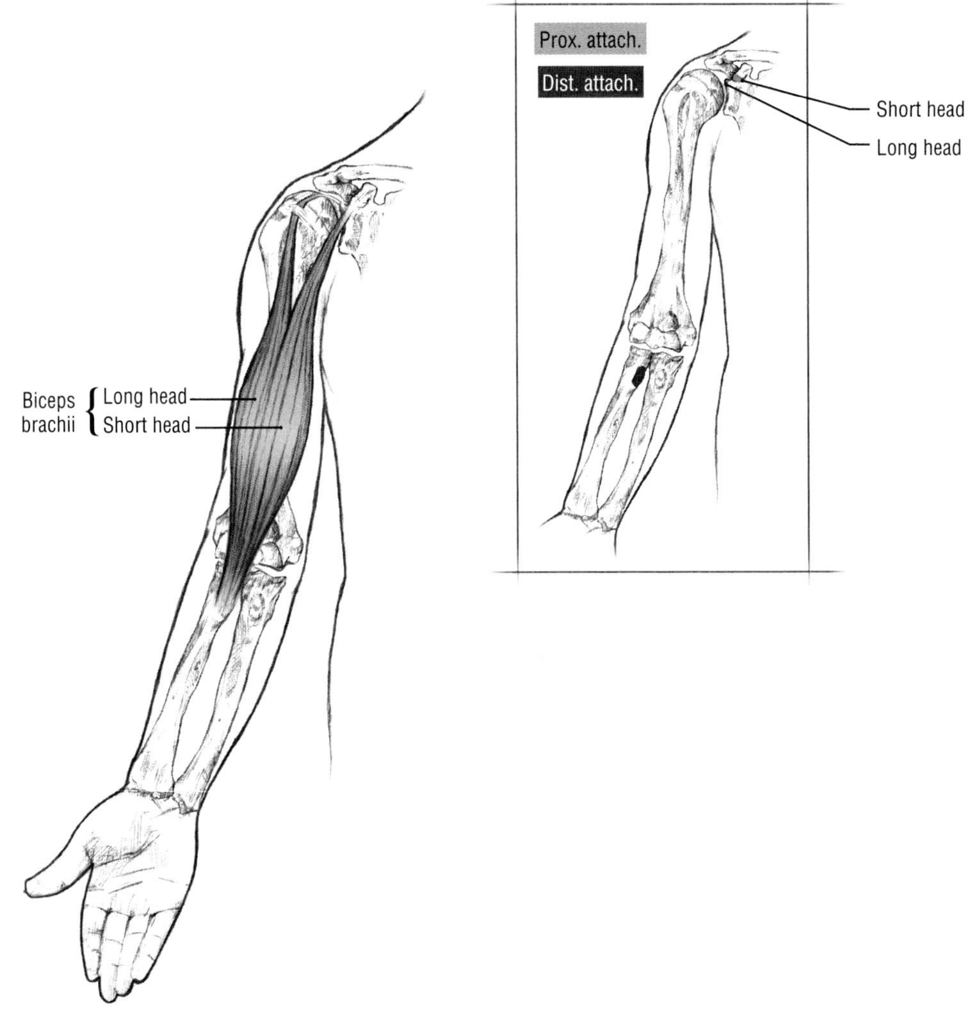

Biceps Brachii

Proximal Attachment:
- Long head: supraglenoid tubercle of the scapula
- Short head: coracoid process of the scapula

Distal Attachment: Bicipital tuberosity of the radius

Innervation: Musculocutaneous nerve

Actions:
- Elbow flexion
- Forearm supination
- Shoulder flexion

Comments: The combined action of elbow flexion and forearm supination provided by the biceps brachii is important in bringing the palm of the hand toward the face such as when eating.

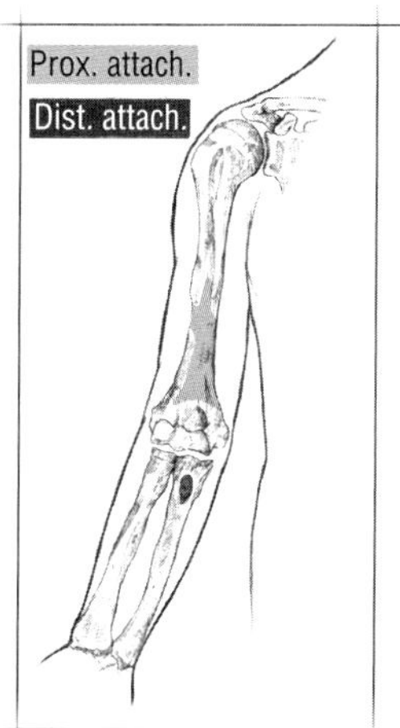

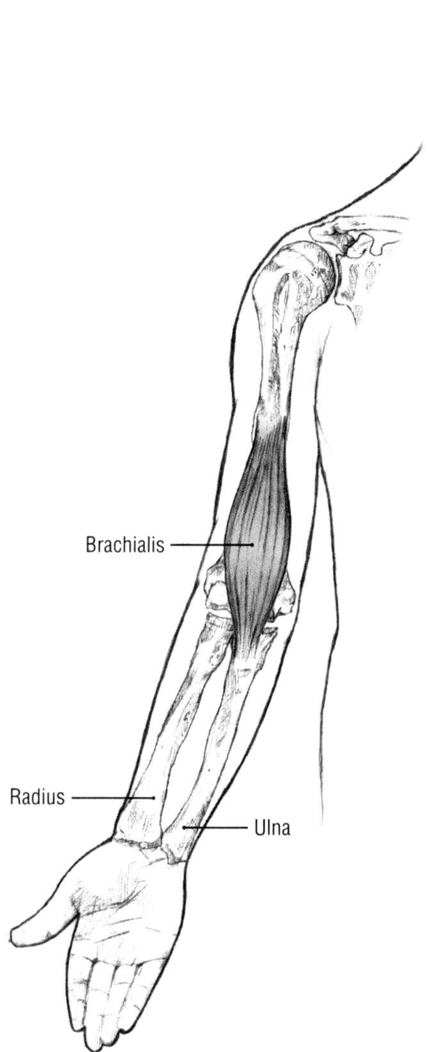

Brachialis

Proximal Attachment: Anterior aspect of the distal humerus

Distal Attachment: Coronoid process of the ulna

Innervation: Musculocutaneous nerve

Action: Elbow flexion

Comments: This muscle is often referred to as the "workhorse" of elbow flexion partially because it has a larger cross-sectional area than its competitor, the biceps, but also because of its distal attachment. By attaching distally to the ulna (and not the radius like the biceps), a pronated or supinated position of the forearm has no influence on the muscle's length or force-producing capability. Furthermore, because its only potential action is elbow flexion, no other stabilizing muscles are necessary to prevent unwanted motion at the forearm, such as is the case when other elbow flexors like the biceps are activated. This brachialis is therefore a favorite choice of the nervous system for virtually any elbow flexion activity, regardless of associated pronation or supination motions.

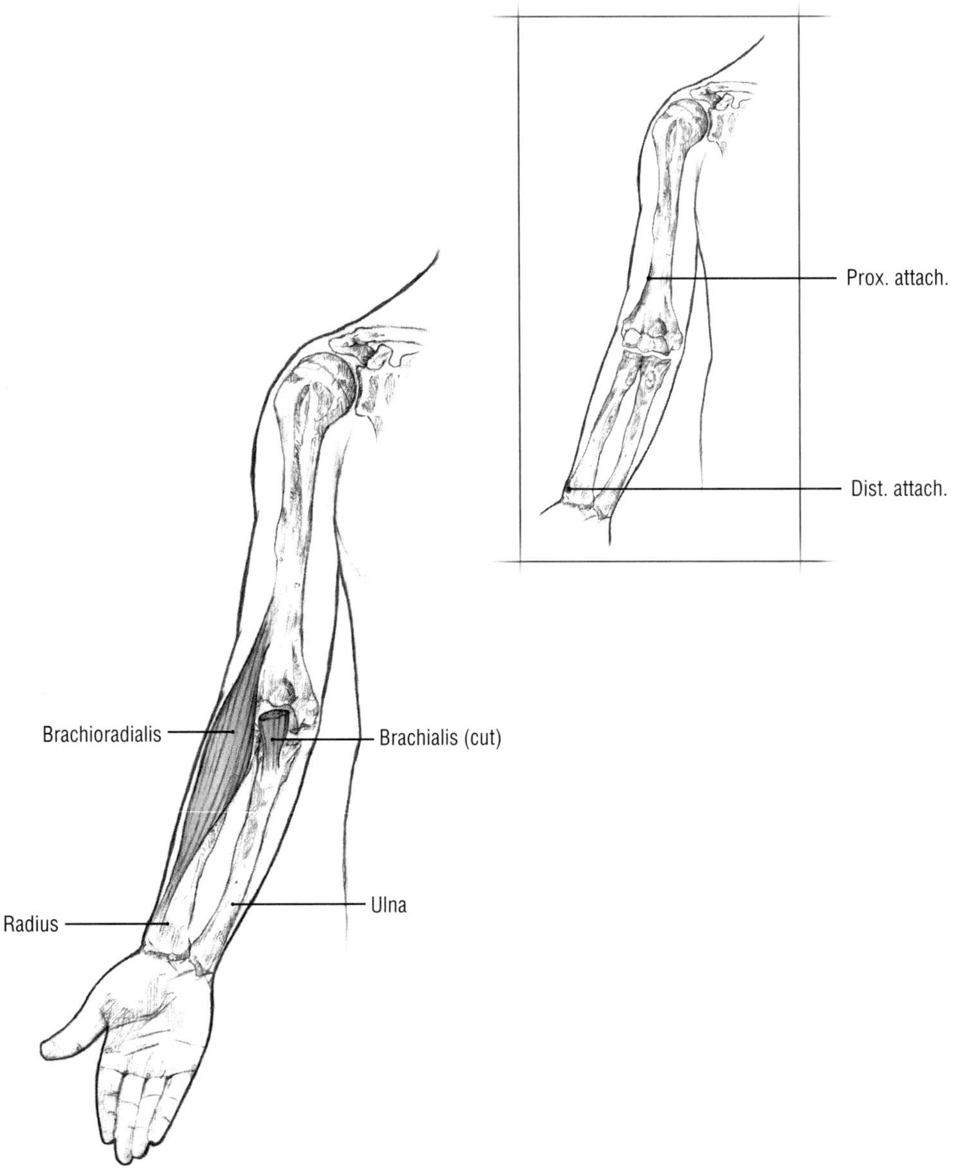

Brachioradialis

Proximal Attachment: Lateral supracondylar ridge of the humerus

Distal Attachment: Near the styloid process of the distal radius

Innervation: Radial nerve

Actions:
- Elbow flexion
- Pronating or supinating the forearm to the neutral (thumb-up position)

Comments: Contraction of the brachioradialis causes the elbow to flex and the forearm to simultaneously rotate to its neutral position (i.e., a position midway between full pronation and supination). The neutral forearm position greatly enhances the flexion leverage of the brachioradialis, thereby amplifying the flexion torque potential of this muscle. Engineers have used this force advantage by positioning handles so that lifting occurs in a position of forearm neutral.

Clinical **INSIGHT**

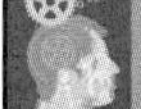

When the Biceps Are Unopposed...

Persons with C5 or C6 quadriplegia, for example, have functioning biceps (elbow flexors) but lack functioning triceps (elbow extensors). Because the biceps are unopposed (lack a functioning antagonist), they are likely to become over-shortened and tight, resulting in a fixed or contracted position of elbow flexion and supination. In order to maximally stretch the biceps, the arm should be placed in a position opposite *all* of its actions: elbow extension, forearm pronation, and shoulder extension.

Important clinical principles include the following:

- A muscle without a functioning antagonist is at high risk for developing a contracture.
- When a muscle becomes tight, over-shortened, or contracted, it will create a posture that reflects *all* of its potential actions.
- To maximally stretch a muscle, it must be placed in a position opposite *all* of its actions.

especially at high power levels. Because the biceps is also a shoulder flexor, a shoulder extensor muscle like the posterior deltoid must also become active to neutralize unwanted shoulder flexion.

Consider this...

Why Multi-Articular Muscles Need Help from Stabilizer Muscles

Simply stated, a contracting muscle attempts to draw its proximal and distal attachments together, thereby potentially expressing *all* of its actions. How then, can a contracting multi-articular muscle express only one action while seeming to ignore others? Unwanted or unexpressed actions of a muscle must be cancelled or offset by opposing muscles or outside forces, not by the muscle itself. Muscles that cancel a given action of another muscle are often referred to as *stabilizers*. Weakness in stabilizer muscles can therefore dramatically influence the expression of a multi-articular muscle.

FUNCTIONAL CONSIDERATIONS

Biceps versus Brachialis

The combined efforts of all the elbow flexors can create large amounts of elbow flexion torque, evident as a person performs a pull-up, for example. However, most everyday activities do not require a maximal level of torque; during ordinary activities, the nervous system selects just the right muscle and optimal amount of force for the specific task.

The brachialis is the muscle of choice for essentially all elbow flexion activities, whether performed against a small or large resistance, or with the forearm held pronated, neutral, or fully supinated. If the flexion movement requires a strong supination component, the nervous system would find it necessary to also recruit the biceps muscle, based on its attachment to the radius. A simple exercise will show this point. While letting gravity keep your forearm fully pronated, slowly and repeatedly flex your elbow. Palpation of your upper arm during this movement should quickly verify that your biceps muscle is *not* active. If it were, your forearm would supinate. The most active muscle is your deeper brachialis—a muscle that cannot pronate or supinate. Next, while continuing to palpate your upper arm as you flex and extend your elbow, quickly and forcefully supinate your forearm. The immediate increase in tension in your biceps while supinating reflects the strong activation of this muscle. The nervous system recruits the biceps muscle because its combined actions exactly match the task at hand. The brachialis likely remains relentlessly active during both scenarios. Realize that a "price" must be paid when the nervous system recruits a multi-articular muscle such as the biceps,

Biceps as a Multi-Articular Muscle: A Closer Look

As stated, the biceps crosses the shoulder, elbow, and forearm joints and is therefore often referred to as being multiarticular. Many movements of the upper extremity can influence the length at which the biceps is activated. Consider the natural motion of pulling, which combines elbow flexion with shoulder extension. Such a motion occurs while attempting to start a lawnmower with a pull cord. By crossing the shoulder and elbow, the biceps, in effect, contracts (and shortens) across the elbow as it simultaneously lengthens across the shoulder. By contracting at one end and lengthening at the other, the muscle actually shortens a small net distance. This offers the physiologic advantage based on the muscle's length-tension relationship.

A muscle is considered more **actively efficient** when a given effort level produces a greater amount of force. This occurs when (1) a muscle contracts, and the muscle fibers shorten a relatively small amount per instant in time; and (2) a muscle remains at a nearly optimal length (to create contractile force) throughout an active movement.

These two principles of active efficiency are favored for the biceps during the pulling motion described earlier. Furthermore, considering that the shoulder extensors are overpowering the shoulder flexion potential of the biceps, the torque created by the biceps is focused solely on elbow flexion and forearm supination—two primary actions involved in effectively pulling the cord of the lawnmower.

Clinical INSIGHT

Reverse Action of the Elbow Flexors

Contraction of the elbow flexor muscles is typically performed to bring the forearm closer to the humerus such as a biceps curl or bringing a bottle of water toward the mouth. However, the elbow flexors can also be used in a closed-chain perspective by bringing the upper arm closer to the forearm. A clinical example of this is shown in Figure 5-24, which depicts a person with C6 quadriplegia using his elbow flexors in *reverse action* to come to a sitting position. Importantly, persons with C6 quadriplegia have functioning elbow flexors but paralysis of triceps or trunk musculature. Without functioning elbow extensors, an independent transition from supine to sitting can be difficult. Many individuals with this impairment will equip their beds with hooks or loops, similar to the one shown in Figure 5-24. This allows the forearm to be fixed so that a contraction of the elbow flexors pulls the upper arm (and therefore the trunk) toward the forearm, assisting the individual to a sitting position.

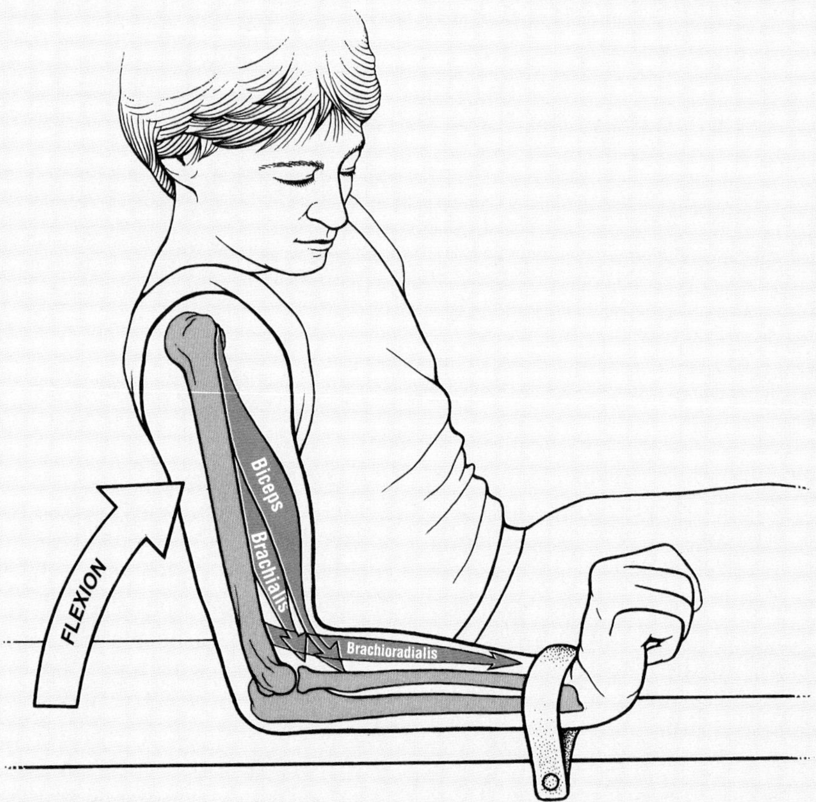

Figure 5-24 A person with C6 quadriplegia (lacking triceps function) is shown using his elbow flexors in reverse to come to a sitting position. With the wrist fixed to the mat via a bed loop, contraction of the elbow flexors brings the humerus toward the forearm, elevating the trunk toward a sitting position. (From Neumann DA: *Kinesiology of the musculoskeletal system: foundations for physical rehabilitation*, St Louis, 2002, Mosby, Figure 6-40.)

Elbow Extensors

The elbow extensor muscles are the triceps brachii and the anconeus. Because extension of the elbow is often associated with pushing motions, the elbow extensor muscles often work in concert with shoulder flexor muscles to achieve the desired action.

Primary Elbow Extensors

- Triceps brachii (all three heads)
- Anconeus

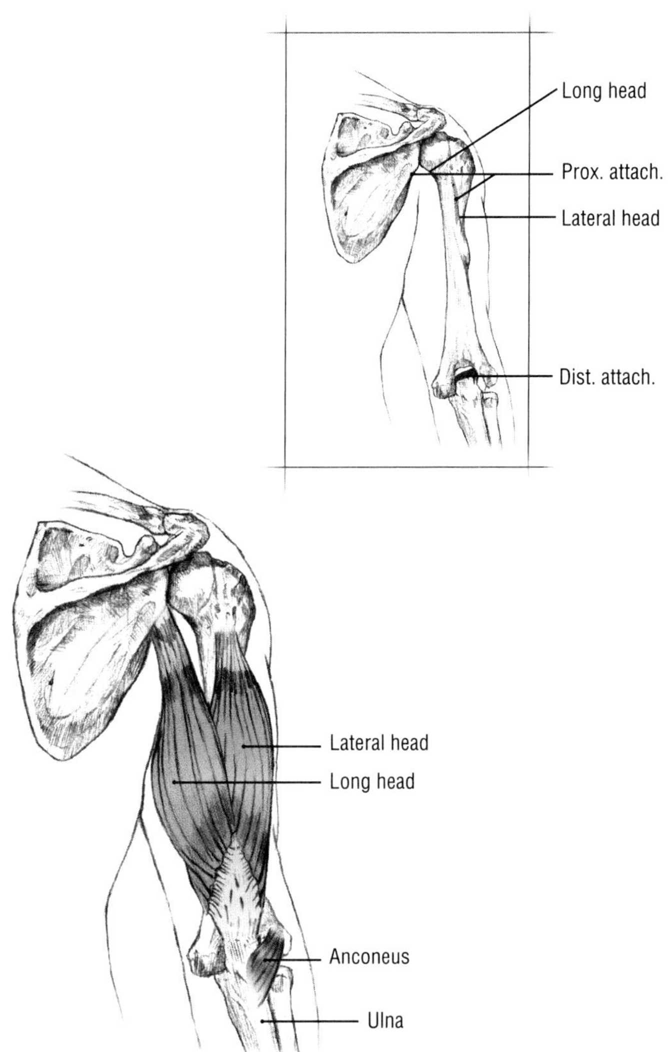

A posterior view of the right arm, showing the long and lateral heads of the triceps, as well as the anconeus.

Triceps Brachii

Proximal Attachment:
- Long head: infraglenoid tubercle of the scapula
- Lateral head: posterior aspect of the superior humerus, lateral to the radial groove
- Medial head (shown on next page): posterior aspect of the superior humerus, medial to the radial groove

Distal Attachment: Olecranon process of the ulna

Innervation: Radial nerve

Actions:
- Elbow extension
- Shoulder extension—long head only

Comments: All heads of the triceps brachii can extend the elbow. The long head, which crosses the shoulder, can also perform shoulder extension. The two-joint nature of this muscle is often used to help maintain an optimal length-tension relationship during pushing activities, such as when pushing open a heavy door.

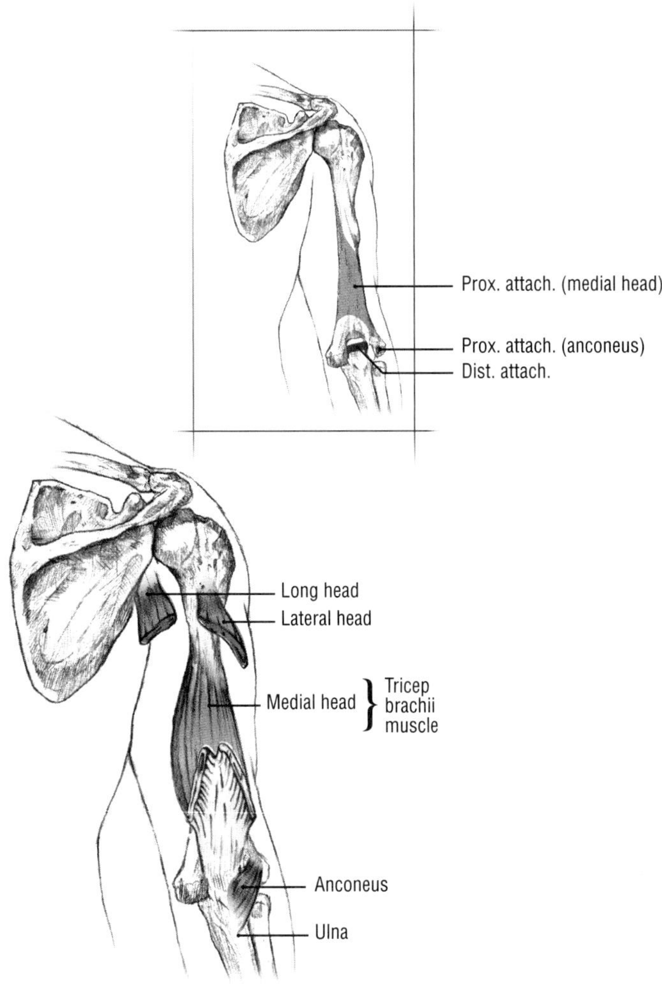

A posterior view of the right arm, showing the medial head of the triceps brachii. The long and lateral heads are partially removed to expose the deeper medial head.

Anconeus

Proximal Attachment:	Posterior aspect of the lateral epicondyle of the humerus
Distal Attachment:	Olecranon process of the ulna
Innervation:	Radial nerve
Action:	Elbow extension
Comments:	The anconeus is a small, triangular-shaped muscle. Its small size and moment arm limit its torque-producing potential; nevertheless it likely helps to stabilize the elbow in medial-lateral directions.

FUNCTIONAL CONSIDERATIONS

One- versus Two-Joint Muscles: Back Again

Functions that require large forces for extending the elbow usually demand strong activation of all three heads of the triceps and the anconeus. These functions include nearly any type of heavy pushing activity such as a push-up or pushing up from a seated position. Many daily functions, however, require relatively low elbow extension force, requiring the nervous system to activate only the one-joint extensor muscles. Extending your arm upward to grab a glass from the cupboard, for example, will likely activate only the lateral or medial heads of the triceps, and possibly the anconeus. These muscles are a logical choice because they are capable of extending just the elbow. Significant activation of the long head of the triceps would be unnecessary and metabolically inefficient because of the muscle's potential to also extend the shoulder. For this example, activating the large, two-joint, long head of the triceps would require more muscular energy than what is absolutely required because other neutralizer muscles would be necessary to cancel the unwanted shoulder extension torque produced by the long head of the triceps.

Clinical INSIGHT

Using Shoulder Muscles to Substitute for Triceps Paralysis

Persons with C6 quadriplegia (and above) have marked or total paralysis of the elbow extensors because these muscles receive most of the nerve root innervation below C6. Loss of elbow extension reduces the ability to reach or push away from the body; therefore activities such as moving up to sit or transferring from a wheelchair become difficult and very labor intensive.

A valuable method of muscle substitution uses innervated proximal shoulder muscles such as the clavicular head of the pectoralis major and the anterior deltoid to actively extend and lock the elbow (Figure 5-25). This ability of a proximal muscle to extend the elbow requires that the hand be firmly fixed or stabilized. Under these circumstances, contraction of the shoulder musculature adducts or horizontally adducts the glenohumeral joint, or both, pulling the humerus toward the midline. Because the hand is "fixed," the forearm must follow the humerus and the elbow is pulled into extension.

Once the arm is locked into extension, it can be used as a stable base for many functional activities such as transferring into or out of a wheelchair.

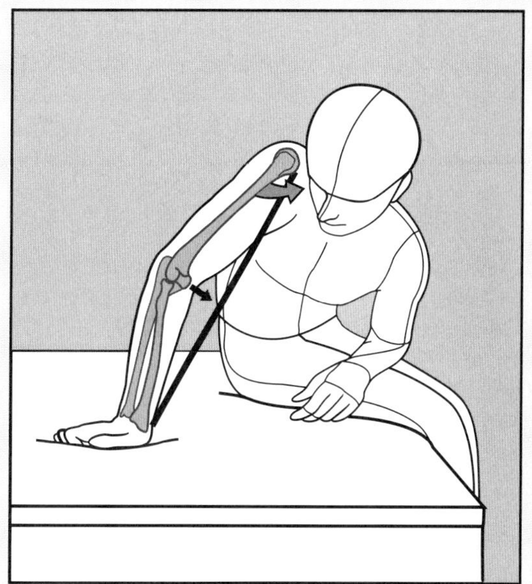

Figure 5-25 A depiction of an individual with C6 quadriplegia using the innervated portion of the pectoralis major and anterior deltoid *(red arrow)* to pull the humerus toward the midline, resulting in elbow extension. (From Neumann DA: *Kinesiology of the musculoskeletal system: foundations for physical rehabilitation*, St Louis, 2002, Mosby, Figure 6-45.)

Normally, the nervous system selects just the right muscles for a given task; however, persons with a brain injury or another disease that affects motor planning may activate more muscles than are necessary for a given task. This inefficient choice of muscular activation can account, in part, for the activity appearing labored or uncoordinated.

Pushing Activities: A "Natural" for the Triceps

A common activity requiring strong activation from all three heads of the triceps is the act of pushing, an activity that involves a combination of elbow extension and shoulder flexion. Consider, for instance, pushing open a heavy steel door as depicted in Figure 5-26. As the triceps strongly contracts to extend the elbow, the shoulder simultaneously flexes by action of the anterior deltoid. The logical question arises: How can the shoulder flex when the long head of the triceps (a shoulder extensor) is active? The answer is that the shoulder flexors such as the anterior deltoid overpower the shoulder extension torque of the long head of the triceps. With the shoulder extension potential of the long head of the triceps neutralized, all of its contractile energy is channeled into elbow extension torque. The end result is a synergistic action, with both the triceps and anterior deltoid cooperating to produce a strongly flexing shoulder and a strongly extending elbow, the exact two actions required for pushing a heavy object.

Forearm Supinators and Pronators

Muscles that supinate or pronate the forearm must meet at least two requirements: (1) The muscles must originate on the humerus or ulna, or both, *and* insert on the radius or hand; and (2) the muscles must have a line of force that intersects (versus parallels) the axis of rotation of the forearm joints (Figure 5-27).

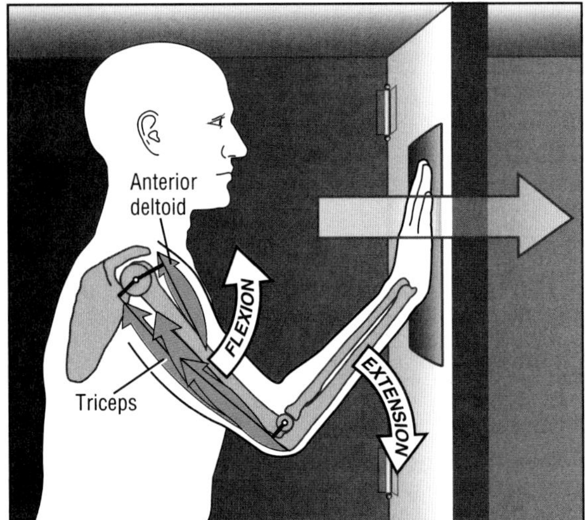

Figure 5-26 The triceps is shown generating an extensor torque across the elbow to rapidly push open a door. Note that the elbow is extending as the anterior deltoid is flexing the shoulder. The anterior deltoid must oppose and exceed the shoulder extensor torque produced by the long head of the triceps. The black lines represent the internal moment arms, originating at the joint's axis of rotation. (From Neumann DA: *Kinesiology of the musculoskeletal system: foundations for physical rehabilitation*, St Louis, 2002, Mosby, Figure 6-43.)

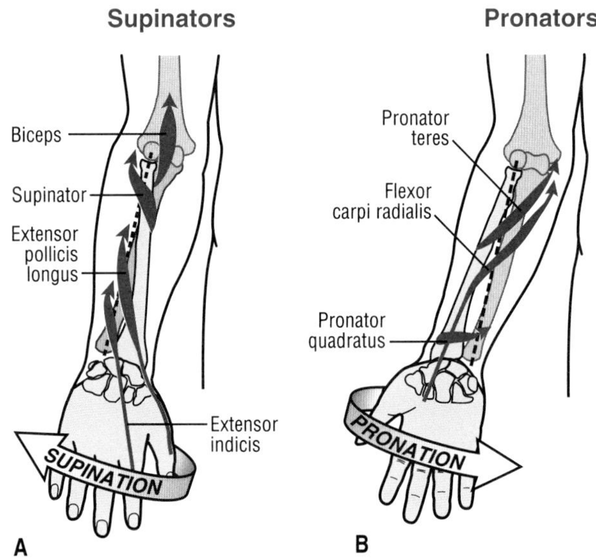

Figure 5-27 The lines of pull of the supinators **(A)** and the pronators **(B).** The dotted line represents the forearm's axis of rotation. (From Neumann DA: *Kinesiology of the musculoskeletal system: foundations for physical rehabilitation*, St Louis, 2002, Mosby, Figure 6-46.)

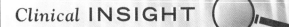

Clinical INSIGHT

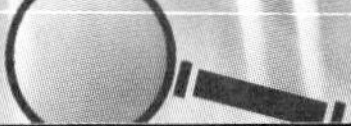

Using Shoulder Position to Help Isolate Muscles of the Elbow during a Manual Muscle Test

The long head of the triceps and biceps brachii muscles each crosses the elbow *and* the shoulder. As with any multi-articular muscle, if the muscle contracts and expresses *all* of its actions at once, it will quickly become too short or **actively insufficient**, significantly decreasing its ability to produce contractile force. Clinicians often use this principle in attempts to partially isolate muscles during a manual muscle test.

For example, performing a manual muscle test of the elbow extensors with the shoulder flexed to 90 degrees places the long head of the triceps at a favorable length to produce elbow extension torque. This test therefore is a relatively good indication of overall elbow extension strength. However, if a manual muscle test of the elbow extensors is performed with the shoulder fully extended, the long head of the triceps becomes relatively short over the elbow *and* the shoulder—effectively reducing its force-producing potential. With the long head of the triceps in a compromised position, the manual muscle test (in the shoulder extended position) reflects the strength of the medial and lateral heads of the triceps.

This same principle can be used to isolate the one-joint elbow flexors such as the brachialis from the multi-articular biceps brachii by performing elbow flexion with the shoulder in a flexed position.

SUPINATORS

The primary supinator muscles are the biceps brachii and the supinator muscle. Secondary supinator muscles include the extensor pollicis longus and the extensor indicis. Although not illustrated in Figure 5-27, A, it should be restated that the brachioradialis can supinate *or* pronate the forearm to the mid position. Whether the brachioradialis is considered a pronator or a supinator depends entirely on the position of the forearm at the start of the muscle contraction.

Primary Supinators

- Biceps brachii
- Supinator

Secondary Supinators

- Extensor pollicis longus
- Extensor indicis

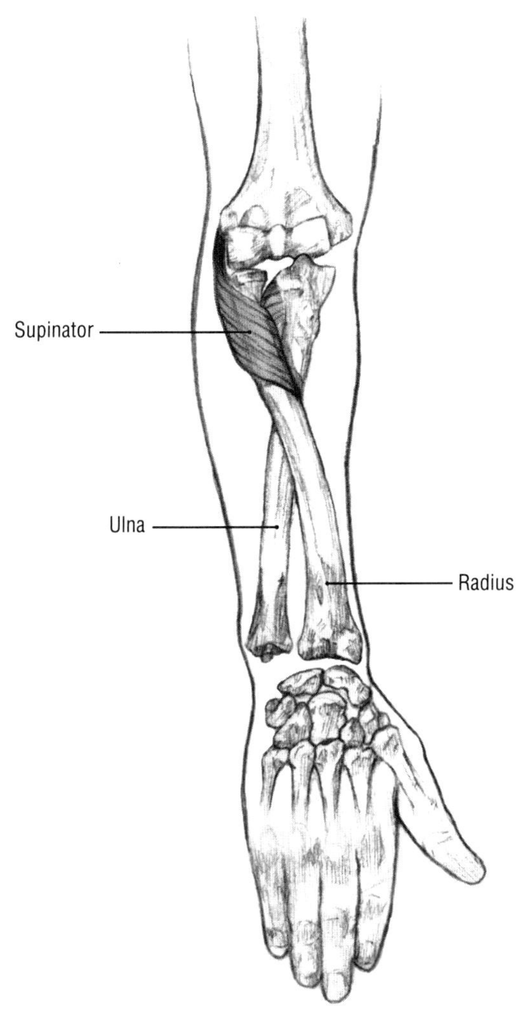

Biceps Brachii

Refer to p. 108 for an illustration and attachments of this muscle.

Supinator

Proximal Attachment:	Lateral epicondyle of the humerus and supinator crest of the ulna
Distal Attachment:	Lateral surface of the proximal radius
Innervation:	Radial nerve
Action:	Forearm supination
Comments:	In a pronated position, the supinator muscle wraps over the top of the radius, giving it the ability to spin the radius back into supination. The supinator muscle is the first muscle to respond to a task that requires a low level of supination force, assuming there is no need to also flex the elbow. The biceps muscle is held in reserve to assist the supinator muscle only when larger supination forces are required.

Functional Considerations: Interaction of the Supinator Muscles

Contraction of the biceps brachii from a pronated position can effectively spin the radius in the direction of supination. The effectiveness of the biceps as a supinator is greatest when the elbow is flexed to near 90 degrees. At this elbow position, the biceps tendon approaches the radius at a 90-degree angle. Similar to pulling a string attached to a toy top or a yo-yo, all the linear force produces rotation and therefore efficiently rotates the radius.

In contrast, with the elbow flexed only 30 degrees, much of the rotational efficiency of the biceps is lost. For example, the biceps can produce only 50% of the supination torque (at 30 degrees) as compared with when the elbow is flexed to 90 degrees. Such a kinesiologic principle is useful in the ergonomic design of tools and workplace environments.

Figure 5-28 shows the action of the biceps and other supinator muscles in an individual who is vigorously tightening a screw with a screwdriver. Note that the direction of rotation for tightening a screw (with the right hand) is clockwise and is produced by all the supinator muscles. Realize that a greater force is required to tighten a screw than to loosen it. Furthermore, the supinator muscles, as a group, are stronger than the pronator muscles. The act of tightening a screw therefore takes full advantage of the force superiority of the supinator muscles—at least when the screwdriver is held by the right hand.

Also shown in Figure 5-28, the action of tightening a screw involves strong activation from both the biceps *and* the triceps. The triceps muscle is essential in this activity because it must neutralize the tendency of a strongly activated biceps to also flex the elbow. Because it attaches to the ulna, the triceps stabilizes the humeroulnar joint but does not interfere with the mechanics of a supination task.

PRONATORS

The primary pronator muscles are the pronator teres and the pronator quadratus. Secondary pronators are the flexor carpi radialis and the palmaris longus (see Figure 5-27, *B*); these muscles are covered in detail in the next chapter.

Primary Pronators

- Pronator teres
- Pronator quadratus

Secondary Pronators

- Flexor carpi radialis
- Palmaris longus

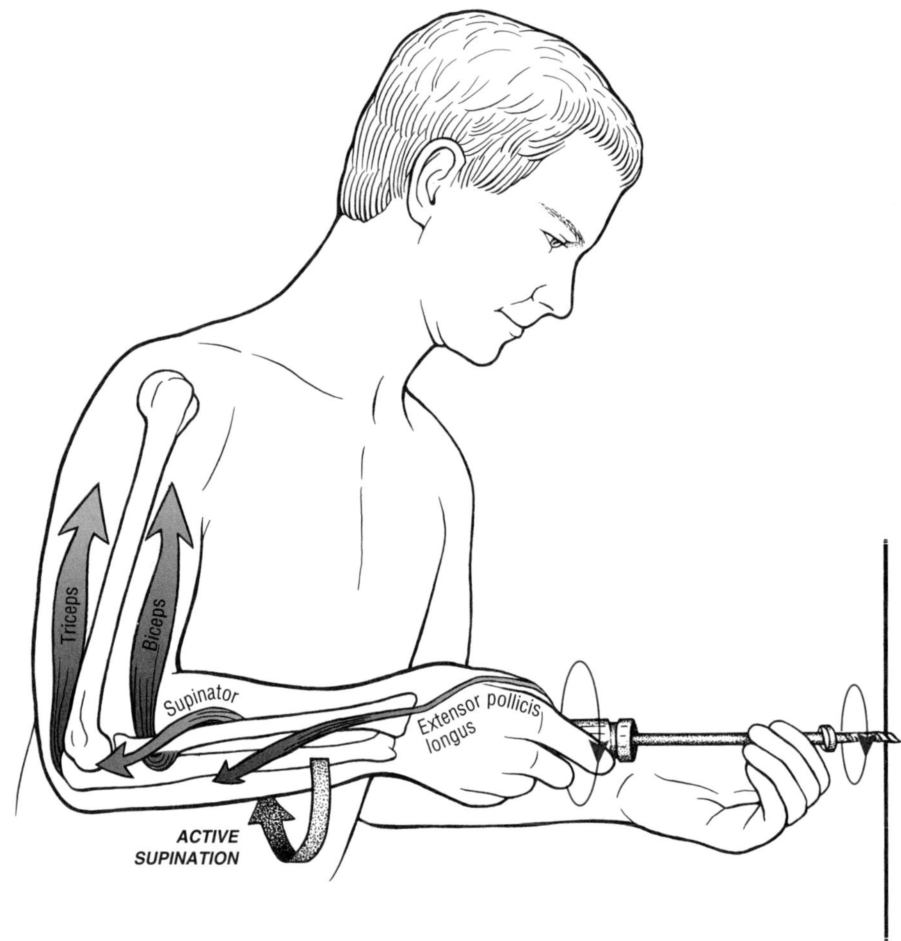

Figure 5-28 The combined supination force of the right biceps, supinator, and extensor pollicis longus muscles is used to tighten a screw in a clockwise rotation with a screwdriver. The triceps muscle is activated isometrically to neutralize the strong elbow flexion tendency of the biceps. (From Neumann DA: *Kinesiology of the musculoskeletal system: foundations for physical rehabilitation*, St Louis, 2002, Mosby, Figure 6-50.)

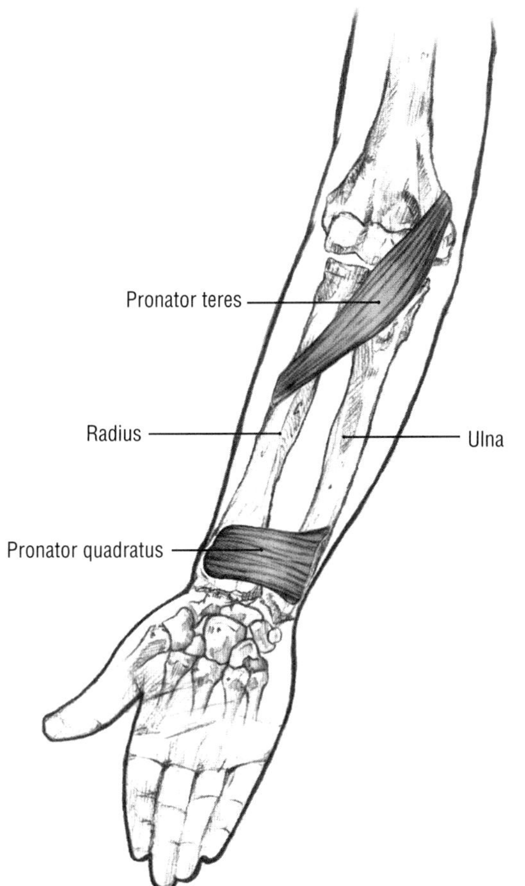

An anterior view of the right pronator teres and pronator quadratus muscles.

Pronator Teres

Proximal Attachment:
- Humeral head: medial epicondyle of the humerus
- Ulnar head: just medial to the tuberosity of the ulna

Distal Attachment: Lateral surface of the mid radius

Innervation: Median nerve

Actions:
- Forearm pronation
- Elbow flexion

Comments: The two heads of the pronator teres converge to attach distally on the lateral surface of the radius near its midpoint. As its name implies, it is a strong pronator but can also flex the elbow because it crosses the anterior aspect of the elbow joint.

Pronator Quadratus

Proximal Attachment: Anterior surface of the distal ulna

Distal Attachment: Anterior surface of the distal radius

Innervation: Median nerve

Action: Forearm pronation

Comments: The pronator quadratus is a short, flat, rectangular-shaped muscle that is in excellent position to stabilize the distal radioulnar joint. Because this muscle intersects the axis of rotation at the forearm at a near perfect right angle, it is a particularly effective pronator.

Functional Considerations: Interaction of the Pronator Muscles

The pronator teres muscle assists the pronator quadratus muscle when larger pronation forces are required or when elbow flexion is also desired. If the pronator teres is activated, the elbow will also flex unless neutralized by the triceps muscles.

By now you may have noticed that the functional relationship between the pronator quadratus and the pronator teres is similar to that between the supinator and biceps. In each case a small one-joint muscle is "on call" to produce low-forearm isolated efforts of the forearm without associated movements of the elbow. Also, in both cases, a larger two-joint muscle is on reserve when more strength (greater torque) is required.

Summary

The elbow and forearm complex contribute highly to the overall function of the upper extremity. Located between the shoulder and the hand, muscles must stabilize the region to allow for the transmission of external forces between the shoulder and hand. These external forces may be large such as during walking with crutches or crawling. In addition to stability, the elbow and forearm complex must supply ample mobility to adjust the functional length of the arm (by flexing and extending the elbow), as well as place the hand in a position of function (by supinating and pronating the forearm). The structure of the four joints of the elbow and forearm complex allows for both mobility and stability needs.

Many of the muscles that cross the elbow also cross other regions such as the shoulder or forearm. The many multi-articular muscles reflect the functional interdependence among all regions of the upper extremity. Muscles work together to augment the overall function of the upper extremity.

Study Questions

1. Which of the following statements is true regarding the interosseous membrane?
   a. It helps bind the radius and ulna together for increased stability.
   b. It helps transmit compression forces from the hand or wrist evenly through the humeroulnar and humeroradial joints of the elbow.
   c. It helps bind the radius to the humerus for increased valgus stability.
   d. A and B
   e. B and C
2. Which of the following muscles becomes maximally stretched in full supination of the forearm and full elbow extension?
   a. Supinator
   b. Long head of the triceps
   c. Pronator teres
   d. Lateral head of the triceps
   e. A and B
3. Injury to the radial nerve will likely result in significant weakness of which action?
   a. Elbow flexion
   b. Elbow extension
   c. Wrist flexion
   d. Shoulder flexion
   e. All of the above
4. How many degrees of freedom are allowed at the humeroulnar joint?
   a. 1
   b. 2
   c. 3
   d. 4
5. Beginning with the forearm in a fully pronated position and the elbow flexed to 90 degrees, which of the following muscles can supinate the forearm?
   a. Brachialis
   b. Brachioradialis
   c. Biceps brachii
   d. A and C
   e. B and C
6. Which of the following statements is true?
   a. Full range of motion of elbow flexion is typically 100 degrees.
   b. Normal cubitus valgus (of the elbow) is approximately 15 degrees.
   c. The brachioradialis is innervated by the musculocutaneous nerve.
   d. A bony end feel at the elbow is usually associated with full elbow flexion.
7. Which of the following statements is true?
   a. With the hand free, supination and pronation of the forearm result from the radius rotating about the ulna.
   b. When pushing down on the hand, most of the compressive force is transmitted directly to the ulna, not the radius.
   c. The pronator quadratus attaches to the distal humerus.
   d. The long head of the triceps is an effective pronator of the forearm.
   e. B and D
8. Which of the following muscles has its distal attachment on the radius?
   a. Brachialis
   b. Brachioradialis
   c. Biceps brachii
   d. A and B
   e. B and C
9. Which of the following muscles is innervated by the radial nerve?
   a. Brachialis
   b. Brachioradialis
   c. Medial head of the triceps
   d. A and B
   e. B and C
10. Which of the following positions maximally elongate the long head of the triceps?
    a. Shoulder flexion and elbow extension
    b. Shoulder flexion and elbow flexion
    c. Shoulder extension and elbow extension
    d. Shoulder extension and elbow flexion
11. The trochlea is a structure on which bone?
    a. Humerus
    b. Radius
    c. Ulna
    d. Scapula
12. The primary function of the annular ligament is to:
    a. Help transmit forces from the ulna to the humerus
    b. Bind the radial head to the proximal ulna
    c. Bind the distal radius to the distal ulna
    d. Serve as an attachment for the triceps
13. For a low-effort elbow extension activity, the nervous system will first "choose" the medial and lateral heads of the triceps over the long head of the triceps because:
    a. The medial and lateral heads also perform shoulder flexion.
    b. The medial and lateral heads also perform shoulder extension.
    c. Activation of the long head requires simultaneous activation of the anterior deltoid to prevent unwanted shoulder extension.
    d. The long head of the triceps has a poor line of pull to perform elbow extension.
14. In the anatomic position:
    a. The radius is medial to the ulna.
    b. The forearm is pronated.
    c. The radius is lateral to the ulna.
    d. The trochlea is lateral to the capitulum.

15. During strong activation of the biceps to perform elbow flexion, the posterior head of the deltoid must be activated to prevent:
    a. Unwanted supination of the forearm
    b. Unwanted flexion of the shoulder
    c. Excessive cubitus valgus
    d. Excessive cubitus varus
16. A *Colles' fracture* refers to:
    a. An impaction fracture of the humeral head
    b. Simultaneous fracture of the proximal radius and ulna
    c. A fracture of the distal radius
    d. A rupture of the interosseous membrane
17. Performing elbow extension with the shoulder in an extended position:
    a. Requires activation of the brachialis
    b. Produces automatic pronation of the forearm
    c. Results in long head of the triceps becoming actively insufficient
    d. Is the strongest position for producing elbow extension torque
18. Individuals with a painful or inflamed elbow:
    a. Typically hold the elbow in a fully extended position to maximally stabilize the surrounding musculature
    b. Typically hold the elbow in 70 to 90 degrees of flexion to help reduce intra-capsular pressure and therefore be in a position of comfort
    c. Are typically unable to extend the shoulder past neutral
    d. Are typically compensating for weakness of the opposite shoulder
19. Injury to the musculocutaneous nerve will most likely result in:
    a. Elbow extensor weakness
    b. Elbow flexor weakness
    c. Pronator weakness
    d. Shoulder extensor weakness
20. A cubitus-valgus producing force is most likely to injure the:
    a. Medial collateral ligament of the elbow
    b. Long head of the biceps
    c. Long head of the triceps
    d. Lateral collateral ligament of the elbow
21. The biceps brachii and the brachialis are both innervated by the musculocutaneous nerve.
    a. True
    b. False
22. The brachialis is an effective supinator of the forearm.
    a. True
    b. False
23. The end feel for elbow extension is typically considered bony.
    a. True
    b. False
24. Excessive valgus-producing force to the elbow will likely result in injury to the lateral collateral ligament of the elbow.
    a. True
    b. False
25. Compressive force through the radius is transferred to the ulna largely by the interosseous membrane.
    a. True
    b. False
26. The lateral head of the triceps courses anterior to the medial-lateral axis of rotation of the elbow.
    a. True
    b. False
27. The first muscle to be chosen for a low-effort level elbow flexion activity is most likely the biceps brachii because it is a multi-articular muscle.
    a. True
    b. False
28. Along with binding the radius and ulna together, the interosseous membrane serves as the site of attachment for many muscles.
    a. True
    b. False
29. In a pronated position of the forearm, the radius is crossed over the top of the ulna.
    a. True
    b. False
30. The three primary actions of the biceps brachii are supination, elbow flexion, and shoulder flexion.
    a. True
    b. False

ADDITIONAL READINGS

Adams JE, Steinmann SP: Nerve injuries about the elbow, *J Hand Surg [Am]* 312:303-313, 2006.

An KN, Hui FC, Morrey BF et al: Muscles across the elbow joint: a biomechanical analysis, *J Biomech* 1410:659-669, 1981.

Basmajian JV, Latif A: Integrated actions and functions of the chief flexors of the elbow: a detailed electromyographic analysis, *J Bone Joint Surg Am* 39-A(5):1106-1118, 1957.

Bozkurt M, Acar HI, Apaydin N et al: The annular ligament: an anatomical study, *Am J Sports Med* 331:114-118, 2005.

Callaway GH, Field LD, Deng XH et al: Biomechanical evaluation of the medial collateral ligament of the elbow, *J Bone Joint Surg Am* 798:1223-1231, 1997.

Funk DA, An KN, Morrey BF et al: Electromyographic analysis of muscles across the elbow joint, *J Orthop Res* 54:529-538, 1987.

Hagert CG: The distal radioulnar joint, *Hand Clin* 31:41-50, 1987.

Kihara H, Short WH, Werner FW et al: The stabilizing mechanism of the distal radioulnar joint during pronation and supination, *J Hand Surg [Am]* 206:930-936, 1995.

Lehmkuhl LD, Smith LK: *Brunnstrom's clinical kinesiology*, ed 4, Philadelphia, 1983, FA Davis.

Loftice J, Fleisig GS, Zheng N et al: Biomechanics of the elbow in sports, *Clin Sports Med* 234:519-530, vii-viii, 2004.

MacConaill MA, Basmajian JV: *Muscles and movements: a basis for human kinesiology*, New York, 1977, Robert E. Krieger Publishing.

O'Driscoll SW, Jupiter JB, King GJ et al: The unstable elbow, *Instr Course Lect* 50:89-102, 2001.

Palmer AK, Werner FW: The triangular fibrocartilage complex of the wrist—anatomy and function, *J Hand Surg [Am]* 62:153-162, 1981.

Paraskevas G, Papadopoulos A, Papaziogas B et al: Study of the carrying angle of the human elbow joint in full extension: a morphometric analysis, *Surg Radiol Anat* 261:19-23, 2004.

Pauly JE, Rushing JL, Scheving LE: An electromyographic study of some muscles crossing the elbow joint, *Anat Rec* 1591:47-53, 1967.

Pfaeffle HJ, Tomaino MM, Grewal R et al: Tensile properties of the interosseous membrane of the human forearm, *J Orthop Res* 145:842-845, 1996.

Skahen JR III, Palmer AK, Werner FW et al: The interosseous membrane of the forearm: anatomy and function, *J Hand Surg [Am]* 226:981-985, 1997.

Sojbjerg JO: The stiff elbow, *Acta Orthop Scand* 676:626-631, 1996.

Takigawa N, Ryu J, Kish VL et al: Functional anatomy of the lateral collateral ligament complex of the elbow: morphology and strain, *J Hand Surg [Br]* 302:143-147, 2005.

Werner FW, An KN: Biomechanics of the elbow and forearm, *Hand Clin* 103:357-373, 1994.

CHAPTER 6

Structure and Function of the Wrist

CHAPTER OUTLINE

OBJECTIVES

- Identify the bones and primary bony features relevant to the wrist complex.
- Describe the supporting structures of the wrist.
- Cite the normal ranges of motion for wrist flexion and extension and radial and ulnar deviation.
- Describe the planes of motion and axes of rotation for the joints of the wrist.
- Cite the proximal and distal attachments and innervation of the primary muscles of the wrist.
- Justify the primary actions of the muscles of the wrist.
- Describe how compressive forces are transferred from the hand through the wrist.
- Explain the function of the wrist extensor muscles when grasping.
- List the structures that travel within the carpal tunnel.
- Explain the synergistic action between the muscles of the wrist when performing flexion-extension and radial and ulnar deviation.

KEY TERMS

avascular necrosis
carpal tunnel
carpal tunnel syndrome
dorsal
lateral epicondylitis
palmar

The wrist contains eight small bones that are located between the distal end of the radius and the hand (Figure 6-1). Although slight, the passive movements that occur within the carpal bones help absorb forces that cross between the hand and the forearm, such as when crawling on all four limbs or when bearing weight through the hands when using crutches or a walker.

The wrist has two major articulations: (1) the radiocarpal joint and (2) the midcarpal joint. As a functional pair, these joints allow the wrist to adequately position the hand for optimal function. The wrist can flex and extend and move in a side-to-side fashion known as radial and ulnar deviation. In addition to these important movements, the wrist must also be a stable platform for the hand. A painful or weak wrist typically cannot provide an adequate base for the muscles to operate the hand. Making a firm grip, for example, is not possible with paralysis of the wrist extensor muscles. As will be presented in this chapter, the kinesiology of the wrist is heavily linked to the kinesiology of the hand.

Several new terms in this chapter describe surfaces of the wrist and hand. **Palmar** is synonymous with the anterior aspect of the wrist and hand; **dorsal** refers to the

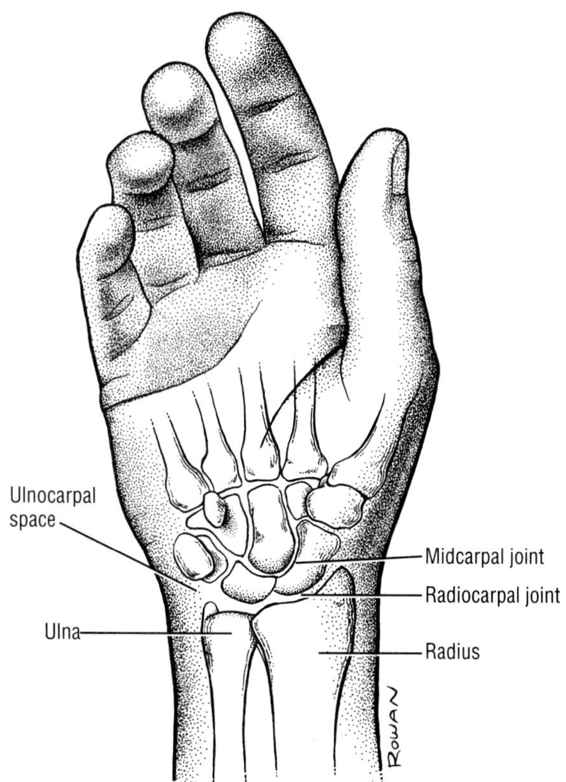

Figure 6-1 The bones and major articulations of the wrist. Note also the ulnocarpal space, just distal to the ulna. (From Neumann DA: *Kinesiology of the musculoskeletal system: foundations for physical rehabilitation*, St Louis, 2002, Mosby, Figure 7-1.)

posterior aspect of the wrist or hand. These terms are used interchangeably throughout this chapter and the next chapter on the hand.

Osteology

Ten bones are involved with the kinesiology of the wrist: the distal radius, distal ulna, and eight carpal bones.

Distal Radius and Ulna

The distal radius and ulna (Figure 6-2) articulate with the proximal row of carpal bones. The distal forearm is bordered laterally by the *radial styloid process* and medially by the *ulnar styloid process*. The *radial tubercle*, also called *Lister's tubercle*, is a small, palpable projection on the dorsal aspect of the distal radius. This ridge of bone helps guide the direction of the tendons of several wrist and thumb extensor muscles.

Carpal Bones

From a radial (lateral) to ulnar direction, the proximal row of carpal bones includes the *scaphoid*, *lunate*, *triquetrum*, and the *pisiform*. The distal row includes the *trapezium*, *trapezoid*, *capitate*, and *hamate* (Figures 6-2 and 6-3). The bones within the proximal row are loosely joined. In contrast, strong ligaments tightly bind the bones of the distal row. The natural stability of the distal row provides an important rigid base for articulations with the metacarpal bones.

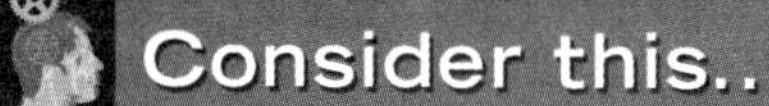

Carpal Bones: A Few Highlights

Scaphoid

The scaphoid is located in the direct pathway of the forces that naturally cross the wrist. For this reason, fracture of the scaphoid occurs more frequently than any other carpal bone. Healing is frequently hindered because blood supply to the fractured component of bone is often poor.

Lunate

Interestingly, no muscles and only few ligaments attach to the lunate. The lunate is therefore loosely articulated and is the most frequently dislocated carpal bone. Like the scaphoid, the blood supply to the lunate is often compromised after trauma, resulting in **avascular necrosis.**

Triquetrum

The triquetrum is named after its triangular appearance.

Pisiform

Strictly speaking, the pisiform is not a true carpal bone. Rather, it is a sesamoid bone that develops within the tendon of the flexor carpi ulnaris. Technically, therefore, the wrist has seven carpal bones, which matches the arrangement of seven tarsal bones of the ankle.

Trapezium

The distal, saddle-shaped surface of the trapezium articulates with the base of the first metacarpal. The resulting carpometacarpal joint is a highly specialized articulation allowing a wide range of motion of the thumb.

Trapezoid

This bone is tightly wedged between the trapezium and capitate, serving as a stable base for the second metacarpal.

Capitate

The capitate is the largest of all carpal bones, occupying a central location within the wrist. The axis of rotation for all wrist motion passes through this bone.

Hamate

The hamate (from Latin, meaning "hook") is named after its prominent hook-like process on its palmer surface.

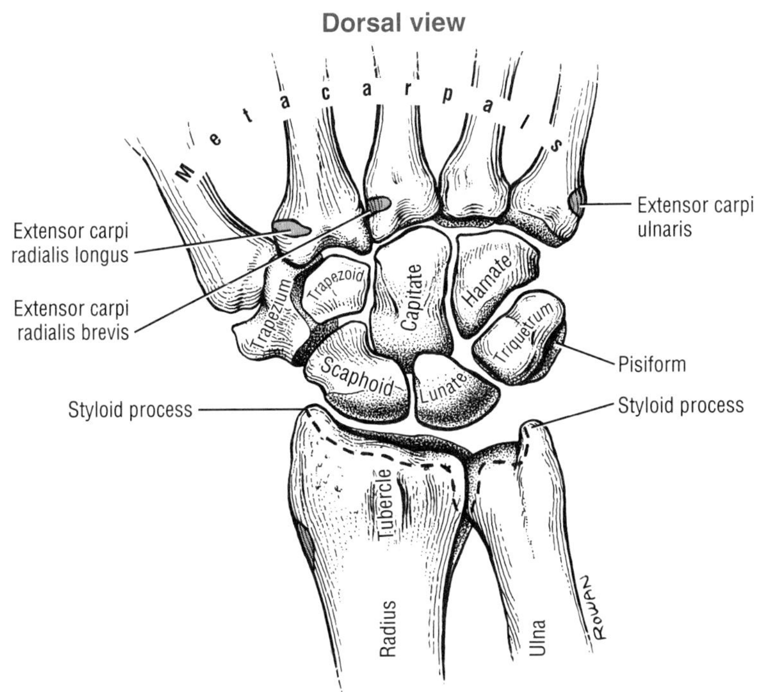

Figure 6-2 The dorsal aspect of the bones of the right wrist. The muscle's distal attachments are shown in gray. The dashed lines show the proximal attachment of the dorsal capsule of the wrist. (From Neumann DA: *Kinesiology of the musculoskeletal system: foundations for physical rehabilitation*, St Louis, 2002, Mosby, Figure 7-2.)

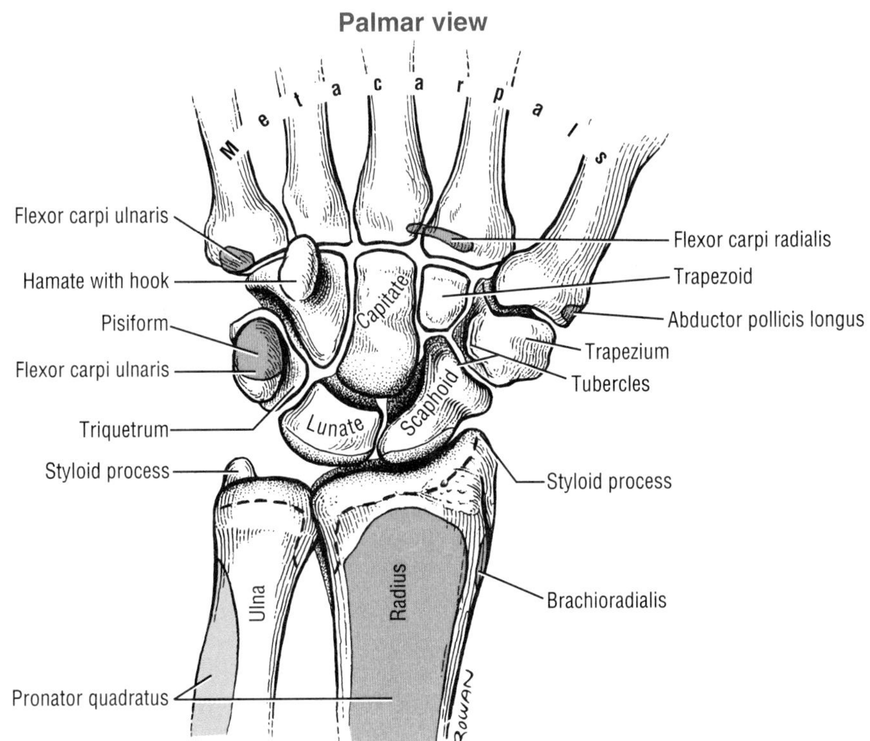

Figure 6-3 The palmar aspect of the bones of the right wrist. The muscle's proximal attachments are shown in red and distal attachments in gray. The dashed lines show the proximal attachment of the palmar capsule of the wrist. (From Neumann DA: *Kinesiology of the musculoskeletal system: foundations for physical rehabilitation*, St Louis, 2002, Mosby, Figure 7-3.)

CARPAL TUNNEL

The transverse carpal ligament bridges the palmar side of the carpal bones, helping to form the **carpal tunnel** (Figure 6-4). The carpel tunnel serves as a passageway that helps protect the median nerve and the tendons of extrinsic flexor muscles of the digits.

> *Clinical* **INSIGHT**
>
> **Carpal Tunnel Syndrome**
>
> All the tendons that flex the digits travel with the median nerve and pass through the tightly packed carpal tunnel (see Figure 6-4). Also traveling within the carpal tunnel are several synovial membranes that help reduce friction between the tendons and surrounding structures. Hand activities that require prolonged and often extreme wrist positions can irritate these tendons and synovial sheaths. Due to the small size of the carpal tunnel, swelling of the synovial membranes can increase the pressure on the median nerve. **Carpal tunnel syndrome**, which is characterized by pain or paresthesia (tingling), or both, over the sensory distribution of the median nerve, may result. In more extreme cases, muscular weakness and atrophy may occur in the intrinsic muscles around the thumb.

Arthrology

Joint Structure

As illustrated in Figure 6-1, the wrist is a double-jointed system, consisting of the radiocarpal and midcarpal joints. Many smaller intercarpal joints also exist between carpal bones. Compared with the large ranges of motion permitted at the radiocarpal and midcarpal joints, motion at the many intercarpal joints is relatively small.

> **Major Joints of the Wrist**
>
> - Radiocarpal joint
> - Midcarpal joint

RADIOCARPAL JOINT

The proximal part of the radiocarpal joint consists of the concave surface of the radius and the adjacent articular disc (Figure 6-5). The distal part of the joint consists primarily of the convex articular surfaces of the scaphoid and the lunate. Approximately 80% of the force that crosses the wrist passes between the scaphoid and the lunate and then to the radius. The large, expanded distal end of the radius is well designed to accept this force. Unfortunately, however, for many persons a fall onto an outstretched hand fractures the distal end of the radius, as well as the

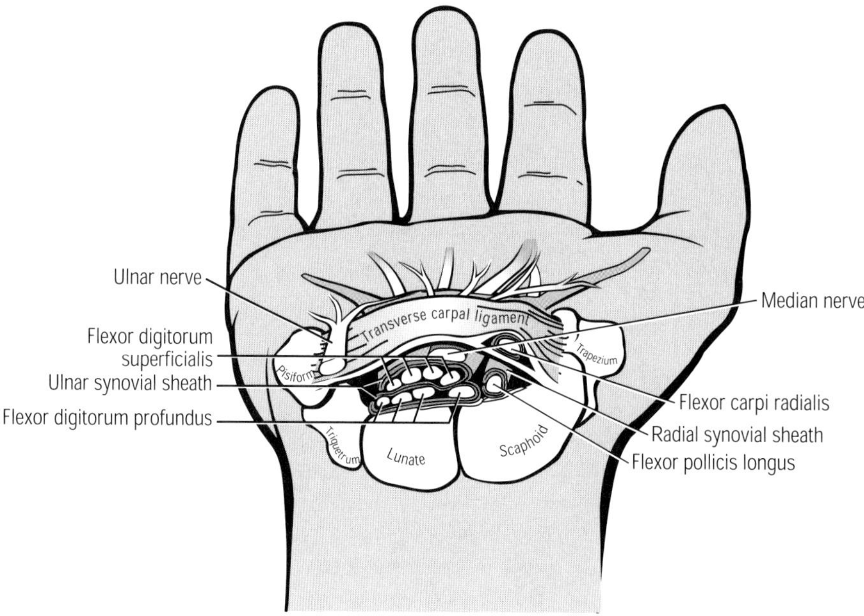

Figure 6-4 The transverse carpal ligament is shown as the roof of the carpal tunnel. Observe the synovial sheaths (*red*) surrounding the tendons of the flexor digitorum superficialis, flexor digitorum profoundus, and flexor pollicis longus. Note that the median nerve is located inside the tunnel, whereas the ulnar nerve is located outside of the tunnel. (From Neumann DA: *Kinesiology of the musculoskeletal system: foundations for physical rehabilitation*, St Louis, 2002, Mosby, Figure 8-39.)

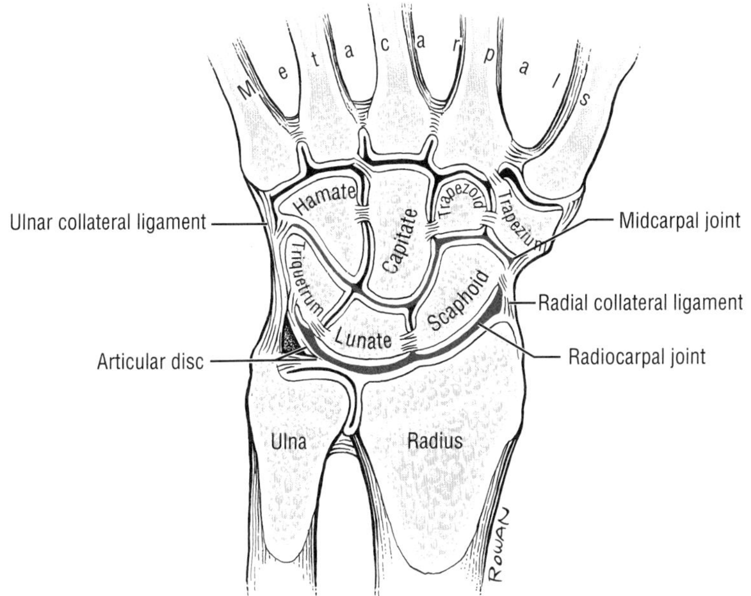

Figure 6-5 A frontal plane cross section through the right wrist and distal forearm showing the shape of the bones and connective tissues. The margins of the radiocarpal and midcarpal joints are highlighted in red. (Modified from Neumann DA: *Kinesiology of the musculoskeletal system: foundations for physical rehabilitation,* St Louis, 2002, Mosby, Figure 7-6.)

scaphoid. Persons with weakened bones due to osteoporosis are particularly susceptible to these fractures.

The ulnar-located carpal bones and the distal ulna are less likely to fracture from such a fall because they are not in the direct path of weight bearing. Furthermore, a relatively wide space exists between the distal ulna and ulnar carpal bones. This space, formally known as the ulnocarpal space (see Figure 6-1), helps buffer the forces that cross the wrist.

MIDCARPAL JOINT

The midcarpal joint separates the proximal and distal rows of carpal bones (see Figure 6-5). Although this joint involves several articulations, the most prominent is formed between the head of the capitate and the socket formed by the distal surfaces of the scaphoid and lunate. Note that the scaphoid and lunate bones are important members of the main two articulations of the wrist.

Ligaments of the Wrist

The joints of the wrist are enclosed within a fibrous capsule. The capsule is thickened by extrinsic and intrinsic ligaments. Extrinsic ligaments have their proximal attachments outside the carpal bones but attach distally within the carpal bones. Intrinsic ligaments, in contrast, have both their proximal and distal attachments located within the carpal bones. Table 6-1 lists the main attachments and primary functions of the four primary extrinsic ligaments: radial collateral, ulnar collateral, dorsal radiocarpal, and palmar radiocarpal. Three of the four primary extrinsic ligaments are indicated by red dots in Figure 6-6, *A* and *B*, and are summarized along with their individual functions in Table 6-1. The detailed anatomy of the intrinsic ligaments is beyond the scope of the text. As a group, however, the intrinsic ligaments (1) interconnect various carpal bones; (2) help transfer forces between the hand and forearm; and (3) maintain the natural shapes of radiocarpal and midcarpal joints, thereby minimizing joint stress during movement.

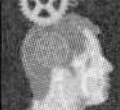

Consider this...

Ulnocarpal Complex

A complex set of connective tissues, known as the ulnocarpal complex, exists near the ulnar border of the wrist (see Figure 6-6, *B*). (This group of tissue is often referred to as the triangular fibrocartilage complex, or TFCC). The ulnocarpal complex includes the articular disc (described in Chapter 5 as an important component of the distal radioulnar joint), ulnar collateral ligament, and palmar ulnocarpal ligament. This set of tissues fills most of the ulnocarpal space between the distal ulna and the carpal bones (see Figure 6-1). The ulnocarpal space allows the carpal bones to follow the pivoting radius during pronation and supination of the forearm, without interference from the distal end of the ulna. Tears in the articular disc, the central component of the ulnocarpal complex, may result in instability and pain of the wrist and the distal radioulnar joint.

WRIST INSTABILITY

Compression forces naturally cross the wrist every time an overlying muscle contracts or weight is placed through the hand. Normally, the wrist remains stable when compressed, even under substantial forces. The resistance from healthy ligaments, muscles and tendons, and the fit of the articulations add an important element of stability to the wrist. However, damage from a large force such as a fall or, in more extreme cases, degeneration associated with rheumatoid arthritis can significantly destabilize this region.

TABLE 6-1 LIGAMENTS OF THE WRIST

Ligament	Function	Comments
Dorsal radiocarpal ligament	Resists extremes of flexion	Attaches between the radius and dorsal side of the carpal bones
Radial collateral ligament	Resists extremes of ulnar deviation	Strengthened by muscles such as the abductor pollicis longus and the extensor pollicis brevis
Palmar radiocarpal ligament	Resists extremes of wrist extension	Thickest ligament of the wrist; consists of three parts
Ulnar collateral ligament	Resists extremes of radial deviation	Part of the ulnocarpal complex; helps stabilize the distal radioulnar joint

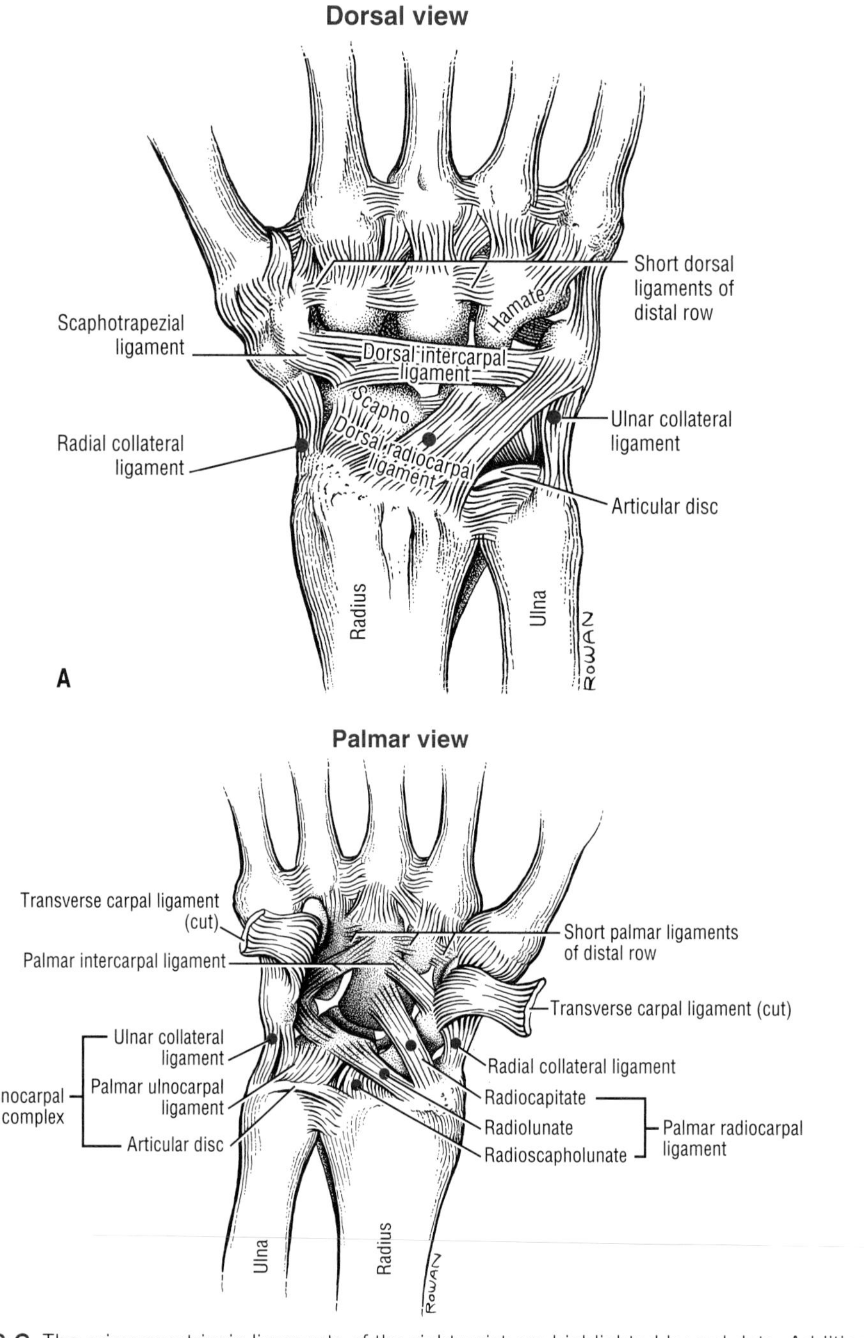

Figure 6-6 The primary extrinsic ligaments of the right wrist are highlighted by red dots. Additional ligaments are listed but not highlighted. **A,** Dorsal view. **B,** Palmer view. The transverse carpal ligament has been cut and reflected to show the underlying ligaments. (Modified from Neumann DA: *Kinesiology of the musculoskeletal system: foundations for physical rehabilitation*, St Louis, 2002, Mosby, Figures 7-8 and 7-9.)

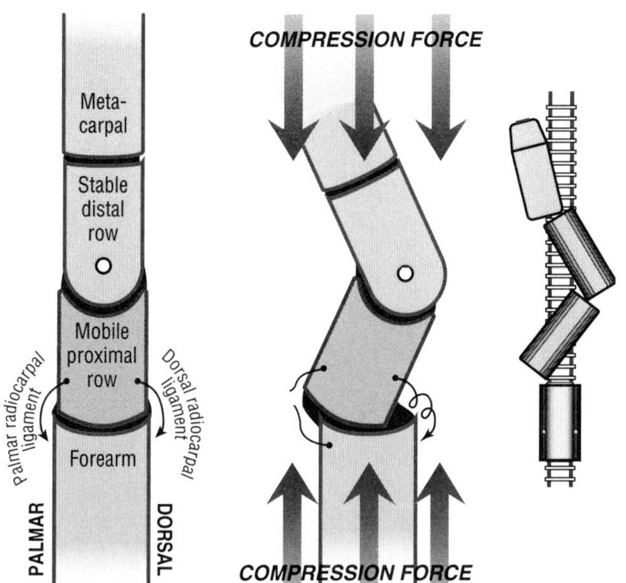

Figure 6-7 A highly diagrammatic depiction of a "zigzag" collapse of the wrist secondary to a large compression force following a fall. Note only selected bones are shown that represent the major joints of the wrist. (From Neumann DA: *Kinesiology of the musculoskeletal system: foundations for physical rehabilitation,* St Louis, 2002, Mosby, Figure 7-17.)

Consider that the loosely articulated proximal row of carpal bones is located between two rigid structures, the radius and distal row of carpal bones. Ligaments weakened by injury or disease often lead to instability of the wrist and even collapse. When compressed strongly from both ends (e.g., from a fall), the proximal row of carpal bones is prone to collapse in a zigzag fashion, much like derailed cars of a freight train (Figure 6-7). An unstable wrist can become painful and is often disabling.

Even a moderately unstable wrist can disrupt the natural arthrokinematics, eventually leading to severe pain and an overall weakening because of atrophy of the surrounding muscles. A painful and weak wrist typically fails to provide a stable platform for the hand. In severe cases surgery is required, often combined with physical therapy. Components of physical therapy typically include strengthening, efforts to relieve pain, education on ways to protect the wrist, and splinting.

Kinematics

OSTEOKINEMATICS

The osteokinematics of the wrist involve flexion and extension and ulnar and radial deviation. Except for minimal accessory motions, the wrist does not spin in a circular motion relative to a fixed radius. The bony fit and ligaments of the radiocarpal joint naturally block this twisting motion. As studied in Chapter 5, pronation and supination involve rotation of the forearm, with the hand and wrist "following" the path of the radius.

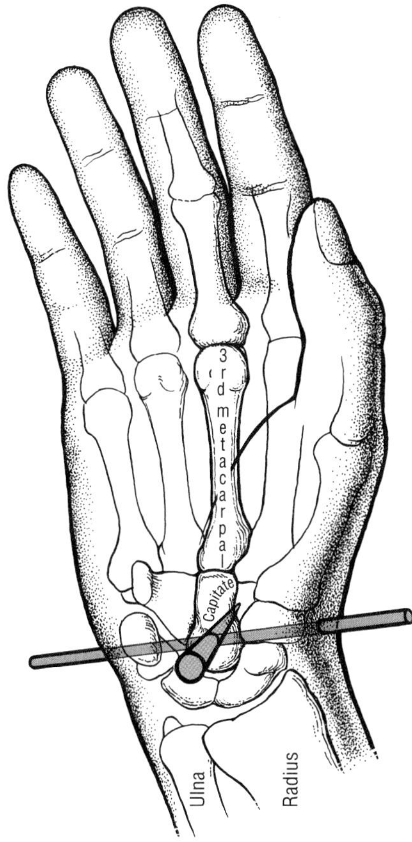

Figure 6-8 The medial-lateral *(gray)* and anterior-posterior *(red)* axes of rotation for wrist movement are shown piercing the base of the capitate bone. (From Neumann DA: *Kinesiology of the musculoskeletal system: foundations for physical rehabilitation,* St Louis, 2002, Mosby, Figure 7-12.)

The axis of rotation for wrist movement pierces the head of the capitate (Figure 6-8). The axis runs in a medial-lateral direction for flexion and extension and in an anterior-posterior direction for radial and ulnar deviation. The firm articulation between the capitate and the base of the third metacarpal bone causes rotation of the capitate to direct the overall path of the entire hand.

Sagittal Plane: Flexion and Extension

On average, from a neutral (0-degree) position, the wrist flexes approximately 70 to 80 degrees and extends approximately 60 to 65 degrees, for a total of approximately 130 to 145 degrees (Figure 6-9, A). Total flexion normally exceeds extension by approximately 15 degrees. Extension is normally limited by tension in the thicker palmar radiocarpal ligaments, as well as the carpal bones contacting the slightly elongated dorsal side of the distal radius.

Frontal Plane: Radial and Ulnar Deviation

On average, from a neutral (0-degree) position, the wrist allows approximately 30 to 35 degrees of ulnar deviation

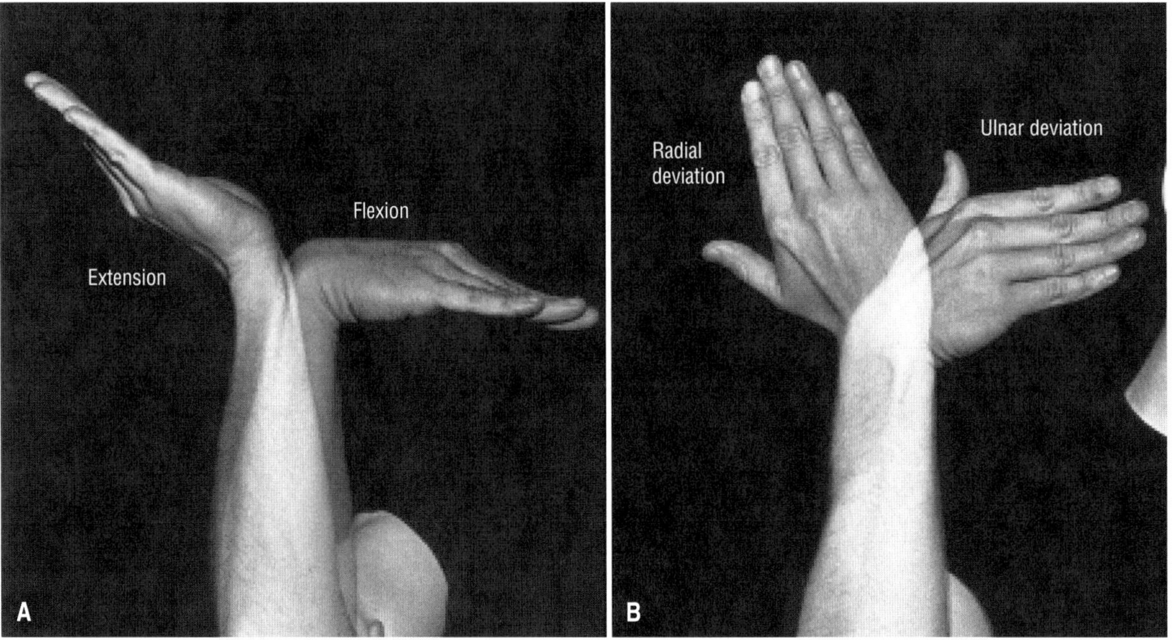

Figure 6-9 Osteokinematics of the wrist. **A**, Flexion and extension. **B**, Ulnar and radial deviation. Note that flexion exceeds extension, and ulnar deviation exceeds radial deviation. (From Neumann DA: *Kinesiology of the musculoskeletal system: foundations for physical rehabilitation*, St Louis, 2002, Mosby, Figure 7-11.)

and approximately 15 to 20 degrees of radial deviations, for a total of about 45 to 55 degrees of motion (Figure 6-9, *B*). Maximum ulnar deviation is normally twice that of radial deviation, mostly because of the void created by the ulnocarpal space. Radial deviation is blocked by contact between the styloid process of the radius and radial side of the carpal bones.

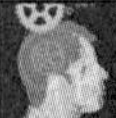

Consider this...

The "Position of Function" of the Wrist

Many common daily activities require about 45 degrees of sagittal plane motion: from 5 to 10 degrees of flexion to 30 to 35 degrees of extension. These same daily activities also require approximately 25 degrees of frontal plane motion: from 15 degrees of ulnar deviation to 10 degrees of radial deviation. Medical management of a severely painful or unstable wrist sometimes requires surgical fusion. To minimize the functional impairment caused by this procedure, the wrist may be fused in an average position of function: approximately 10 to 15 degrees of extension and 10 degrees of ulnar deviation.

ARTHROKINEMATICS

Wrist movements occur simultaneously at both the radiocarpal and midcarpal joints. The upcoming discussion on the arthrokinematics focuses on the dynamic relationship between these two joints.

Central Column of the Wrist

The essential kinematics of the wrist can be well appreciated by observing motion occurring through the central column of the wrist—the series of articulations, or links, among the radius, lunate, capitate, and third metacarpal bone (Figure 6-10, *middle*). Although this central column does not include all the bones of the wrist, it does provide excellent insight into an otherwise complex movement. Within this column the radiocarpal joint is represented by the articulation between radius and lunate, and the midcarpal joint is represented by the articulation between the lunate and the capitate. The carpometacarpal joint indicated in Figure 6-10 (*middle*) is a relatively rigid articulation between the capitate and the base of the third metacarpal; this allows movement of the hand to "follow" the third metacarpal bone.

Extension and Flexion

The arthrokinematics of wrist extension are based on simultaneous convex-on-concave rotations at both radiocarpal and midcarpal joints (see Figure 6-10, *left*). As expected by the convex-concave rules of arthrokinematics (see Chapter 1), the kinematics occur as a roll and slide in opposite directions. What complicates matters, however, is that these kinematics occur simultaneously at two joints: radiocarpal and midcarpal. These compound arthrokinematics are illustrated in Figure 6-10 (*left*) by the red and gray "roll-and-slide" arrows.

Full wrist extension elongates (stretches) the palmar radiocarpal ligaments, palmar capsule, and wrist and

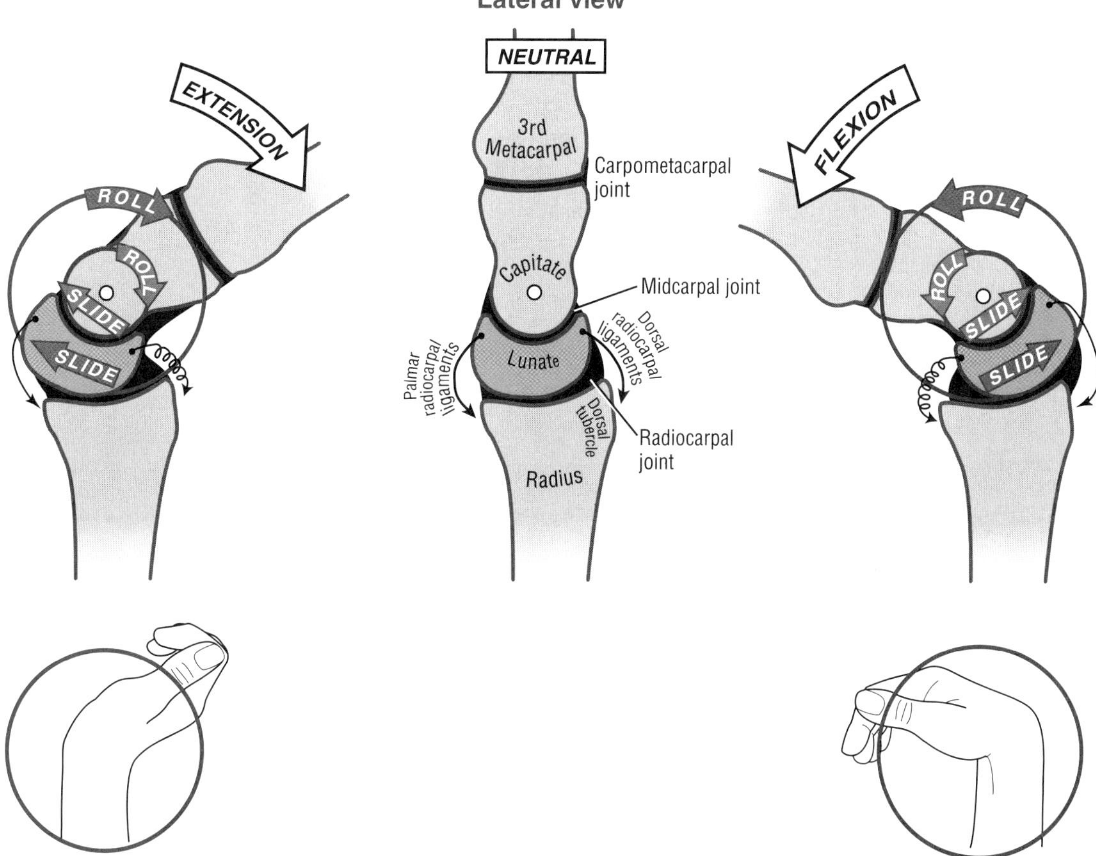

Figure 6-10 A mechanical model of the central column of the right wrist showing the arthrokinematics of flexion and extension. The wrist in the center is shown at rest, in a neutral position. The roll-and-slide arthrokinematics are shown in red for the radiocarpal joint and in gray for the midcarpal joint. During wrist extension *(left)*, the dorsal radiocarpal ligaments become slackened and the palmar radiocarpal ligaments taut. The reverse arthrokinematics occur during wrist flexion *(right)*. (From Neumann DA: *Kinesiology of the musculoskeletal system: foundations for physical rehabilitation*, St Louis, 2002, Mosby, Figure 7-14.)

finger flexor muscles. This helps stabilize the wrist in an extended position, which is useful when bearing weight through the upper extremity.

The arthrokinematics of wrist flexion are similar to that described for extension, but they occur in a reverse fashion (see Figure 6-10, *right*).

Ulnar and Radial Deviation of the Wrist

Like flexion and extension, ulnar and radial deviation can be studied by observing selected bones that represent both the radiocarpal and midcarpal joints (Figure 6-11, *middle*). The motions of ulnar and radial deviation also occur through simultaneous convex-on-concave rotations, at both the radiocarpal joint and the midcarpal joint. The arthrokinematics are shown for ulnar deviation in Figure 6-11 *(left)*. Note that the roll and slide occurs in opposite directions, at both joints. Radial deviation at the wrist occurs through similar arthrokinematics, as just described for ulnar deviation (see Figure 6-11, *right*); however, the amount of radial deviation is far less than ulnar deviation. The radial sides of the nearby carpal bones quickly abut against the styloid process of the radius, thereby limiting the extent of radial deviation across the wrist.

Muscle and Joint Interaction

Innervation of the Wrist Muscles

The radial nerve courses down the posterior aspect of the forearm and supplies all the muscles that extend the wrist (Figure 6-12, A). The median and ulnar nerves travel down the anterior aspect of the forearm and innervate all the primary wrist flexor muscles (see Figure 6-12, *B* and C).

Function of the Wrist Muscles

Wrist muscles can be classified into (1) a primary set that attaches to the wrist or nearby regions and (2) a secondary set that bypasses the wrist and attaches more distally to the digits. The secondary set of muscles is also referred to as

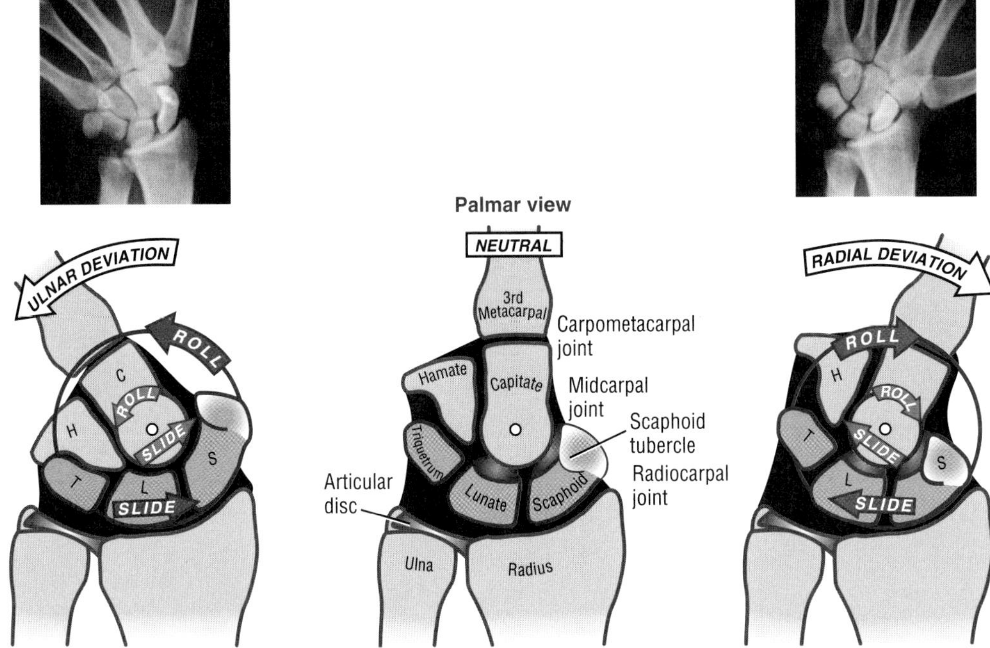

Figure 6-11 Radiographs and a mechanical model of the right wrist showing the arthrokinematics of ulnar and radial deviation. The wrist in the center is shown at rest, in a neutral position. The roll-and-slide arthrokinematics are shown in red for the radiocarpal joint and in gray for the midcarpal joint. *C*, Capitate; *H*, hamate; *L*, lunate; *S*, scaphoid; *T*, triquetrum. (From Neumann DA: *Kinesiology of the musculoskeletal system: foundations for physical rehabilitation*, St Louis, 2002, Mosby, Figure 7-15. Arthrokinetics are based on observations made from cineradiography conducted at Marquette University, Milwaukee, Wis, in 1999.)

the extrinsic muscles to the hand, the detailed anatomy of which is described in Chapter 7.

By necessity, all muscles of the wrist cross the axes of rotation located at the capitate bone and therefore produce movement at the wrist. The two axes of rotation that correspond to the two planes of motion at the wrist are shown in Figure 6-8. Flexion and extension occur about the medial-lateral axis of rotation; radial and ulnar deviation occurs about an anterior-posterior axis of rotation. The specific action of each wrist muscle is determined by the location of its tendon relative to each axis of rotation. For example, the extensor carpi ulnaris is a wrist extensor because it passes posterior to the medial-lateral axis of the wrist. As described later, the extensor carpi ulnaris is also an ulnar deviator of the wrist because it passes ulnar (or medial) to the anterior-posterior axis of the wrist.

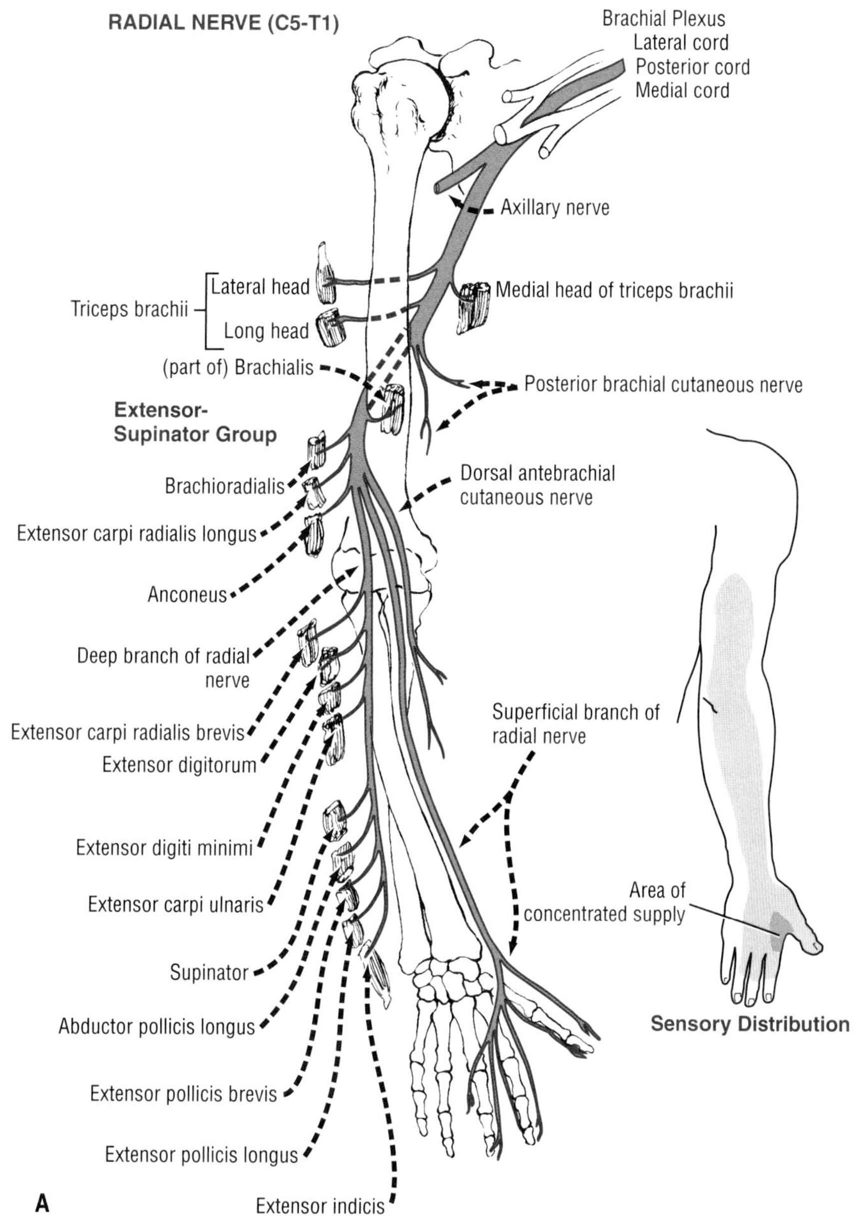

Figure 6-12 Innervations to the muscles of the wrist and hand. **A**, Radial nerve. (From Neumann DA: *Kinesiology of the musculoskeletal system: foundations for physical rehabilitation*, St Louis, 2002, Mosby, Figure 6-33, *B-D*. Modified from Waxman S: *Correlative neuroanatomy*, ed 24, New York, 2000, Lange Medical Books/McGraw-Hill.)

Continued

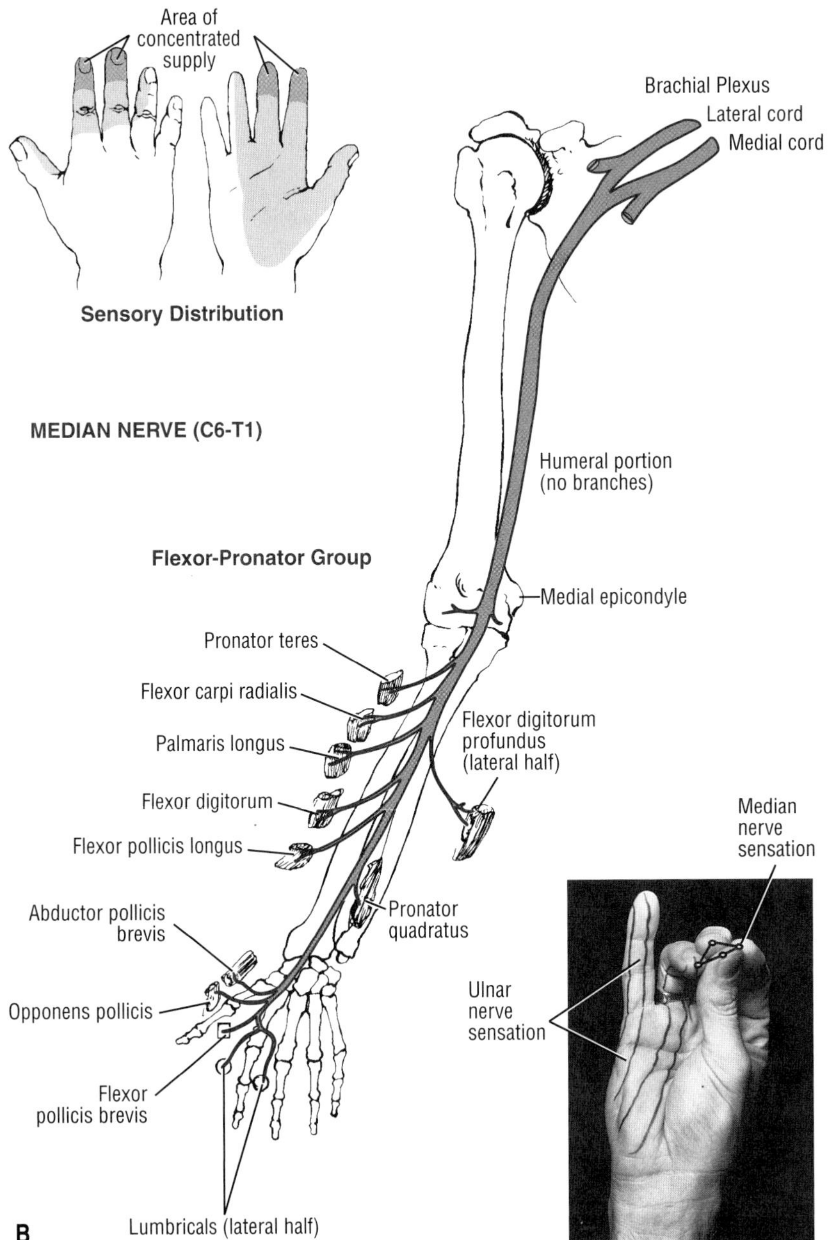

Figure 6-12, cont'd B, Median nerve. (From Neumann DA: *Kinesiology of the musculoskeletal system: foundations for physical rehabilitation*, St Louis, 2002, Mosby, Figure 6-33, *B-D*. Modified from Waxman S: *Correlative neuroanatomy,* ed 24, New York, 2000, Lange Medical Books/McGraw-Hill. Photograph by Donald A. Neumann, PT, PhD, Milwaukee, Wis.)

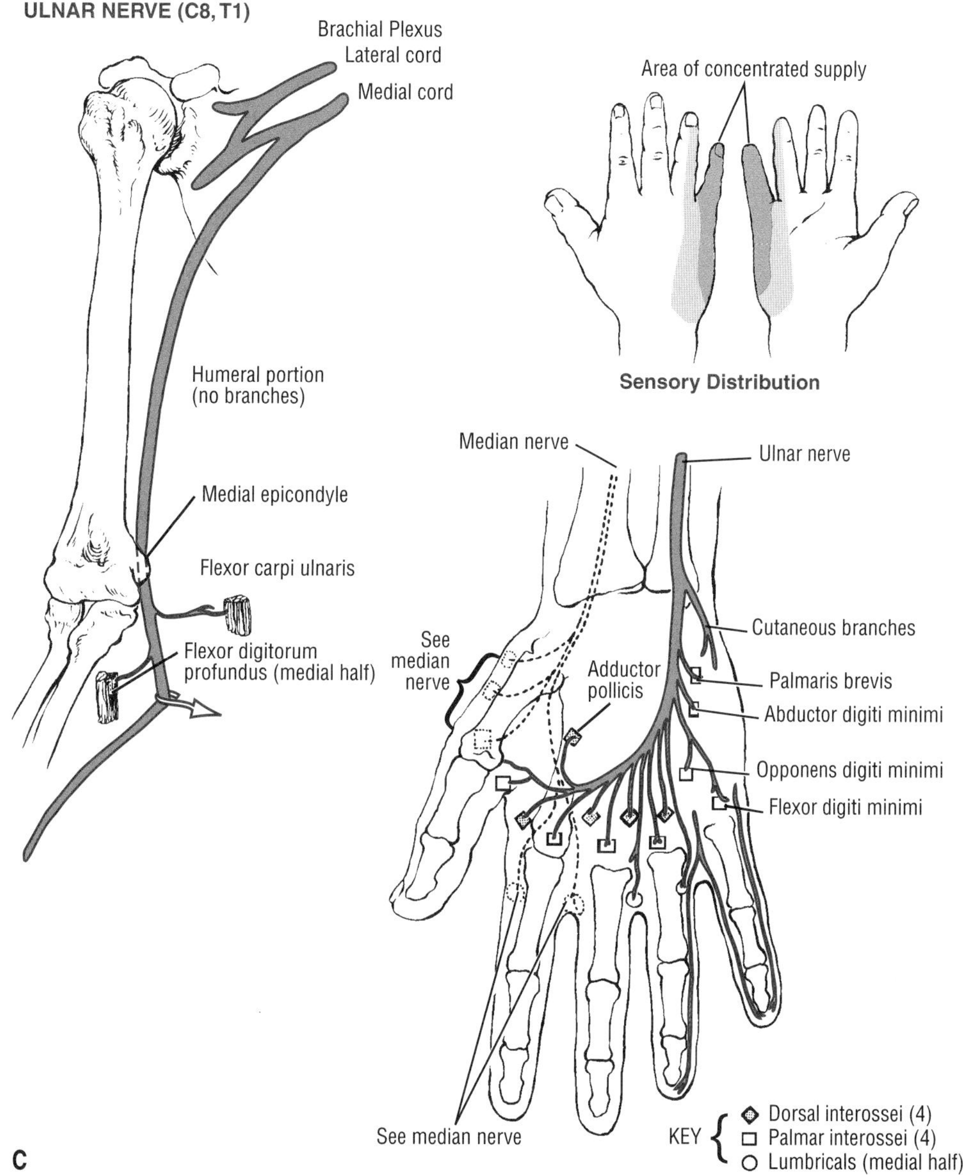

Figure 6-12, cont'd C, Ulnar nerve. (From Neumann DA: *Kinesiology of the musculoskeletal system: foundations for physical rehabilitation*, St Louis, 2002, Mosby, Figure 6-33, *B-D*. Modified from Waxman S: *Correlative neuroanatomy*, ed 24, New York, 2000, Lange Medical Books/McGraw-Hill.)

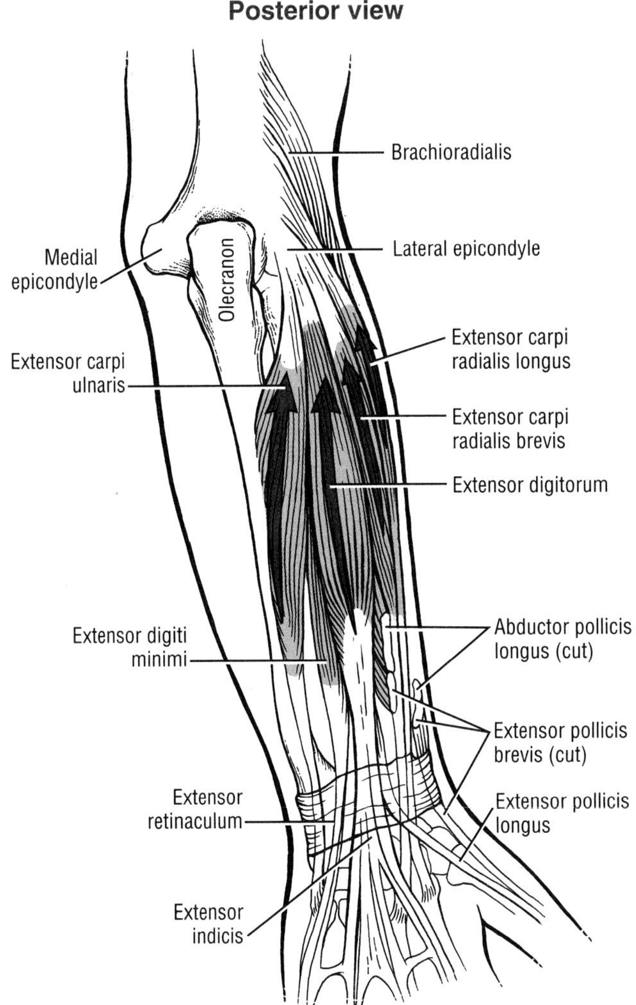

Figure 6-13 Posterior view of the right forearm highlighting the muscles within the primary set of wrist extensors: extensor carpi radialis longus, extensor carpi radialis brevis, and extensor carpi ulnaris. Many of the muscles of the secondary set of wrist extensors are also shown. (From Neumann DA: *Kinesiology of the musculoskeletal system: foundations for physical rehabilitation,* St Louis, 2002, Mosby, Figure 7-22.)

WRIST EXTENSORS

Anatomy

The primary set of wrist extensors includes the extensor carpi radialis longus, extensor carpi radialis brevis, and extensor carpi ulnaris (Figure 6-13). The secondary set of wrist extensors are the extensor digitorum, extensor indicis, extensor digiti minimi, and extensor pollicis longus—muscles that are studied in greater detail in Chapter 7.

Wrist Extensors

Primary Set
- Extensor carpi radialis longus
- Extensor carpi radialis brevis
- Extensor carpi ulnaris

Secondary Set
- Extensor digitorum
- Extensor indicis
- Extensor digiti minimi
- Extensor pollicis longus

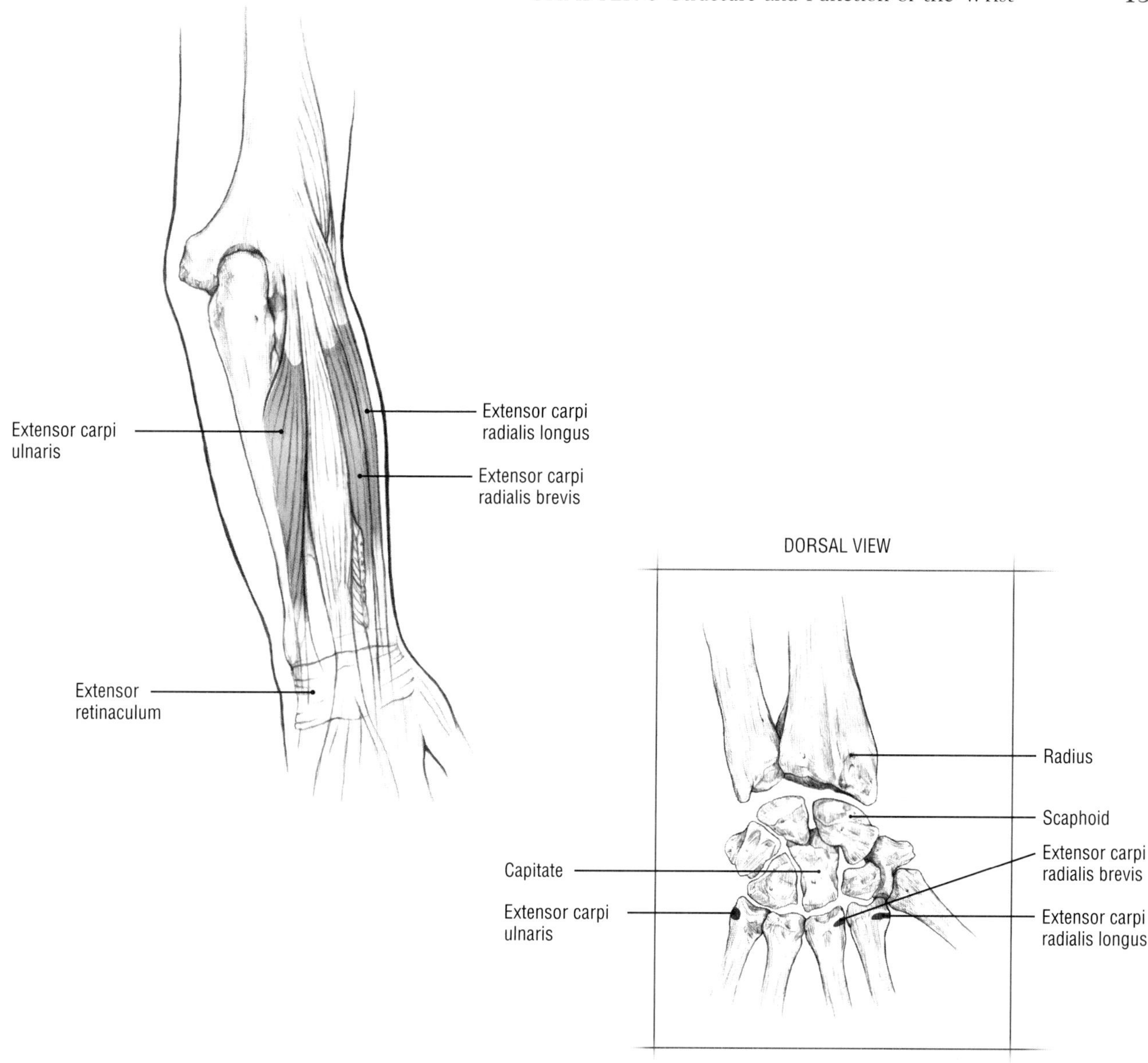

Extensor Carpi Radialis Brevis

Proximal Attachment: Lateral epicondyle of humerus—common extensor tendon

Distal Attachment: Base of the third metacarpal—dorsal aspect

Innervation: Radial nerve

Actions:
- Wrist extension
- Radial deviation

Comments: The extensor carpi radialis longus and brevis attach distally to the bases of the second and third metacarpals, respectively. Not coincidentally, these two metacarpals are rigidly attached to the distal set of carpal bones. This resulting stability helps transfer the wrist extensor forces across the entire regions of the wrist.

Extensor Carpi Radialis Longus

Proximal Attachment: Lateral epicondyle of humerus—common extensor tendon

Distal Attachment: Base of the second metacarpal—dorsal aspect

Innervation: Radial nerve

Actions:
- Wrist extension
- Radial deviation

Comments: The extensor carpi radialis longus is a more effective radial deviator of the wrist than its partner, the extensor carpi radialis brevis. The long radial wrist extensor exceeds in this function because of its farther distance from the anterior-posterior axis of rotation (through the capitate). In other words, the long radial wrist extensor has greater leverage for radial deviation than the short radial wrist extensor.

Continued

Extensor Carpi Ulnaris

Proximal Attachment: Lateral epicondyle of humerus—common extensor tendon and posterior border of the middle one third of the ulna

Distal Attachment: Base of the fifth metacarpal—dorsal aspect

Innervation: Radial nerve

Actions:
- Wrist extension
- Ulnar deviation

Comments: During active wrist extension, the extensor carpi ulnaris has the important job of neutralizing the radial deviation action of two muscles: the extensor carpi radialis longus and brevis. Once neutralized, the wrist can be extended, if desired, in the pure sagittal plane. With a ruptured tendon of the extensor carpi ulnaris, for example, wrist extension is still possible, but only when combined with radial deviation.

Functional Consideration: Wrist Extensor Activity While Making a Grasp

The main function of the wrist extensors is to position and stabilize the wrist for activities involving the fingers, especially while making a strong grasp or fist. The common muscle belly of the wrist extensors can be felt contracting on the dorsal side of the proximal forearm while rapidly tightening and releasing your fist. Contraction of the wrist extensors is necessary to prevent the wrist from collapsing into flexion because of the strong flexion pull of the extrinsic finger flexor muscles, namely the flexor digitorum profundus and flexor digitorum superficialis (Figure 6-14). Because these two strong finger flexors cross palmar (anterior) to the wrist, they generate a strong flexion torque at the wrist while they are flexing the fingers. The wrist extensor muscles, therefore, must contract every time a grasp is made; if not, the wrist collapses into unwanted flexion.

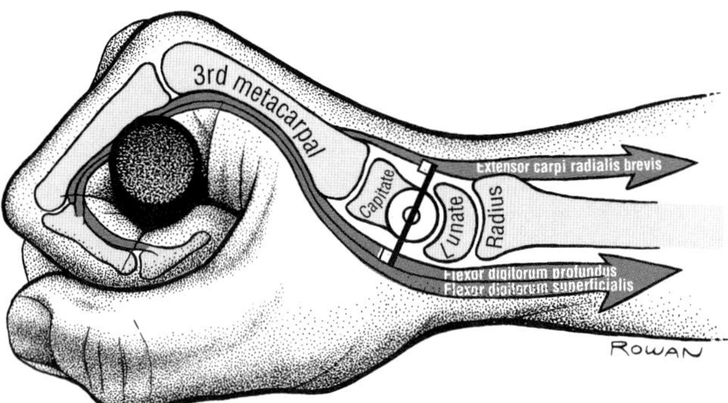

Figure 6-14 An illustration showing the importance of the wrist extensor muscles while making a strong grasp. Activation of the wrist extensors, such as the extensor carpi radialis brevis, is necessary to rule out the wrist flexion tendency caused by the activated finger flexors (flexor digitorum superficialis and profundus). In this manner, the wrist extensors are able to maintain the optimal length of the finger flexors to effectively flex the fingers. The internal moment arms for the extensor carpi radialis brevis and finger flexors are shown in dark bold lines. (From Neumann DA: *Kinesiology of the musculoskeletal system: foundations for physical rehabilitation,* St Louis, 2002, Mosby, Figure 7-24.)

Combining full wrist flexion with active flexion of the fingers results in a very ineffective grasp—something that can be verified on yourself. Normally the wrist extensor muscles hold the wrist in about 30 to 35 degrees of extension while making a grasp—a position that maintains the finger flexors at a length that is conducive to producing a strong force.

> **Clinical INSIGHT**
>
> **What Is "Tennis Elbow"?**
>
> Activities requiring repetitive forceful grasp such as hammering or playing tennis may overwork the wrist extensors, especially the extensor carpi radialis brevis. A condition known as **lateral epicondylitis**, or tennis elbow, occurs from stress and resultant inflammation of the proximal attachment of the wrist extensors. (More recently, the term *lateral epicondylalgia*—the suffix *-algia* meaning "pain"—is used in the medical literature to suggest that this painful condition may not always involve inflammation.) The small common insertion point of the wrist extensors concentrates a large force on a small area near the bony ridge of the lateral epicondyle. The large stress created at this small point is likely involved in the pathology of this painful syndrome.
>
> Clinically this condition is often treated by controlling inflammation, integrating proper stretching and strengthening regimens, and limiting the muscular activation of this group. Overuse of this group may be effectively prevented by wearing a brace that limits excessive wrist motions or a cuff that wraps around the belly of the muscles involved.

A person with paralyzed wrist extensor muscles usually has a great deal of difficulty making a grip, even when the finger flexor muscles possess normal strength. Figure 6-15 shows a person with a damaged radial nerve attempting to produce a maximum grip force on a held-hand dynamometer. Because the wrist extensors are paralyzed, attempts at producing a grip result in a posture of *combined* finger flexion and wrist flexion. This unstable and awkward position is actively inefficient for the finger flexors. Until strength is returned in the wrist extensor muscles, a wrist extension splint is usually required to brace the wrist in extension. Once braced in extension (even applied manually, as shown in Figure 6-15, *B*), the finger flexor muscles are more effective at gripping.

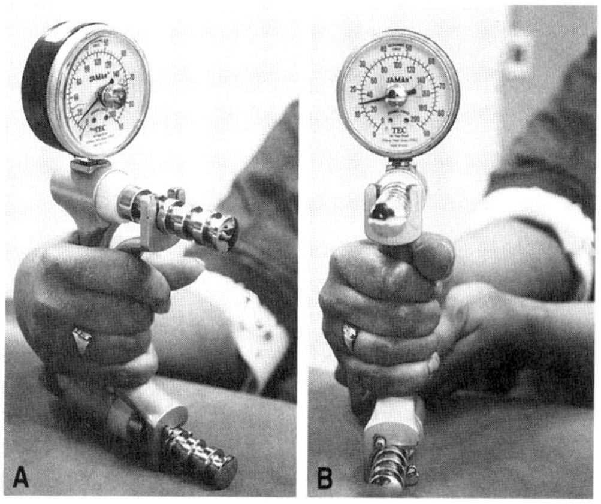

Figure 6-15 **A**, A person with paralysis of the right wrist extensor muscles, following a radial nerve injury, is performing a maximal effort grip using a dynamometer. Despite normally innervated finger flexor muscles, maximal grip strength measures only about 10 lb. **B**, With the wrist stabilized in a neutral position (by the individual's other hand), grip strength nearly triples. (From Neumann DA: *Kinesiology of the musculoskeletal system: foundations for physical rehabilitation*, St Louis, 2002, Mosby, Figure 7-26.)

WRIST FLEXORS

Anatomy

The primary set of wrist flexors includes the flexor carpi radialis, flexor carpi ulnaris, and, when present and fully formed, the palmaris longus (Figure 6-16). The tendons of these muscles are easily identified on the anterior distal wrist (Figure 6-17), especially during strong isometric activation.

The secondary set of wrist flexor muscles includes the extrinsic flexors to the digits (i.e., the flexor digitorum profundus, flexor digitorum superficialis, and flexor pollicis longus).

> **Wrist Flexors**
>
> **Primary Set**
> - Flexor carpi radialis
> - Flexor carpi ulnaris
> - Palmaris longus
>
> **Secondary Set**
> - Flexor digitorum profundus
> - Flexor digitorum superficialis
> - Flexor pollicis longus

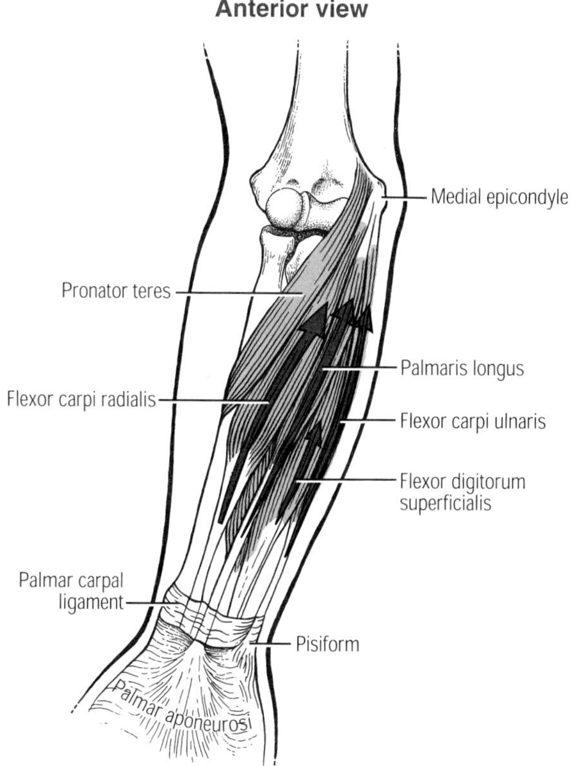

Figure 6-16 Anterior view of the right forearm highlighting the muscles within the primary set of wrist flexors: flexor carpi radialis, palmaris longus, and flexor carpi ulnaris. The flexor digitorum superficialis, a muscle of the secondary set of wrist flexors, is also shown. The pronator teres muscle is shown but does not flex the wrist. (From Neumann DA: *Kinesiology of the musculoskeletal system: foundations for physical rehabilitation*, St Louis, 2002, Mosby, Figure 7-27.)

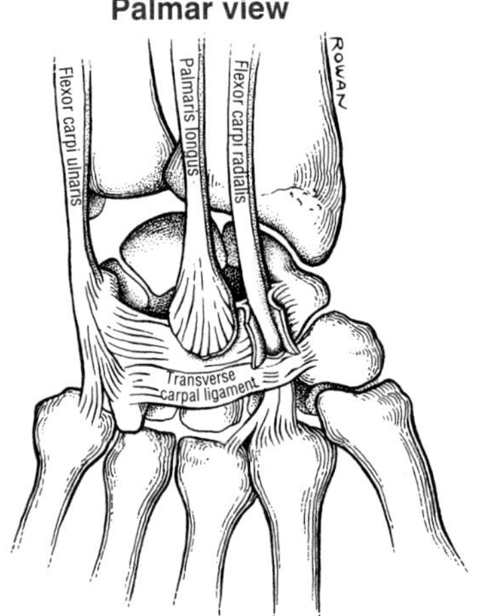

Figure 6-17 The palmar aspect of the right wrist showing the distal attachments of the three important wrist flexor muscles. Note that the tendon of the flexor carpi radialis courses through a sheath located within the superficial fibers of the transverse carpal ligament. Most of the distal attachment of the palmaris longus has been removed with the palmar aponeurosis. (From Neumann DA: *Kinesiology of the musculoskeletal system: foundations for physical rehabilitation*, St Louis, 2002, Mosby, Figure 7-28.)

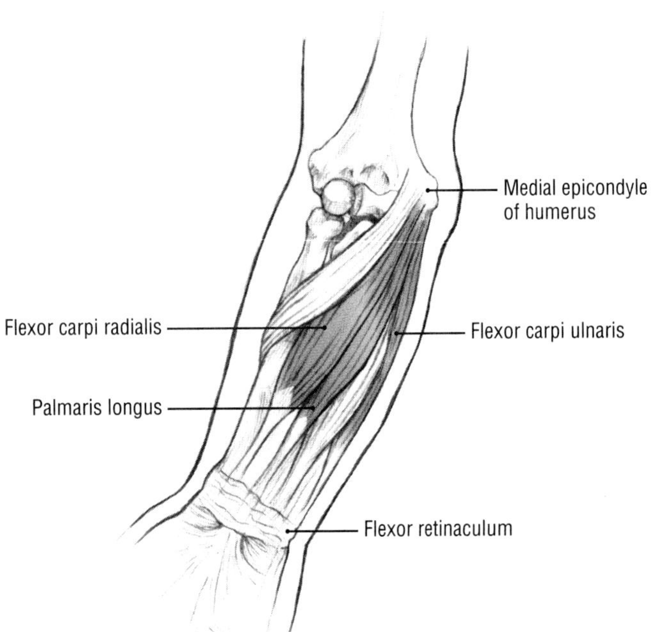

Flexor Carpi Radialis

Proximal Attachment: Medial epicondyle of humerus—common flexor tendon

Distal Attachment: Base of the second metacarpal—palmar aspect

Innervation: Median nerve

Actions:
- Wrist flexion
- Radial deviation

Comments: Interestingly, the tendon of the flexor carpi radialis does *not* reside in the carpal tunnel. How does this tendon, therefore, get to its distal attachment on the palmar side of the base of the second metacarpal? As shown in Figure 6-17, the tendon of this muscle courses in a special groove located within the transverse carpal ligament.

Flexor Carpi Ulnaris

Proximal Attachment: Medial epicondyle of humerus—common flexor tendon and posterior border of the middle one third of the ulna

Distal Attachment: Base of the fifth metacarpal and pisiform—palmar aspect

Innervation: Ulnar nerve

Actions:
- Wrist flexion
- Ulnar deviation

Comments: The distal tendon of flexor carpi ulnaris contains a palpable sesamoid bone known as the pisiform. Similar to the patella in the quadriceps muscle at the knee, the sesamoid bone at the wrist improves the leverage of the flexor carpi ulnaris during the combined action of wrist flexion and ulnar deviation.

Palmaris Longus

Proximal Attachment:	Medial epicondyle of humerus—common flexor tendon
Distal Attachment:	Transverse carpal ligament and palmar aponeurosis
Innervation:	Median nerve
Action:	Wrist flexion
Comments:	The palmaris longus is a small, thin muscle that can flex the wrist but is more often cited for its ability to tense the palmar fascia of the hand. Interestingly, about 10% of the population does not possess this muscle on one or both hands. When present, its tendon is generally visible in the middle of the palmar surface of the wrist as one strongly flexes the wrist while also cupping the palm.

Functional Consideration: Synergistic Action of the Wrist Muscles

Strong activation of all three wrist flexors is usually required while making a power grip, such as when lifting or pulling heavy objects. In this case, isometric activation of the wrist flexor muscles helps stabilize the wrist, especially against the strong activation of the wrist extensor muscles. The palmaris longus also helps stabilize the proximal attachment of many of the intrinsic muscles of the hand.

In addition to flexing the wrist, the flexor carpi radialis is a radial deviator and the flexor carpi ulnaris is an ulnar deviator. Simultaneous activity of both muscles is required to flex the wrist in the pure sagittal plane.

RADIAL AND ULNAR DEVIATORS

Muscles belonging to the primary set of radial deviators are the extensor carpi radialis longus and the extensor carpi radialis brevis (see the earlier discussion on wrist extensors). Muscles in the secondary set are the extensor pollicis longus, extensor pollicis brevis, flexor carpi radialis, abductor pollicis longus, and the flexor pollicis longus. Muscles in both sets radially deviate the wrist because their tendons pass radial (or lateral) to the anterior-posterior axis of rotation at the wrist. The extensor pollicis brevis has the greatest moment arm of all radial deviators; however, due to its small cross-sectional area, this muscle's torque production is likely small. The abductor pollicis longus and extensor pollicis brevis provide important stability to the radial side of the wrist, in conjunction with the radial collateral ligament.

The two muscles within the primary set of ulnar deviators are the extensor carpi ulnaris and the flexor carpi ulnaris.

Radial Deviators of the Wrist

Primary Set
- Extensor carpi radialis longus
- Extensor carpi radialis brevis

Secondary Set
- Extensor pollicis longus
- Extensor pollicis brevis
- Flexor carpi radialis
- Abductor pollicis longus
- Flexor pollicis longus

Ulnar Deviators of the Wrist

Primary Set
- Extensor carpi ulnaris
- Flexor carpi ulnaris

Functional Consideration: The Radial and Ulnar Deviators' Function in Grasping and Controlling Objects in the Hand

The radial and ulnar deviator muscles are frequently used for activities that involve the grasp and control of objects held within the hand. Consider the demands placed on these muscles while using a tennis racquet, casting a fishing rod, or pushing oneself in a wheelchair. Consider, also, hammering a nail into a piece of wood. Figure 6-18 shows the radial deviator muscles contracting to prepare to strike a nail with a hammer. All the muscles shown pass lateral to the wrist's anterior-posterior axis of rotation. The action of the extensor carpi radialis longus and the flexor carpi radialis (shown with moment arms) illustrates a fine example of two muscles cooperating as synergists for one action and acting as agonists or antagonists in another. By opposing each other's flexion and extension actions, the two muscles stabilize the wrist in an extended position necessary to grasp the hammer.

Figure 6-19 shows both ulnar deviator muscles contracting to strike the nail with the hammer. Both the flexor and extensor carpi ulnaris contract synergistically to perform the ulnar deviation but also stabilize the wrist in a slightly extended position. Because of the strong functional association between the flexor and extensor

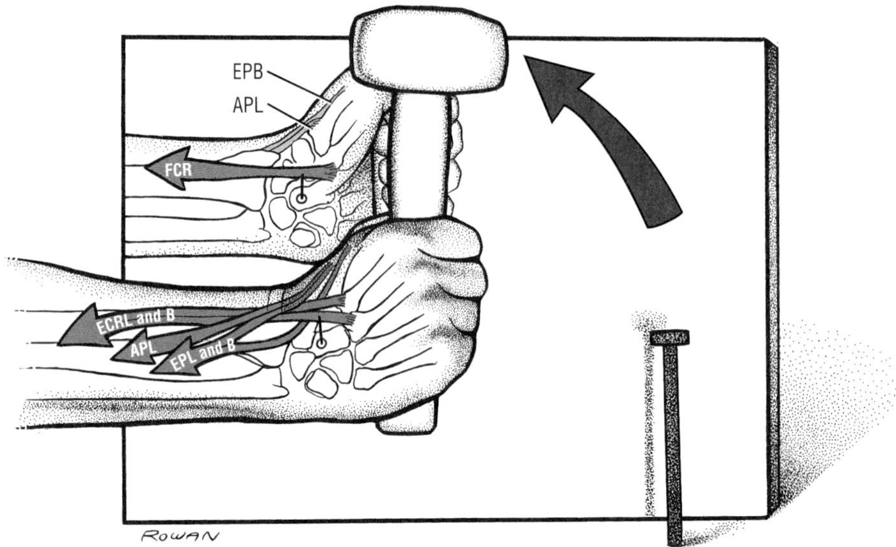

Figure 6-18 Illustration of selected muscles performing radial deviation of the wrist in preparation of striking a nail with a hammer. Image in the background is a mirror reflection of the palmar surface of the wrist. The axis of rotation is through the capitate, with the internal moment arms shown for the extensor carpi radialis brevis and the flexor carpi radialis *(FCR)* only. *APL,* Abductor pollicis longus; *ECRL and B,* extensor carpi radialis longus and brevis; *EPB,* extensor pollicis brevis; *EPL and B,* extensor pollicis longus and brevis. (From Neumann DA: *Kinesiology of the musculoskeletal system: foundations for physical rehabilitation,* St Louis, 2002, Mosby, Figure 7-29.)

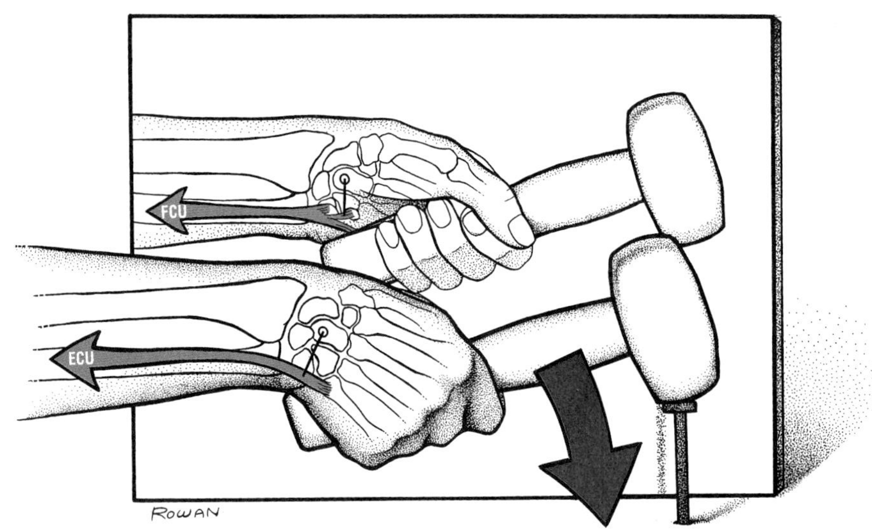

Figure 6-19 Illustration of selected muscles performing ulnar deviation of the wrist while striking a nail with a hammer. Image in the background is a mirror reflection of the palmar surface of the wrist. The axis of rotation is through the capitate, with the internal moment arms shown for the flexor carpi ulnaris *(FCU)* and the extensor carpi ulnaris *(ECU).* (From Neumann DA: *Kinesiology of the musculoskeletal system: foundations for physical rehabilitation,* St Louis, 2002, Mosby, Figure 7-30.)

carpi ulnaris muscles, injury to either muscle can disrupt the overall muscular action of ulnar deviation. For example, rheumatoid arthritis often causes inflammation and pain in the extensor carpi ulnaris tendon. Attempts at active ulnar deviation with minimal to no activation in this painful extensor muscle allow the flexion action of the flexor carpi ulnaris to go unchecked. The resulting flexed posture of the wrist is not suitable for an effective grasp.

Summary

The wrist joint is actually composed of two separate joints: the radiocarpal joint and the midcarpal joint. Although only 2 degrees of freedom are allowed at the wrist, a simple flexion/extension or radial/ulnar deviation motion requires motion at both joints.

The primary muscles of the wrist effectively stabilize and mobilize the wrist for a variety of different functions;

however, most often these muscles are responsible for positioning the hand. As presented in Chapter 7, the muscles of the wrist work in concert with the muscles of the hand to optimize the overall function of the upper extremity.

Study Questions

1. Which of the following is *not* in the proximal row of carpal bones?
   a. Scaphoid
   b. Lunate
   c. Capitate
   d. Pisiform
2. The wrist allows motion in:
   a. One plane
   b. Two planes
   c. All three planes
3. Which of the following statements is true?
   a. Complete range of motion for wrist extension is typically 0 to 25 degrees.
   b. Complete range of motion for wrist flexion is typically 0 to 80 degrees.
   c. Complete range of motion for wrist radial deviation is typically 0 to 60 degrees.
   d. Complete range of motion for wrist extension is typically 0 to 15 degrees.
4. Radial and ulnar deviation occur about:
   a. An anterior-posterior axis of rotation
   b. A medial-lateral axis of rotation
   c. A longitudinal axis of rotation
5. The wrist extensor muscles are activated when making a strong grip:
   a. To prevent the fingers from moving into an ulnar drift
   b. To prevent the wrist from collapsing into unwanted flexion
   c. To help expand the diameter of the carpal tunnel
   d. To prevent the elbow from rotating into a flexed position
6. A person with paralysis of the wrist extensor muscles would most likely display weakness of a grasping or gripping activity because:
   a. The long finger flexors are innervated by the same nerves as the wrist extensors.
   b. The wrist and the fingers will be in a flexed position, causing the long finger flexors to become actively insufficient.
   c. The wrist extensors are innervated by the same nerve as the intrinsic muscles of the hand.
   d. The wrist will likely end up in a hyperextended position.
7. The ulnar deviator muscles of the wrist:
   a. All course on the ulnar side of the anterior-posterior axis of rotation of the wrist
   b. All course on the posterior side of the medial-lateral axis of rotation of the wrist
   c. All prevent excessive flexion of the wrist
   d. All course on the radial side of the anterior-posterior axis of rotation of the wrist
8. The most pure antagonist of the flexor carpi ulnaris is the:
   a. Flexor carpi radialis
   b. Extensor carpi ulnaris
   c. Extensor carpi radialis longus
   d. Palmaris longus
9. Which of the following nerves innervates all of the wrist extensor muscles?
   a. Median nerve
   b. Ulnar nerve
   c. Radial nerve
   d. Hypothenar nerve
10. The flexor carpi radialis, flexor carpi ulnaris, and palmaris longus:
    a. Attach proximally to the lateral epicondyle of the humerus
    b. Are innervated by the ulnar nerve
    c. Attach proximally to the medial epicondyle of the humerus
    d. Are innervated by the median nerve
11. Which of the following is *not* an action of the extensor carpi radialis longus?
    a. Extension of the metacarpophalangeal joints of all four fingers
    b. Radial deviation
    c. Wrist extension
12. The axis of rotation for all motions of the wrist is through which bone?
    a. Lunate
    b. Scaphoid
    c. Capitate
    d. Trapezium
13. The median nerve travels through the carpal tunnel.
    a. True
    b. False
14. Overuse and resultant inflammation of the wrist extensors may result in lateral epicondylitis.
    a. True
    b. False
15. Most muscles that originate off the lateral epicondyle of the humerus are innervated by the radial nerve.
    a. True
    b. False
16. All of the wrist extensors course anterior to the medial-lateral axis of rotation of the wrist.
    a. True
    b. False
17. The wrist is a double-jointed system, consisting of the radiocarpal and midcarpal joints.
    a. True
    b. False
18. About 80% of the compressive force from the hand is transferred directly to the ulna.
    a. True
    b. False

19. During radial and ulnar deviation, the roll-and-slide arthrokinematics occur in opposite directions.
    a. True
    b. False
20. The sesamoid bone located within the set of carpal bones is located on which side of the wrist?
    a. Ulnar
    b. Radial

ADDITIONAL READINGS

Adams BD: Total wrist arthroplasty, *Orthopedics* 27(3):278-284, 2004.

Berger RA: The anatomy and basic biomechanics of the wrist joint, *J Hand Ther* 9(2):84-93, 1996.

Berger RA: The anatomy of the ligaments of the wrist and distal radioulnar joints, *Clin Orthop* (383):32-40, 2001.

Brumfield RH, Champoux JA: A biomechanical study of normal functional wrist motion, *Clin Orthop* (187):23-25, 1984.

Cassidy C, Ruby LK: Carpal instability, *Instr Course Lect* 52:209-220, 2003.

De Smet L: The distal radioulnar joint in rheumatoid arthritis, *Acta Orthop Belg* 72(4):381-386, 2006.

Delp SL, Grierson AE, Buchanan TS: Maximum isometric moments generated by the wrist muscles in flexion-extension and radial-ulnar deviation, *J Biomech* 29(10):1371-1375, 1996.

Kauer JM: Functional anatomy of the wrist, *Clin Orthop* (149):9-20, 1980.

Kaufmann RA, Pfaeffle HJ, Blankenhorn BD et al: Kinematics of the midcarpal and radiocarpal joint in flexion and extension: an in vitro study, *J Hand Surg [Am]* 31(7):1142-1148, 2006.

LaStayo PC, Chidgey LK: The mysterious wrist, *J Hand Ther* 9(2):81-83, 1996.

Linscheid RL: Kinematic considerations of the wrist, *Clin Orthop* (202):27-39, 1986.

MacConaill MA, Basmajian JV: *Muscles and movements: a basis for human kinesiology*, New York, 1977, Robert E. Krieger Publishing.

MacDermid JC, Wessel J: Clinical diagnosis of carpal tunnel syndrome: a systematic review, *J Hand Ther* 17(2):309-319, 2004.

Nathan RH: The isometric action of the forearm muscles, *J Biomech Eng* 114(2):162-169, 1992.

Nirschl RP, Pettrone FA: Tennis elbow: the surgical treatment of lateral epicondylitis, *J Bone Joint Surg Am* 61(6A):832-839, 1979.

Norkin CC, White DJ: *Measurement of joint motion: a guide to goniometry*, ed 2, Philadelphia, 1995, FA Davis.

Palmer AK, Werner FW, Murphy D et al: Functional wrist motion: a biomechanical study, *J Hand Surg [Am]* 10(1):39-46, 1985.

Radonjic D, Long C: Kinesiology of the wrist, *Am J Phys Med* 50(2):57-71, 1971.

Standring S: *Gray's anatomy: the anatomical basis of clinical practice*, ed 39, New York, 2005, Churchill Livingstone.

Stanley JK, Trail IA: Carpal instability, *J Bone Joint Surg Br* 76(5):691-700, 1994.

CHAPTER 7

Structure and Function of the Hand

CHAPTER OUTLINE

OBJECTIVES

- Identify the bones and primary bony features of the hand.
- Identify the carpometacarpal, metacarpophalangeal, proximal interphalangeal, and distal interphalangeal joints of the hand.
- Describe the supporting structures of the hand.
- Describe the planes of motion and axes of rotation for the motions of the hand.
- Cite the proximal and distal attachments, as well as the innervation of the muscles of the hand.
- Justify the primary actions of the muscles of the hand.
- Describe the primary mechanism that causes an ulnar drift deformity.
- Describe the mechanics of a "tenodesis" grasp action of the wrist.
- Explain the interaction between the intrinsic and extrinsic muscles when opening and closing the hand.
- Explain why the fourth and fifth digits cannot be fully extended across all interphalangeal joints following a severance of the ulnar nerve.
- Identify which active motions are lost (or severely weakened) following a cut of the median nerve at the level of the wrist.
- Explain why an injury to the radial nerve would reduce the effectiveness and strength of one's grasp.

KEY TERMS

arthritis
extensor mechanism
opposition
reposition
tenodesis action
ulnar drift

When functioning normally, the 19 bones and 19 joints of the hand produce amazingly diverse functions. The hand may be used in a primitive fashion such as a hook or a club or, more often, as a highly specialized instrument performing complex manipulations requiring multiple levels of force and precision. A hand that is totally incapacitated by **arthritis**, pain, stroke, or nerve injury, for instance, can dramatically reduce the overall function of the entire upper limb. The function of the entire upper limb depends strongly on the function of the hand.

This chapter describes the basic anatomy of the bones, joints, and muscles of the hand—information essential to understanding the impairments of the hand, as well as the treatments used to help restore its function following injury or disease.

The digits of the hand are designated numerically from one to five, or as the thumb and the index, middle, ring, and

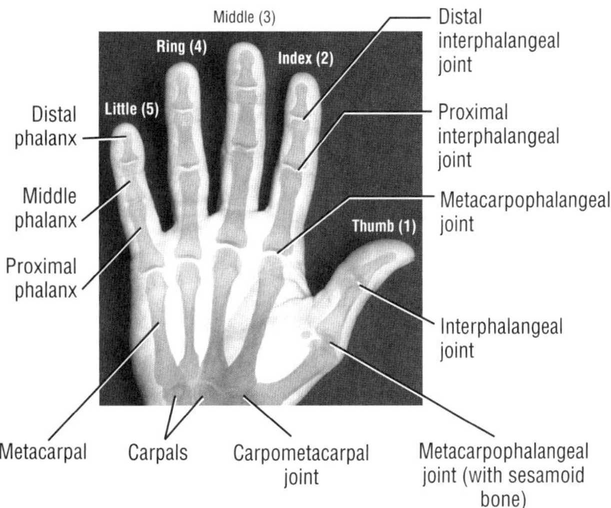

Figure 7-1 A palmar view of the major bones and joints of the hand. (From Neumann DA: *Kinesiology of the musculoskeletal system: foundations for physical rehabilitation,* St Louis, 2002, Mosby, Figure 8-3, A.)

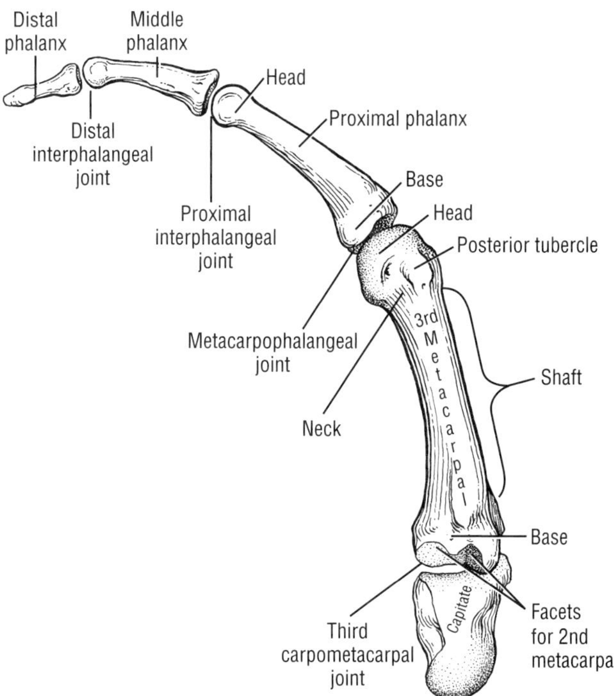

Figure 7-2 A radial view of the bones of the third ray (metacarpal and associated phalanges) including the capitate bone of the wrist. (From Neumann DA: *Kinesiology of the musculoskeletal system: foundations for physical rehabilitation,* St Louis, 2002, Mosby, Figure 8-6.)

little (small) fingers (Figure 7-1). Each of the five digits contains one metacarpal and a group of phalanges. A *ray* describes one metacarpal bone and its associated phalanges.

The articulations between the proximal end of the metacarpals and the distal row of carpal bones form the carpometacarpal joints (see Figure 7-1). The articulations between the distal end of the metacarpals and the proximal phalanges form the metacarpophalangeal joints. Each finger has two interphalangeal joints: a proximal interphalangeal and a distal interphalangeal joint. The thumb has only two phalanges and therefore only one interphalangeal joint.

Articulations Common to Each Ray of the Hand

- Carpometacarpal joint
- Metacarpophalangeal joint
- Interphalangeal joints
  - Thumb has one interphalangeal joint.
  - Fingers have a proximal interphalangeal joint and a distal interphalangeal joint.

Osteology

Metacarpals

The metacarpals, like the digits, are designated numerically as one through five, beginning on the radial (lateral) side.

Each metacarpal has the following similar anatomic characteristics: *base*, *shaft*, *head*, and *neck*. These characteristics are shown for the third ray in Figure 7-2. As indicated in Figures 7-3 and 7-4, the first (thumb) metacarpal is the shortest and thickest, and the length of the remaining bones generally decreases from the radial to ulnar (medial) direction.

Osteologic Features of a Metacarpal

- *Shaft:* Slightly concave palmarly (anteriorly)
- *Base:* Proximal end; articulates with carpal bones
- *Head:* Distal end: forms the "knuckles" on the dorsal side of a clenched fist
- *Neck:* Slightly constricted region just proximal to the head; common site for fracture, especially the fifth digit

With the hand at rest in the anatomic position, the thumb's metacarpal is oriented in a different plane than the other digits. The second through the fifth metacarpals are aligned generally side by side, with their palmar surfaces facing anteriorly. The position of the thumb's metacarpal, however, is rotated almost 90 degrees medially (i.e., internally), relative to the other digits (see Figure 7-1). This rotated position places the sensitive palmar surface of the thumb toward the midline of the hand. In addition, the thumb's metacarpal is positioned well anterior, or palmar,

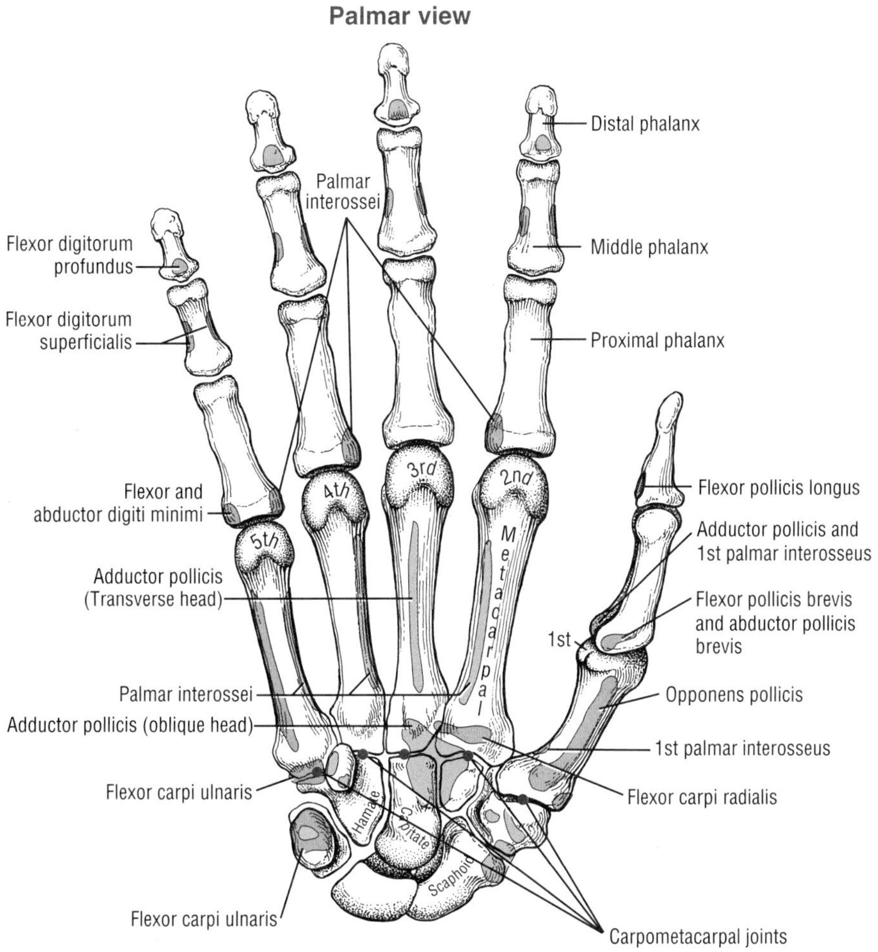

Palmar view

Distal phalanx
Palmar interossei
Flexor digitorum profundus
Middle phalanx
Flexor digitorum superficialis
Proximal phalanx
3rd
4th
2nd
Flexor and abductor digiti minimi
Flexor pollicis longus
5th
Metacarpal
Adductor pollicis and 1st palmar interosseus
Adductor pollicis (Transverse head)
Flexor pollicis brevis and abductor pollicis brevis
1st
Palmar interossei
Opponens pollicis
Adductor pollicis (oblique head)
1st palmar interosseus
Flexor carpi ulnaris
Flexor carpi radialis
Hamate
Capitate
Scaphoid
Flexor carpi ulnaris
Carpometacarpal joints

Figure 7-3 A palmar view of the bones of the right wrist and hand. Proximal attachments of muscle are indicated in red, and distal attachments in gray. (Modified from Neumann DA: *Kinesiology of the musculoskeletal system: foundations for physical rehabilitation*, St Louis, 2002, Mosby, Figure 8-4.)

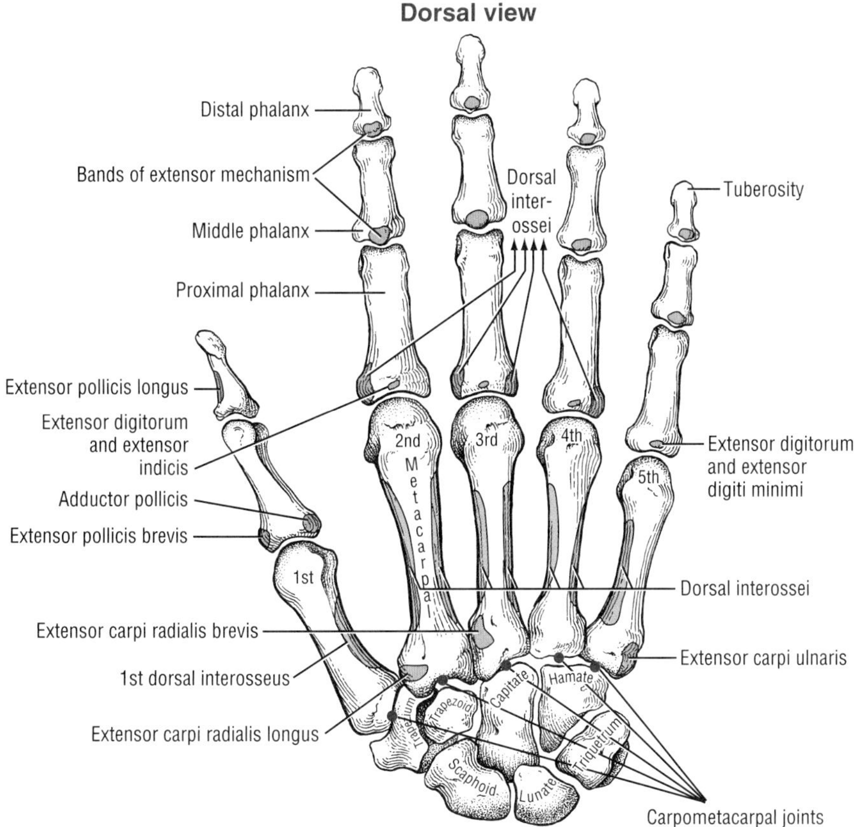

Figure 7-4 A dorsal view of the bones of the right wrist and hand. Proximal attachments of muscle are indicated in red, and distal attachments in gray. (Modified from Neumann DA: *Kinesiology of the musculoskeletal system: foundations for physical rehabilitation*, St Louis, 2002, Mosby, Figure 8-5.)

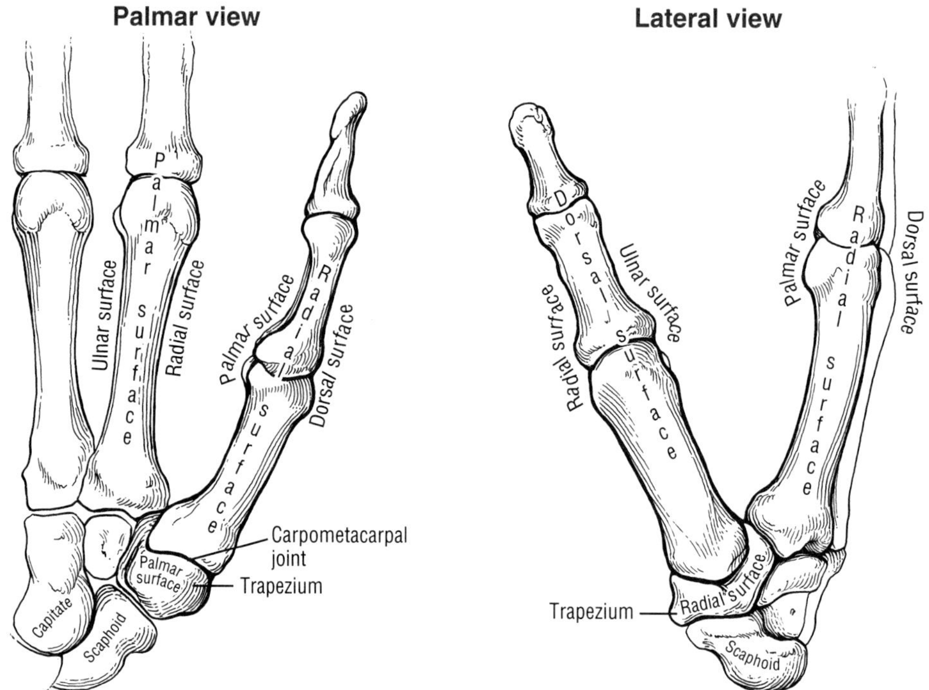

Figure 7-5 Palmar and lateral views of the hand showing the orientation of the bony surfaces of the right thumb. Note that the bones of the thumb are rotated 90 degrees relative to the other bones of the wrist and the hand. (From Neumann DA: *Kinesiology of the musculoskeletal system: foundations for physical rehabilitation*, St Louis, 2002, Mosby, Figure 8-8.)

to the other metacarpals. This can be verified by observing your own relaxed hand. The location of the first metacarpal allows the entire thumb to sweep freely across the palm toward the fingers. Virtually all motions of the hand require the thumb to interact with the fingers. Without a healthy and mobile thumb, the overall function of the hand is significantly reduced.

The medially rotated thumb requires unique terminology to describe its movement and position. In the anatomic position the dorsal surface of the bones of the thumb (i.e., the surface where the thumbnail resides) faces laterally (Figure 7-5). Therefore the palmar surface faces medially, the radial surface anteriorly, and the ulnar surface posteriorly. The terminology to describe the surfaces of the carpal bones and all the bones of the fingers is standard: The palmar surface faces anteriorly, radial surface faces laterally, and so forth.

Phalanges

The hand has 14 phalanges. The phalanges within each finger are referred to as *proximal*, *middle*, and *distal* (see Figures 7-3 and 7-4). The thumb has only a proximal and a distal phalanx. Except for differences in sizes, all phalanges within a particular digit have similar morphology (see Figure 7-2).

> **Osteologic Features of a Phalanx**
>
> - Base: Proximal end; articulates with the head of the more proximal-located bone
> - Shaft
> - Head (proximal and middle phalanx only)
> - Tuberosity (distal phalanx only)

Arches of the Hand

Observe the natural arched curvature of the palmar surface of your relaxed hand. Control of this concavity allows the human hand to securely hold and manipulate objects of many and varied shapes and sizes. This palmar concavity is supported by three integrated arch systems: two transverse and one longitudinal (Figure 7-6). The *proximal transverse arch* is formed by the distal row of carpal bones. This is a static, rigid arch that forms the *carpal tunnel*, permitting passage of the median nerve and many flexor tendons coursing toward the digits. Like most arches in buildings and bridges, the arches of the hand are supported by a central *keystone* structure. The capitate bone is the keystone of the proximal transverse arch.

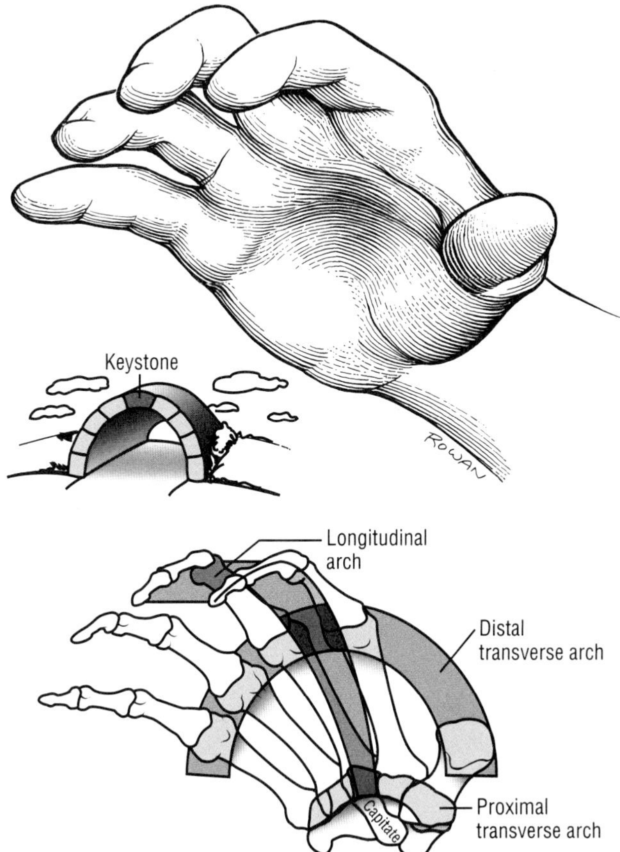

Figure 7-6 The natural concavity of the palm of the hand is supported by three integrated arch systems: one longitudinal and two transverse. (From Neumann DA: *Kinesiology of the musculoskeletal system: foundations for physical rehabilitation*, St Louis, 2002, Mosby, Figure 8-9.)

The *distal transverse arch* of the hand passes through the metacarpophalangeal joints. In contrast to the rigid proximal arch, the ulnar and radial sides of the distal arch are relatively mobile. To appreciate this mobility, imagine transforming your completely flat hand into a cup shape that surrounds a baseball. Transverse flexibility within the hand occurs as the peripheral metacarpals (first, fourth, and fifth) fold around the more stable central (second and third) metacarpals. The keystone of the distal transverse arch is formed by the metacarpophalangeal joints of these central metacarpals.

The *longitudinal arch* of the hand follows the general shape of the second and third rays. These relatively rigid articulations provide an important element of longitudinal stability to the hand.

Arthrology

Before progressing to the study of the joints, the terminology that describes the movement of the digits must be defined. The following descriptions assume that a particular movement starts from the anatomic position, with the elbow extended, forearm fully supinated, and wrist in a neutral position. Movement of the fingers is described in the standard fashion using the cardinal planes of the body: Flexion and extension occur in the sagittal plane, and abduction and adduction occur in the frontal plane (Figure 7-7, *A-D*). In most other regions of the body, abduction and adduction describe movement of a bony segment toward or away from the midline of the body; however, abduction and adduction of the fingers is described as motion toward (adduction) or away (abduction) from the middle finger.

Because the entire thumb is rotated almost 90 degrees in relation to the fingers, the terminology used to describe thumb movement is different from that for the fingers (Figure 7-7, *E-I*). Flexion is the movement of the palmar surface of the thumb in the frontal plane across and parallel with the palm. Extension returns the thumb back towards its anatomic position. Abduction is the forward movement of the thumb away from the palm in a sagittal plane. Adduction returns the thumb to the plane of the hand. Opposition is a special term describing the movement of the thumb across the palm, making direct contact with the tips of any of the fingers. This special terminology used to define the movement of the thumb serves as the basis for the naming of the "pollicis" (thumb) muscles; for example, the opponens pollicis, extensor pollicis longus, and the adductor pollicis.

Carpometacarpal Joints

OVERVIEW

The carpometacarpal (CMC) joints of the hand form the articulation between the distal row of carpal bones and the bases of the five metacarpal bones. These joints are positioned at the extreme proximal region of the hand (see Figures 7-3 and 7-4).

The basis for all movements within the hand starts at the CMC joints—at the most proximal region of each ray. Figure 7-8 shows a simplified illustration of the relative mobility at the CMC joints. The joints of the second and third digits shown in gray are rigidly joined to the distal row of carpal bones, forming a stable central pillar throughout the hand. In contrast, the peripheral CMC joints (shown in red) form mobile radial and ulnar borders, which are capable of folding around the hand's central pillar.

The first CMC joint (known as the thumb's saddle joint) is the most mobile, especially during the movement of opposition. (The CMC joint of the thumb is extremely important and is described separately in a subsequent section.) The fourth and fifth CMC joints are the next most mobile CMC joints, allowing a cupping motion of the ulnar border of the hand. The increased mobility of the fourth and fifth CMC joints improves the effectiveness of grasp and enhances the functional interaction with the opposing thumb.

The CMC joints of the hand transform the palm into a gentle concavity, greatly improving dexterity. This feature

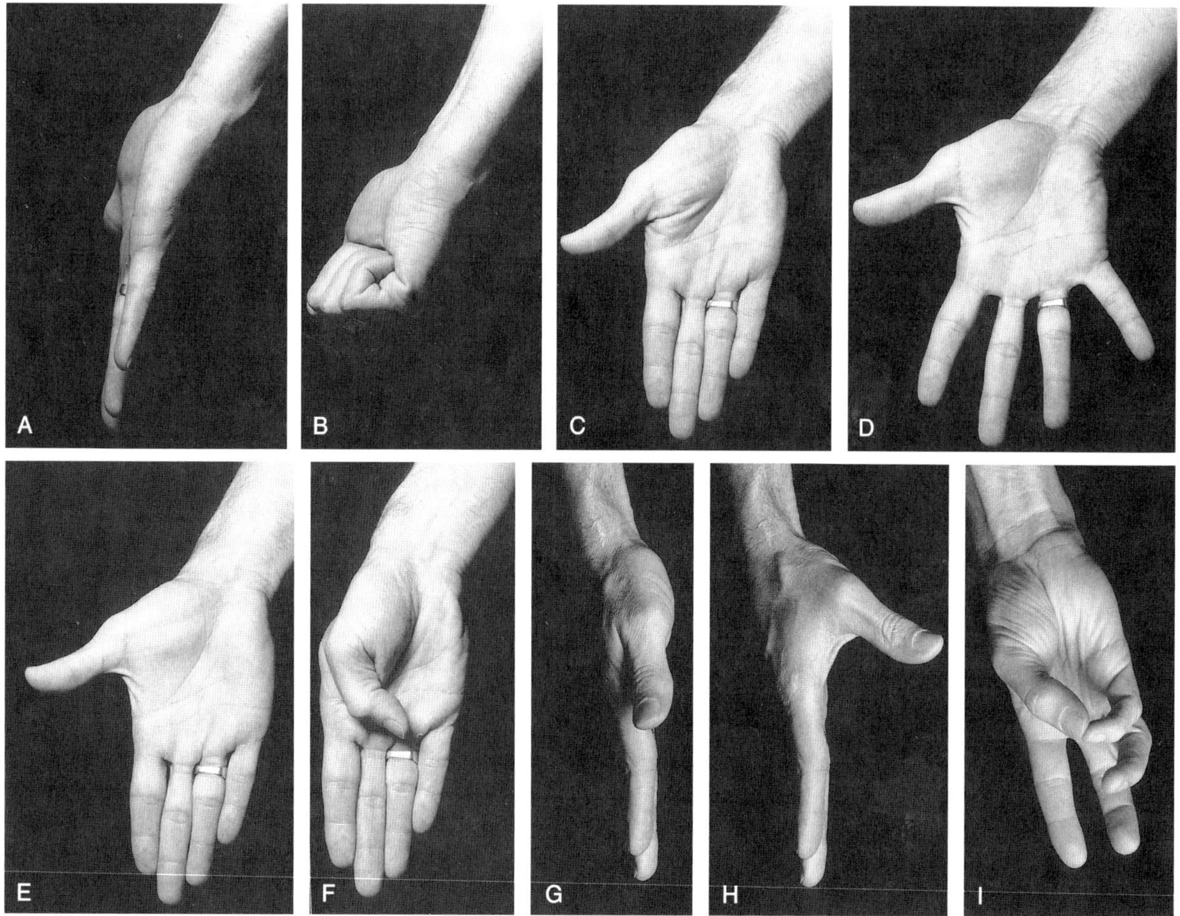

Figure 7-7 The system for naming the movements within the hand. **A-D**, Finger motion. **E-I**, Thumb motion. (**A**, Finger extension; **B**, finger flexion; **C**, finger adduction; **D**, finger abduction; **E**, thumb extension; **F**, thumb flexion; **G**, thumb adduction; **H**, thumb abduction; and **I**, thumb opposition.) (From Neumann DA: *Kinesiology of the musculoskeletal system: foundations for physical rehabilitation*, St Louis, 2002, Mosby, Figure 8-10.)

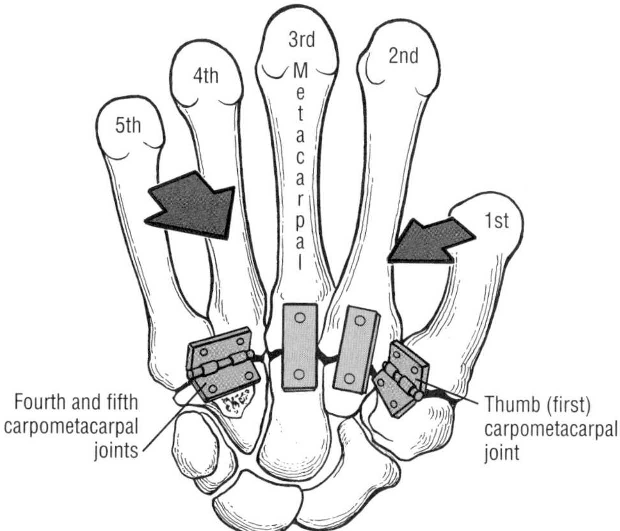

Figure 7-8 Palmar view of the right hand showing a highly mechanical depiction of the mobility across the five carpometacarpal joints. The peripheral joints—the first, fourth, and fifth *(red)*—are much more mobile than the central two joints *(gray)*. (From Neumann DA: *Kinesiology of the musculoskeletal system: foundations for physical rehabilitation*, St Louis, 2002, Mosby, Figure 8-11.)

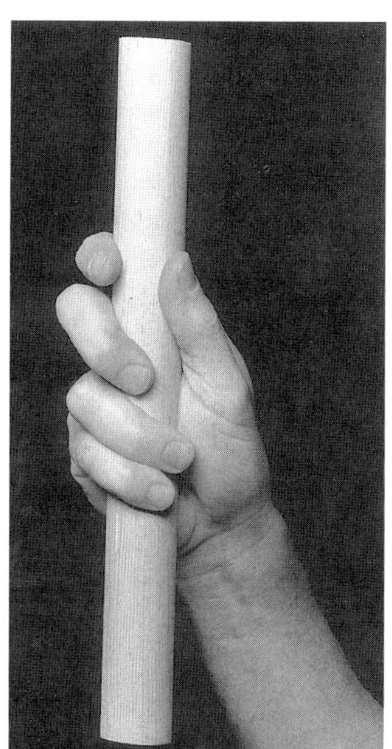

Figure 7-9 The mobility of the carpometacarpal joints of the hand enhances the security of grasping objects such as this cylindrical pole. (From Neumann DA: *Kinesiology of the musculoskeletal system: foundations for physical rehabilitation*, St Louis, 2002, Mosby, Figure 8-12.)

is one of the most impressive functions of the human hand. Cylindrical objects, for example, can fit snugly into the palm, with the index and middle digits positioned to reinforce grasp (Figure 7-9). Without this ability, the dexterity of the hand is reduced to a primitive hinge-like grasping motion.

CARPOMETACARPAL JOINT OF THE THUMB

The CMC joint of the thumb is located at the base of the first ray, between the metacarpal and the trapezium (see Figure 7-5). This joint is by far the most complex and likely most important of the CMC joints, enabling extensive movements of the thumb. Its unique saddle shape allows the thumb to fully oppose, thereby easily contacting the tips of the other digits. Through this action, the thumb is able to encircle objects held within the palm.

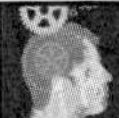

Consider this...

Osteoarthritis at the Base of the Thumb

The large functional demand placed on the carpometacarpal (CMC) joint of the thumb often results in a painful condition called basilar joint osteoarthritis. The term *basilar* refers to the CMC joint being located at the base of the entire thumb. This common condition receives more surgical attention than any other osteoarthritis-related condition of the upper limb. Arthritis may develop at this joint secondary to acute injury or, more likely, from normal wear and tear associated with a physical occupation or hobby. Interestingly, persons who needlepoint or milk cows for many years frequently develop painful arthritis at the base of their thumb.

Persons who require medical attention for basilar joint arthritis typically present foremost with pain, but also with functional limitations, ligamentous laxity (looseness), and instability of the joint. The loss of pain-free function of the thumb markedly reduces the functional potential of the entire hand and thus the entire upper extremity. Persons with advanced arthritis of the base of the thumb demonstrate severe pain (made worse by pinching actions), weakness, swelling, dislocation, and crepitation (abnormal popping or clicking sounds that occur with movement). This condition occurs with a disproportionately greater frequency in females, typically in their fifth and sixth decades.

The more common conservative therapeutic intervention for basilar joint arthritis includes splinting, careful use of nonstrenuous exercise, physical modalities such as cold and heat, non-steroidal anti-inflammatory drugs, and corticosteroid injections. In addition, patients are instructed in ways to modify their activities of daily living to protect the base of their thumb from unnecessarily large forces.

Surgical intervention is typically used when conservative therapy is unable to retard the progression of pain or the instability.

The capsule that surrounds the CMC joint of the thumb is naturally loose to allow a large range of motion. The capsule, however, is strengthened by stronger ligaments and by the forces produced by the over-riding musculature. Rupture of ligaments secondary to trauma, overuse, or arthritis often causes a dislocation of the joint, forming a characteristic hump at the base of the thumb.

Saddle Joint Structure

The CMC joint of the thumb is the classic saddle joint of the body (Figure 7-10). The characteristic feature of a saddle joint is that each articular surface is convex in one dimension and concave in the other—just like the saddle on a horse. This shape allows maximal mobility *and* stability.

Kinematics

The motions at the CMC joint occur primarily in 2 degrees of freedom (Figure 7-11). Abduction and adduction occur generally in the sagittal plane, and flexion and extension occur generally in the frontal plane. **Opposition** and **reposition** of the thumb are special movements that incorporate the two primary planes of motion. The kinematics of opposition and reposition are discussed following the description of the two primary motions.

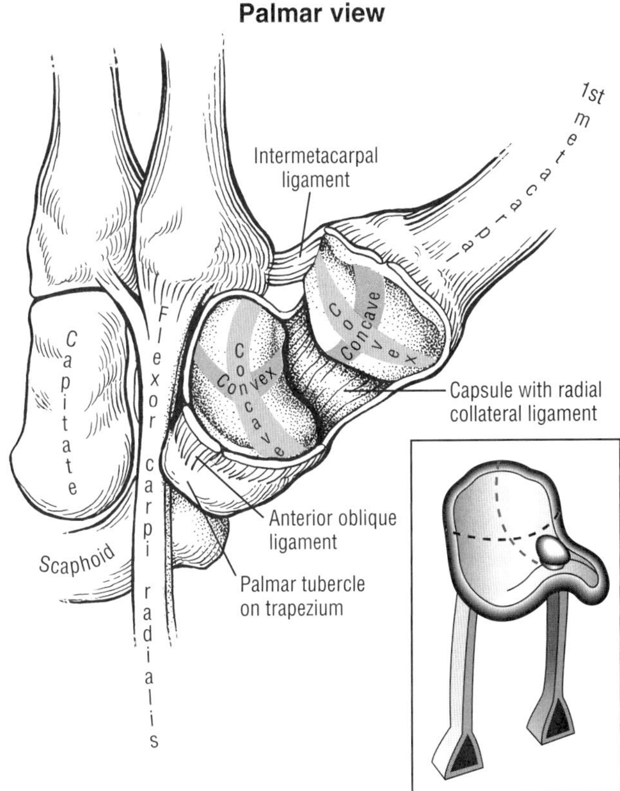

Figure 7-10 The carpometacarpal of the right thumb is opened to expose the saddle shape of the joint. The longitudinal diameters are shown in gray, and the transverse diameters in red. (From Neumann DA: *Kinesiology of the musculoskeletal system: foundations for physical rehabilitation*, St Louis, 2002, Mosby, Figure 8-17.)

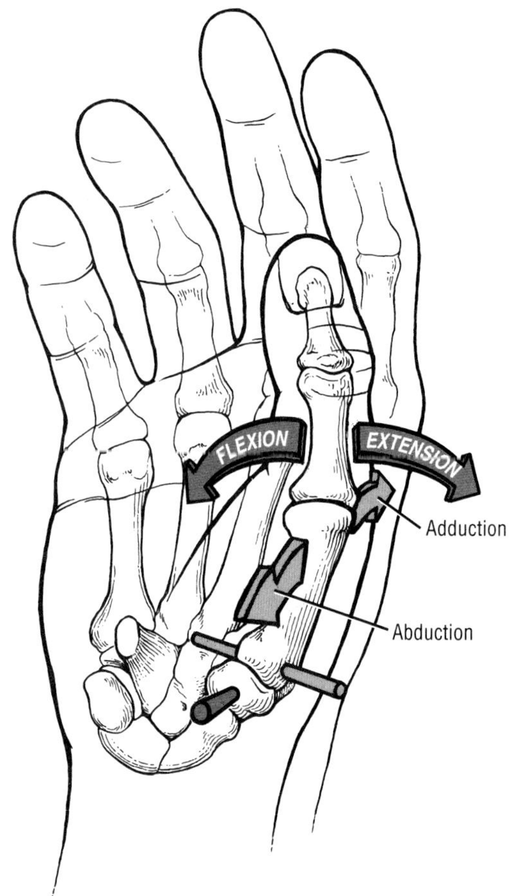

Figure 7-11 The primary biplanar osteokinematics at the carpometacarpal joint of the right thumb. Note that abduction and adduction occur about a medial-lateral axis of rotation *(gray);* flexion and extension occur about an anterior-posterior axis of rotation *(red).* The more complex motion of opposition requires a combination of these two primary motions. (From Neumann DA: *Kinesiology of the musculoskeletal system: foundations for physical rehabilitation,* St Louis, 2002, Mosby, Figure 8-18.)

Abduction and Adduction. In the (neutral) position of adduction of the CMC joint, the thumb lies within the plane of the hand. Maximum abduction, in contrast, positions the thumb metacarpal about 45 degrees anterior to the plane of the palm. Full abduction opens the web space of the thumb, forming a wide concave curvature useful for grasping objects like a coffee cup (Figure 7-12).

Flexion and Extension. Actively performing flexion and extension of the CMC joint of the thumb is associated with varying amounts of axial rotation (spinning) of the metacarpal. During flexion, the metacarpal rotates slightly medially (i.e., toward the third digit); during extension, the metacarpal rotates slightly laterally (i.e., away from the third digit). The axial rotation is evident by watching the change in orientation of the nail of the thumb between full extension and full flexion.

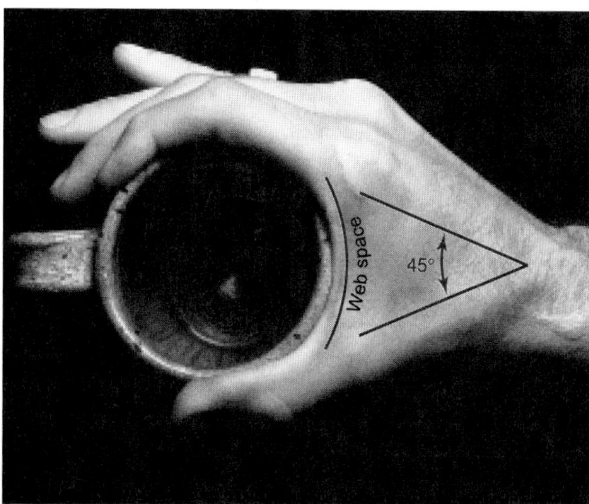

Figure 7-12 Maximum abduction of the carpometacarpal joint of the thumb opens the web space of the thumb. (From Neumann DA: *Kinesiology of the musculoskeletal system: foundations for physical rehabilitation,* St Louis, 2002, Mosby, Figure 8-19 *A.*)

In the anatomic position the CMC joint can be extended an additional 10 to 15 degrees. From full extension, the thumb metacarpal flexes across the palm about 45 to 50 degrees.

Opposition. The ability to precisely oppose the thumb to the tips of the other fingers is perhaps the ultimate expression of functional health of this digit and, arguably, of the entire hand. This complex motion is a composite of the other primary motions already described for the CMC joint.

For ease of discussion, Figure 7-13, *A,* shows the full arc of opposition divided into two phases. In phase 1, the thumb metacarpal abducts. In phase 2, the abducted metacarpal flexes and medially rotates across the palm toward the small finger. Figure 7-13, *B,* shows the detail of the kinematics of this complex movement. Muscle force, especially from the opponens pollicis, helps guide and rotate the metacarpal to the extreme medial side of the articular surface of the trapezium.

As evident by the change in orientation of the thumbnail, full opposition incorporates at least 45 to 60 degrees of medial rotation of the thumb. The small finger contributes indirectly to opposition through a cupping motion at the fifth CMC joint. This motion allows the tip of the thumb to more easily contact the tip of the little finger.

Metacarpophalangeal Joints

FINGERS

General Features and Ligaments

The metacarpophalangeal (MCP) joints, or knuckles, of the fingers are relatively large articulations formed between the convex heads of the metacarpals and the shallow concave proximal surfaces of the proximal phalanges (Figure 7-14). Motion at the MCP joint occurs predominantly in two

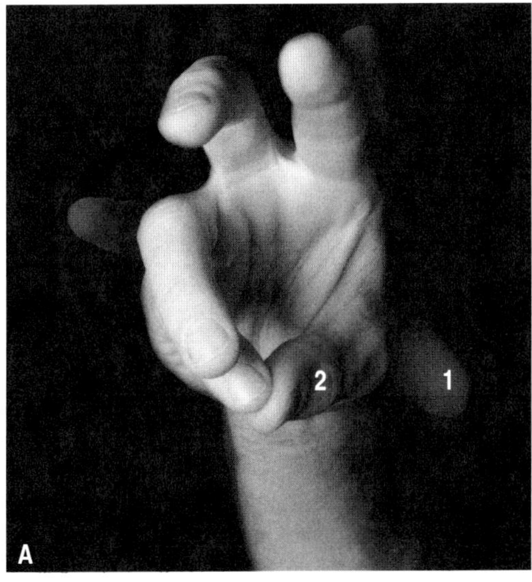

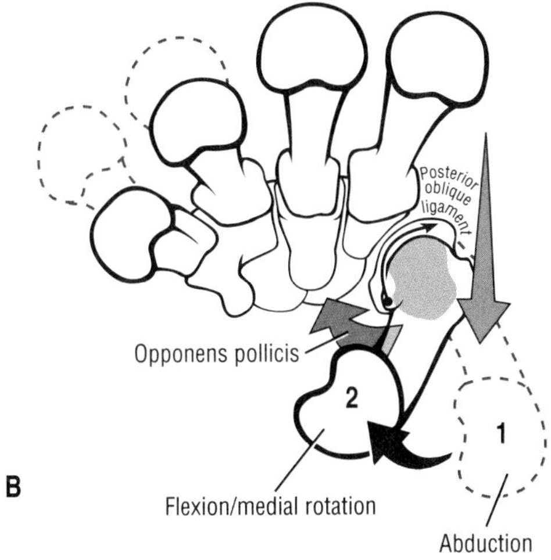

Figure 7-13 The kinematics of opposition of the carpometacarpal joint of the thumb. **A**, Two phases of opposition are shown: *(1)* abduction and *(2)* flexion with medial rotation. **B**, The detailed kinematics of the two phases of opposition: The posterior oblique ligament is shown taut, and the opponens pollicis is shown contracting *(red)*. (From Neumann DA: *Kinesiology of the musculoskeletal system: foundations for physical rehabilitation*, St Louis, 2002, Mosby, Figure 8-22.)

planes: (1) flexion and extension in the sagittal plane and (2) abduction and adduction in the frontal plane

Mechanical stability at the MCP joint is critical to the overall biomechanics of the hand. As discussed earlier, the MCP joints serve as keystones that support the mobile arches of the hand. In the healthy hand, stability at the MCP joints is achieved by an elaborate set of interconnecting connective tissues (Figure 7-15).

Supporting Structures

Figure 7-15 illustrates many of the supporting structures of MCP joints.

- *Capsule*: Connective tissue that surrounds and stabilizes the MCP joint

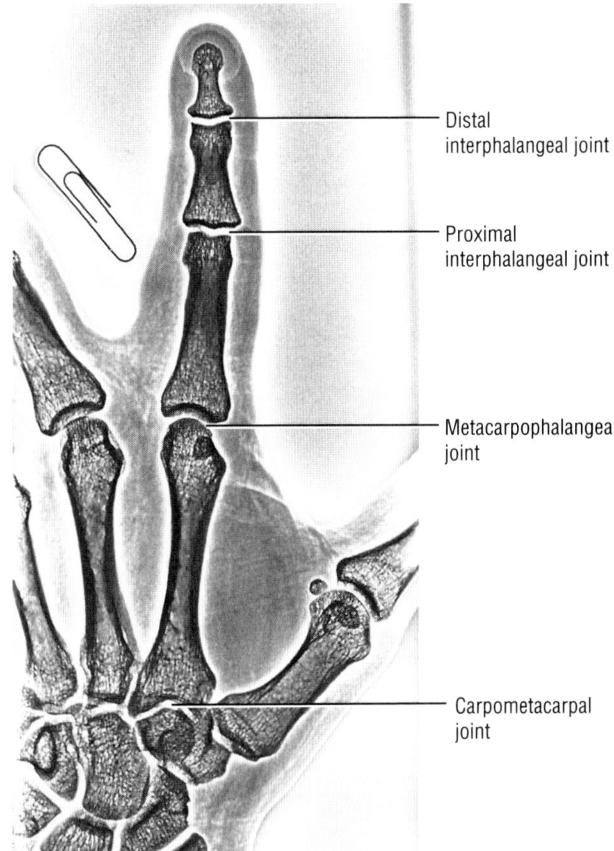

Figure 7-14 The joints of the index finger. (From Neumann DA: *Kinesiology of the musculoskeletal system: foundations for physical rehabilitation*, St Louis, 2002, Mosby, Figure 8-23.)

- *Radial and Ulnar Collateral Ligaments*: Cross the MCP joints in an oblique palmar direction; limit abduction and adduction; become taut on flexion
- *Fibrous Digital Sheaths*: Form tunnels or pulleys for the extrinsic finger flexor tendons; contain synovial sheaths to help lubrication
- *Palmar (or Volar) Plates*: Thick fibrocartilage ligaments or "plates" that cross the palmar side of each MCP joint; these structures limit hyperextension of the MCP joints
- *Deep Transverse Metacarpal Ligaments*: These three ligaments merge into a wide, flat structure that interconnects and loosely binds the second through the fifth metacarpals

As shown in Figure 7-15, the concave component of an MCP joint is extensive, formed by the articular surface of the proximal phalanx, the collateral ligaments, and the dorsal surface of the palmar plate. These tissues form a three-sided receptacle aptly suited to accept the large metacarpal head. This structure adds to the stability of the joint and also increases the area of articular contact.

KINEMATICS

In addition to the motions of flexion and extension and abduction and adduction at the MCP joints, substantial

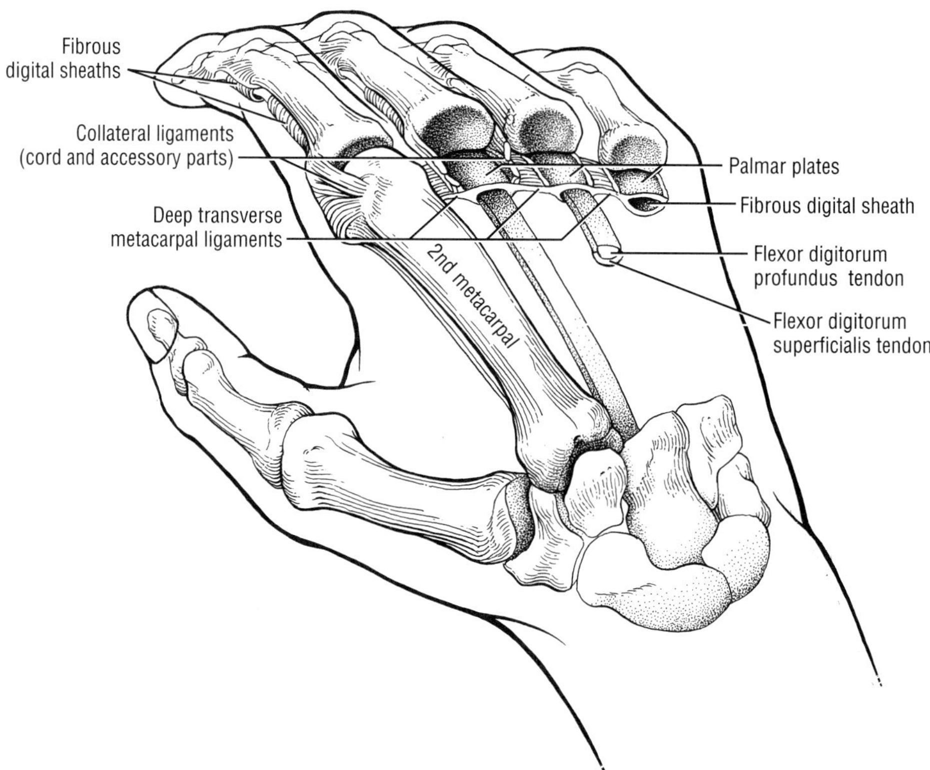

Figure 7-15 A dorsal view of the hand with emphasis on the periarticular connective tissues at the metacarpophalangeal joints. Several metacarpal bones have been removed to expose various joint structures. (From Neumann DA: *Kinesiology of the musculoskeletal system: foundations for physical rehabilitation,* St Louis, 2002, Mosby, Figure 8-25.)

accessory motions are possible. With the MCP joint relaxed and nearly extended, appreciate on your own hand the amount of passive mobility of the proximal phalanx relative to the head of the metacarpal. These accessory motions permit the fingers to better conform to the shapes of held objects, thereby increasing control of grasp (Figure 7-16).

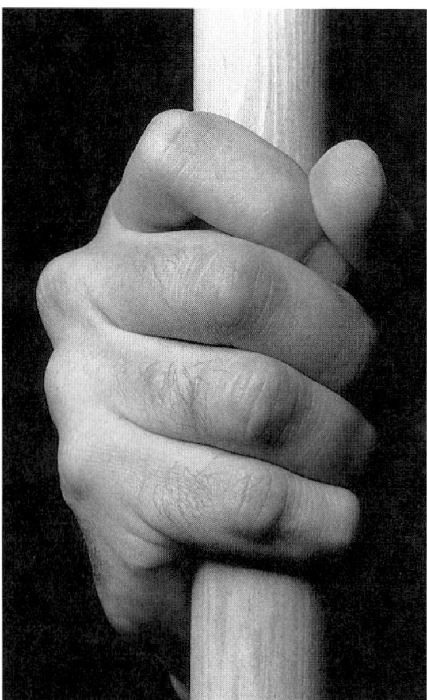

Figure 7-16 The passive accessory motions at the metacarpophalangeal joints during the grasp of a cylinder. Axial rotation of the index finger is most notable. (From Neumann DA: *Kinesiology of the musculoskeletal system: foundations for physical rehabilitation,* St Louis, 2002, Mosby, Figure 8-26.)

Metacarpophalangeal Joints of the Fingers Permit Volitional Movements Primarily in 2 Degrees of Freedom

- Flexion and extension occur in the sagittal plane about a medial-lateral axis of rotation.
- Abduction and adduction occur in the frontal plane about an anterior-posterior axis of rotation.

Figure 7-17 shows the kinematics of flexion of the MCP joints, controlled by two finger flexor muscles: flexor digitorum superficialis and flexor digitorum profundus. Flexion stretches and therefore increases tension in both the dorsal part of the capsule and the collateral ligaments. In the healthy state, this passive tension helps guide the joint's natural arthrokinematics. The increased tension in the dorsal capsule and collateral ligaments stabilizes the joint in flexion, which is useful during grasp. The kinematics of extension of the MCP joints occurs in reverse fashion as that described for flexion.

Because the proximal surface of the proximal phalanx is concave and the head of the metacarpal is convex, the arthrokinematics of flexion and extension occur as a roll and slide in similar directions.

The overall range of flexion and extension at the MCP joints increases gradually from the second (index finger) to

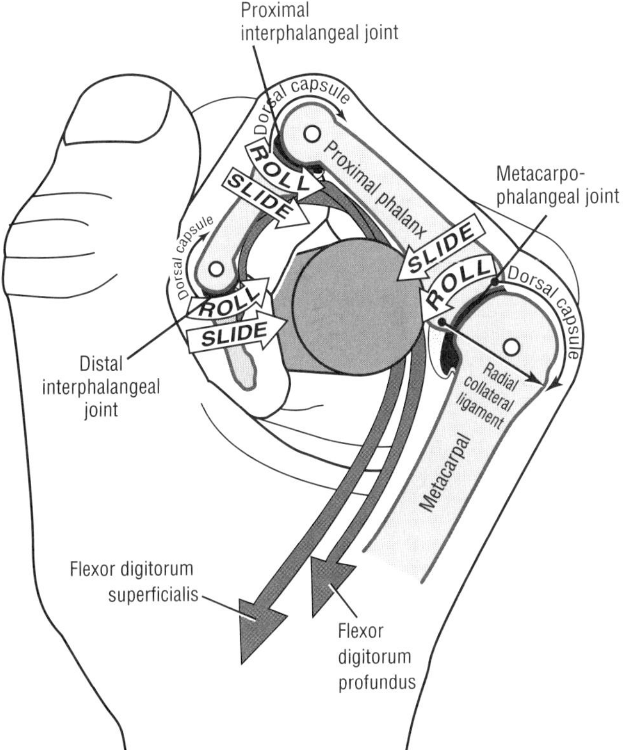

Figure 7-17 The arthrokinematics of active flexion at the metacarpophalangeal (MCP), proximal interphalangeal, and distal interphalangeal joints of the index finger. The radial collateral ligament at the MCP joint is pulled taut in flexion. Flexion elongates the dorsal capsule and other associated connective tissues. The joints are shown flexing under the power of the flexor digitorum superficialis and the flexor digitorum profundus. The axis of rotation for flexion and extension at all three finger joints is in the medial-lateral direction, through the convex member of the joint. (From Neumann DA: *Kinesiology of the musculoskeletal system: foundations for physical rehabilitation*, St Louis, 2002, Mosby, Figure 8-29.)

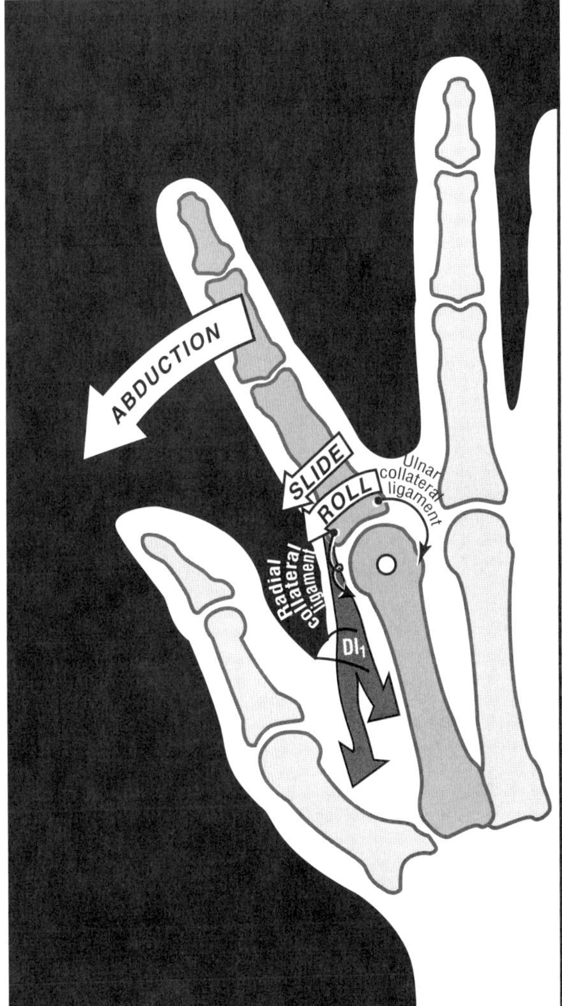

Figure 7-18 The arthrokinematics of active abduction at the metacarpophalangeal joint. Abduction is shown powered by the first dorsal interosseus muscle (DI_1). At full abduction, the ulnar collateral ligament is taut and the radial collateral ligament is slack. Note that the axis of rotation for this motion is in an anterior-posterior direction, through the head of the metacarpal. (From Neumann DA: *Kinesiology of the musculoskeletal system: foundations for physical rehabilitation*, St Louis, 2002, Mosby, Figure 8-30.)

the fifth digit: The second finger flexes to about 90 degrees, and the fifth to about 110 to 115 degrees. The MCP joints can be passively extended beyond the neutral (0-degree) position for a considerable range of 30 to 45 degrees.

Figure 7-18 shows the kinematics of abduction of the MCP joint of the index finger, controlled by the first dorsal interosseus muscle. During abduction, the proximal phalanx rolls and slides in a radial direction: The radial collateral ligament becomes slack, and the ulnar collateral ligament is stretched. The kinematics of adduction of the MCP joints occur in a reverse fashion. Abduction and adduction at the MCP joints occur to about 20 degrees on either side of the midline reference formed by the third metacarpal.

THUMB

The MCP joint of the thumb consists of the articulation between the convex head of the first metacarpal and the concave proximal surface of the proximal phalanx of the thumb (Figure 7-19). The basic structure of the MCP joint of the thumb is similar to that of the fingers. Active and passive motions at the MCP joint of the thumb are significantly less than those at the MCP joints of the fingers. For all practical purposes, the MCP joint of the thumb allows only 1 degree of freedom: flexion and extension within the frontal plane. Unlike the MCP joints of the fingers, extension of the thumb MCP joint is usually limited to just a few degrees. From full extension, the proximal phalanx of the thumb can actively flex about 60 degrees across the palm toward the middle digit (Figure 7-20). Active abduction and adduction of the thumb MCP joint is limited and therefore considered an accessory motion.

Consider this...

Flexion of the Metacarpophalangeal Joint: Placing Useful Tension in the Collateral Ligaments

Flexion of the metacarpophalangeal joints places a stretch within the collateral ligaments. Like a stretched rubber band, the increased tension in these ligaments reduces the passive motion at the joints. (This can be appreciated by noting how abduction and adduction of the fingers is much less in full flexion compared with full extension.) The increased tension in the collateral ligaments can be useful because it lends natural stability to the base of the fingers, especially useful during flexion movements such as holding a hand of playing cards. Furthermore, clinicians often use the increased tension in the collateral ligaments to prevent joint stiffness or deformity. This strategy is commonly used with a hand that must be held immobile in a cast (or splint) for extended time following, for example, a fractured metacarpal. Maintaining the metacarpophalangeal joints in flexion (with interphalangeal joints usually close to full extension) increases the passive tension within the ligaments just enough to reduce the likelihood of their undergoing permanent shortening and developing a contracture.

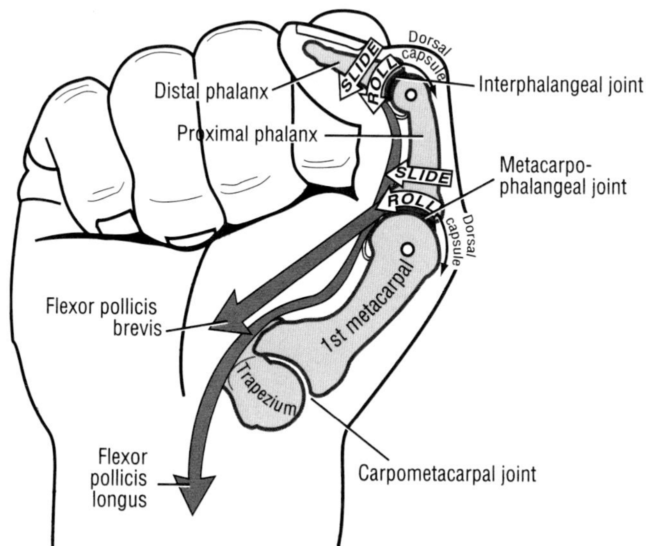

Figure 7-20 The arthrokinematics of active flexion at the metacarpophalangeal and interphalangeal joints of the thumb. Flexion is shown powered by the flexor pollicis longus and the flexor pollicis brevis. The axis of rotation for flexion and extension at these joints is in the anterior-posterior direction, through the convex member of the joints. (From Neumann DA: *Kinesiology of the musculoskeletal system: foundations for physical rehabilitation,* St Louis, 2002, Mosby, Figure 8-33.)

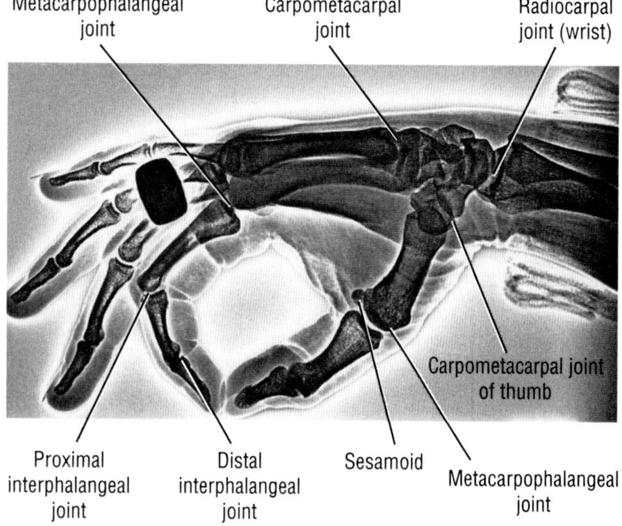

Figure 7-19 A side view showing the shape of many joint surfaces in the wrist and hand. Note the sesamoid bone on the palmar side of the metacarpophalangeal joint of the thumb. (From Neumann DA: *Kinesiology of the musculoskeletal system: foundations for physical rehabilitation*, St Louis, 2002, Mosby, Figure 8-32.)

Interphalangeal Joints

FINGERS

The proximal and distal interphalangeal joints of the fingers are located distal to the MCP joints (see Figure 7-19). Each joint allows only 1 degree of freedom: flexion and extension. From both a structural and functional perspective, these joints are simpler than the MCP joints.

General Features and Ligaments

The proximal interphalangeal (PIP) joints are formed by the articulation between the heads of the proximal phalanges and the bases of the middle phalanges (Figure 7-21). The distal interphalangeal (DIP) joints are formed through the articulation between the heads of the middle phalanges and the bases of the distal phalanges. The articular surfaces of these joints appear as a tongue-in-groove articulation similar to that used in carpentry to join planks of wood. This articulation helps limit the motion at the PIP and DIP joints to flexion and extension only.

Except for being smaller, the same ligaments that surround the MCP joints also surround the PIP and DIP joints. The capsule at each interphalangeal (IP) joint is strengthened by radial and ulnar collateral ligaments and a palmar plate. The collateral ligaments restrict any side-to-side movements, and the palmar (volar) plate limits hyperextension. In addition, the fibrous digital sheaths house the tendons of the extrinsic finger flexor muscles (see index and small finger in Figure 7-15).

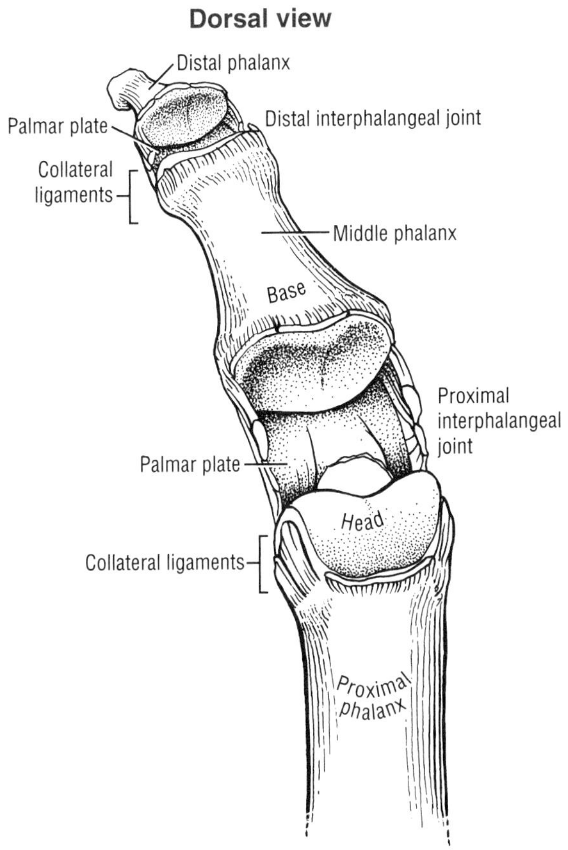

Figure 7-21 A dorsal view of the proximal interphalangeal and distal interphalangeal joints opened to expose the shape of the articular surfaces. (Modified from Neumann DA: *Kinesiology of the musculoskeletal system: foundations for physical rehabilitation,* St Louis, 2002, Mosby, Figure 8-34.)

Kinematics

The PIP joints flex to about 100 to 120 degrees. The DIP joints allow less flexion, to about 70 to 90 degrees. Like the MCP joints, flexion at the PIP and DIP joints is greater in the more ulnar digits. Minimal hyperextension is usually allowed at the PIP and DIP joints.

Figure 7-17 shows the kinematics of flexion of the PIP and DIP joints, controlled by two finger flexor muscles: flexor digitorum superficialis and flexor digitorum profundus. Similarities in joint structure cause similar roll-and-slide arthrokinematics at the PIP and DIP joints. In contrast to the MCP joints, passive tension in the collateral ligaments at the IP joints remains relatively constant throughout the range of motion.

THUMB

The structure and function of the IP joint of the thumb are similar to that of the IP joints of the fingers. Motion is limited primarily to 1 degree of freedom, allowing active flexion to about 70 degrees (see Figure 7-20). The IP joint of the thumb can be passively hyperextended beyond neutral to about 20 degrees. This motion is often employed to apply a force between the pad of the thumb and an object, such as in pushing a thumbtack into a wall.

Table 7-1 summarizes the joints of the hand and their associated allowable motions, planes of motion, and ranges of motion.

> **Consider this...**
>
> **Position of Function of the Wrist and Hand**
>
> Some medical conditions such as a traumatic head injury, stroke, or high-level quadriplegia can result in a permanent deformity of the wrist and hand. The deformity is caused by a combination of long-term paralysis, disuse, or abnormal tone in the muscles. Clinicians therefore often use splints that favor a position of the wrist and hand that maximally preserves its functional potential. This position, often called the position of function, is shown in Figure 7-22. This position provides a slightly opened and cupped hand, with the wrist extended 20 degrees to maintain optimal length of the finger flexor muscles.
>
> 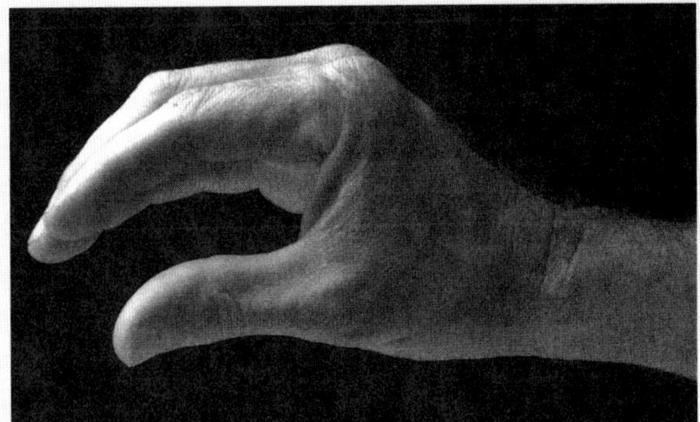
>
> **Figure 7-22** The position of function of the wrist and hand. (From Neumann DA: *Kinesiology of the musculoskeletal system: foundations for physical rehabilitation,* St Louis, 2002, Mosby, Figure 8-35.)

Muscle and Joint Interaction

Innervation of the Hand

The highly complex and coordinated functions of the hand require a rich source of nerve supply to the region's muscles, skin, and joints. Normal sensory innervation is essential for the protection of the hand against mechanical and thermal injury. Persons with peripheral neuropathy, spinal cord injury,

TABLE 7-1 JOINTS OF THE HAND

Joint	Motions Allowed	Planes of Motion	Range of Motion (from Anatomic Position)	Comments
CMC digits 2-5	Allow the palm to change its shape to securely hold a large number of different-shaped objects	Variable	Variable	Second and third CMC joints are the most stable
CMC of the thumb	Flexion/extension	Frontal	10-15 degrees of extension to 45 degrees of flexion	Most common joint for arthritis of the hand
	Abduction/adduction	Sagittal	0-45 degrees of abduction	
	Opposition	Triplanar	Full range allows the tip of the thumb to touch the tip of the little finger	
MCP digits 2-5	Flexion/extension Abduction/adduction	Sagittal Frontal	0-100 degrees of flexion 0-35 degrees of hyperextension 0-20 degrees of abduction	Form the keystone of the distal transverse arch; collapse causes a flattened hand
MCP of the thumb	Flexion/extension	Frontal	0-60 degrees of flexion	
PIP digits 2-5	Flexion/extension	Sagittal	0-110 degrees of flexion	Allows just one plane of motion
DIP digits 2-5	Flexion/extension	Sagittal	0-90 degrees of flexion	Allows just one plane of motion
IP of the thumb	Flexion/extension	Frontal	0-70 degrees of flexion 0-20 degrees of hyperextension	May allow considerable hyperextension

CMC, Carpometacarpal; *DIP*, distal interphalangeal; *IP*, interphalangeal; *MCP*, metacarpophalangeal; *PIP*, proximal interphalangeal.

and uncontrolled diabetes, for example, often lack sensation in their extremities, making them vulnerable to injury.

The radial, median, and ulnar nerves supply the innervation to the skin, joints, and muscles of the hand. The path of these nerves is illustrated in Chapter 6, Figure 6-12.

Muscular Function in the Hand

Muscles that operate the digits are divided into two broad sets: (1) extrinsic or (2) intrinsic (Box 7-1). Extrinsic muscles have their proximal attachment in the forearm or arm and attach distally within the hand. Intrinsic muscles, in contrast, have both proximal and distal attachments within the hand.

The following sections describe the basic anatomy and individual actions of the extrinsic and intrinsic muscles. A thorough understanding of the kinesiology of the hand, however, requires an appreciation of how the extrinsic muscles work simultaneously with the intrinsic muscles. This important concept is a recurring theme throughout this chapter.

EXTRINSIC FLEXORS OF THE DIGITS

Anatomy and Isolated Action

The extrinsic flexor muscles of the digits are the flexor digitorum superficialis, flexor digitorum profundus, and flexor pollicis longus (see the figures on p. 160). These muscles originate primarily from the medial epicondyle of the humerus and palmar surfaces of the radius and ulna. The bellies of these muscles are located in the mid to deeper regions of the forearm, often indistinguishable from the muscle bellies of the wrist flexor muscles. The flexor digitorum superficialis and flexor digitorum profundus each transmit a set of four tendons to the hand. After crossing the palmar side of the wrist within the carpal tunnel (see the first figure on p. 160), each tendon attaches to the palmar surface of a particular phalanx. The tendons of the flexor digitorum superficialis attach to the base of the middle phalanx; the deeper tendons of the flexor digitorum profundus continue distally to attach to the base of the distal phalanx. On the basis of distal attachments, the flexor digitorum superficialis causes isolated flexion of the PIP joints; the flexor digitorum profundus causes isolated flexion of the DIP joints.

Extrinsic Flexors of the Digits

- Flexor digitorum superficialis
- Flexor digitorum profundus
- Flexor pollicis longus

0010 **BOX 7-1**

Extrinsic and Intrinsic Muscles of the Hand

Extrinsic Muscles

Flexors of the Digits
- Flexor digitorum superficialis
- Flexor digitorum profundus
- Flexor pollicis longus

Extensors of the Fingers
- Extensor digitorum
- Extensor indicis
- Extensor digiti minimi

Extensors of the Thumb
- Extensor pollicis longus
- Extensor pollicis brevis
- Abductor pollicis longus

Intrinsic Muscles

Thenar Eminence
- Abductor pollicis brevis
- Flexor pollicis brevis
- Opponens pollicis

Hypothenar Eminence
- Abductor digiti minimi
- Flexor digiti minimi
- Opponens digiti minimi

Adductor Pollicis
- (Two heads)

Lumbricals
- (Four)

Interossei
- Palmar (four)
- Dorsal (four)

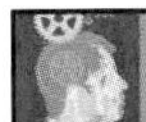

Consider this...

Let the Muscle's Name Do Some of the Work for You!

Many of the muscles of the hand have long and seemingly complicated names. However, if you spoke Latin or Greek, the names would be quite simple. The names of most hand muscles describe either the actions or anatomic location of the muscle. For example, the flexor pollicis longus would literally translate to "long muscle that flexes the thumb," and the abductor digiti minimi would mean "small muscle that abducts the little finger." With knowledge of a few Latin and Greek root words, the name of the muscle can tell you a lot about the location and actions of the muscle in question.

The flexor pollicis longus sends a single tendon to the palmar surface of the distal phalanx of the thumb, therefore causing isolated flexion of the IP joint of the thumb. Simultaneous contraction of all three sets of digital flexor muscles (flexor digitorum superficialis, flexor digitorum profundus, and flexor pollicis longus) flexes all the hand joints used for activities such as gripping or holding the strap of a handbag. As described later, simultaneous contraction of the intrinsic muscles of the fingers is necessary to perform more precise movements.

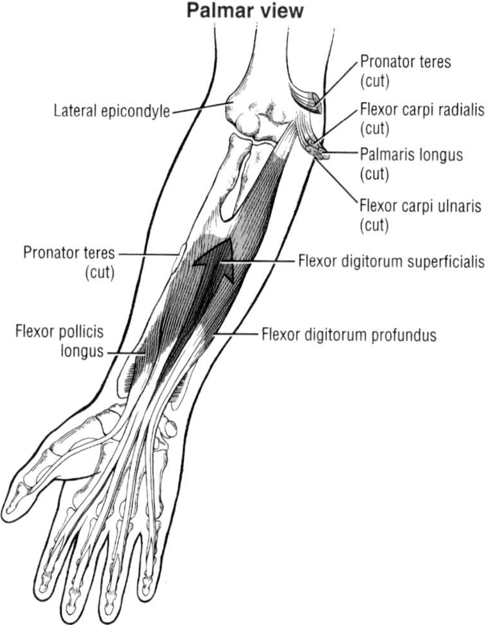

An anterior view of the right forearm highlighting the flexor digitorum superficialis muscle. Note the cut proximal ends of the wrist flexors and pronator teres muscles. (From Neumann DA: *Kinesiology of the musculoskeletal system: foundations for physical rehabilitation,* St Louis, 2002, Mosby, Figure 8-36.)

Flexor Digitorum Superficialis

Proximal Attachments: Common flexor tendon on the medial epicondyle of the humerus, coronoid process of the ulna, and radius—just lateral to the bicipital tuberosity

Distal Attachment: By four tendons, each to the sides of the middle phalanges of the fingers

Innervation: Median nerve

Actions:
- MCP and PIP joint flexion
- Wrist flexion

Comments: The flexor digitorum superficialis divides into four tendons, each coursing to one of the four fingers. Interestingly, each tendon splits as it inserts to both sides of the middle phalanx. The split in each tendon creates a "tunnel" that allows the deeper profundus tendon to pass distally to attach to the base of the distal phalanx.

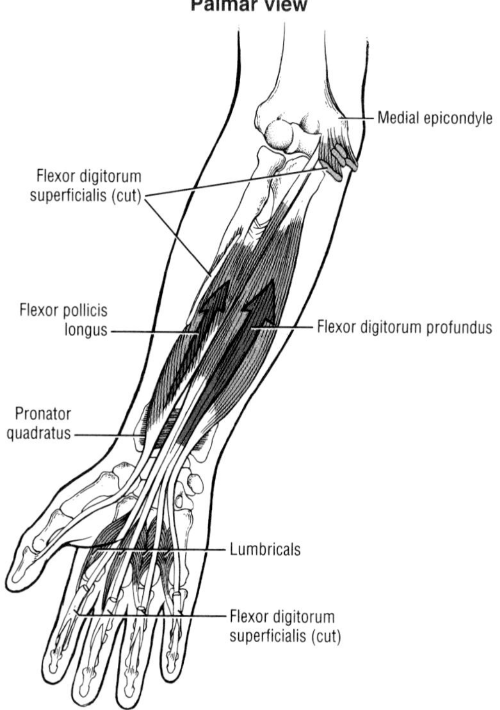

An anterior view of the right forearm highlighting the flexor digitorum profundus and the flexor pollicis longus muscles. The lumbrical muscles are shown attaching to the tendons of the flexor profundus. Note the cut proximal and distal ends of the flexor digitorum superficialis muscle. (From Neumann DA: *Kinesiology of the musculoskeletal system: foundations for physical rehabilitation,* St Louis, 2002, Mosby, Figure 8-37.)

Flexor Digitorum Profundus

Proximal Attachments: Anterior ulna and interosseous membrane

Distal Attachment: By four tendons, each to the base of the distal phalanx of digits 2 to 5

Innervation: *Medial half:* Ulnar nerve
Lateral half: Median nerve

Actions:
- MCP, PIP, and DIP joint flexion
- Wrist flexion

Comments: Because the tendons of the deeper flexor digitorum profundus cross all joints of the finger, it is active during most simple gripping motions. The flexor digitorum superficialis, in contrast, is more active during complex motions or those that involve only the PIP joints.

Flexor Pollicis Longus

Proximal Attachments: Middle anterior portion of the radius and interosseous membrane

Distal Attachment: Base of the distal phalanx of the thumb

Innervation: Median nerve

Actions:
- CMC, MCP, and IP joint flexion of the thumb
- Wrist flexion

Comments: Because the flexor pollicis longus attaches to the distal phalanx of the thumb, this muscle is functionally identical to the flexor digitorum profundus of the fingers.

Functional Consideration

Flexor Pulleys. The extrinsic flexor tendons of the digits travel distally throughout the hand in protective tunnels known as fibrous digital sheaths (Figure 7-23, *small finger*). Embedded within each digital sheath are bands of tissues called flexor pulleys (see Figure 7-23, labeled A_{1-5}, C_{1-3} in ring finger). These pulleys surround the flexor tendons, providing them with nutrition and lubrication. Synovial fluid secreted within the inner walls of the pulleys reduces friction as the tendons slide past one another during muscle contraction. Following a tendon injury, adhesions may develop between the tendon and adjacent digital sheath or between adjacent tendons. A hand therapist usually initiates a closely monitored exercise program to facilitate gliding of the tendons, often following a surgical repair.

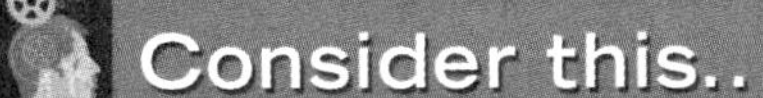

"Trigger Finger"

The extrinsic flexor tendons and surrounding synovial membranes may become inflamed. Associated swelling limits the space within the pulley and thereby restricts the smooth gliding of the tendons. The inflamed region of the tendon may also develop a nodule that occasionally becomes wedged within the narrowed region of the fibrous digital sheath, thereby blocking movement of the digit. With additional force, the tendon may suddenly slip through the constriction with a snap, a condition often referred to as trigger finger. Conservative management including activity modification, splinting, and cortisone injection may be effective in early stages, but surgical release of the constricted region of the sheath is usually required in chronic cases.

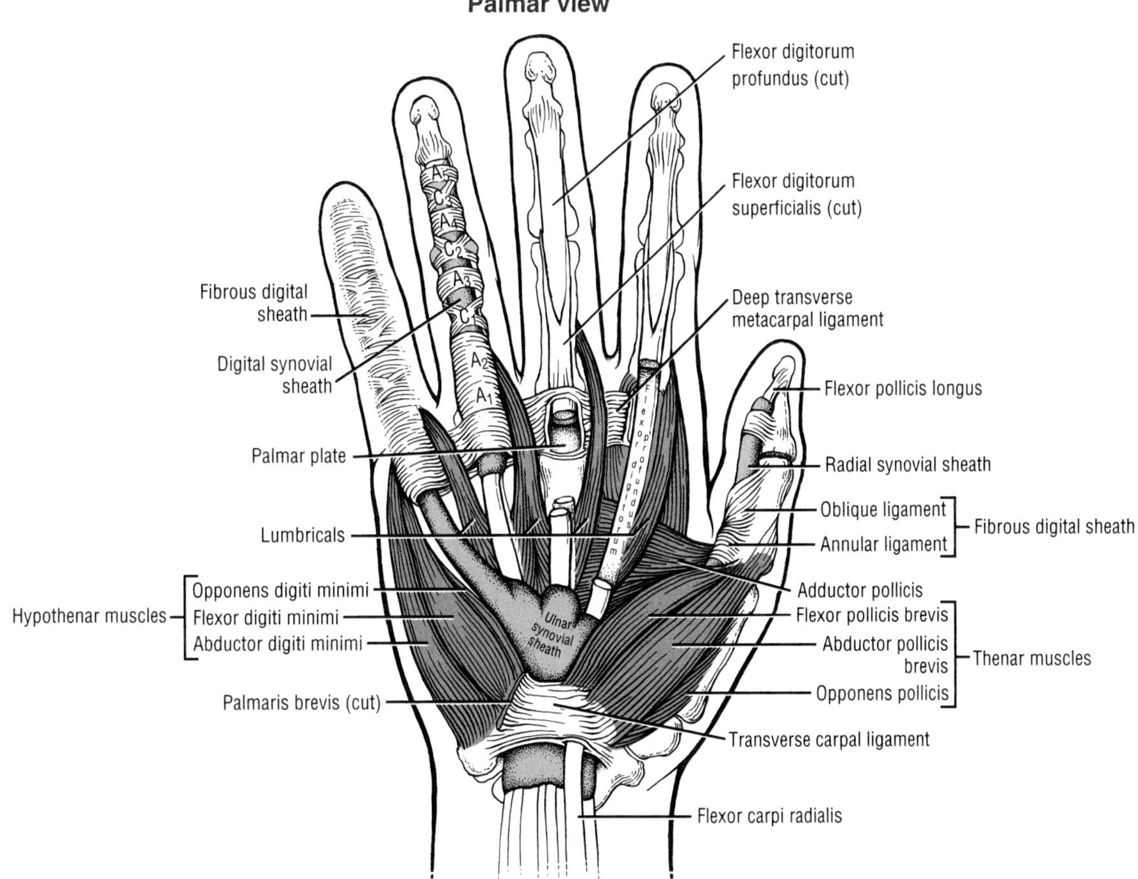

Figure 7-23 A palmar view illustrates several important structures of the hand. Note the little finger showing the fibrous digital sheath and ulnar synovial sheath encasing the extrinsic flexor tendons. The ring finger has the digital sheath removed, thereby highlighting the digital synovial sheath *(red)* and the annular (A_{1-5}) and cruciate (C_{1-3}) pulleys. The middle finger shows the pulleys removed to expose the distal attachments of the flexor digitorum superficialis and flexor digitorum profundus. The index finger has a portion of flexor digitorum superficialis tendon removed, thereby exposing the deeper tendon of the flexor digitorum profundus and attached lumbrical. The thumb highlights the oblique and annular pulleys along with the radial synovial sheath, surrounding the tendon of the flexor pollicis longus. (From Neumann DA: *Kinesiology of the musculoskeletal system: foundations for physical rehabilitation,* St Louis, 2002, Mosby, Figure 8-38.)

Passive Finger Flexion via Tenodesis Action of the Extrinsic Digital Flexors. The extrinsic flexors of the digits—namely the flexor digitorum profundus, flexor digitorum superficialis, and flexor pollicis longus—cross over the anterior side of the wrist. The position of the wrist therefore significantly alters the amount of stretch placed on these muscles. One implication of this arrangement can be appreciated by actively extending the wrist and observing the passive flexion of the fingers and thumb (Figure 7-24). Try this on yourself. The digits automatically flex due to the increased passive tension in the stretched finger flexor muscles. Stretching a multi-articular muscle at one joint that subsequently creates passive movement at another joint is referred to as a **tenodesis action** of a muscle. When stretched, essentially all multi-articular muscles in the body demonstrate some degree of tenodesis action. Importantly, the clinician must not be fooled by assuming that a tenodesis response from a stretched muscle is actually an active or volitional movement; in fact, the movement is passive and generated only by the elastic nature of the stretched muscle.

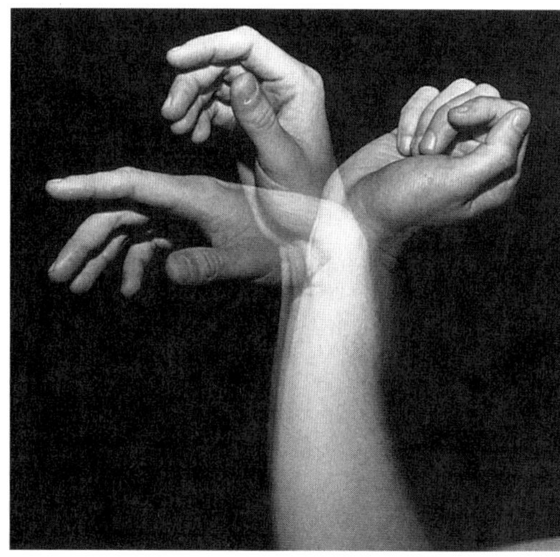

Figure 7-24 Tendosis action of the finger flexors in a healthy person. As the wrist is extended, the thumb and fingers automatically flex due to the stretch placed on the extrinsic digital flexors. The flexion occurs passively, without effort from the subject. (From Neumann DA: *Kinesiology of the musculoskeletal system: foundations for physical rehabilitation,* St Louis, 2002, Mosby, Figure 8-42.)

EXTRINSIC EXTENSORS OF THE FINGERS

The extrinsic extensors of the fingers are the extensor digitorum, extensor indicis, and extensor digiti minimi (see the first figure on p.164). These muscles originate primarily from the lateral epicondyle of the humerus and dorsal surfaces of the radius and ulna. The bellies of these muscles are located close to the bellies of the wrist extensor muscles.

Extrinsic Extensors of the Fingers

- Extensor digitorum
- Extensor indicis
- Extensor digiti minimi

Tendons of the extensor digitorum, extensor indicis, and extensor digiti minimi cross the wrist in synovial-lined compartments, located within the extensor retinaculum (Figure 7-26). Distal to the extensor retinaculum, the tendons of the extensor digitorum course to the dorsal side of the fingers (one to each finger). As the name implies, the extensor indicis sends one tendon to the index finger. The extensor digiti minimi is a small muscle interconnected with the extensor digitorum. As shown in Figure 7-26 the tendons of the extensor digitorum are interconnected by several juncturae tendinae. These thin strips of connective tissue stabilize the tendons to the base of the MCP joints.

The extensor tendons do not attach directly to the phalanges, as is the case for the distal attachments of the extrinsic finger flexor muscles. Instead, the extensor tendons blend with a special set of connective tissues called the **extensor mechanism** (see Figure 7-26). The complex set of connective tissues extends the entire length of each finger. The proximal end of the extensor mechanism is called the dorsal hood. The sides of dorsal hood wrap completely around the MCP joint, joining palmarly at the palmar plate. Through central and lateral bands, the extensor mechanism ultimately attaches to the dorsal side of the distal phalanx. The extensor mechanism is important because it serves as the primary distal attachment for both the extensor muscle tendons and the intrinsic muscles of the fingers (lumbricals and interossei). As explained later, co-contraction of the extensor muscles of the fingers *and* the intrinsic muscles are required to fully and smoothly extend all the joints of the fingers.

Clinical **INSIGHT**

Usefulness of Tenodesis Action in Persons with Quadriplegia

The natural tenodesis action of the extrinsic digital flexor muscles can help produce a functional grip, or grasp, for some patients. One example involves a person with C6 quadriplegia who has near or complete paralysis of his or her finger flexors but well innervated and strong wrist extensor muscles. Persons with this level of spinal cord injury often employ a tenodesis action for many functions such as holding a cup of water (Figure 7-25).

Active contraction of the wrist extensor muscles, shown in red in Figure 7-25, stretches the paralyzed finger flexor muscles such as the flexor digitorum profundus. The stretch in these flexor muscles creates enough passive tension to effectively flex the digits and grasp the cup. The amount of passive tension (passive gripping force) in the digital flexors is controlled indirectly by the degree of active wrist extension. Someone with paralyzed wrist extensor muscles cannot perform such a useful tenodesis action to substitute for paralyzed grasp—a wrist extension splint is often required in this case.

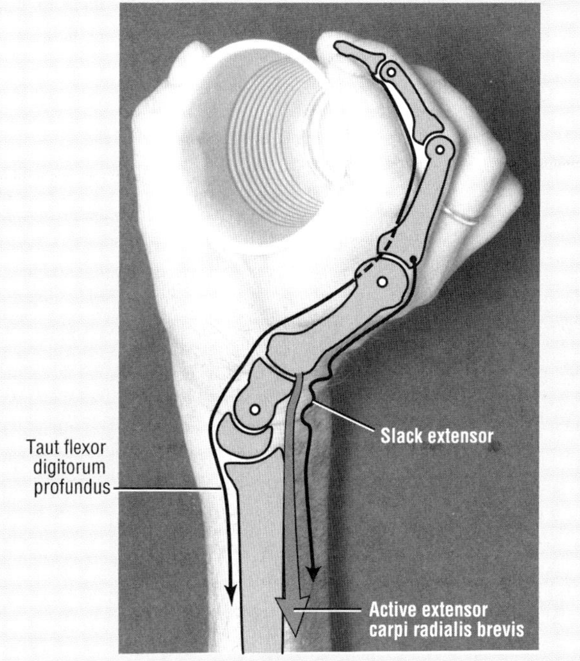

Figure 7-25 A person with C6-level quadriplegia using tenodesis action to grasp a cup of water. Active wrist extension by contraction of the innervated extensor carpi radialis brevis *(red)* creates useful passive tension in the paralyzed digital flexors needed to hold the cup of water. (From Neumann DA: *Kinesiology of the musculoskeletal system: foundations for physical rehabilitation*, St Louis, 2002, Mosby, Figure 8-43, *B*.)

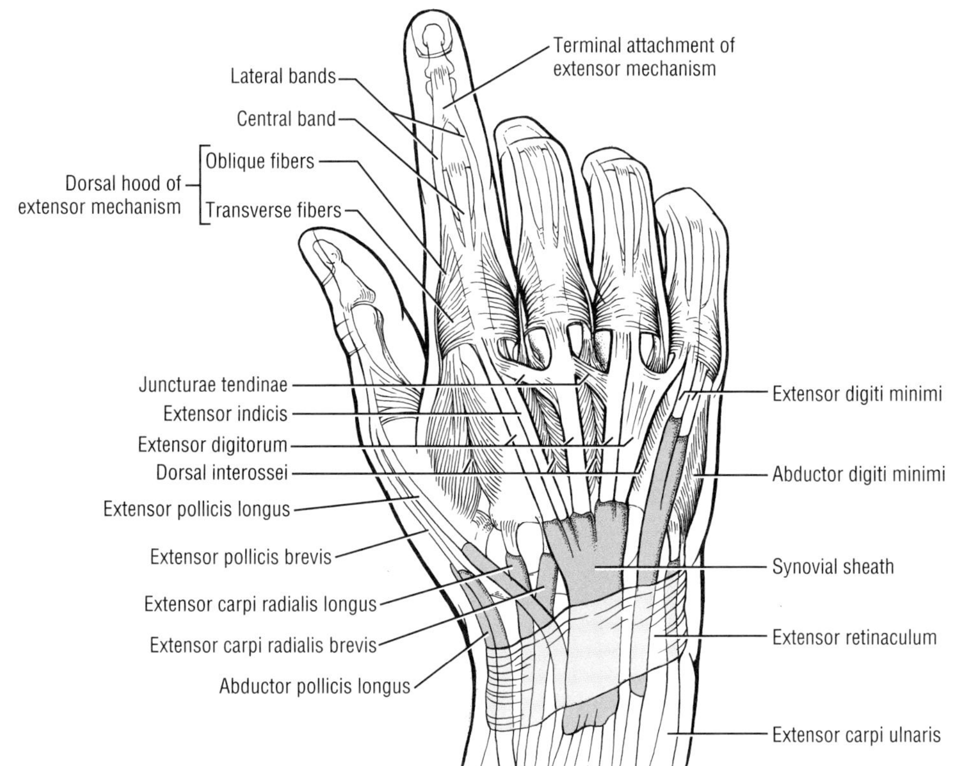

Figure 7-26 A dorsal view of the muscles, tendons, and extensor mechanism of the right hand. The synovial sheaths are indicated in darker red, the extensor retinaculum in lighter red. (From Neumann DA: *Kinesiology of the musculoskeletal system: foundations for physical rehabilitation*, St Louis, 2002, Mosby, Figure 8-45.)

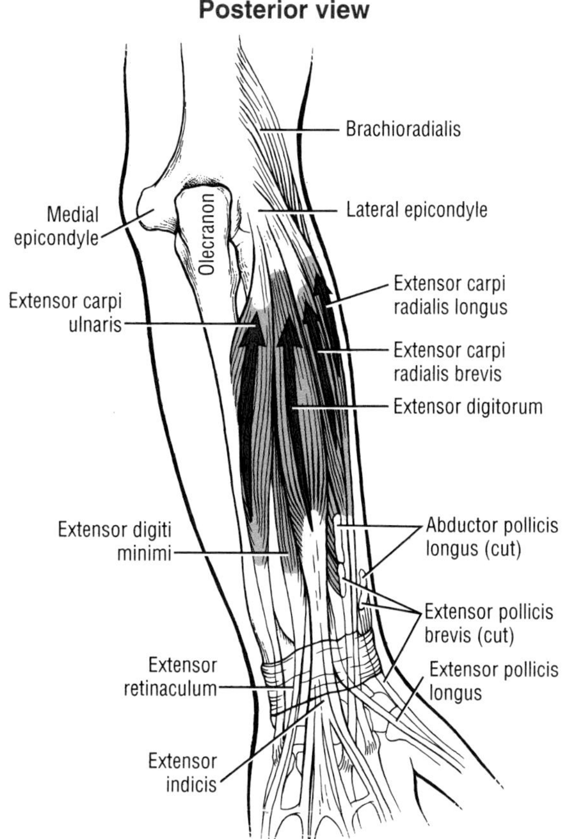

Dorsal view of the right upper extremity highlighting several muscles, including the extensor digitorum, extensor indicis, and extensor digiti minimi. (From Neumann DA: *Kinesiology of the musculoskeletal system: foundations for physical rehabilitation*, St Louis, 2002, Mosby, Figure 7-22.)

Extensor Digitorum

Proximal Attachments:	Lateral epicondyle of the humerus—common extensor tendon
Distal Attachment:	By four tendons, each to the base of the extensor mechanism and base of the proximal phalanx of all four fingers
Innervation:	Radial nerve
Action:	Extension of the fingers
Comments:	Isolated contraction of only the extensor digitorum muscle causes hyperextension of the MCP joints. Activation of the intrinsic muscles (lumbricals and interossei) is needed to completely extend *all* the joints of the each finger.

Extensor Indicis

Proximal Attachments:	Posterior surface of distal ulna and interosseous membrane
Distal Attachment:	Blends with the index tendon of the extensor digitorum
Innervation:	Radial nerve
Action:	Extension of the index finger
Comments:	The tendon of the extensor indicis can usually be visualized during a strong hyperextension movement of the MCP joint of the index finger, with the PIP joint remaining fully flexed. The tendon of the extensor indicis is located just ulnar to the tendon of the extensor digitorum.

Extensor Digiti Minimi

Proximal Attachments:	Ulnar side of the belly of the extensor digitorum
Distal Attachment:	Joins the tendon of the extensor digitorum to the little finger
Innervation:	Radial nerve
Action:	Extension of the little finger
Comments:	This muscle is often considered a fifth tendon of the extensor digitorum.

EXTRINSIC EXTENSORS OF THE THUMB

The extrinsic extensors of the thumb are the extensor pollicis longus, extensor pollicis brevis, and abductor pollicis longus (see the figure on p.165). These three muscles each have their proximal attachments on the dorsal region of the forearm. The tendons of these muscles compose the "anatomic snuff box" located on the radial side of the wrist (Figure 7-27).

Extrinsic Extensors of the Thumb

- Extensor pollicis longus
- Extensor pollicis brevis
- Abductor pollicis longus

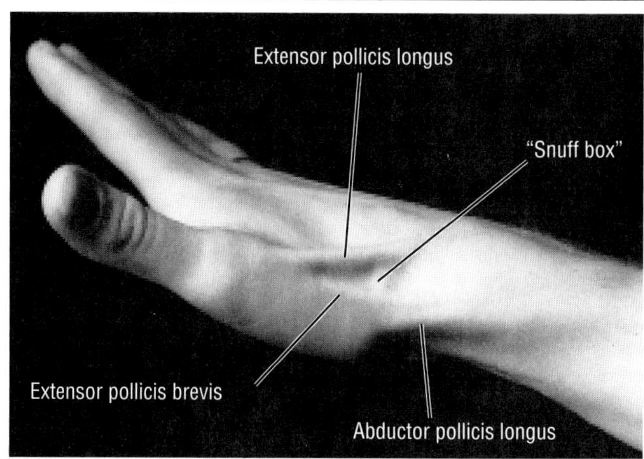

Figure 7-27 Muscles of the "anatomic snuff box" are shown. (From Neumann DA: *Kinesiology of the musculoskeletal system: foundations for physical rehabilitation*, St Louis, 2002, Mosby, Figure 8-49.)

The tendons of the three extensors of the thumb attach to different regions of the dorsal side of the thumb. On the basis of their attachments, the abductor pollicis longus abducts and extends the CMC joint, the extensor pollicis brevis extends the MCP joint, and the extensor pollicis longus extends the IP joint. Realize, however, that each muscle can also exert a secondary action over each joint it crosses. Because each of the three muscles also crosses the wrist, each may have a secondary action, most notably in extension and radial deviation.

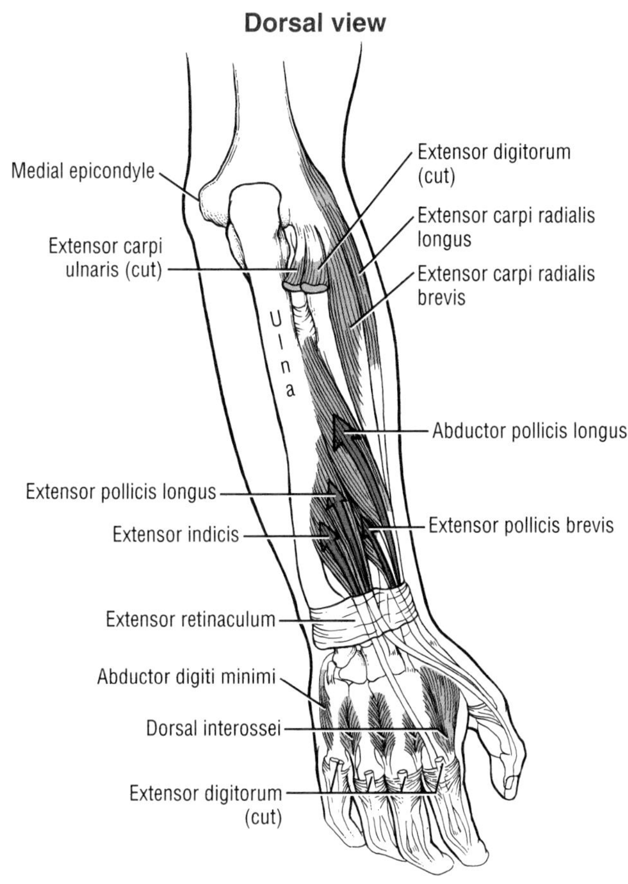

Dorsal-radial view of the right hand highlighting the abductor pollicis longus and the extensor pollicis longus and brevis. (From Neumann DA: *Kinesiology of the musculoskeletal system: foundations for physical rehabilitation*, St Louis, 2002, Mosby, Figure 8-44.)

Extensor Pollicis Longus

Proximal Attachments: Posterior surface of ulna and interosseous membrane

Distal Attachment: Dorsal base of the distal phalanx of thumb

Innervation: Radial nerve

Action: Extension of the IP, MCP, and CMC joints of the thumb

Comments: This is the only muscle that can actively extend the IP joint of the thumb, making it one of the most reliable muscles to test the function of the radial nerve.

Extensor Pollicis Brevis

Proximal Attachments: Posterior aspect of the radius and interosseous membrane

Distal Attachment: Dorsal base of the proximal phalanx of thumb

Innervation: Radial nerve

Action: Extension of the MCP and CMC joints of the thumb

Comments: This muscle is often small and may have several tendons.

Abductor Pollicis Longus

Proximal Attachments: Posterior surface of the radius, ulna, and interosseous membrane

Distal Attachment: Base of the metacarpal of the thumb

Innervation: Radial nerve

Action: Abduction and extension of the CMC joint of the thumb

Comments: Due to this muscle's distal attachment, it is an equally effective abductor and extensor of the base of the thumb.

INTRINSIC MUSCLES OF THE HAND

The hand contains 20 intrinsic muscles. Despite their relatively small size, these muscles are essential to the fine control of the digits. The intrinsic muscles are divided into the following four sets:

1. Muscles of the Thenar Eminence
   - Abductor pollicis brevis
   - Flexor pollicis brevis
   - Opponens pollicis
2. Muscles of the Hypothenar Eminence
   - Flexor digiti minimi
   - Abductor digiti minimi
   - Opponens digiti minimi
3. Adductor Pollicis
4. Lumbricals and Interossei (Intrinsic Muscles of the Fingers)

   Figure 7-28 highlights these muscle groups.

Muscles of the Thenar Eminence

The abductor pollicis brevis, flexor pollicis brevis, and opponens pollicis make up the bulk of the thenar eminence

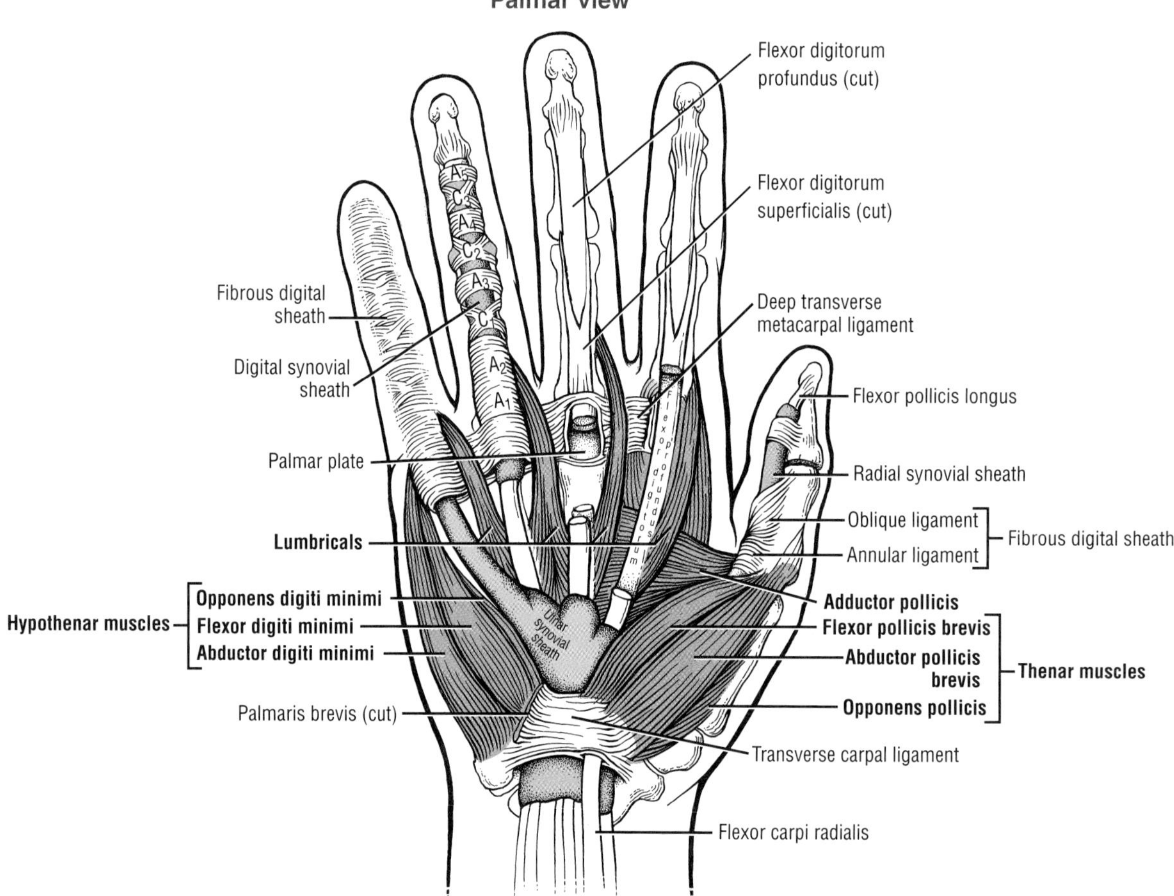

Figure 7-28 A palmar view of the right hand highlighting the many intrinsic muscles *(red)*. (Modified from Neumann DA: *Kinesiology of the musculoskeletal system: foundations for physical rehabilitation,* St Louis, 2002, Mosby, Figure 8-38.)

(see Figure 7-28). All three thenar muscles have their proximal attachments on the transverse carpal ligament and adjacent carpal bones. The short abductor and flexor attach to the base of the proximal phalanx of the thumb; the deeper opponens muscle, however, attaches along the radial border of the first metacarpal, proximal to the MCP joint (Figure 7-29). The following table summarizes each of these muscles and their associated attachments, actions, and innervations.

A primary responsibility of the muscles of the thenar eminence is to position the thumb in varying amounts of opposition, usually to facilitate grasping (see Figure 7-29). As discussed previously, opposition combines elements of CMC joint abduction, flexion, and medial rotation. Each muscle within the thenar eminence is a prime mover for at least one component of opposition. The opponens pollicis is especially important in its ability to medially rotate the thumb toward the fingers—an essential part of opposition.

MUSCLES OF THE THENAR EMINENCE

Muscle	Proximal Attachment	Distal Attachment	Actions	Innervation
Abductor pollicis brevis	Transverse carpal ligament and adjacent carpal bones	Base of the proximal phalanx of the thumb	Abduction and flexion of the CMC joint of the thumb; flexion of the MCP joint	Median nerve
Flexor pollicis brevis	Transverse carpal ligament and adjacent carpal bones	Base of the proximal phalanx of the thumb	Flexion of the MCP and CMC joints of the thumb	Median nerve
Opponens pollicis	Transverse carpal ligament and adjacent carpal bones	Radial surface of the shaft of the thumb metacarpal	Opposition of the CMC joint (medial rotation) of the thumb	Median nerve

CMC, Carpometacarpal; *MCP*, metacarpophalangeal.

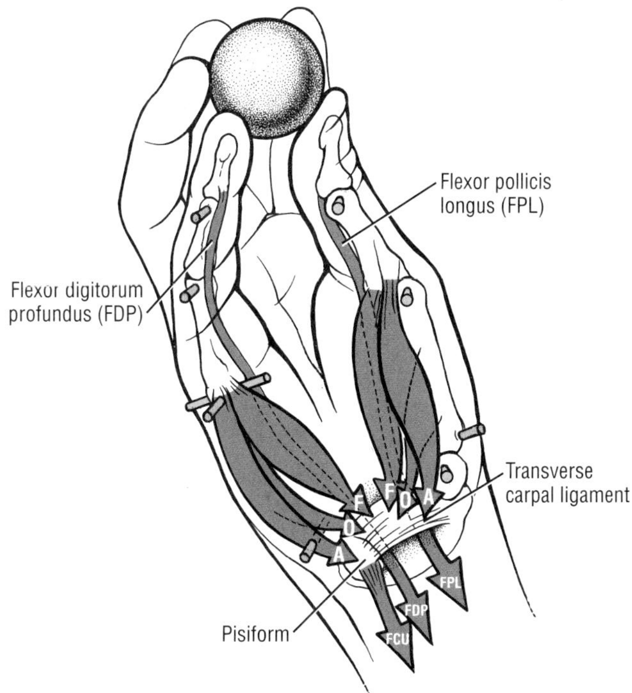

Figure 7-29 The action of the thenar and hypothenar muscles during opposition of the thumb and cupping of the little finger. Muscle function is based on the muscles' line of force relative to each joint's axes of rotation. Medial-lateral axes are in gray; anterior-posterior axes are in red. Other muscles shown in an active state are the flexor pollicis longus and flexor digitorum profundus of the little finger. The flexor carpi ulnaris *(FCU)* stabilizes the pisiform bone for the abductor digiti minimi. *A*, Abductor pollicis brevis and abductor digiti minimi; *F*, flexor pollicis brevis and flexor digiti minimi; *O*, opponens pollicis and opponens digiti minimi. (From Neumann DA: *Kinesiology of the musculoskeletal system: foundations for physical rehabilitation*, St Louis, 2002, Mosby, Figure 8-51.)

Muscles of the Hypothenar Eminence

The muscles of the hypothenar eminence consist of the flexor digiti minimi, abductor digiti minimi, and opponens digiti minimi (see Figure 7-28). The overall anatomic plan of the hypothenar muscles is similar to that of the muscles of the thenar eminence. The three muscles have their proximal attachments on the transverse carpal ligament and adjacent carpal bones. The short abductor and flexor both have their distal attachments on the base of the proximal phalanx of the small finger. The opponens digiti minimi has its distal attachment along the ulnar border of the fifth metacarpal, proximal to the MCP joint (see Figure 7-29). The following table summarizes each of these muscles and their associated attachments, actions, and innervations.

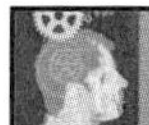

Consider this...

Implications of Median Nerve Injury

A severance or other trauma of the median nerve paralyzes all three muscles of the thenar eminence, namely the opponens pollicis, flexor pollicis brevis, and abductor pollicis brevis. Consequently, opposition of the thumb is essentially lost. The thenar eminence region of the hand also becomes flat due to muscle atrophy. The functional loss of opposition, in conjunction with the anesthesia (loss of sensation) of the tips of the thumb and radial fingers, greatly reduces precision grip and other manipulative functions of the hand.

A common function of the hypothenar muscles is to raise and curl the ulnar border of the hand, such as that used when cupping the hand to collect water. This action deepens the distal transverse arch and enhances contact with held objects (see Figure 7-29). When needed, the abductor digiti minimi can spread the small finger for greater control of grasp.

Injury to the ulnar nerve can completely paralyze the hypothenar muscles. The hypothenar eminence becomes flat due to muscle atrophy. Raising, or cupping, of the ulnar border of the hand is significantly reduced. Anesthesia over the entire small finger can contribute to a loss of dexterity.

Adductor Pollicis

The adductor pollicis is a two-headed muscle lying deep in the web space of the thumb (Figure 7-30; see also Figure 7-28). The muscle has its proximal attachments

MUSCLES OF THE HYPOTHENAR EMINENCE

Muscle	Proximal Attachment	Distal Attachment	Actions	Innervation
Flexor digiti minimi	Transverse carpal ligament and adjacent carpal bones	Base of the proximal phalanx of the small finger	Flexion of the MCP joint of the small finger	Ulnar nerve
Abductor digiti minimi	Pisiform and tendon of the flexor carpi ulnaris	Base of the proximal phalanx of the small finger	Abduction of the MCP joint of the small finger	Ulnar nerve
Opponens digiti minimi	Transverse carpal ligament and hook of the hamate	Shaft of the fifth metacarpal—ulnar side	Opposition of the CMC joint of the small finger	Ulnar nerve

CMC, Carpometacarpal; *MCP*, metacarpophalangeal.

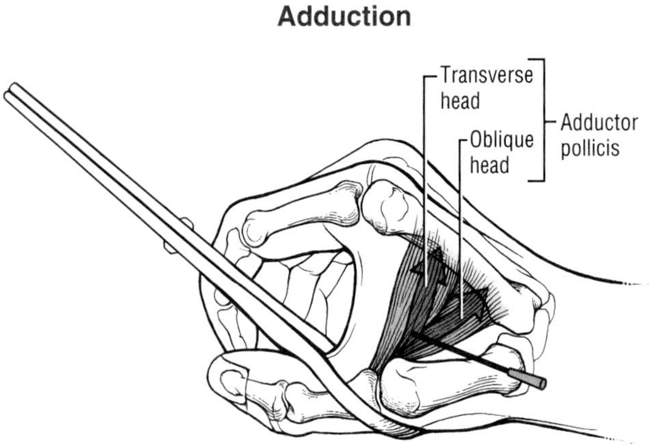

Adduction

Transverse head
Oblique head
Adductor pollicis

Figure 7-30 The powerful adduction action of the adductor pollicis muscle is illustrated using a pair of scissors. Note that the transverse head of the adductor pollicis produces a significant torque due to its long moment arm about a medial-lateral axis *(gray)*. (From Neumann DA: *Kinesiology of the musculoskeletal system: foundations for physical rehabilitation*, St Louis, 2002, Mosby, Figure 8-52, *B*.)

on the most stable skeletal regions of the hand: the capitate bone and second and third metacarpals. Both the transverse and oblique heads join and form a common distal attachment on the base of the proximal phalanx of the thumb.

Located deep to the thenar muscles, the adductor pollicis is not readily palpable and therefore often underappreciated. This muscle, however, is the most powerful adductor and flexor of the base of the thumb (CMC joint). The muscle is important for activities involving pinching objects between the thumb and index finger and for actions used to close a pair of scissors.

Lumbricals and Interossei: Intrinsic Muscles of the Fingers

The lumbricals (meaning "earthworms") are four slender muscles originating from the tendons of the flexor digitorum profundus (see Figure 7-28). Distally, the lumbricals attach not directly to bone, but to the lateral bands of the extensor mechanism. This distal attachment of the lumbricals allows these muscles to flex the MCP joints and extend the PIP and DIP joints. This action is possible because the lumbricals pass palmar to the MCP joints but dorsal to the PIP and DIP joints (Figure 7-31).

The lumbricals are active during activities that require combined flexion at the MCP joint and extension of the PIP and DIP joint such as holding a hand of cards. The muscles are also active along with the extensor digitorum during extension of all joints of the fingers.

The interosseus muscles are named according to their location between the metacarpal bones (Figure 7-32). Two sets of interossei exist: palmar and dorsal. Both sets contain four individual muscles, originating on the medial or lateral shafts of the metacarpals. The dorsal interossei are larger and slightly more dorsally located; therefore they are responsible for the fullness of shape of the dorsal side of the hand. All eight interosseus muscles are innervated by the ulnar nerve, traveling deep within the hand (see Chapter 6, Figure 6-12, C).

The primary function of the interosseous muscles is to abduct or adduct the fingers. As a set, the dorsal interossei *abduct* the fingers at the MCP joint away from an imaginary reference line through the middle digit. Note that the middle digit has two dorsal interosseous muscles: one that radial deviates and one that ulnar deviates. The palmar interossei *adduct* the fingers at the MCP joints toward the middle digit. (Because of the special terminology used to describe thumb movements, the first palmar interosseous technically flexes the thumb.)

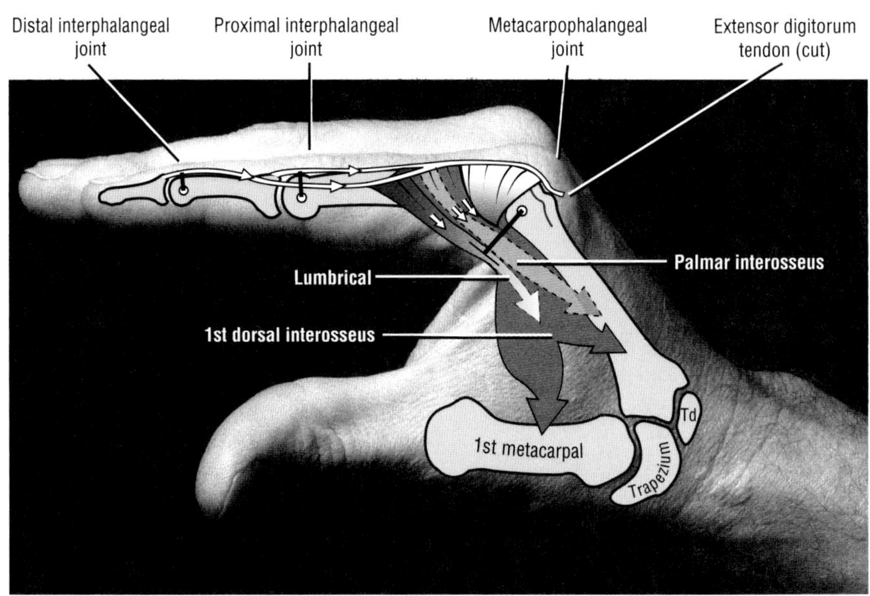

Figure 7-31 The combined action of the lumbricals and interossei is shown as flexors at the metacarpophalangeal (MCP) joint and extensors at the interphalangeal joints. The lumbrical is shown with the greatest moment arm for flexion at the MCP joint. *Td*, Trapezoid bone. (From Neumann DA: *Kinesiology of the musculoskeletal system: foundations for physical rehabilitation*, St Louis, 2002, Mosby, Figure 8-53.)

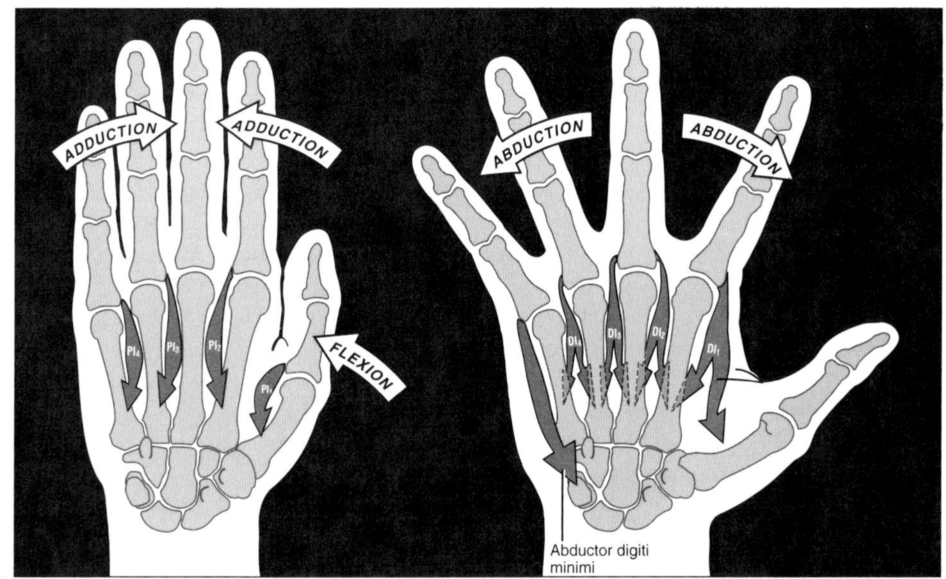

Figure 7-32 A palmar view of the frontal plane action of the palmar interossei (PI_1 *to* PI_4) and dorsal interossei (DI_1 *to* DI_4) at the metacarpophalangeal joints of the hand. The abductor digiti minimi is shown abducting the little finger. (From Neumann DA: *Kinesiology of the musculoskeletal system: foundations for physical rehabilitation,* St Louis, 2002, Mosby, Figure 8-54.)

The palmar and dorsal interossei have a line of force that passes palmar to the MCP joints. Because the interossei attach partially into the extensor mechanism, they (like the lumbricals) flex the MCP joints and extend the PIP and DIP joints (see the palmar and dorsal interossei to the index finger in Figure 7-31).

The following table summarizes the attachments, actions, and innervations of the adductor pollicis, lumbricals, and interossei.

Interaction of Extrinsic and Intrinsic Muscles of the Fingers

The joints of the fingers can perform many different combinations of movements. Two of the most useful combinations, however, combine: (1) simultaneous extension at the MCP, PIP, and DIP joints for opening the hand and (2) simultaneous flexion at the MCP, PIP, and DIP joints for closing the hand. These two important actions are described separately.

ADDUCTOR POLLICIS, LUMBRICALS, AND INTEROSSEI

Muscle	Proximal Attachment	Distal Attachment	Actions	Innervation
Adductor pollicis	Oblique head: capitate, bases of the second and third metacarpals Transverse head: Palmar surface of the third metacarpal	Base of the proximal phalanx of the thumb—ulnar side	Adduction and flexion of the CMC joint of the thumb; flexion of the MCP joint	Ulnar nerve
Lumbricals	Tendons of the flexor digitorum profundus	Lateral band of the extensor mechanism of the fingers	Flexion of the MCP joint and extension of the PIP and DIP joints of the fingers	Medial two: ulnar nerve Lateral two: median nerve
Dorsal interossei	Adjacent sides of all metacarpals	Base and sides of the proximal phalanx and the lateral bands of the extensor mechanism of digits 2-4	Abduction of the MCP joints of digits 2-4 (radial and ulnar deviation of middle finger)	Ulnar nerve
Palmar interossei	Metacarpals of the thumb, index, ring, and little finger	Base and sides of the proximal phalanx of digits one, two, four, and five plus extensor mechanism of the fingers	Adduction of the MCP joints of the second, fourth, and fifth digits (first palmar interossei weakly flexes the thumb)	Ulnar nerve

CMC, Carpometacarpal; *DIP*, distal interphalangeal; *MCP*, metacarpophalangeal; *PIP*, proximal interphalangeal.

OPENING THE HAND: FINGER EXTENSION

Opening the hand is often performed in preparation for grasp. The primary extensors of the fingers are the extensor digitorum and the intrinsic muscles of the fingers, specifically the lumbricals and interossei. Figure 7-33, *A*, shows the extensor digitorum exerting a force on the extensor mechanism, pulling the MCP joint toward extension. The intrinsic muscles furnish both direct and indirect effects on the mechanics of extension of the IP joints (Figure 7-33, *B* and *C*). The direct effect is provided by the proximal pull placed on the bands of the extensor mechanism; the indirect effect is provided by the production of a flexion torque at the MCP joint. This flexion torque prevents the extensor digitorum from hyperextending the MCP joint—an action that would prematurely dissipate most of its contractile force. Only with the MCP joint blocked from being hyperextended can the extensor digitorum effectively tense the bands of the extensor mechanism sufficiently to completely extend the IP joints. This relationship becomes apparent by observing a person with an injury of the ulnar nerve (Figure 7-34). Without active contraction of the lumbricals and interossei of the fourth and fifth digits (which are innervated by the ulnar nerve), contraction of the extensor digitorum causes a characteristic "clawing" of the fingers: The MCP joints hyperextend, and the IP joints remain partially flexed. This is often called the intrinsic-minus posture because of the lack of intrinsic-innervated muscles.

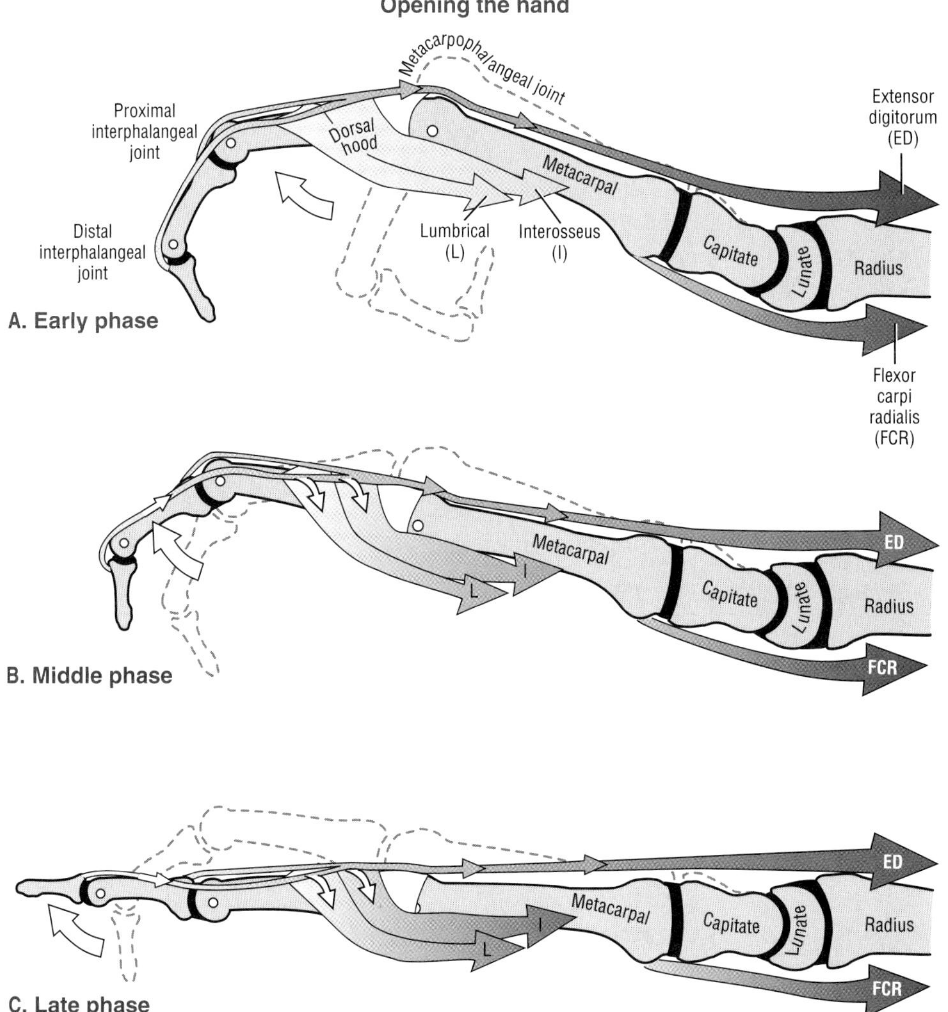

Figure 7-33 A lateral view of the intrinsic and extrinsic muscular interactions at one finger during the opening of the hand. The dotted outlines depict starting positions. **A**, Early phase: The extensor digitorum is shown extending primarily the metacarpophalangeal (MCP) joint. **B**, Middle phase: The intrinsic muscles (lumbricals and interossei) assist the extensor digitorum with extension of the proximal and distal interphalangeal joints. The intrinsic muscles also produce a flexion torque at the MCP joint that prevents the extensor digitorum from hyperextending the MCP joint. **C**, Late phase: Muscle activation continues through full finger extension. (The intensity of the red indicates the relative intensity of the muscle activity.) (From Neumann DA: *Kinesiology of the musculoskeletal system: foundations for physical rehabilitation*, St Louis, 2002, Mosby, Figure 8-58.)

CLOSING THE HAND: FINGER FLEXION

Primary Muscle Action

The muscles used to close the hand depend in part on the specific joints that need to be flexed and on the force requirements of the action. Flexing the fingers against resistance or at relatively high speed requires activation of the flexor digitorum profundus, flexor digitorum superficialis, and, to a lesser extent, the interossei muscles (Figure 7-35). Force produced by both the long finger flexors flexes all three joints of the fingers. The lumbricals may exert a passive flexion torque at the MCP joint as the small muscles are stretched in opposing directions.

Functional Consideration: Wrist Extensors during Finger Flexion

Making a strong fist or grasp requires equally strong synergistic activation from the wrist extensor muscles (see Figure 7-35, *extensor carpi radialis brevis*). Wrist extensor activity can be verified by palpating the dorsum of the forearm while making a fist. As explained in Chapter 6, the primary

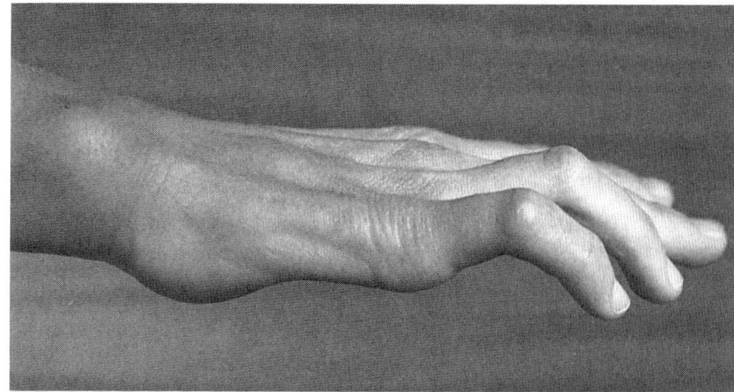

Figure 7-34 Attempts to extend the fingers with an ulnar nerve lesion and a paralysis of the most intrinsic muscles of the fingers. The medial (ulnar) fingers show the claw position with metacarpophalangeal joints hyperextended and fingers partially flexed. Note the atrophy in the hypothenar eminence and interosseous spaces. (From Neumann DA: *Kinesiology of the musculoskeletal system: foundations for physical rehabilitation*, St Louis, 2002, Mosby, Figure 8-59, *A*.)

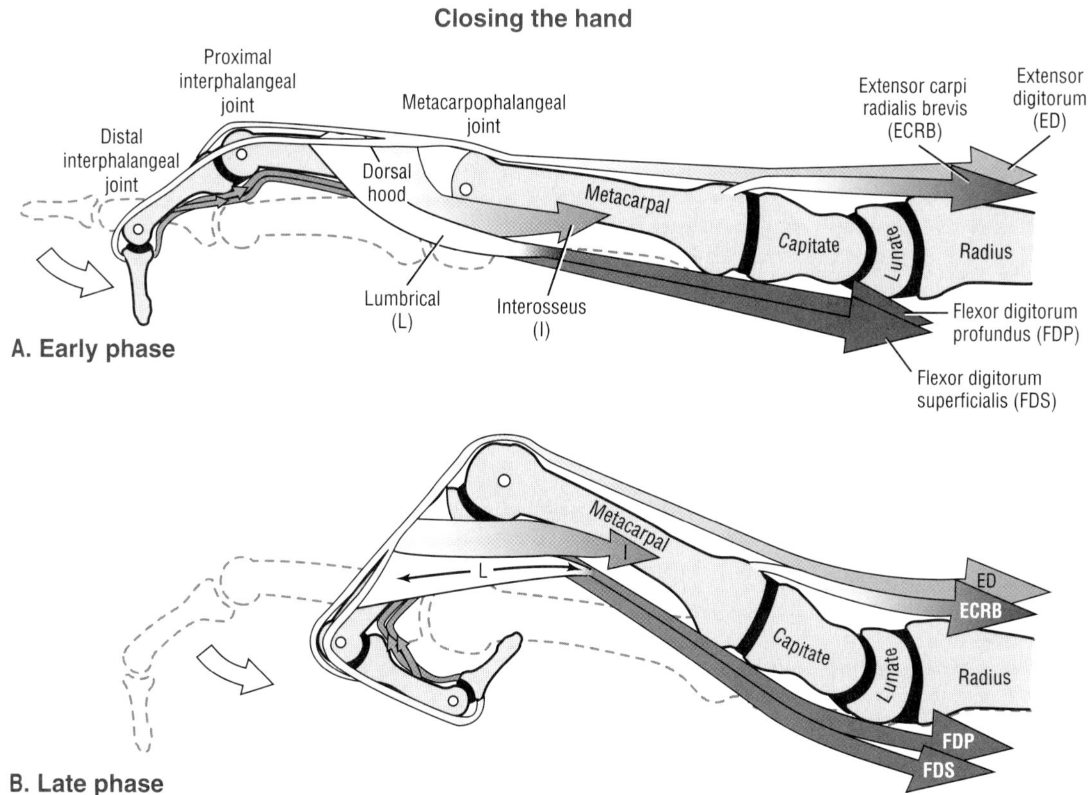

Figure 7-35 A side view of the intrinsic and extrinsic muscular interaction at one finger during a "high-powered" closing of the hand. The dotted outlines depict the starting positions. **A**, Early phase: The flexor digitorum profundus, flexor digitorum superficialis, and interossei muscles actively flex the joints of the finger. The lumbrical is shown as being inactive *(white)*. **B**, Late phase: Muscle activation continues essentially unchanged through full flexion. The lumbrical *(L)* remains inactive but is stretched across both ends. The extensor carpi radialis brevis *(ECRB)* is shown extending the wrist slightly. (The intensity of the red indicates the relative intensity of the muscle activity.) (From Neumann DA: *Kinesiology of the musculoskeletal system: foundations for physical rehabilitation*, St Louis, 2002, Mosby, Figure 8-61.)

function of the wrist extensors is to prevent the wrist from simultaneously flexing by action of the activated extrinsic finger flexor muscles. If the wrist extensors are paralyzed, attempts at making a fist result in a posture of wrist flexion *and* finger flexion—a weak and ineffective action. This weakness can be appreciated by trying to make a strong fist with your wrist held in full flexion.

Joint Deformities of the Hand

Common Deformities

Deformity of the hand is often caused by disease or trauma that disrupts the balance of forces around the joints. This imbalance often results from muscle paralysis, altered muscle tone (e.g., spasticity), increased resistance from ligaments and other connective tissues, or weakened or disrupted connective tissues. Long-term poor positioning of the hand can also contribute to its deformity.

This discussion highlights deformities that typically result from chronic and severe rheumatoid arthritis—a disease that involves chronic synovitis (inflammation of the synovial lining in the joints) and an eventual loss of strength of the connective tissues. Without the normal restraint provided by these tissues, external contact from the environment and, equally important, from muscle contraction can eventually destroy the mechanical integrity of a joint. In worst cases the joint may become misaligned, unstable, and frequently deformed permanently. Knowledge of the underlying cause of the hand deformities is often the basis for physical therapy and surgery.

Three types of deformities are typical in the hand with severe rheumatoid arthritis: ulnar drift, swan-neck deformity, and boutonniere deformity (Figure 7-36). The following section focuses only on the pathomechanics of ulnar drift.

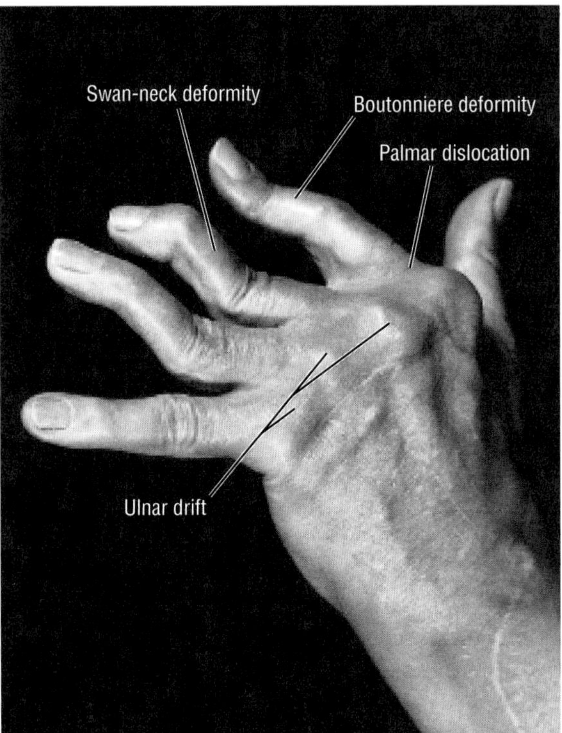

Figure 7-36 A hand showing the common deformities caused by severe rheumatoid arthritis. Particularly evident are the following: palmar dislocation of the metacarpophalangeal joint; ulnar drift; swan-neck deformity; and boutonniere deformity. (See text for further details.) (Courtesy Teri Bielefeld, PT, CHT, Zablocki VA Hospital, Milwaukee, Wis.)

Ulnar Drift

An **ulnar drift** deformity at the MCP joint consists of an excessive ulnar deviation and ulnar translation (slide) of the proximal phalanx relative to the head of the metacarpal. Persons with severe ulnar drift are typically concerned about appearance and reduced function, especially related to pinching and gripping.

To fully understand the pathomechanics of ulnar drift, it is important to realize that all hands—healthy or otherwise—are constantly subjected to factors that favor an ulnar-deviated posture of the fingers. Perhaps the most important factor stems from the almost constant ulnar-directed forces applied against the fingers by hand-held objects, often combined with pinching forces from the thumb. Figure 7-37, A, shows an example of these ulnar-directed forces pushing the index finger in an ulnar direction. The subsequent ulnar deviation of the MCP joint increases the ulnar deflection, or bend, in the extensor digitorum tendon as it crosses the dorsal side of the joint. The deflection creates a potentially destabilizing "bowstringing" force on the tendon. In the healthy hand, however, the extensor mechanism and radial collateral ligament maintain the extensor tendon close to the axis of rotation, thereby minimizing ulnar deviation torque.

The previous description reinforces the important role that healthy connective tissue plays in maintaining the stability of a joint. Often in severe cases of rheumatoid arthritis, the transverse bands of the dorsal hood (part of the extensor mechanism) may rupture or over-stretch, allowing the tendon of the extensor digitorum to slip toward the ulnar side of the joint's axis of rotation (Figure 7-37, *B*). In this position the force produced by the extensor digitorum acts with a moment arm that amplifies the ulnar-deviated posture. This situation initiates a self-perpetuating process: The greater the ulnar deviation, the greater the associated moment arm and the greater the deforming ulnar deviation torque. In time a weakened and over-stretched radial collateral ligament may rupture, allowing the proximal phalanx to rotate and slide ulnarly, leading to complete joint dislocation (Figure 7-37, C).

Treatment for ulnar drift typically includes optimizing the alignment of the joint and, when possible, minimizing the underlying mechanics that caused the instability or deformity. Common non-surgical treatment includes the

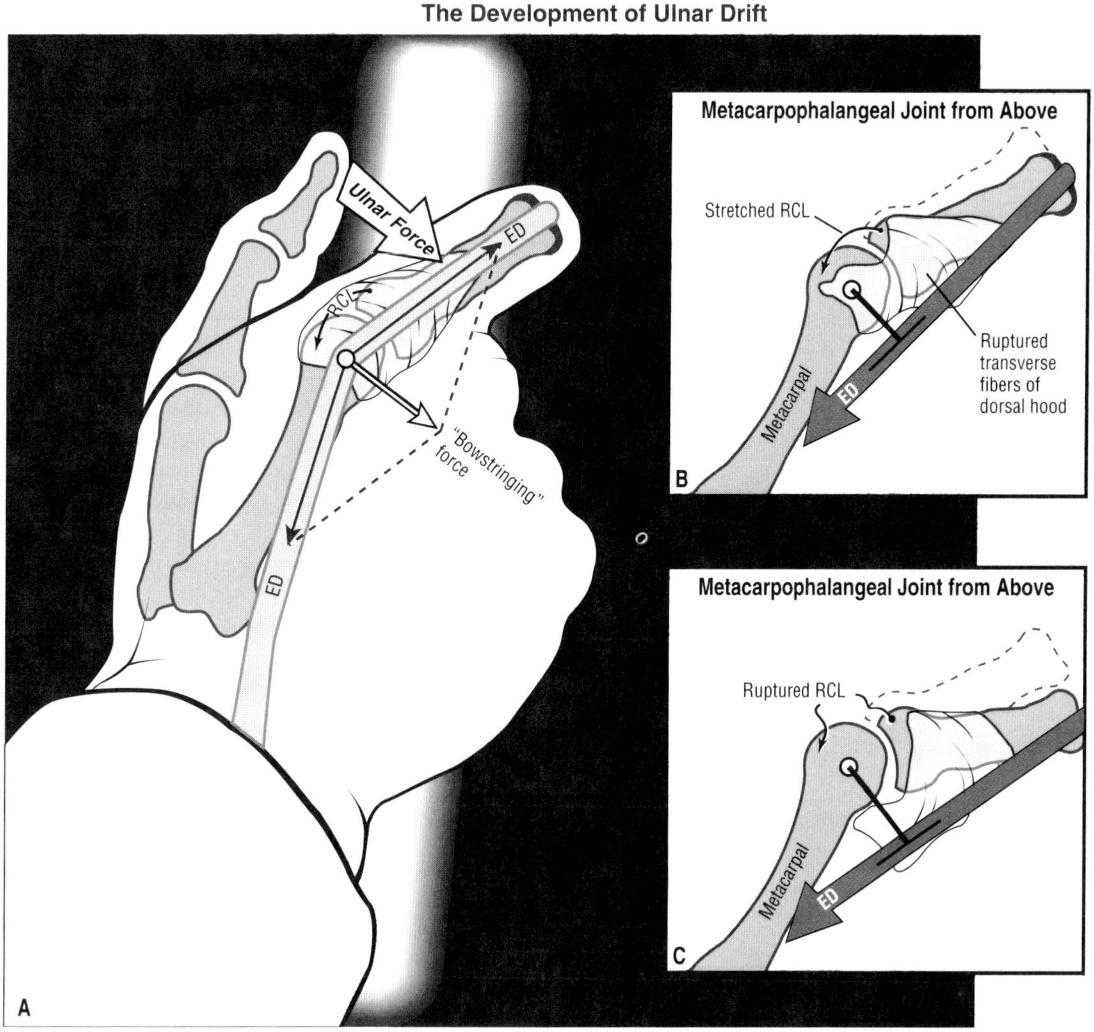

The Development of Ulnar Drift

Figure 7-37 Developmental stages of ulnar drift at the metacarpophalangeal (MCP) joint of the index finger. **A**, Ulnar forces from the thumb produce a natural bowstringing force on the deflected tendon of the extensor digitorum *(ED)*. **B**, In rheumatoid arthritis, rupture of the transverse fibers of the dorsal hood (part of extensor mechanism) allows the extensor tendon to act with a moment arm that increases the ulnar deviation torque at the MCP joint. **C**, Over time, the radial collateral ligament *(RCL)* may rupture, resulting in the ulnar drift deformity. (From Neumann DA: *Kinesiology of the musculoskeletal system: foundations for physical rehabilitation*, St Louis, 2002, Mosby, Figure 8-67.)

use of splints and advising patients on how to minimize the deforming forces across the MCP joint. Consider the strong ulnar deviation torque placed on the MCP joints of the right hand while tightening the lid of a jar or holding a pitcher of water. This torque may, over time, encourage ulnar drift. In general, patients are advised to avoid most heavy gripping and forceful key pinch activities, especially during the acute inflammation or painful stage of rheumatoid arthritis.

Summary

The joints of the hand are organized into three sets of articulations: carpometacarpal (CMC), metacarpophalangeal (MCP), and interphalangeal (IP). Located most proximally within the hand, the CMC joints are responsible for adjusting the curvature of the palm, from flat to deeply cup shaped. The first and fifth CMC joints are particularly important in this regard because they oppose the thumb toward the other digits and raise the ulnar border of the hand, respectively. Trauma or disease involving these joints can deprive the hand of many postures that are unique to human prehension.

The relatively large MCP joints form the base of each digit. The MCP joints of the fingers move in 2 degrees of freedom: abduction and adduction, and flexion and extension. The action of extension and abduction maximizes the functional width of the hand, which is especially useful for holding broad objects of varying curvatures.

The IP joints flex and extend only; the other potential planes of motion are blocked by the bony fit of the joint and by periarticular connective tissues. Flexion range of motion is nevertheless extensive at the IP joints, from 70 degrees at the IP joint of the thumb to 120 degrees at the more ulnarly located PIP joints of the fingers. Such motion is necessary to fully close the fist, hold a handbag, or otherwise maximize digital contact with objects. Full extension at these joints is equally important to open the hand in preparation for grasp.

The 29 muscles of the hand have been classified into extrinsic and intrinsic groups. As described earlier in this chapter, simultaneous extension of all three joints of the fingers requires a coordinated interplay among the extensor digitorum *and* the intrinsic muscles such as the lumbricals and interossei. More complex and rapid movements of the digits demands an even greater functional interdependence between the intrinsic and extrinsic muscles.

Study Questions

1. Which of the following joints are most proximal within the hand?
   a. MCP joints
   b. PIP joints
   c. DIP joints
   d. CMC joints
2. Which of the following statements is true regarding abduction of the index finger?
   a. This motion occurs in the frontal plane.
   b. This motion describes the index finger moving away from the middle finger (toward the thumb).
   c. This motion describes the index finger moving toward the middle finger.
   d. A and B
   e. B and C
3. Flexion of the thumb:
   a. Occurs in the sagittal plane
   b. Occurs in the frontal plane
   c. Occurs in the horizontal plane
   d. Occurs about a longitudinal axis of rotation
   e. C and D
4. Which of the following joints can perform flexion *and* abduction?
   a. CMC joint of the thumb
   b. DIP joints of digits 2 to 5
   c. MCP joints of digits 2 to 5
   d. A and B
   e. A and C
5. The motion of touching the thumb to the other fingertips is called:
   a. Abduction
   b. Hypothenar flexion
   c. Opposition
   d. Reposition
6. The tendons of the extrinsic finger extensors:
   a. All course posterior to the medial-lateral axis of rotation of the MCP joints
   b. All course anterior to the medial-lateral axis of rotation of the wrist
   c. All blend with a special set of connective tissues called the extensor mechanism
   d. A and B
   e. A and C
7. Which of the following muscles is *not* part of the hypothenar eminence?
   a. Flexor digiti minimi
   b. Abductor digiti minimi
   c. Opponens pollicis
   d. Opponens digiti minimi
8. The primary function of the muscles of the thenar eminence is:
   a. Curl the ulnar border of the hand such as when cupping
   b. Position the thumb in varying amounts of opposition to facilitate grasping
   c. Extend the thumb and ulnarly deviate the wrist
   d. Flex the MCP joints of digits 2 to 5
9. Which of the following is *not* an action of the lumbrical muscles?
   a. Flexion of the MCP joints of the fingers
   b. Extension of the DIP joints of the fingers
   c. Flexion of the PIP joints of the fingers
   d. Extension of the PIP joints of the fingers
10. The primary function of the dorsal interossei muscles is:
    a. Abduction of the fingers
    b. Adduction of the fingers
    c. Flexion of the PIP and DIP joints
    d. Flexion of the DIP joints
11. Injury or paralysis of the ulnar nerve will significantly affect the muscles of the hypothenar eminence.
    a. True
    b. False
12. *Basilar joint osteoarthritis* refers to arthritis of the CMC joint of the thumb.
    a. True
    b. False
13. Injury or paralysis to the median nerve will likely result in an inability to oppose the thumb.
    a. True
    b. False
14. An individual without functional finger flexors may perform a tenodesis grip through activation of the wrist extensors.
    a. True
    b. False
15. Paralysis of the radial nerve will primarily result in an inability to oppose the thumb.
    a. True
    b. False
16. The structure of the CMC joint of the thumb is that of a hinge joint.
    a. True
    b. False

17. Hyperextension of the MCP joints of the fingers is primarily limited by tension in the palmar (volar) plates.
    a. True
    b. False
18. A strong pinching activity such as when cutting with scissors involves strong activation of the adductor pollicis muscle.
    a. True
    b. False
19. Extrinsic muscles of the hand have their proximal attachments on the forearm or arm but attach distally to a structure within the hand.
    a. True
    b. False
20. Without activation of the lumbricals and interossei muscles, contraction of the extensor digitorum results in clawing of the fingers.
    a. True
    b. False

ADDITIONAL READINGS

Allison DM: Anatomy of the collateral ligaments of the proximal interphalangeal joint, *J Hand Surg [Am]* 30(5):1026-1031, 2005.

Bettinger PC, Linscheid RL, Berger RA et al: An anatomic study of the stabilizing ligaments of the trapezium and trapeziometacarpal joint, *J Hand Surg [Am]* 24(4):786-798, 1999.

Bielefeld T, Neumann DA: The unstable metacarpophalangeal joint in rheumatoid arthritis: anatomy, pathomechanics, and physical rehabilitation considerations, *J Orthop Sports Phys Ther* 35(8): 502-520, 2005.

Boatright JR, Kiebzak GM: The effects of low median nerve block on thumb abduction strength, *J Hand Surg [Am]* 22(5):849-852, 1997.

Brand PW: *Clinical biomechanics of the hand*, St Louis, 1985, Mosby.

Brand PW: Biomechanics of tendon transfers, *Hand Clin* 4(2):137-154, 1988.

Dubousset JF: The digital joints. In Tubiana R, editor: *The hand*, Philadelphia, 1981, Saunders.

Dvir Z: Biomechanics of muscle. In Dvir Z, editor: *Clinical biomechanics*, Philadelphia, 2000, Churchill Livingstone.

Flatt AE: Ulnar drift, *J Hand Ther* 9(4):282-292, 1996.

Jenkins M, Bamberger HB, Black L et al: Thumb joint flexion. What is normal?, *J Hand Surg [Br]* 23(6):796-797, 1998.

Kapandji IA: *The physiology of the joints*, ed 5, Edinburgh, 1982, Churchill Livingstone.

Katarincic JA: Thumb kinematics and their relevance to function, *Hand Clin* 17(2):169-174, 2001.

Momose T, Nakatsuchi Y, Saitoh S: Contact area of the trapeziometacarpal joint, *J Hand Surg [Am]* 24(3):491-495, 1999.

Neumann DA, Bielefeld T: The carpometacarpal joint of the thumb: stability, deformity, and therapeutic intervention, *J Orthop Sports Phys Ther* 33(7):386-399, 2003.

Omokawa S, Ryu J, Tang JB et al: Trapeziometacarpal joint instability affects the moment arms of thumb motor tendons, *Clin Orthop* (372):262-271, 2000.

Pagalidis T, Kuczynski K, Lamb DW: Ligamentous stability of the base of the thumb, *Hand* 13(1):29-36, 1981.

Seradge H, Jia YC, Owens W: In vivo measurement of carpal tunnel pressure in the functioning hand [see comment], *J Hand Surg [Am]* 22(5):855-859, 1997.

Tubiana R: *The hand*, Philadelphia, 1981, Saunders.

Valentin P: The interossei and the lumbricals. In Tubinia R, editor: *The hand*, Philadelphia, 1981, Saunders.

Wilton JC: *Hand splinting: principles of design and fabrication*, Philadelphia, 1997, Saunders.

CHAPTER 8

Structure and Function of the Vertebral Column

CHAPTER OUTLINE

OBJECTIVES

- Identify the normal curvatures of the vertebral column, and explain how these curves provide spinal stability.
- Identify the bones and bony features of the vertebral column and cranium.
- Describe the ligaments and soft tissues of the vertebral column and important features of an intervertebral disc.
- Describe the unique features of the cervical, thoracic, lumbar, and sacral vertebrae.
- Cite the normal ranges of motion allowed for flexion and extension, lateral flexion, and axial rotation at the craniocervical and thoracolumbar regions of the vertebral column.
- Explain how the orientation of the facet joints helps determine the primary movements of the various regions of the vertebral column.
- Describe the motions of the spine that decrease and increase the diameter of the intervertebral foramen.
- Describe the effect of flexion, extension, and lateral flexion on the potential migration of the intervertebral disc.
- Justify the actions of the muscles within the anterior and posterior craniocervical region of the vertebral column.
- Justify the actions of the muscles within the anterior and posterior thoracolumbar region of the vertebral column.
- Differentiate between segmental and gross stabilization of the vertebral column.
- Describe the factors that contribute to safe and unsafe lifting techniques.

KEY TERMS

anterior pelvic tilt
anterior spondylolisthesis
cauda equina
core stabilization
counternutation
herniated nucleus pulposus
kyphosis
line of gravity
lordosis
neutral spine
nutation
posterior pelvic tilt
scoliosis
spinal nerve
stenosis
thoracic outlet syndrome
Wolff's Law

The spine, or vertebral column, consists of 33 vertebral segments, divided into 5 regions: cervical, thoracic, lumbar, sacral, and coccygeal. Normally there are 7 cervical, 12 thoracic, 5 lumbar, 5 sacral, and 4 coccygeal segments. The sacral and coccygeal segments are fused in the adult, forming individual sacral and coccygeal bones. This text focuses primarily on the kinesiology of the cervical, thoracic, and lumbar regions. Each of these three regions allows flexion and extension, lateral flexion, and horizontal plane (axial) rotation. The amount of motion allowed at any particular region is largely dictated by the shapes and functions of local bony, muscular, and ligamentous structures. The movement that occurs between two vertebrae is typically only a few degrees; however, when added across several vertebrae, the motion allowed at any particular region can be quite substantial.

Disease, trauma, or reaching an advanced age can lead to a host of neuromuscular and musculoskeletal problems that involve the spine. These problems may be associated with pain or other impairments because of the close anatomic relationship among the spinal cord, nerve roots, bony structures, and connective tissues of the vertebral column. For example, a herniated (bulging) intervertebral disc can press on the adjacent nerve roots, causing pain, weakness, and reduced reflexes. Furthermore, poor posture and certain movements of the spinal column can increase the likelihood of impinging the adjacent neural structures.

This chapter presents an overview of the important anatomic structures and kinematic interactions required for normal posture and spinal motion. This material is intended to provide a sound basis for understanding common impairments of the back and neck, as well as the rehabilitation principles involved in treatment of these conditions.

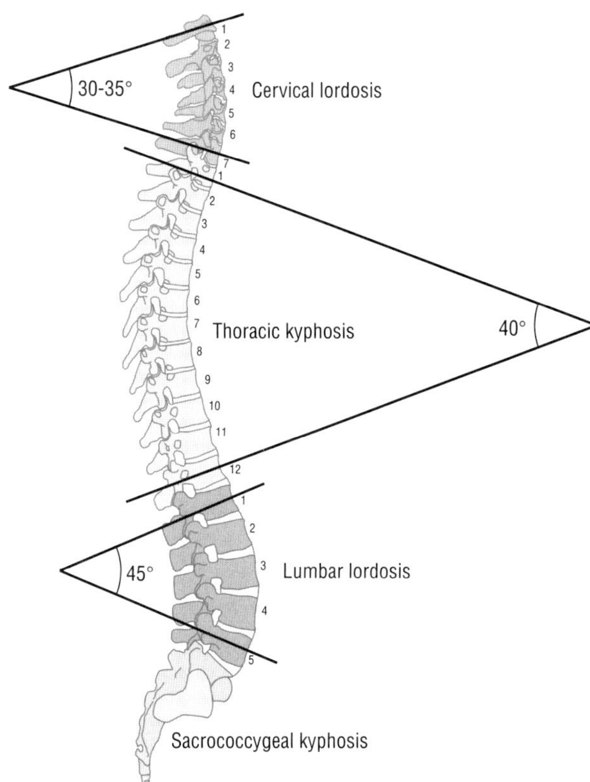

Figure 8-1 The normal curvatures of the vertebral column. These curvatures represent the normal resting posture of each region. (From Neumann DA: *Kinesiology of the musculoskeletal system: foundations for physical rehabilitation,* St Louis, 2002, Mosby, Figure 9-40.)

Normal Curvatures

The human vertebral column is composed of a set of natural curves, illustrated in Figure 8-1. These reciprocal curves are responsible for the normal resting, or neutral, posture of the spine. The cervical and lumbar regions display a natural **lordosis**, or slightly extended posture, in the sagittal plane. In contrast, the thoracic and sacrococcygeal regions exhibit a natural **kyphosis**, or slightly flexed, posture. The anterior concavity of the thoracic and sacral regions provides space for the important vital organs within the chest and pelvis.

The natural curvatures of the vertebral column are not fixed; they are dynamic and flexible to accommodate a wide variety of different postures and movements (Figure 8-2). For example, extension increases the lordosis of the cervical and lumbar regions but reduces the thoracic kyphosis (see Figure 8-2, *B*). Flexion, in contrast, reduces the lordosis of the lumbar and cervical regions and accentuates the kyphotic curve of the thoracic region (see Figure 8-2, *C*).

The normal curvatures of the spine provide strength and stability to the entire axial skeleton. Interestingly, a vertebral column that possesses these natural curves can support more compressive force than one that is straight. When these natural curvatures are maintained, compressive forces can be shared by the tension produced from the stretched connective tissues and muscles located along the convex side of each curve. Also, the flexible nature of the spinal curvatures allows the vertebral column to "give" slightly under a load, rather than support large forces statically.

Disease, trauma, genetically loose ligaments, or habitual poor posture can lead to an exaggeration (or reduction) of the normal spinal curvatures. These variations of the natural spinal curves can stress the local muscles and joints, as well as reduce the volume in the thorax for expansion of the lungs.

Line of Gravity

Although highly variable, the **line of gravity** acting on a person with ideal posture passes through the mastoid process of the temporal bone, anterior to the second sacral

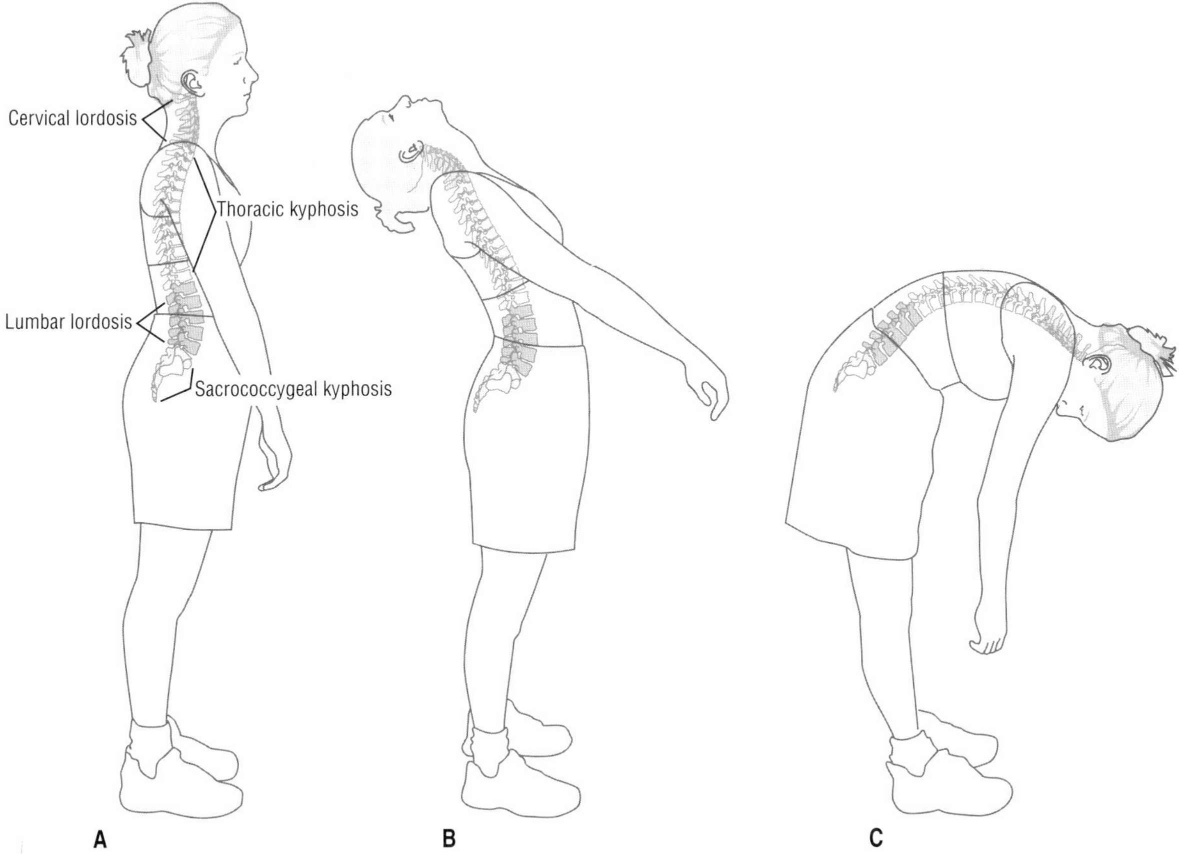

Figure 8-2 A side view of the normal sagittal plane curvatures of the vertebral column. **A,** Neutral position of the vertebral column during standing. **B,** Extension of the vertebral column increases the cervical and lumbar lordosis but decreases (straightens) the thoracic kyphosis. **C,** Flexion of the vertebral column decreases the cervical and lumbar lordosis but increases the thoracic kyphosis. (From Neumann DA: *Kinesiology of the musculoskeletal system: foundations for physical rehabilitation,* St Louis, 2002, Mosby, Figure 9-8.)

vertebrae, slightly posterior to the hip, and slightly anterior to the knee and ankle (Figure 8-3). As indicated in Figure 8-3, the line of gravity courses just to the concave side of each vertebral region's curvature. Consequently, in ideal posture, gravity produces a torque that helps maintain the optimal shape of each spinal curvature, allowing one to stand at ease with minimal muscular activation and minimal stress on the surrounding connective tissues. These ideal biomechanics significantly reduce the energy of maintaining postures such as standing and sitting.

Many persons exhibit poor posture due to muscular tightness or weakness, trauma, poor habit, body-fat distribution, disease, or heredity. Figure 8-4 displays five commonly observed abnormal or "faulty" postures. Over time, these postures may significantly destabilize the spine and require compensatory strategies that alter normal motion of the trunk, extremities, or the body as a whole. For example, the swayback posture illustrated in Figure 8-4, C, is often associated with significant tightness of the lumbar extensor muscles and excessive stretch (and potentially weakness) of the abdominal muscles. This posture can increase the shear forces on the intervertebral discs and joints that interconnect the lumbar spine. Clinicians who treat people with back and neck pain often attempt to correct faulty postures as a primary component of the rehabilitation process.

Osteology

Cranium

The cranium, or skull, is the bony encasement that protects the brain. Many of the bony features described herein serve as attachments for muscles and ligaments. Numerous other important features of the cranium are not described but are labeled in Figures 8-5 and 8-6.

The *external occipital protuberance* (often referred to as the *"bump of knowledge"*) is a palpable landmark located at the midpoint of the posterior skull serving as an attachment for the ligamentum nuchae and upper trapezius. The *superior nuchal line* is a ridge of bone that extends laterally from the occipital protuberance to the mastoid process. The *inferior nuchal line* resides just

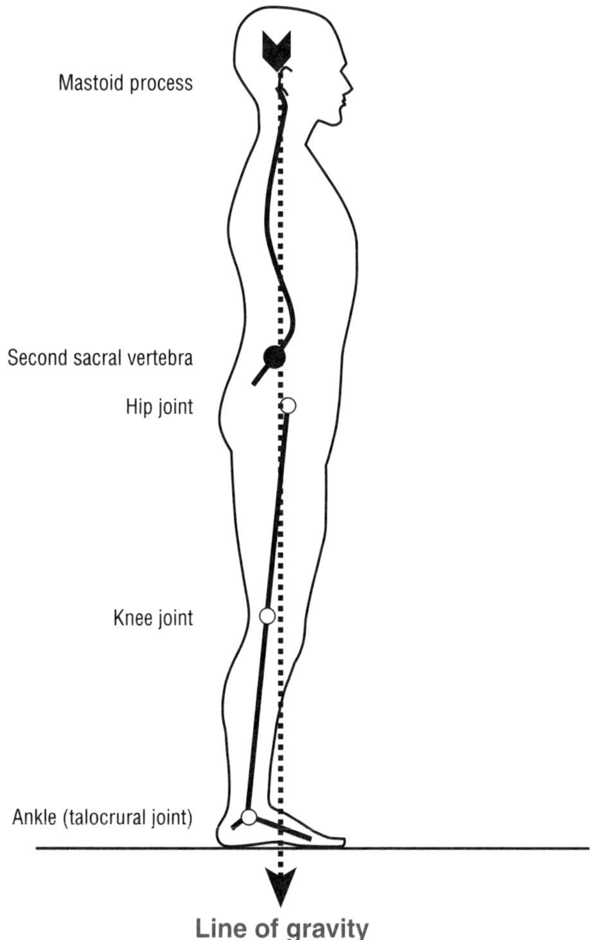

Figure 8-3 The line of gravity in a person with ideal standing posture. (Modified from Neumann DA: Arthrokinesiologic considerations for the aged adult. In Guccione AA, editor: *Geriatric physical therapy*, ed 2, Chicago, 2000, Mosby.)

below the superior nuchal line, near the base of the skull. The nuchal lines provide the cranial attachments for numerous muscles and ligaments.

Literally meaning "large hole," the *foramen magnum* is located at the base of the skull, providing a passage for the spinal cord to meet the brain (see Figure 8-6). The prominent *occipital condyles* project from the anterior-lateral margins of the foramen magnum. These convex structures articulate with the atlas (first cervical vertebrae), forming the atlanto-occipital joint. Just posterior to each ear are the large, palpable *mastoid processes*, which serve as the cranial attachment for numerous muscles of the head and neck, most notably the sternocleidomastoid.

Typical Vertebrae

All vertebrae have several common features, many of which are evident by examining different views of a thoracic vertebra (Figure 8-7). The *body* of a vertebra is the large cylindrical mass of bone that serves as the primary weight-bearing structure throughout the vertebral column. The *intervertebral disc* is the thick fluid-filled ring of fibrocartilage that serves as a shock absorber throughout the vertebral column. The specific anatomy of intervertebral discs is covered in the next section. The *interbody joint* is formed by the junction of two vertebral bodies and the interposed intervertebral disc.

Posterior to the body of each vertebra is the *vertebral canal*, which houses and protects the delicate spinal cord. *Pedicles* are short, thick projections of bone that connect the body of the vertebrae to each *transverse process*. The *laminae* are thin plates of bone that form the posterior wall of the vertebral canal, connecting each transverse process to the base of the *spinous process*.

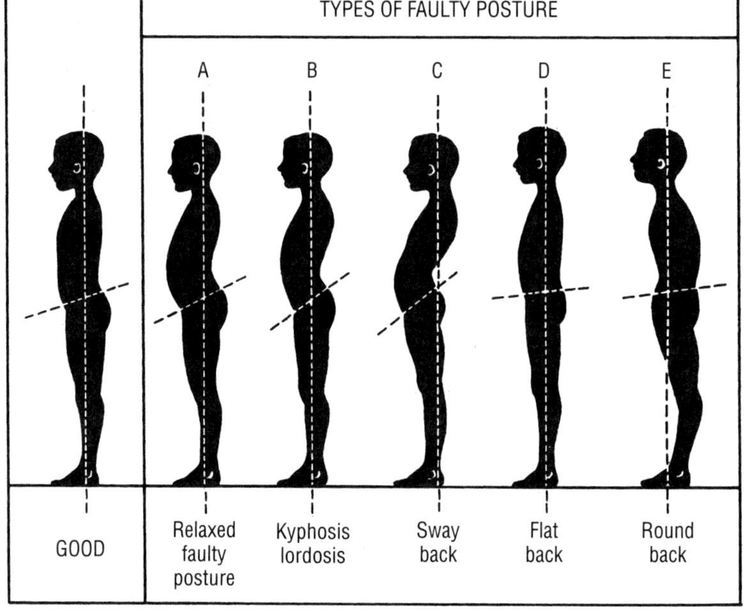

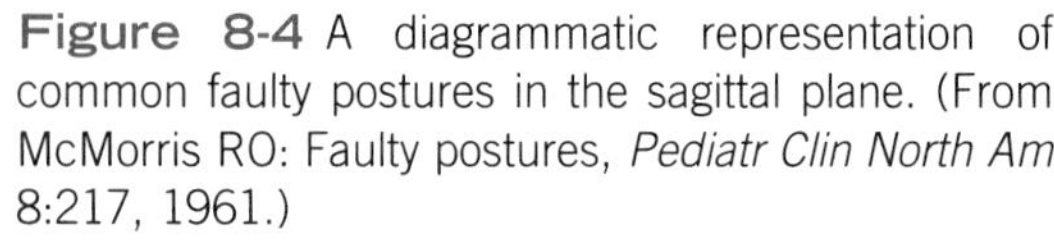
Figure 8-4 A diagrammatic representation of common faulty postures in the sagittal plane. (From McMorris RO: Faulty postures, *Pediatr Clin North Am* 8:217, 1961.)

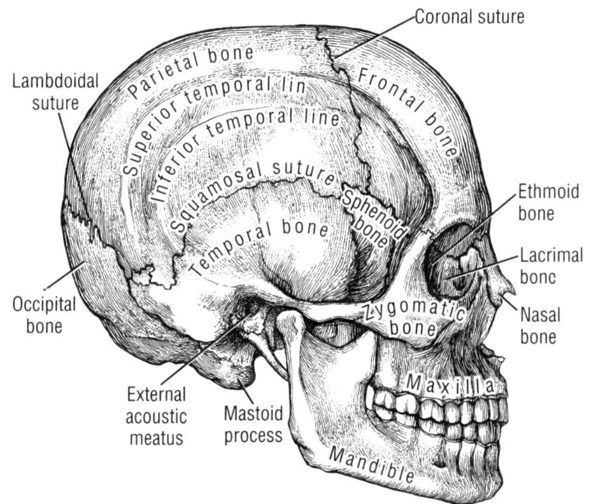

Figure 8-5 Lateral view of the skull. (From Neumann DA: *Kinesiology of the musculoskeletal system: foundations for physical rehabilitation*, St Louis, 2002, Mosby, Figure 9-2.)

Each vertebra has matching pairs of *superior and inferior articular facets*. The inferior facets of one vertebra articulate with the superior facets of the vertebra below it, composing a pair of *apophyseal joints*. These joints, more commonly referred to as *facet joints*, help guide the direction of vertebral motion.

Right and left *intervertebral foramina* exist between adjacent vertebrae, forming passageways for nerve roots entering or exiting the vertebral column. Because the intervertebral foramen is formed *between* two vertebrae, spinal movement naturally alters its diameter. This important point is revisited later in this chapter.

Intervertebral Discs

Intervertebral discs play an extremely important role in absorbing and transmitting compression and shear forces throughout the spinal column. Each intervertebral disc is composed of three primary components: the nucleus pulposus, the annulus fibrosus, and the vertebral end plate (Figure 8-8).

The *nucleus pulposus* is the gelatinous center of the disc. Composed of 70% to 90% water, the nucleus pulposus serves as a hydraulic shock absorber, dissipating and transferring forces between consecutive vertebrae. The *annulus fibrosus* is composed of 10 to 20 concentric rings of fibrocartilage that, in essence, encase the nucleus pulposus. As illustrated in Figure 8-9, the rings of fibrocartilage form a crisscross pattern that strengthens the walls of the annulus. When two vertebrae are compressed from the pressure of body weight or muscular forces, the nucleus pulposus is squeezed outward, producing tension within the annulus fibrosus (Figure 8-10). This tension stabilizes the spongy disc, converting it to a stable weight-bearing structure. The *vertebral end plate* connects the intervertebral disc to the vertebrae above and below and helps provide the disc with nutrition.

Specifying Vertebrae and Intervertebral Discs

Individual vertebrae are numbered by region in a cranial-to-sacral direction. For example, C3 indicates the third cervical vertebrae from the top of the cervical spine. T8 indicates the eighth thoracic vertebrae (from the top), L4 describes

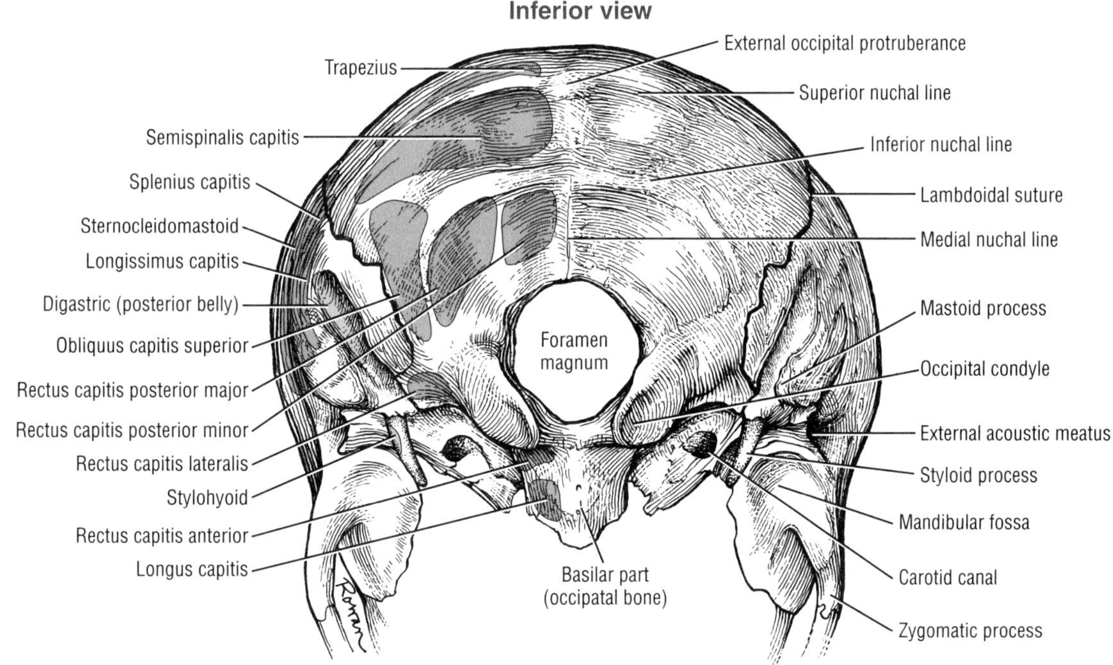

Figure 8-6 An inferior view of the skull. Distal muscular attachments are indicated in gray, proximal attachments in red. (From Neumann DA: *Kinesiology of the musculoskeletal system: foundations for physical rehabilitation*, St Louis, 2002, Mosby, Figure 9-3.)

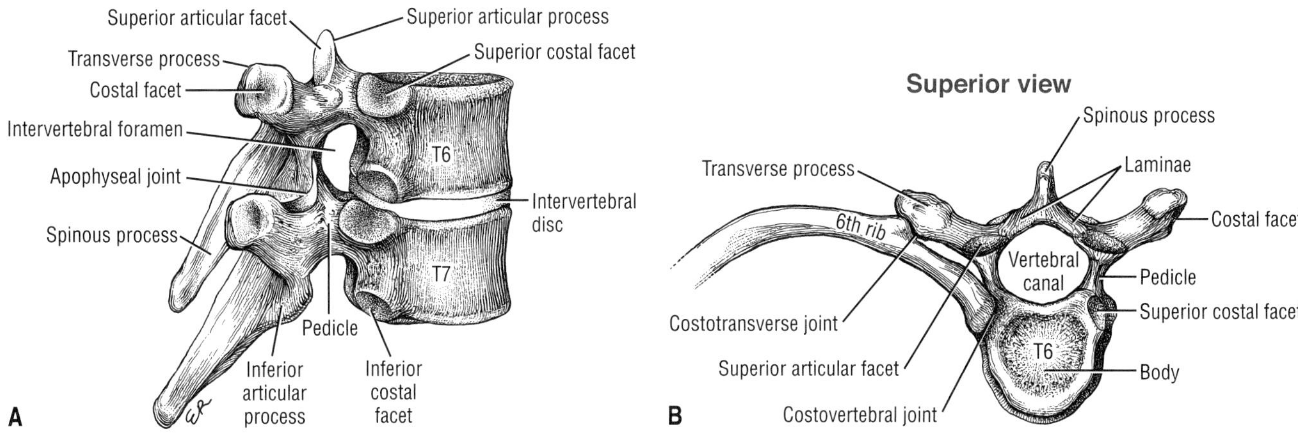

Figure 8-7 The essential characteristics of a typical vertebra. **A,** Lateral view of two thoracic vertebrae. **B,** Superior view of the sixth thoracic vertebra. (From Neumann DA: *Kinesiology of the musculoskeletal system: foundations for physical rehabilitation*, St Louis, 2002, Mosby, Figure 9-5.)

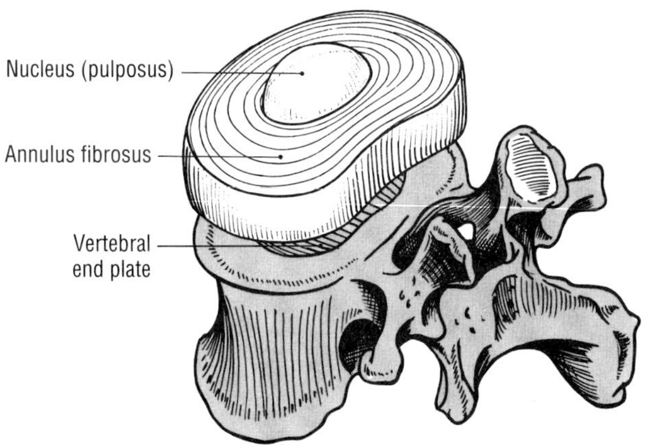

Figure 8-8 The intervertebral disc is shown lifted away from the underlying vertebra. (Modified from Kapandji IA: *The physiology of joints*, vol 3, New York, 1974, Churchill Livingstone.)

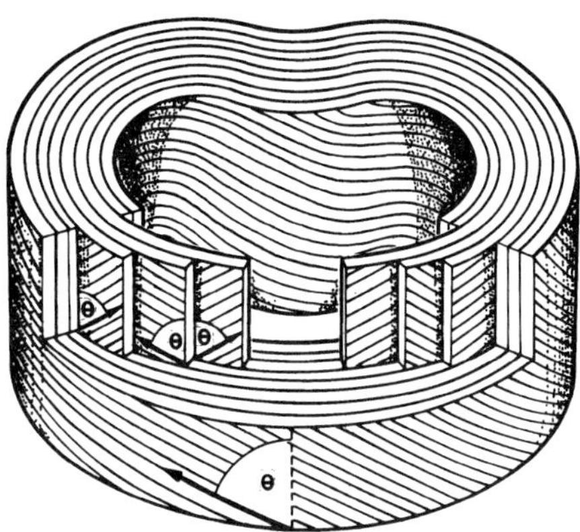

Figure 8-9 An illustration of an intervertebral disc with the nucleus pulposus removed, highlighting the crisscross pattern of the annulus fibrosus. (From Bogduk N: *Clinical anatomy of the lumbar spine*, ed 3, New York, 1997, Churchill Livingstone.)

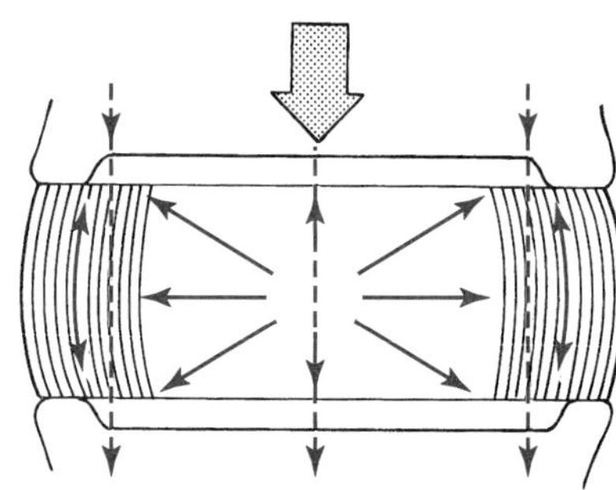

Figure 8-10 The mechanism of force transmission through an intervertebral disc. The pressure within the nucleus converts the annulus fibrosus to a stable weight-bearing structure. (From Bogduk N: *Clinical anatomy of the lumbar spine*, ed 3, New York, 1997, Churchill Livingstone.)

the fourth lumbar vertebrae, and so on (see Figure 8-22 on p. 189).

Intervertebral discs are described by their position *between* two vertebrae. For example, the L4-L5 disc describes the intervertebral disc located between the fourth and fifth lumbar vertebrae, and the C6-C7 disc indicates the intervertebral disc between the sixth and seventh cervical vertebrae.

Spinal nerves are described in much the same way as the vertebrae. Realize, however, that cervical spinal nerves exit *above* their respective cervical vertebrae; in contrast, thoracic and lumbar spinal nerves exit *below* their respective thoracic or lumbar vertebrae.

Comparison of Vertebrae at Different Regions

Although all vertebrae have common anatomic characteristics, they also possess distinct features that reflect the unique function of a particular region. The following section, along with Table 8-1, highlights osteologic features that are specific to each region of the vertebral column.

TABLE 8-1 OSTEOLOGIC FEATURES OF THE VERTEBRAL COLUMN

	Body	Superior Articular Facets	Inferior Articular Facets	Spinous Processes	Vertebral Canal	Transverse Processes	Comments
Atlas (C1)	None	Concave, face generally superior	Flat to slightly concave, face generally inferior	None, replaced by a small posterior tubercle	Triangular, largest of cervical region	Largest of cervical region	Appears as two large lateral masses, joined by anterior and posterior arches
Axis (C2)	Tall with a vertical projecting dens	Flat to slightly convex, face generally superior	Flat, face anterior and inferior	Largest and bifid (i.e., double)	Large and triangular	Form anterior and posterior tubercles	Contains large spinous process
C3-6	Wider than deep; have uncinate processes	Flat, face posterior and superior	As above	Bifid	Large and triangular	End as anterior and posterior tubercles	Considered typical cervical vertebrae
C7	Wider than deep	As above	Transition to typical thoracic vertebrae	Large and prominent, easily palpable	Triangular	Thick and prominent, may have a large anterior tubercle forming an "extra rib"	Often called vertebral prominens due to large spinous process
T2-9	Equal width and depth Costal facets for attachment of the heads of ribs 2-9	Flat, face mostly posterior	Flat, face mostly anterior	Long and pointed, slant inferiorly	Round, smaller than cervical	Project horizontally and slightly posterior, have costal facets for tubercles of ribs	Considered typical thoracic vertebrae
T1 and T10-12	Equal width and depth T1 has a full costal facet for rib 1 and a partial facet for rib 2 T10-12 each has a full costal facet	As above	As above	As above	As above	T10-12 may lack costal facets	Considered atypical thoracic vertebrae primarily by the manner of rib attachment
L1-5	Wider than deep; L5 is slightly wedged (i.e., higher height anteriorly than posteriorly)	Slightly concave, face medial to posterior-medial	L1-4 slightly convex, face lateral to anterior-lateral L5: flat, face anterior and slightly lateral	Stout and rectangular	Triangular, contains cauda equina	Slender, project laterally	Superior articular processes have mamillary bodies
Sacrum	Fused Body of first sacral vertebra most evident	Flat, face posterior and slightly medial	None	None, replaced by multiple spinous tubercles	As above	None, replaced by multiple transverse tubercles	
Coccyx	Fusion of four rudimentary vertebrae	Rudimentary	Rudimentary	Rudimentary	Ends at the first coccyx	Rudimentary	

From Neumann DA: *Kinesiology of the musculoskeletal system: foundations for physical rehabilitation*, St Louis, 2002, Mosby, Table 9-4.

CERVICAL VERTEBRAE

The seven cervical vertebrae are the smallest and most mobile of all vertebrae, reflecting the wide range of motion available to the head and neck (Figure 8-11).

The first two cervical vertebrae, called the atlas (C1) and the axis (C2), are unique even to the cervical region. The rest of the cervical vertebrae (C3-C7) are considered typical and are described as follows.

Typical Cervical Vertebrae (C3-C7)

The transverse processes of the cervical vertebrae possess *transverse foramina*, which are holes within the transverse processes (see Figure 8-11) that serve as conduits for each vertebral artery coursing toward the brain. The small rectangular bodies of the cervical vertebrae are bordered posterior-laterally by *uncinate processes* (see Figure 8-11). The articulation of these hook-like uncinate processes with the adjacent vertebrae make the cervical vertebrae appear like a set of stackable shelves. Most of the *spinous processes* in the cervical region are bifid, or two-pronged, and provide attachments for muscles from both sides of the body.

Observe that the apophyseal (facet) joints throughout C3-C7 are oriented like shingles on a sloped roof in a plane that is about 45 degrees between the horizontal and frontal planes (Figure 8-12). This orientation has an important impact on the kinematics of this region—a point that is revisited later in this chapter.

Atlas (C1)

The Greek god Atlas is said to have supported the weight of the world on his back. The first cervical vertebra is also called the atlas, reflecting its function in supporting the weight of the cranium. The atlas is essentially two large lateral masses connected by *anterior and posterior arches* (Figure 8-13). Two large concave *superior facets* sit on top of these lateral masses to accept the large convex occipital condyles, forming the *atlanto-occipital joint*. Other distinguishing features include large *transverse processes*, the largest in the cervical region.

Axis (C2)

The axis derives its name from the large pointed projection of bone, called the dens, which literally functions as the vertical axis of rotation for rotary movements between the

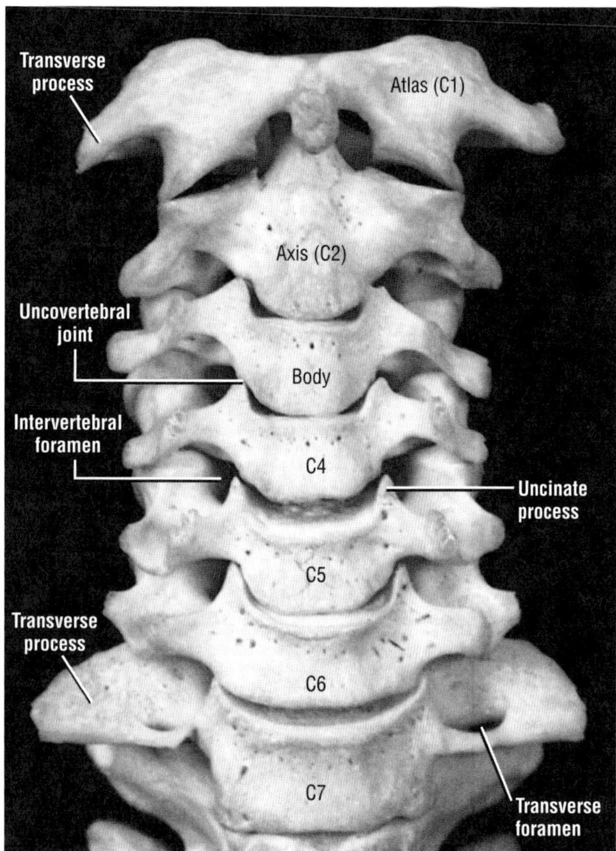

Figure 8-11 An anterior view of the cervical vertebral column. (Modified from Neumann DA: *Kinesiology of the musculoskeletal system: foundations for physical rehabilitation*, St Louis, 2002, Mosby, Figure 9-18.)

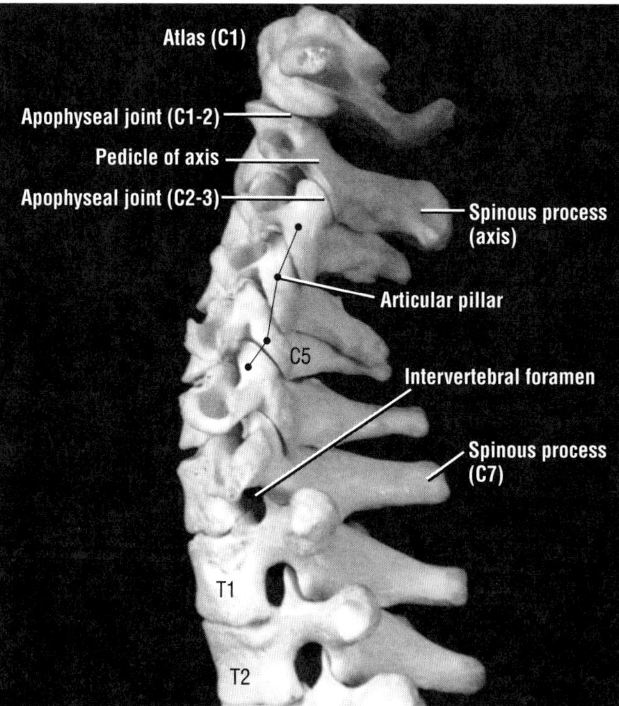

Figure 8-12 A lateral view of the cervical vertebral column. (Modified from Neumann DA: *Kinesiology of the musculoskeletal system: foundations for physical rehabilitation*, St Louis, 2002, Mosby, Figure 9-21.)

Clinical INSIGHT

Osteophytes and Degenerative Disc Disease

Due to excessive wear, arthritis, or advanced age, some intervertebral discs become dehydrated and lose their ability to act as shock absorbers and functional spacers within the cervical region. Figure 8-14 shows a portion of the cervical spine. The disc between C3 and C4 is healthy and well hydrated, designed to prevent bone-on-bone compression of the vertebrae. The C4-C5 intervertebral disc, however, is degenerated and almost flat. As a result, there is bone-on-bone compression of the uncinate processes, which has stimulated the formation of osteophytes (bone spurs).

Osteophytes develop in accordance with **Wolff's Law,** which states that "bone is laid down in areas of high stress and reabsorbed in areas of low stress." As indicated in Figure 8-14, an osteophyte may encroach on a spinal nerve root. Most often, this results in pain and weakness throughout the pinched nerve's peripheral distribution.

Degeneration of an intervertebral disc can also reduce the size of the intervertebral foramen; often this can cause painful impingement on the exiting nerve.

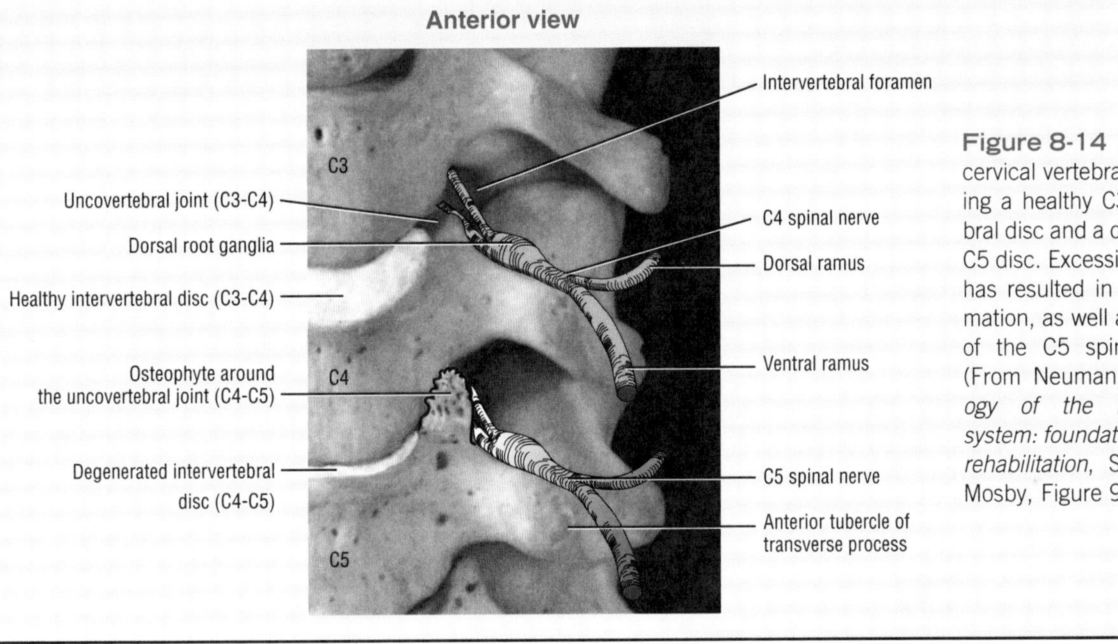

Figure 8-14 A portion of the cervical vertebral column showing a healthy C3-C4 intervertebral disc and a degenerated C4-C5 disc. Excessive compression has resulted in osteophyte formation, as well as impingement of the C5 spinal nerve root. (From Neumann DA: *Kinesiology of the musculoskeletal system: foundations for physical rehabilitation*, St Louis, 2002, Mosby, Figure 9-19.)

head and upper cervical region (Figure 8-15, *A*). The superior facets of the axis (C2) are relatively flat, matching the flattened inferior facets of the atlas. This conformation is well designed to allow the atlas (and head) to freely rotate in the horizontal plane over the axis, such as when turning the head to the left or right. The bifid *spinous process* of C2 is broad and palpable (Figure 8-15, *B*).

THORACIC VERTEBRAE

The 12 thoracic vertebrae are characterized by their sharp, inferiorly projected spinous processes and large posterior, laterally projected transverse processes. The body and transverse processes of most thoracic vertebrae have *costal facets* for articulation with the posterior aspect of the ribs (Figure 8-16). The anterior portion of most ribs attaches either directly or indirectly to the sternum. Therefore the ribs, thoracic vertebrae, and sternum define the volume of the thoracic cavity. Of note is that the apophyseal

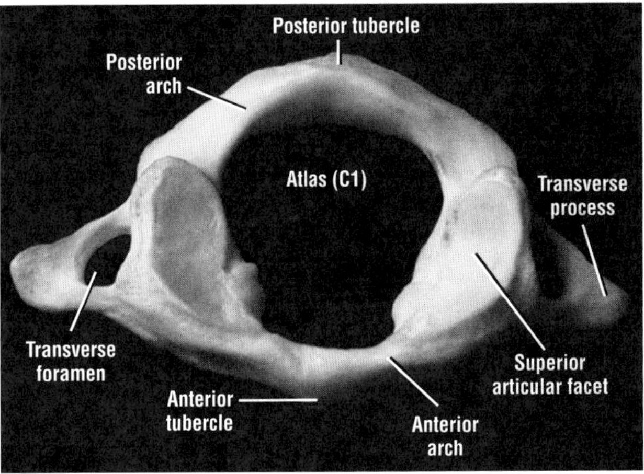

Figure 8-13 Superior view of the atlas (C1). (From Neumann DA: *Kinesiology of the musculoskeletal system: foundations for physical rehabilitation,* St Louis, 2002, Mosby, Figure 9-22, *A*.)

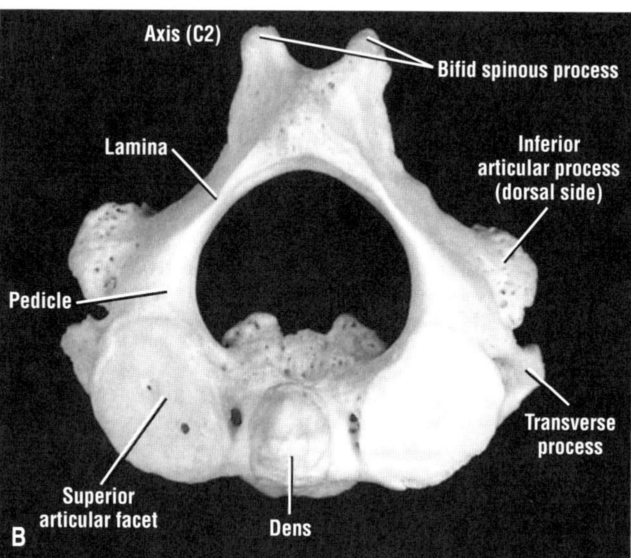

Figure 8-15 The axis (C2). **A,** Anterior view. **B,** Superior view. (From Neumann DA: *Kinesiology of the musculoskeletal system: foundations for physical rehabilitation,* St Louis, 2002, Mosby, Figure 9-23.)

joints of the thoracic vertebrae are aligned nearly in the frontal plane.

LUMBAR VERTEBRAE

The lumbar vertebrae have massive, wide bodies, suitable for supporting the entire superimposed weight of the body (Figure 8-17). The spinous processes are broad and rectangular, connected to the body of the vertebrae through stout, thick laminae and pedicles. The facet joints of the upper lumbar region are oriented close to the sagittal plane but transition toward the frontal plane in the lower regions (L4 and L5) (see Figure 8-17).

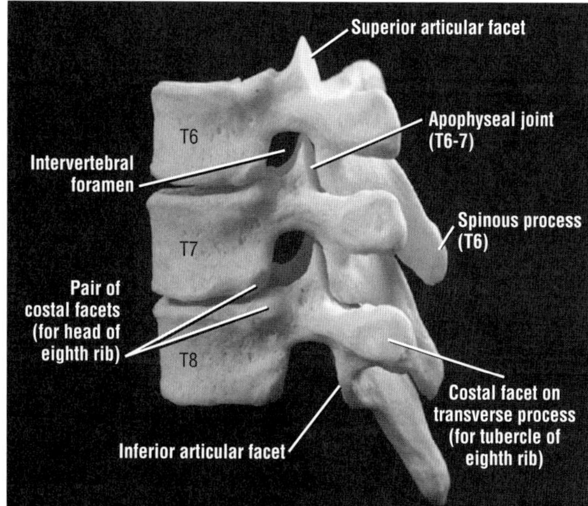

Figure 8-16 Lateral view of the sixth through eighth thoracic vertebrae. (From Neumann DA: *Kinesiology of the musculoskeletal system: foundations for physical rehabilitation,* St Louis, 2002, Mosby, Figure 9-25.)

SACRUM

The sacrum is a triangular bone that transmits the weight of the vertebral column to the pelvis. The wide flat *sacral promontory* (Figure 8-18) articulates with L5, forming the *lumbosacral junction*. The posterior or dorsal surface of the sacrum is convex and rough, reflecting the numerous ligamentous and muscular attachments. The *sacral canal* (see Figure 8-18) houses and protects the cauda equina (peripheral nerves extending from the bottom end of the spinal cord). Four paired *dorsal sacral foramina* transmit the dorsal rami of sacral nerves. On the anterior or pelvic aspect of the sacrum, four paired *ventral sacral foramina* (Figure 8-19) transmit the ventral rami of spinal nerves that form much of the sacral plexus.

COCCYX

Sometimes referred to as the tailbone, the coccyx is a small triangular bone consisting of four fused vertebrae (see Figure 8-19). The base of the coccyx articulates with the inferior sacrum, forming the *sacrococcygeal* joint.

Superior view

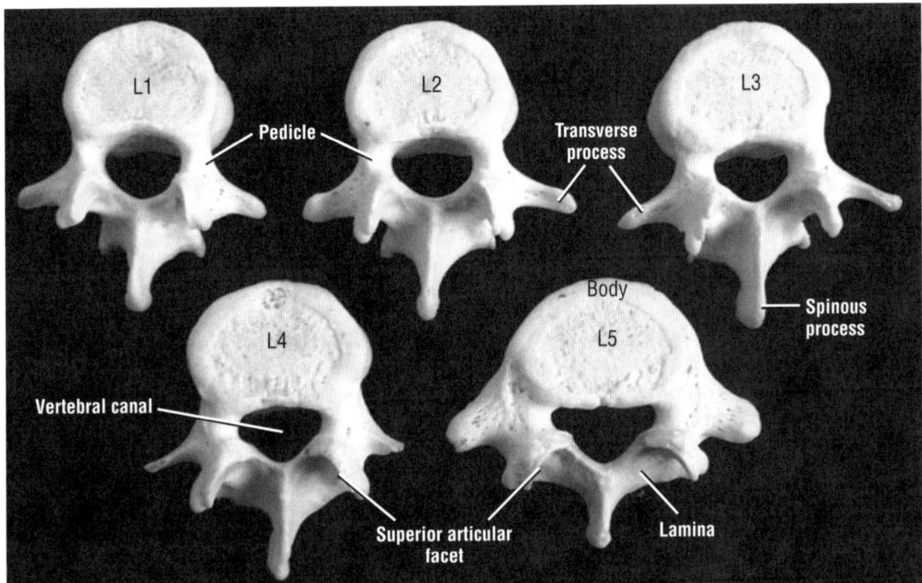

Figure 8-17 A superior view of the five lumbar vertebrae. (From Neumann DA: *Kinesiology of the musculoskeletal system: foundations for physical rehabilitation*, St Louis, 2002, Mosby, Figure 9-26.)

Superior view

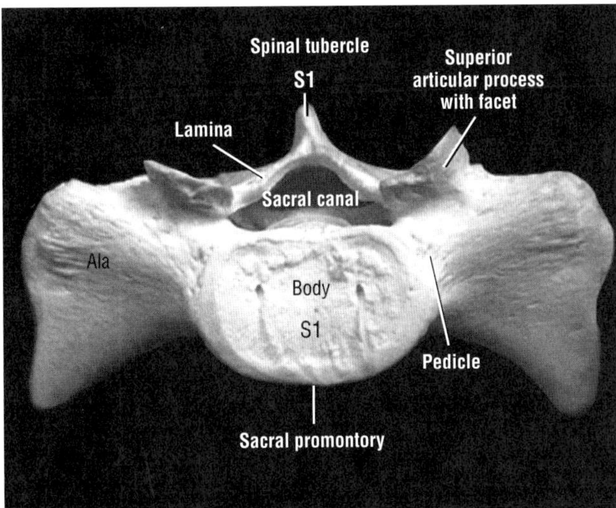

Figure 8-18 A superior view of the sacrum. (From Neumann DA: *Kinesiology of the musculoskeletal system: foundations for physical rehabilitation*, St Louis, 2002, Mosby, Figure 9-32.)

Anterior view

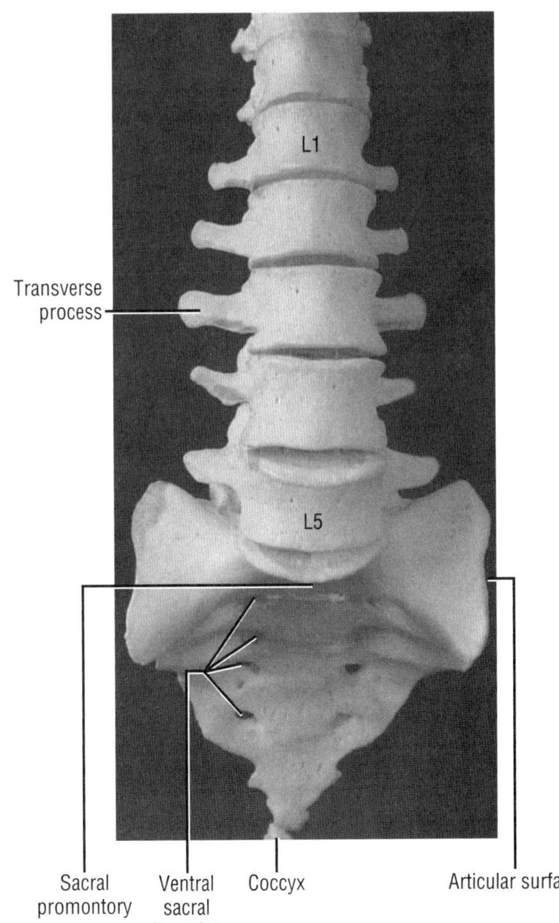

Figure 8-19 An anterior view of the lumbosacral region. (Modified from Neumann DA: *Kinesiology of the musculoskeletal system: foundations for physical rehabilitation*, St Louis, 2002, Mosby, Figure 9-30.)

Supporting Structures of the Vertebral Column

Like any other joint in the body, the joints of the spine are supported by ligaments that (1) prevent unwanted or excessive movements and (2) protect underlying structures (Figures 8-20 and 8-21). Both functions are particularly important in the vertebral column because the soft and vulnerable spinal cord relies on the integrity of the vertebral column for protection. The primary supporting structures of the vertebral column are described within Table 8-2. As will be described later in this chapter, forces from activated muscle also play an essential role in stabilizing and protecting the vertebral column.

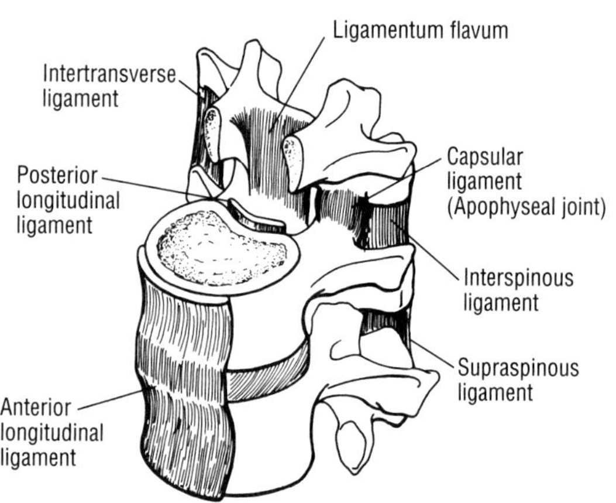

Figure 8-20 Primary ligaments that stabilize the vertebral column. (Modified from White AA, Panjabi MM: *Clinical biomechanics of the spine*, ed 2, Philadelphia, 1990, JB Lippincott.)

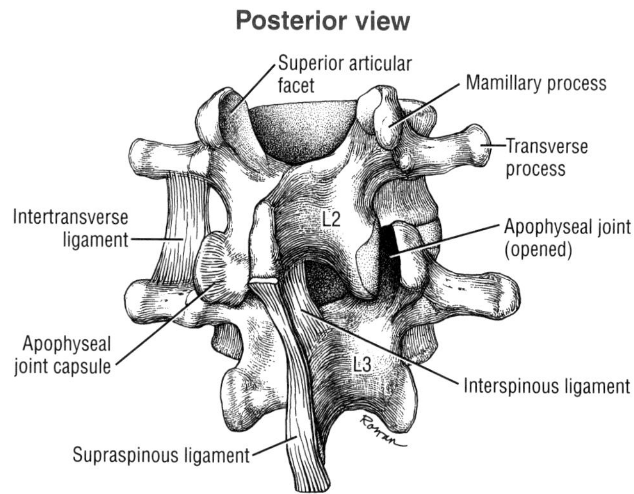

Figure 8-21 Posterior view of the second and third lumbar vertebrae showing the supraspinous and intertransverse ligaments. (From Neumann DA: *Kinesiology of the musculoskeletal system: foundations for physical rehabilitation*, St Louis, 2002, Mosby, Figure 9-15.)

TABLE 8-2 MAJOR LIGAMENTS OF THE VERTEBRAL COLUMN

Name	Attachments	Function	Comment
Ligamentum flavum	Between the anterior surface of one lamina and the posterior surface of the lamina below	Limits flexion	Contains a high percentage of elastin Lies just posterior to the spinal cord Thickest in the lumbar region
Supraspinous and interspinous ligaments	Between the adjacent spinous processes from C7 to the sacrum	Limits flexion	Ligamentum nuchae is the cervical and cranial extension of the supraspinous ligaments, providing a midline structure for muscle attachments, and passive support for the head
Intertransverse ligaments	Between adjacent transverse processes	Limits contralateral lateral flexion	Few fibers exist in the cervical region. In the thoracic region, the ligaments are rounded and intertwined with local muscle. In the lumbar region, the ligaments are thin and membranous.
Anterior longitudinal ligament	Between the basilar part of the occipital bone and the entire length of the anterior surfaces of all vertebral bodies, including the sacrum	Adds stability to the vertebral column Limits extension or excessive lordosis in the cervical and lumbar regions	
Posterior longitudinal ligament	Throughout the length of the posterior surfaces of all vertebral bodies, between the axis (C2) and the sacrum	Stabilizes the vertebral column Limits flexion Reinforces the posterior annulus fibrosus	Lies within the vertebral canal, just anterior to the spinal cord
Capsule of the apophyseal joints	Margin of each apophyseal joint	Strengthens and supports the apophyseal joint	Becomes taut at the extremes of all intervertebral motions

From Neumann DA: *Kinesiology of the musculoskeletal system: foundations for physical rehabilitation*, St Louis, 2002, Mosby, Table 9-3.

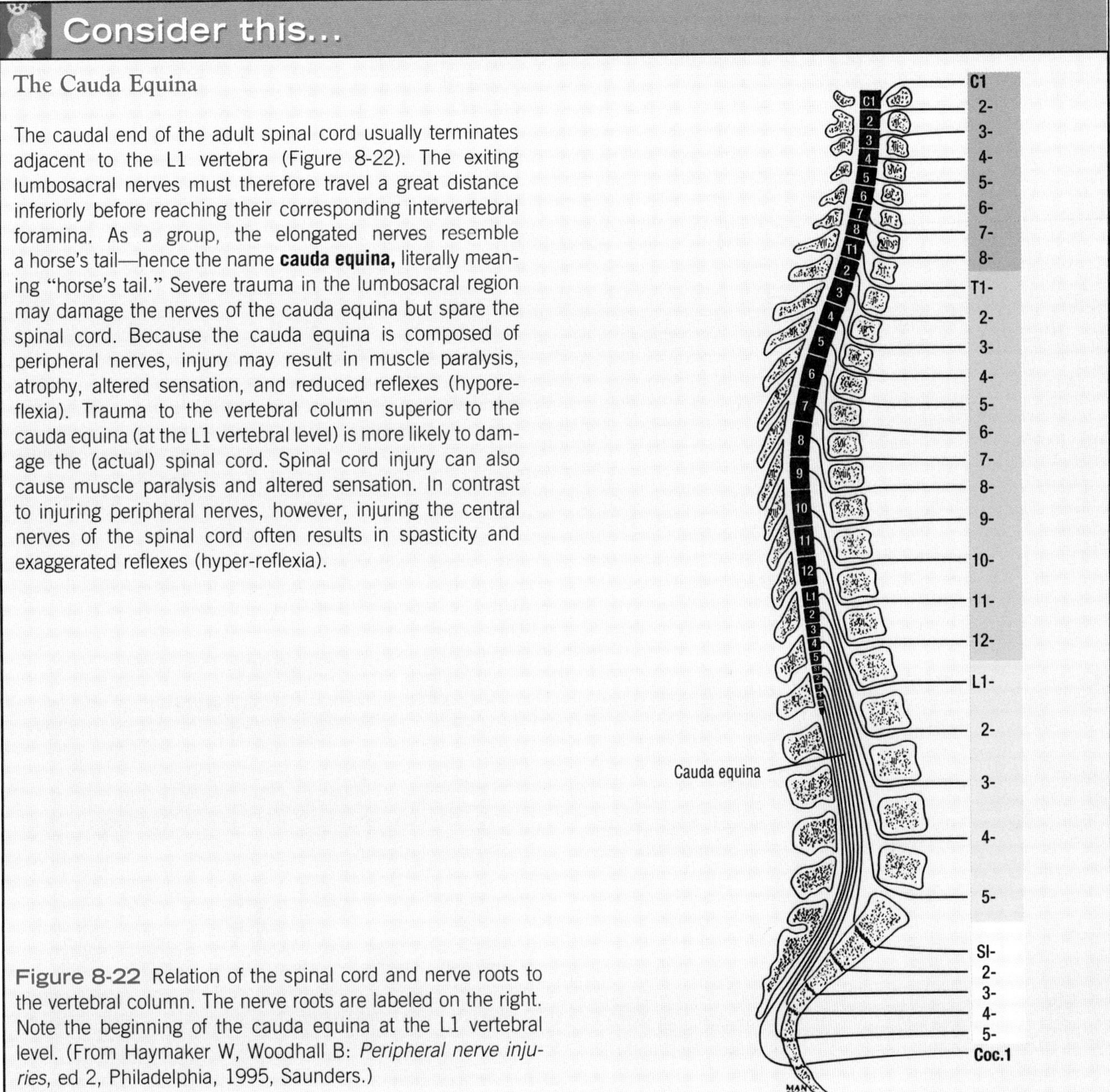

The Cauda Equina

The caudal end of the adult spinal cord usually terminates adjacent to the L1 vertebra (Figure 8-22). The exiting lumbosacral nerves must therefore travel a great distance inferiorly before reaching their corresponding intervertebral foramina. As a group, the elongated nerves resemble a horse's tail—hence the name **cauda equina,** literally meaning "horse's tail." Severe trauma in the lumbosacral region may damage the nerves of the cauda equina but spare the spinal cord. Because the cauda equina is composed of peripheral nerves, injury may result in muscle paralysis, atrophy, altered sensation, and reduced reflexes (hyporeflexia). Trauma to the vertebral column superior to the cauda equina (at the L1 vertebral level) is more likely to damage the (actual) spinal cord. Spinal cord injury can also cause muscle paralysis and altered sensation. In contrast to injuring peripheral nerves, however, injuring the central nerves of the spinal cord often results in spasticity and exaggerated reflexes (hyper-reflexia).

Figure 8-22 Relation of the spinal cord and nerve roots to the vertebral column. The nerve roots are labeled on the right. Note the beginning of the cauda equina at the L1 vertebral level. (From Haymaker W, Woodhall B: *Peripheral nerve injuries,* ed 2, Philadelphia, 1995, Saunders.)

Kinematics of the Vertebral Column

By convention, movement at any spinal region is defined by the direction of the motion of a point on the *anterior* side of the vertebrae. For example, rotation to the right indicates that the anterior side (body) of the vertebrae is rotating to the right. This can be confusing because the more visible (and palpable) spinous process rotates to the left—in the opposite direction. Furthermore, movement occurs within a plane relative to an associated axis of rotation coursing through the vertebral body (Table 8-3).

For the sake of organization, this text examines the motions of the spine in two regions: *craniocervical* and *thoracolumbar*. Each region permits flexion and extension, lateral flexion, and axial rotation—rotation in the horizontal plane. As introduced earlier, the motion of a particular spinal region is the summation of relatively small motions between individual vertebrae. Furthermore, these movements are guided primarily by the spatial orientation of the surfaces within the facet joints.

TABLE 8-3 TERMINOLOGY DESCRIBING THE MOVEMENTS OF THE AXIAL SKELETON

Common Terminology	Plane of Movement	Axis of Rotation	Other Terminology
Flexion and extension	Sagittal	Medial-lateral	Forward and backward bending
Lateral flexion to the right or left	Frontal	Anterior-posterior	Side bending to the right or left
Axial rotation to the right or left*	Horizontal	Vertical	Rotation, torsion

From Neumann DA: *Kinesiology of the musculoskeletal system: foundations for physical rehabilitation*, St Louis, 2002, Mosby, Table 9-6.
*Axial rotation of the spine is defined by the direction of movement of a point on the *anterior* side of the vertebral body.

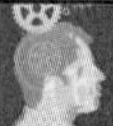

Consider this...

Facet Joints throughout the Vertebral Column: Different Orientations, Different Primary Motions

Facet (apophyseal) joints are formed by the articulation between the inferior facets of one vertebra and the superior facets of the vertebra below. The spatial orientation of the facet joints largely determines the direction and extent of motion allowed across a particular region of the vertebral column. The facet joints act like railroad tracks, guiding the direction of motion of a train.

A vertebra naturally moves in the direction of least bony resistance, which is strongly dictated by the specific plane of the articular surfaces of the facet joints. This concept is useful to the understanding of the kinematics across the vertebral column.

Figure 8-23 shows the spatial orientation of a sample of vertebrae (indicated in red). The superior facet surfaces of the axis (C2) are oriented closest to the horizontal plane. The freest motion between C1 and C2 (atlanto-axial joint) is therefore in the horizontal plane, which occurs while turning the head fully to the left or right.

The facet surfaces C2-C7 are oriented about halfway between the horizontal plane and the frontal plane (see Figure 8-23). This alignment allows nearly equal and ample amounts of horizontal plane rotation and lateral flexion.

The facet surfaces of thoracic vertebrae are oriented closest to the frontal plane (see Figure 8-23). This alignment would allow ample lateral flexion, but this potential of movement is limited by the attachment of the ribs.

As indicated in Figure 8-23, the facet surfaces of the upper lumbar vertebrae are oriented closest to the sagittal plane, which favors sagittal plane motions of flexion and extension. The facet surfaces of the lower lumbar vertebrae transition toward the frontal plane. This alignment favors lateral flexion and may help accommodate the natural "hip-hiking" motions that occur during walking and running. Likely more important, this near frontal plane alignment between L5 and S1 helps prevent the lower lumbar vertebra from sliding anteriorly relative to the sacrum.

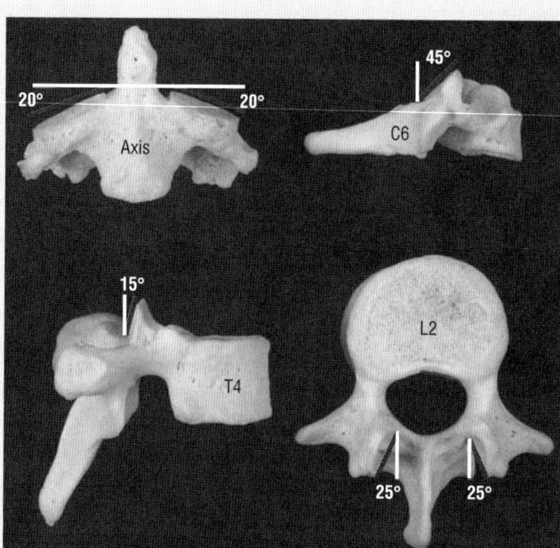

Figure 8-23 Typical spatial orientations for selected superior facet surfaces of the cervical, thoracic, and lumbar vertebrae. (From Neumann DA: *Kinesiology of the musculoskeletal system: foundations for physical rehabilitation*, St Louis, 2002, Mosby, Figure 9-34.)

Craniocervical Region

The terms *craniocervical region* and *neck* are used interchangeably. Both terms refer to the combined set of three articulations: atlanto-occipital joint, atlanto-axial joint, and the intracervical region—referring to the cervical joints between C2 and C7. The craniocervical region is the most mobile area of the entire vertebral column. The individual joints within this region function in a highly coordinated manner to facilitate positioning of the head, which plays a large role in vision, hearing, hand-eye coordination, and equilibrium. Table 8-4 summarizes the average ranges of motion contributed by each area within the craniocervical region.

FLEXION AND EXTENSION

Figure 8-24 illustrates an individual in full 85 degrees of craniocervical extension. Full craniocervical flexion of 45 to 50 degrees is pictured in Figure 8-25. About 25% of the

TABLE 8-4 APPROXIMATE RANGE OF MOTION FOR THE THREE PLANES OF MOVEMENT FOR THE JOINTS OF THE CRANIOCERVICAL REGION

Joint or Region	Flexion and Extension (Sagittal Plane, Degrees)	Axial Rotation (Horizontal Plane, Degrees)*	Lateral Flexion (Frontal Plane, Degrees)*
Atlanto-occipital joint	Flexion: 5 Extension: 10 TOTAL: 15	Negligible	Approximately 5
Atlanto-axial joint	Flexion: 5 Extension: 10 TOTAL: 15	40-45	Negligible
Intracervical region (C2-C7)	Flexion: 35 Extension: 70 TOTAL: 105	45	35
Total across craniocervical region	Flexion: 45-50 Extension: 85 TOTAL: 130-135	90	Approximately 40

From Neumann DA: *Kinesiology of the musculoskeletal system: foundations for physical rehabilitation*, St Louis, 2002, Mosby, Table 9-10.
*The horizontal and frontal plane motions are to one side only.

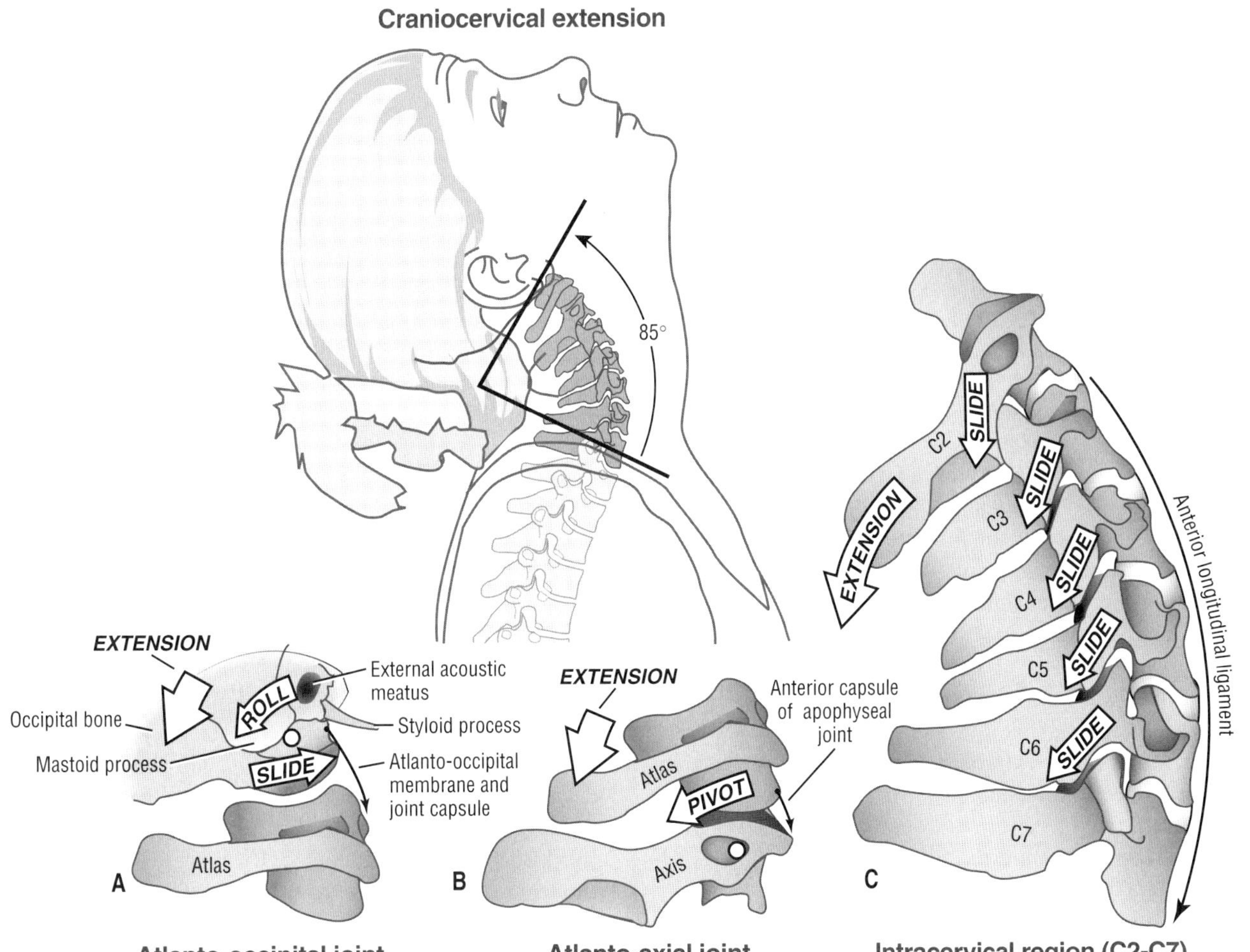

Figure 8-24 Kinematics of craniocervical extension. **A,** Atlanto-occipital joint. **B,** Atlanto-axial joint. **C,** Intracervical region (C2-C7). Elongated and taut tissues are indicated by thin black arrows. (From Neumann DA: *Kinesiology of the musculoskeletal system: foundations for physical rehabilitation*, St Louis, 2002, Mosby, Figure 9-46.)

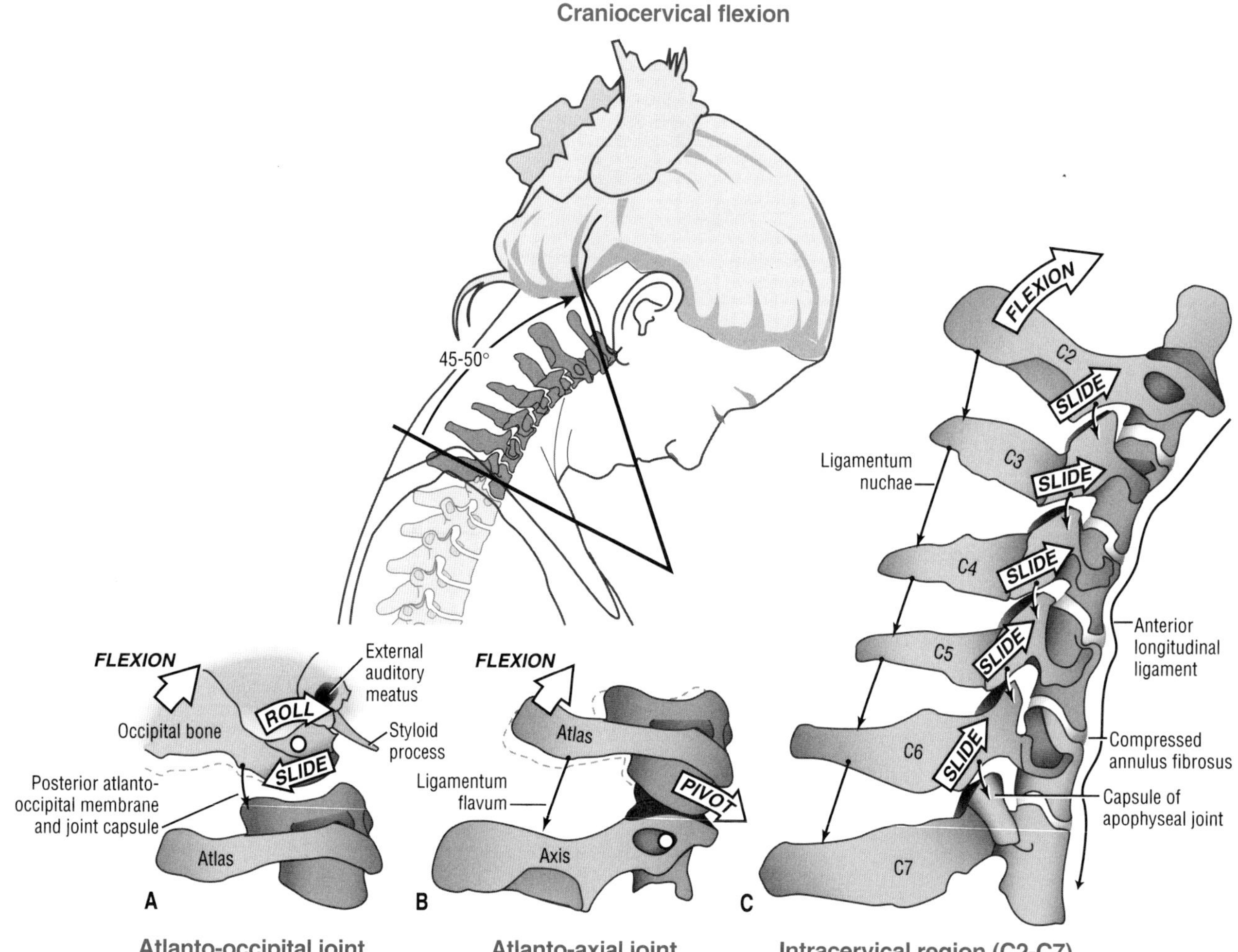

Figure 8-25 Kinematics of craniocervical flexion. **A,** Atlanto-occipital joint. **B,** Atlanto-axial joint. **C,** Intracervical region (C2-C7). Elongated and taut tissues are indicated by thin black arrows; slackened tissues are indicated by a wavy black arrow. (From Neumann DA: *Kinesiology of the musculoskeletal system: foundations for physical rehabilitation,* St Louis, 2002, Mosby, Figure 9-47.)

total sagittal plane motion occurs by the combined motions of the atlanto-occipital and atlanto-axial joints; the remaining motion occurs across the intracervical (C2-C7) region.

The atlanto-occipital joints are well designed to produce flexion and extension because the convex occipital condyles and corresponding concave facet surfaces of the atlas fit like rockers on a rocking chair: the occipital condyles roll backward during extension (see Figure 8-24, *A*) and forward during flexion (see Figure 8-25, *A*). In accordance with the arthrokinematic rules described in Chapter 1, the roll and slide occur in opposite directions.

The atlanto-axial joint, although primarily designed for horizontal plane motion, allows about 10 degrees of extension and 5 degrees of flexion (see Figures 8-24, *B*, and 8-25, *B*).

Flexion and extension of the intracervical region (C2-C7) result in an arc of motion determined by the oblique plane of the cervical facet joints. As described earlier, these joints are oriented in a plane about 45 degrees between the horizontal and the frontal planes. During extension, the inferior facets of the superior vertebra slide posteriorly and inferiorly—relative to the vertebra below it (see Figure 8-24, *C*). The mechanics of flexion are the reverse of extension (see Figure 8-25, *C*).

AXIAL ROTATION

Rotation of the head and neck in the horizontal plane is an important motion, integral to vision and hearing. As shown in Figure 8-26, the craniocervical region rotates about 90 degrees to each side, allowing nearly 180 degrees of rotational motion. With an additional 150 to 160 degrees of total horizontal plane motion of the eyes, the visual field approaches 360 degrees without moving the trunk.

The atlanto-axial joint is responsible for about half of the rotation that occurs in the craniocervical region. The vertical dens and nearly horizontal superior facets of the axis (C2) allow the ring-shaped atlas (C1) to rotate freely and securely about 45 degrees in either direction (see Figure 8-26, *A*). Note that the head does *not* rotate

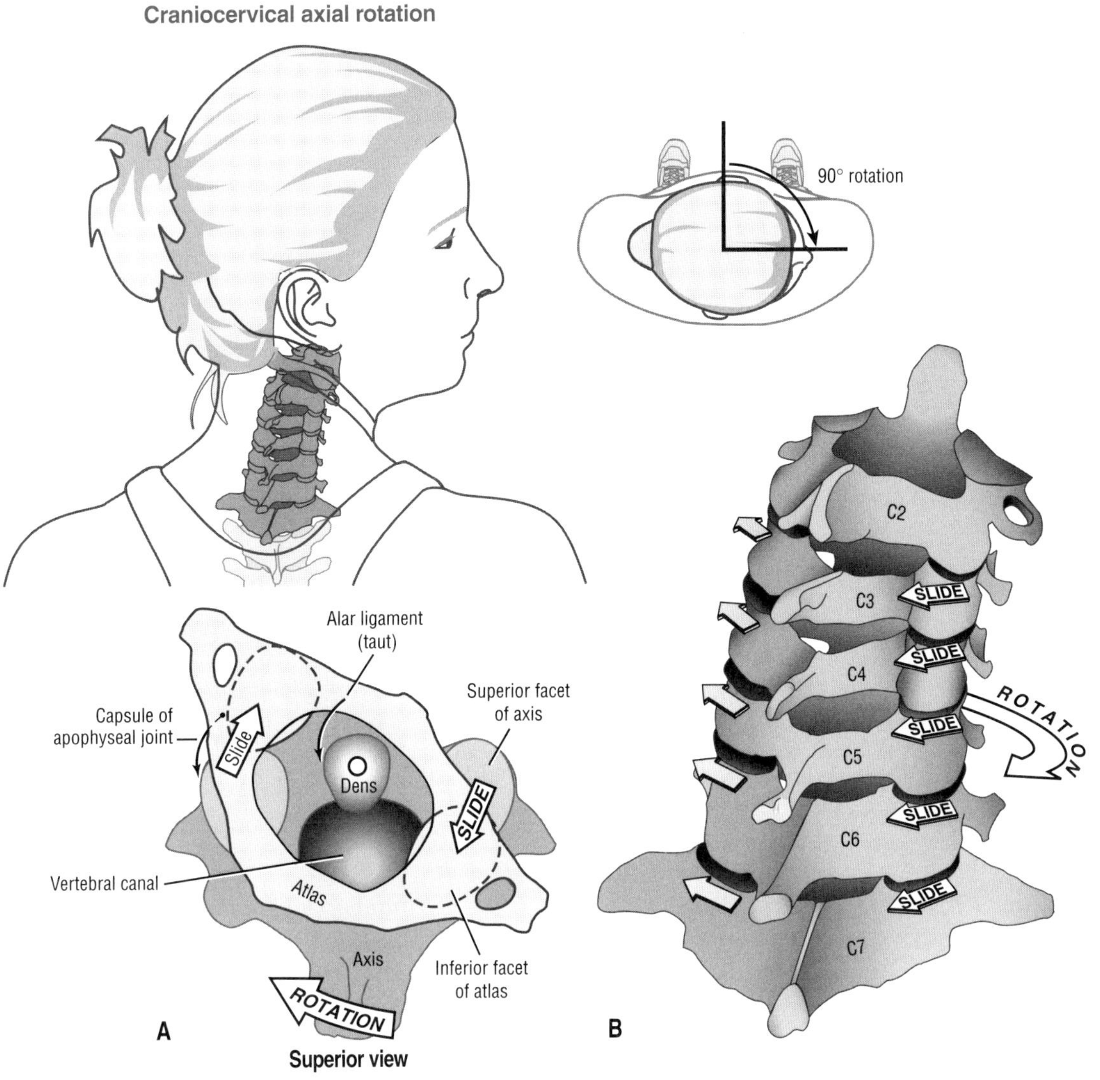

Craniocervical axial rotation

90° rotation

Alar ligament (taut)

Capsule of apophyseal joint

Slide

Dens

Superior facet of axis

SLIDE

Vertebral canal

Atlas

Axis

Inferior facet of atlas

ROTATION

A

Superior view

Atlanto-axial joint (C1-C2)

C2 C3 C4 C5 C6 C7

SLIDE

ROTATION

B

Intracervical region (C2-C7)

Figure 8-26 Kinematics of craniocervical axial rotation. **A,** Atlanto-axial joint. **B,** Intracervical region (C2-C7). (From Neumann DA: *Kinesiology of the musculoskeletal system: foundations for physical rehabilitation*, St Louis, 2002, Mosby, Figure 9-51.)

independent of the ring-shaped atlas. The deeply seated atlanto-occipital joint strongly resists rotation; rotation of the head therefore is the result of the atlas and the attached cranium rotating as a fixed unit relative to the axis (see Figure 8-26, *A*).

Rotation of C2-C7 is guided primarily by the oblique orientation of the facet joints. The combined motion of these joints allows about 45 degrees of rotation in either direction and is mechanically coupled with very slight amounts of lateral flexion secondary to the orientation of the facet joints (see Figure 8-26, *B*). The arthrokinematic movements involved with rotation to the right are illustrated in Figure 8-26, *B*.

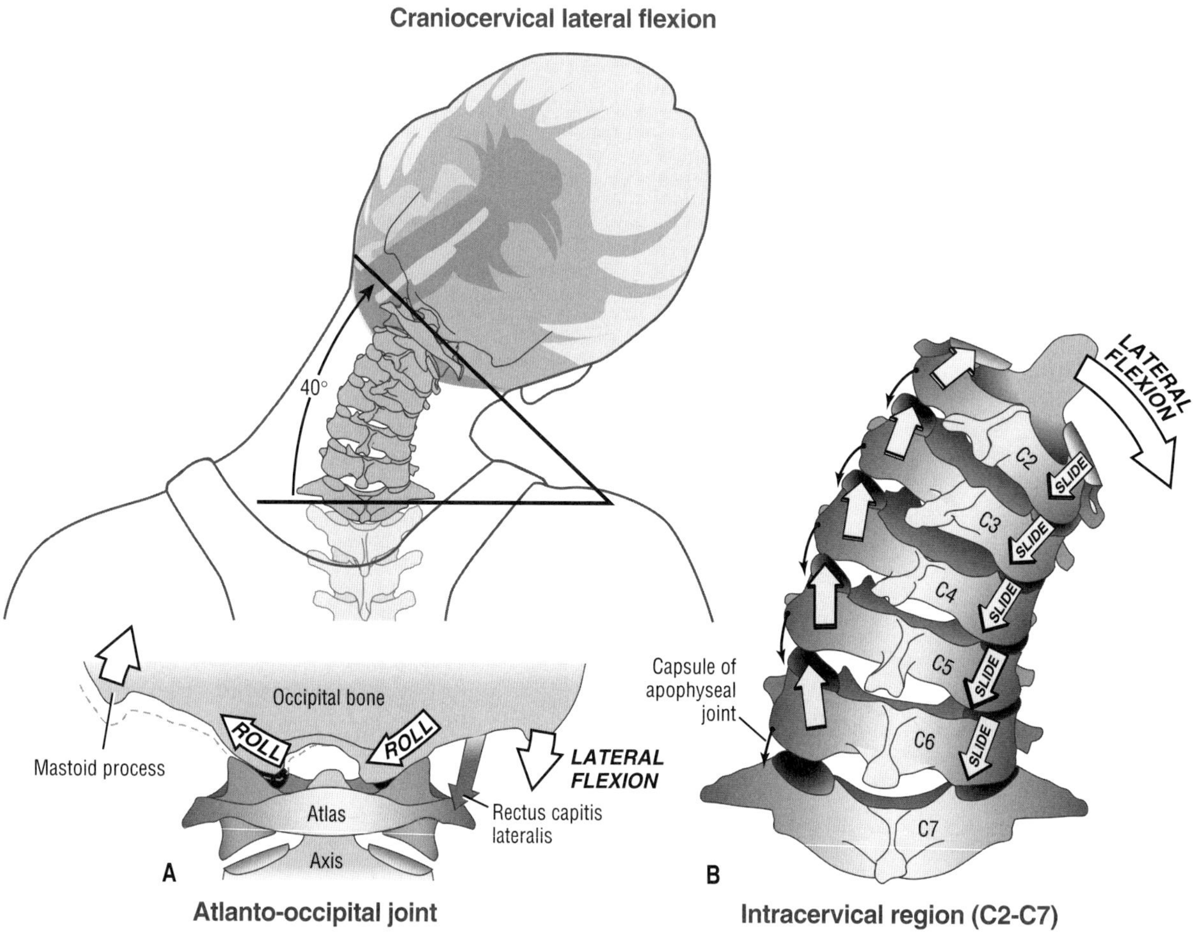

Craniocervical lateral flexion

Atlanto-occipital joint

Intracervical region (C2-C7)

Figure 8-27 Kinematics of craniocervical lateral flexion. **A,** Atlanto-occipital joint. **B,** Intracervical region. (From Neumann DA: *Kinesiology of the musculoskeletal system: foundations for physical rehabilitation*, St Louis, 2002, Mosby, Figure 9-52.)

LATERAL FLEXION

The craniocervical region allows about 40 degrees of lateral flexion to each side. Although minimal, the atlanto-occipital joint contributes about 5 degrees of lateral flexion in either direction (Figure 8-27, A). Most of the motion occurs between C2 and C7.

The arthrokinematic motion between C2-C7 is illustrated in Figure 8-27, B. Once again, this motion is guided by the 45-degree incline of the facet joints. Due to the orientation of the facet surfaces, sight horizontal plane rotation is mechanically coupled with lateral flexion.

Clinical INSIGHT

Flexion and Extension and the Effect on the Diameter of the Intervertebral Foramina

Intervertebral foramina allow protected passage of spinal nerves to and from the spinal cord. As the name implies, an intervertebral foramen is created by the approximation of two adjacent vertebrae. Consequently, the motion or position of either vertebra can alter the shape and therefore size of the foramen.

Flexion increases the diameter of the intervertebral foramen; extension, in contrast, decreases it (Figure 8-28). This has clinical relevance in cases of stenosed (narrowed) intervertebral foramen. For example, osteophyte formation within the intervertebral foramen may cause compression of a **spinal nerve** as it passes through this space. This can result in symptoms such as tingling, numbness, muscle weakness, reduced reflexes, and radiating pain.

Individuals with a narrowed intervertebral foramen or osteophyte formation may develop a chronically flexed neck or "forward head" posture in an attempt to alleviate pressure on the spinal nerve roots. The flexed position of the lower cervical vertebrae increases the space of the intervertebral foramen, allowing the nerves to exit with less chance of impingement.

Treatment of cervical nerve root compression often includes cervical traction with the neck in partial flexion to decompress the irritated nerve root and reduce painful symptoms.

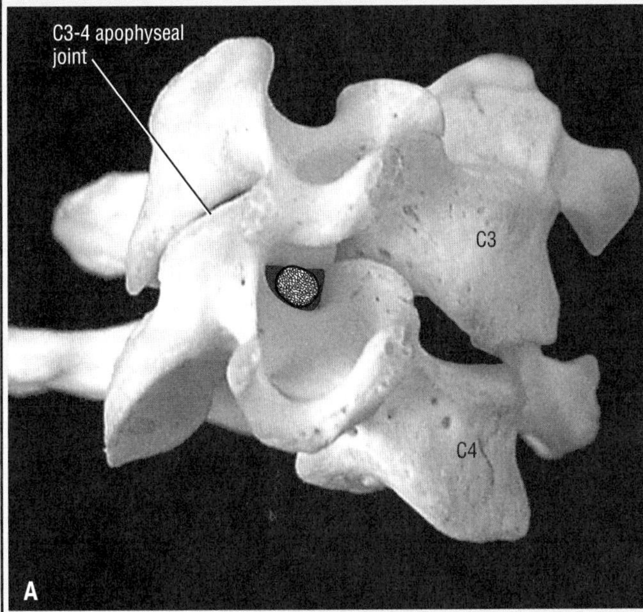

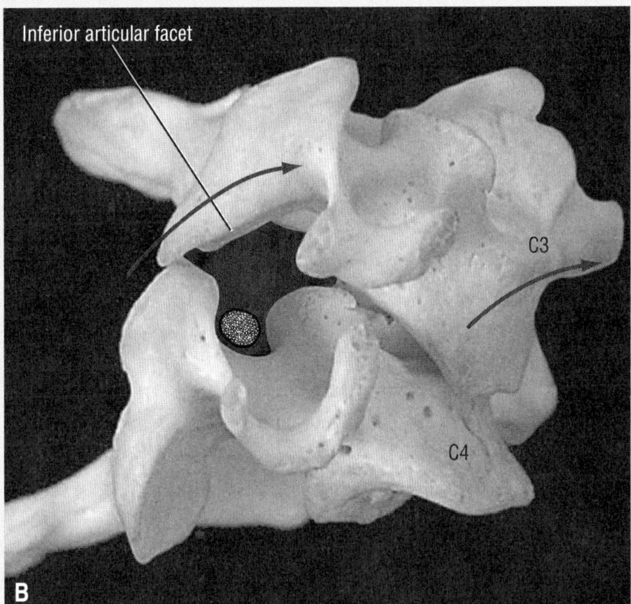

Neutral position **Fully flexed**

Figure 8-28 Comparison of the intervertebral foramen in neutral **(A)** and flexion **(B)**. Flexion significantly increases the space within the intervertebral foramen (indicated in red). (From Neumann DA: *Kinesiology of the musculoskeletal system: foundations for physical rehabilitation*, St Louis, 2002, Mosby, Figure 9-49.)

Clinical INSIGHT

Forward-Head Posture: Treating Poor Posture through Active Chin Tucks

A forward-head posture is one of the most commonly observed faulty postures of the craniocervical region. Typically this posture occurs from holding the head in an excessively forward position for extended periods such as when reading a textbook resting on a table. Protraction of the head is the result of flexion of the lower cervical vertebrae and extension—and typically hyperextension—of the upper craniocervical region (Figure 8-29, *A*). Over time, the muscles and ligaments of the upper cervical region shorten, adapting to the close proximity of the bony structures in this area. (Note the proximity of the C1 and C2 spinous processes to the base of the skull in Figure 8-29, *A*.)

One technique to treat forward-head posturing is known as a chin-tuck maneuver (Figure 8-29, *B*). A chin tuck is actually retraction of the head. This motion reverses the forward head posture by bringing the lower cervical vertebrae into extension and the upper craniocervical region into greater flexion. When performed regularly, chin tucks can often yield good results in correcting a forward-head posture.

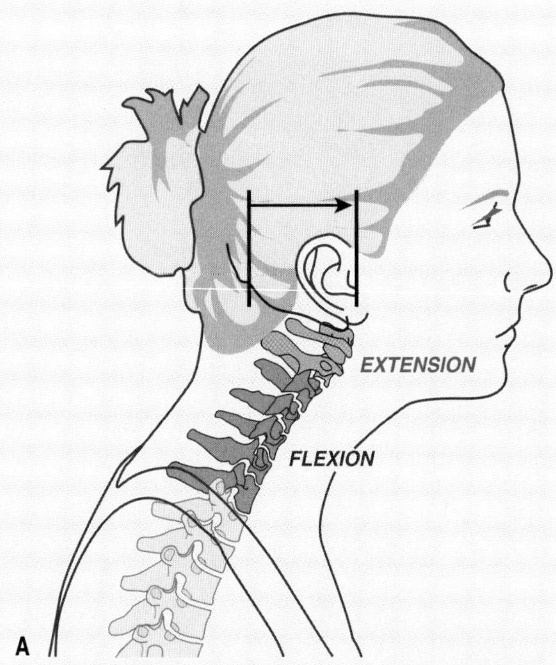

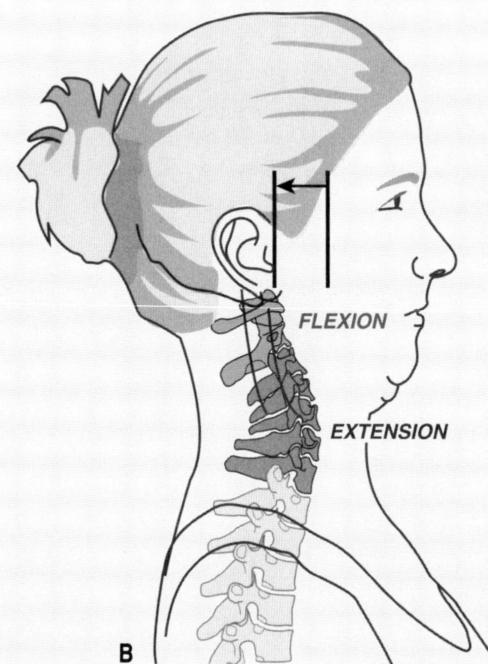

Figure 8-29 Protraction and retraction of the head. **A,** During protraction, the lower cervical spine flexes as the upper craniocervical region extends. **B,** During retraction, in contrast, the lower cervical spine extends as the upper craniocervical region flexes. (From Neumann DA: *Kinesiology of the musculoskeletal system: foundations for physical rehabilitation*, St Louis, 2002, Mosby, Figure 9-50.)

Thoracolumbar Region

Although anatomically distinct, the thoracic and lumbar vertebrae typically work together to allow the wide ranges of trunk motion relative to the pelvis and lower extremities. The kinematics of the thoracic and lumbar regions are described together. The average ranges of motion for the thoracic and lumbar regions are summarized in Table 8-5.

FLEXION AND EXTENSION

Flexion of the thoracolumbar region is pictured in Figure 8-30. The combined motion of the thoracic and lumbar vertebrae allows about 85 degrees of forward flexion. About 50 degrees of this forward bend occurs at the lumbar region, which is extraordinary considering that this region consists of only five vertebrae. The large amount of flexion permitted in the lumbar region is mechanically linked to the near sagittal plane orientation of the facet joints. Large amounts of flexion are functionally important, allowing activities such as bending forward to pick an object off the floor. Paradoxically, this freedom of motion may be partially responsible for the high incidence of herniated discs in the lumbar region. The arthrokinematic motions of flexion of the thoracic and lumbar regions are shown in Figure 8-30.

Approximately 35 to 40 degrees of extension occur across the thoracolumbar region (Figure 8-31). Extension in the thoracic region is limited by the potential contact of the inferiorly slanting spinous processes, as well as tension in the anterior longitudinal ligament (see Figure 8-31).

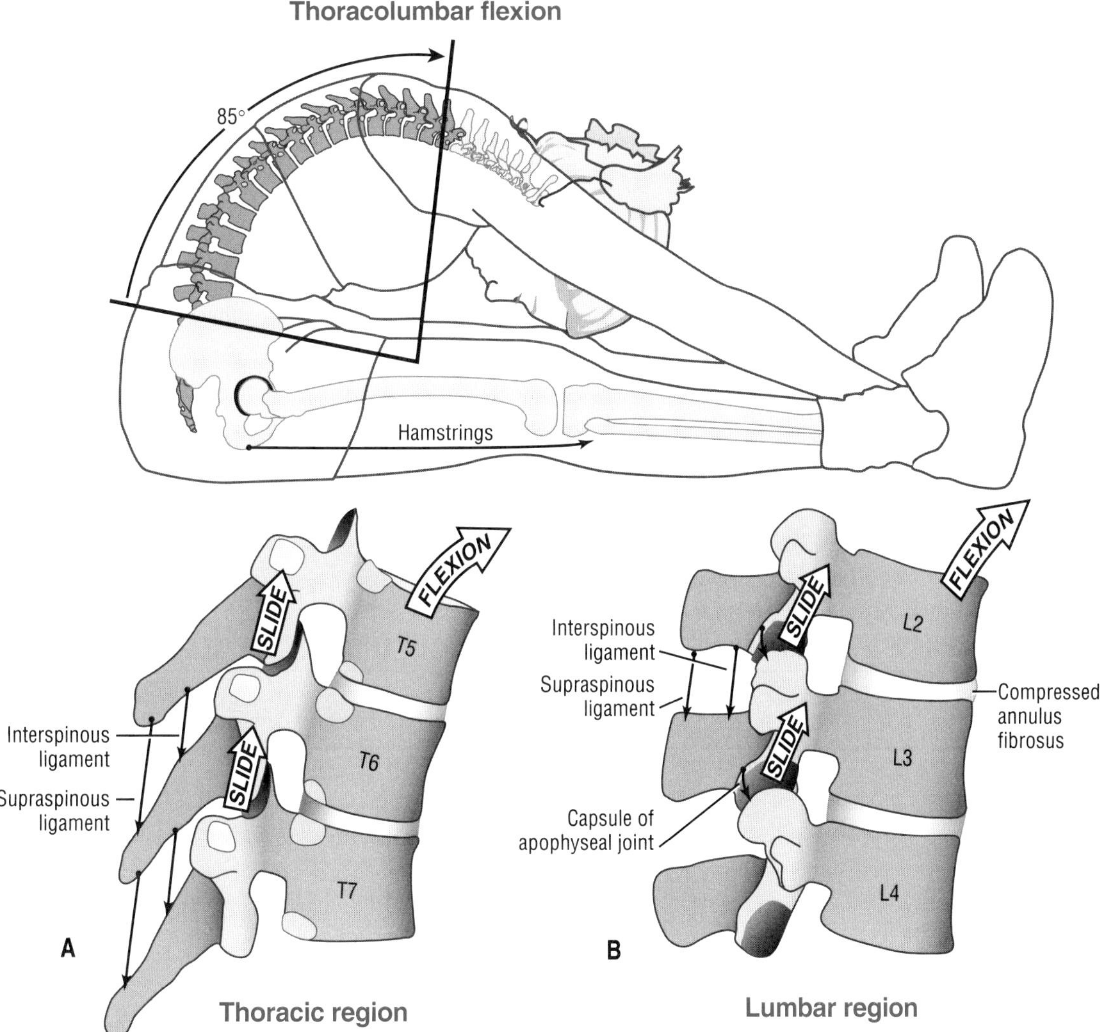

Figure 8-30 Kinematics of thoracolumbar flexion. **A,** Kinematics at the thoracic region. **B,** Kinematics at the lumbar region. (From Neumann DA: *Kinesiology of the musculoskeletal system: foundations for physical rehabilitation*, St Louis, 2002, Mosby, Figure 9-54.)

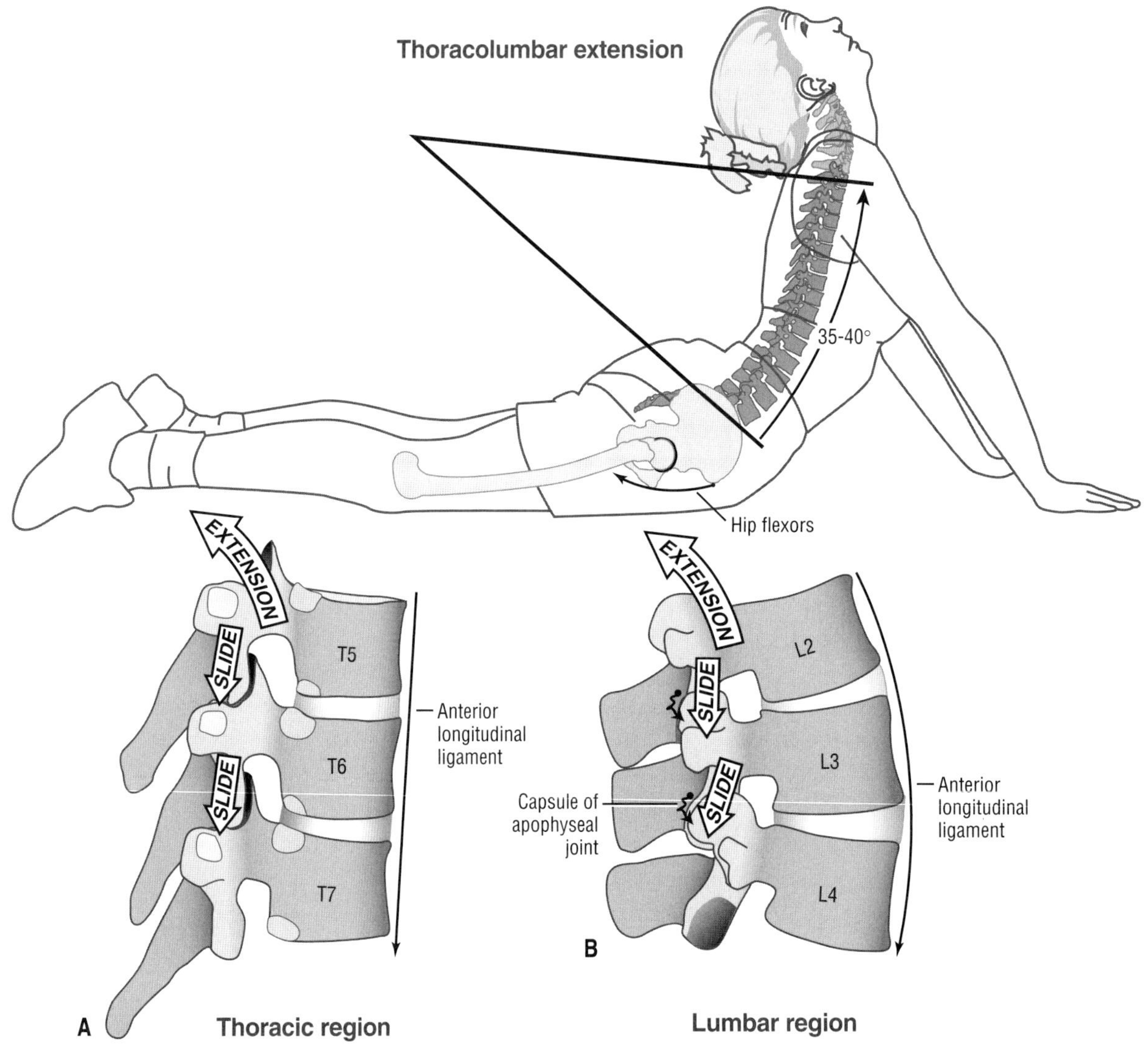

Figure 8-31 Kinematics of thoracolumbar extension. **A,** Kinematics at the thoracic region. **B,** Kinematics at the lumbar region. (From Neumann DA: *Kinesiology of the musculoskeletal system: foundations for physical rehabilitation,* St Louis, 2002, Mosby, Figure 9-55.)

TABLE 8-5 APPROXIMATE RANGES OF MOTION FOR THE THORACIC AND LUMBAR REGIONS

Flexion and Extension (Sagittal Plane, Degrees)	Rotation (Horizontal Plane, Degrees)*	Lateral Flexion (Frontal Plane, Degrees)*
Thoracic Region		
Flexion: 30-40	30	25
Extension: 20-25		
Total: 50-65		
Lumbar Region		
Flexion: 50	5	20
Extension: 15		
Total: 65		

From Neumann DA: *Kinesiology of the musculoskeletal system: foundations for physical rehabilitation*, St Louis, 2002, Mosby, Tables 9-11 (thoracic) and 9-12 (lumbar).

*Horizontal and frontal plane motions are to one side only.

AXIAL ROTATION

The thoracolumbar region permits only about 35 degrees of horizontal plane rotation in either direction, most of which occurs at the thoracic region (Figure 8-32). The limited rotation permitted in the lumbar region is explained by the near sagittal plane orientation of the facet joint surfaces, which physically block the rotation of the vertebrae. As shown in Figure 8-32, *A* and *B*, rotation to the right causes the facet joint surfaces on the left (opposite the side of the rotational action) to quickly collide. The immediate compression of the facet surfaces is very limiting; in fact, the average amount of rotation between two lumbar vertebrae averages slightly more than 1 degree. The kinematic design of the lumbar region truly favors flexion at the expense of horizontal plane rotation. Fortunately, however, the limited rotation in the lumbar region is partially offset by the available rotation in the thoracic region. Thoracolumbar rotation adds up over 17 vertebral segments (12 thoracic and 5 lumbar), enabling the entire region to rotate nearly 35 degrees in either direction. However, when compared with the 90 degrees of rotation available to the craniocervical region, rotation of the thoracolumbar region remains relatively limited.

LATERAL FLEXION

Lateral flexion (or side bending) of the thoracolumbar region is typically limited to about 45 degrees in either direction (Figure 8-33). The arthrokinematic motions involved between vertebrae are illustrated in Figure 8-33, *A* and *B*.

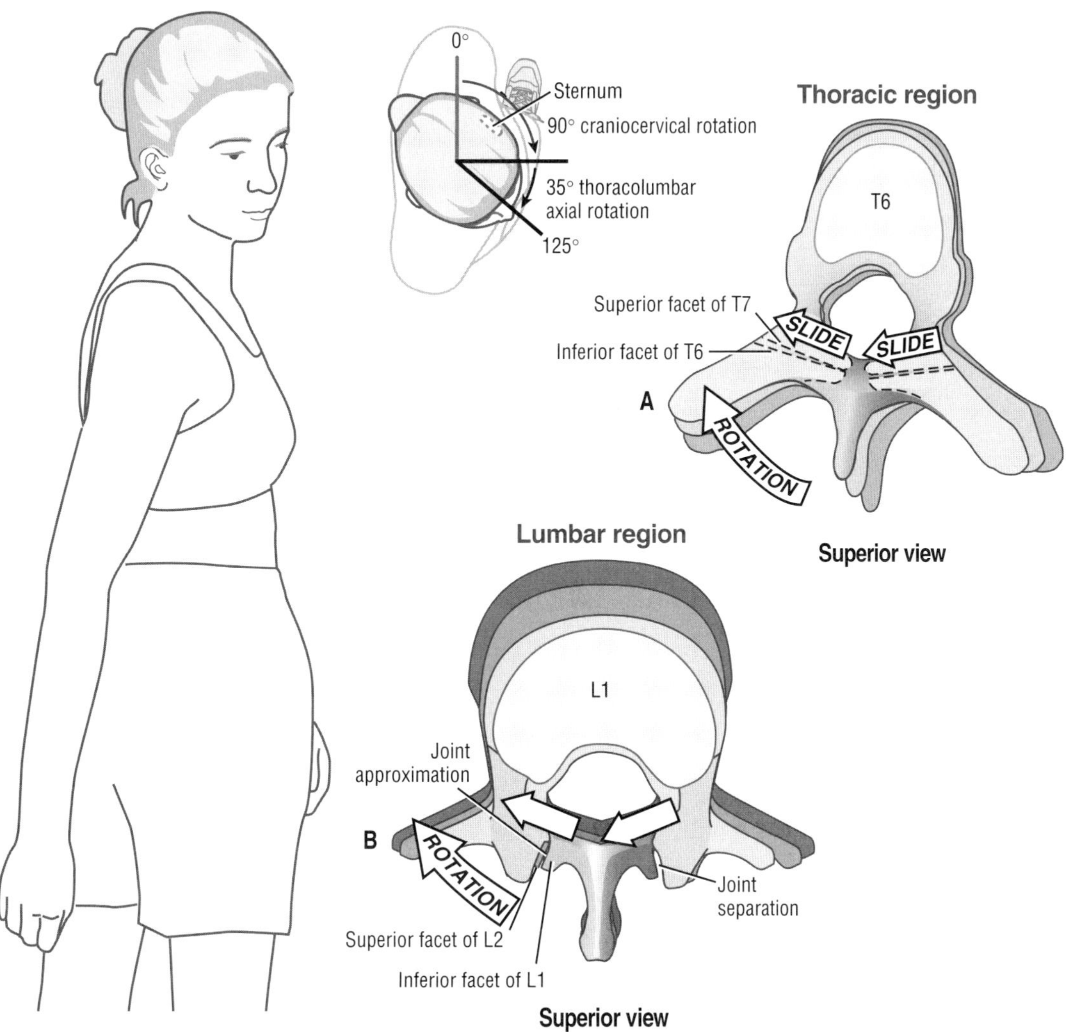

Figure 8-32 Kinematics of thoracolumbar axial rotation. **A,** Kinematics at the thoracic region. **B,** Kinematics at the lumbar region. (From Neumann DA: *Kinesiology of the musculoskeletal system: foundations for physical rehabilitation,* St Louis, 2002, Mosby, Figure 9-56.)

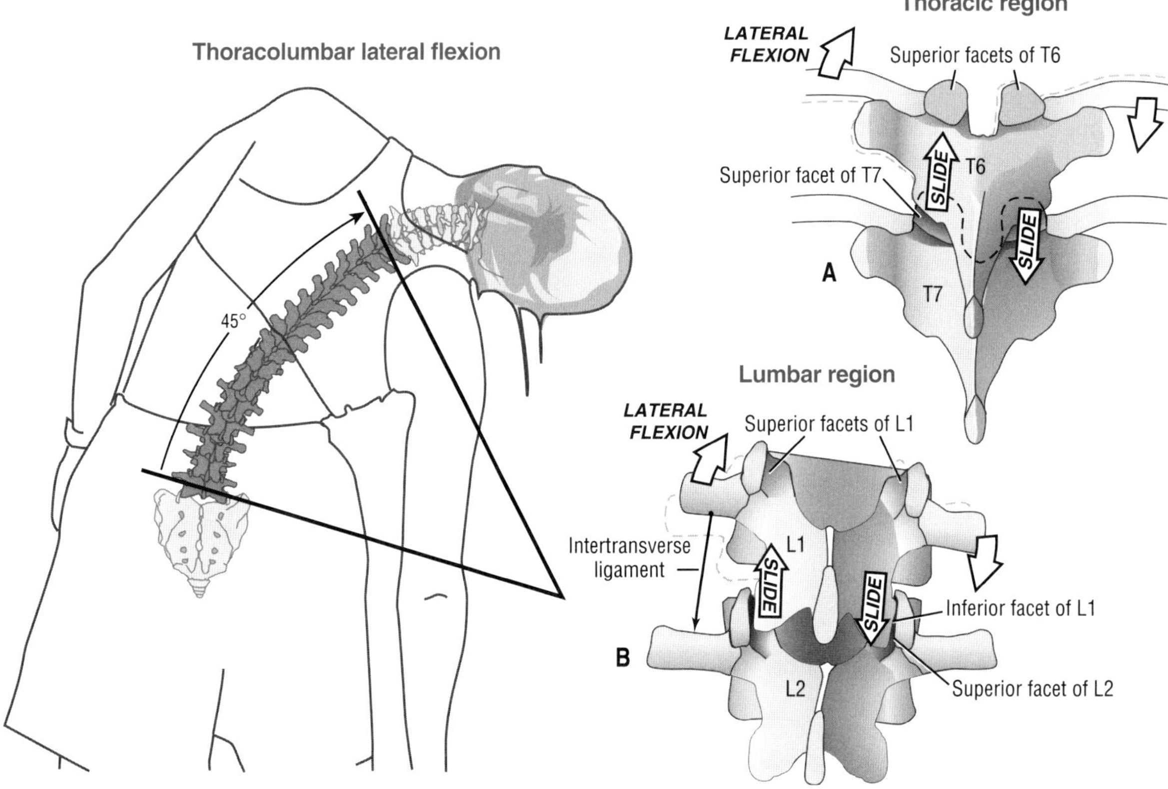

Figure 8-33 Kinematics of thoracolumbar lateral flexion. **A,** Kinematics at the thoracic region. **B,** Kinematics at the lumbar region. (From Neumann DA: *Kinesiology of the musculoskeletal system: foundations for physical rehabilitation*, St Louis, 2002, Mosby, Figure 9-57.)

Clinical INSIGHT

Herniated Nucleus Pulposus

The formal name for a bulging or slipped disc is a herniated nucleus pulposus. Most painful disc herniations involve a posterior-lateral or posterior migration of the nucleus pulposus toward the spinal cord or spinal nerve roots. The radiating pain and numbness typically reported by patients is due to the pressure of the disc against neural elements.

Generally four categories of disc herniation result in varying degrees of pain and impairment (Figure 8-34):

- *Protrusion:* Displaced nucleus pulposus remains within the annulus fibrosus but may create a pressure bulge on the neural tissues.
- *Prolapse:* Displaced nucleus pulposus reaches the posterior edge of the disc but remains confined within the outer layers of the annulus fibrosus.
- *Extrusion:* Annulus fibrosus ruptures, allowing the nucleus pulposus to completely escape from the disc into the epidural space.
- *Sequestration:* Parts of the nucleus pulposus and fragments of the annulus fibrosus become lodged within the epidural space.

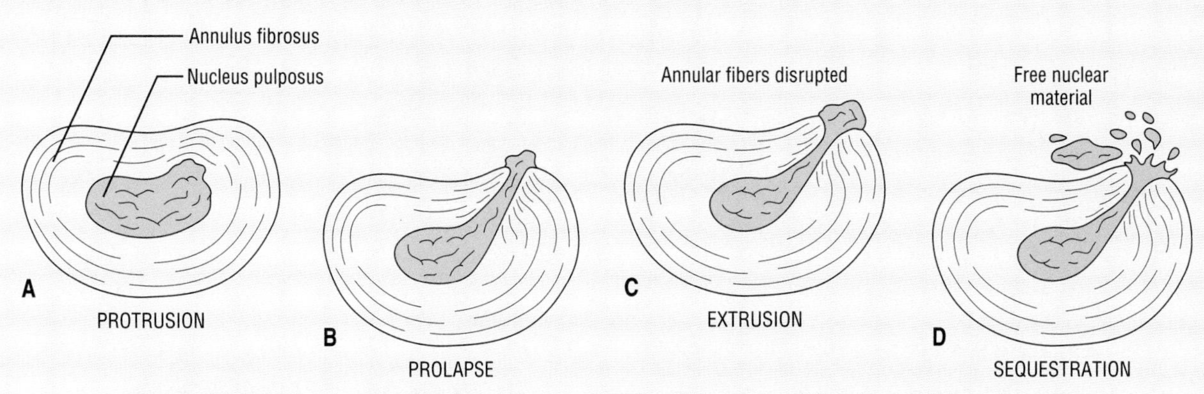

Figure 8-34 Four types of disc herniations: protrusion **(A),** prolapse **(B),** extrusion **(C),** and sequestration **(D).** (From Magee DL: *Orthopedic physical assessment*, ed 5, Philadelphia, 2008, Saunders.)

Functional Considerations

POTENTIAL MIGRATION OF THE INTERVERTEBRAL DISC

Movement between any two vertebrae results in a relatively small displacement, or migration, of the nucleus pulposus within the intervertebral disc. Recall that the nucleus pulposus is the gelatinous center of the disc, encased by the annulus fibrosus. Because the nucleus pulposus is mostly fluid, it tends to migrate *away* from the compressed regions of adjacent vertebrae (Figure 8-35). For example, extension of the lumbar spine compresses the posterior aspects of the vertebral bodies but separates the anterior aspect (see Figure 8-35, *A*). As a result, the nucleus pulposus is pushed anteriorly, where the pressure is least. Flexion, on the contrary, pushes the nucleus pulposus posteriorly (see Figure 8-35, *B*). As a general rule, the nucleus pulposus of the disc is pushed in a direction opposite that of the spinal motion.

The small migrations of the nucleus pulposus with spinal movement are considered normal. Over time or combined with excessive pressure, however, the nucleus pulposus may ooze through small cracks created within a fragmented annulus fibrosis and may lead to a herniated nucleus pulposus (see Figure 8-34). A **herniated nucleus pulposus** occurs most commonly in the lumbar region and, furthermore, most often occurs in a posterior direction, in the direction of the spinal cord or cauda equina. Such a herniation may cause local or radiating pain, or both, down into the buttocks and leg.

Most often a herniated disc in the lumbar region migrates posteriorly—toward the neural elements. Often the herniation is associated with poor sitting posture or improper lifting technique. Slouching—sitting with a rounded, flexed, low back—reduces the natural lordosis in the lumbar spine. Such a posture, especially if chronic, can increase the likelihood of the nucleus pulposus migrating posteriorly. Over time, the posterior wall of annulus fibrosis may weaken from being over-stretched. When weakened, the annulus fibrosis is not able to restrict the posterior migration of the nucleus pulposus. Posterior herniation of the nuclear material can also occur from a more sudden or isolated event such as when lifting. For example, lifting a box off the floor requires forward bending of the trunk. If the forward bend occurs from over-flexing the lumbar spine, rather than being shared by flexing forward at the hips, the nucleus pulposus is under pressure to slide posteriorly. Upon lifting the object, muscular forces further compress the disc and can generate even larger pressures. Figure 8-36 illustrates the many types of forward flexed postures that can create relatively high pressures on the nucleus pulposus with the disc. Note that the least pressure occurs while lying down, which is often a relatively comfortable position chosen by someone who has recently experienced a herniated nucleus pulposus.

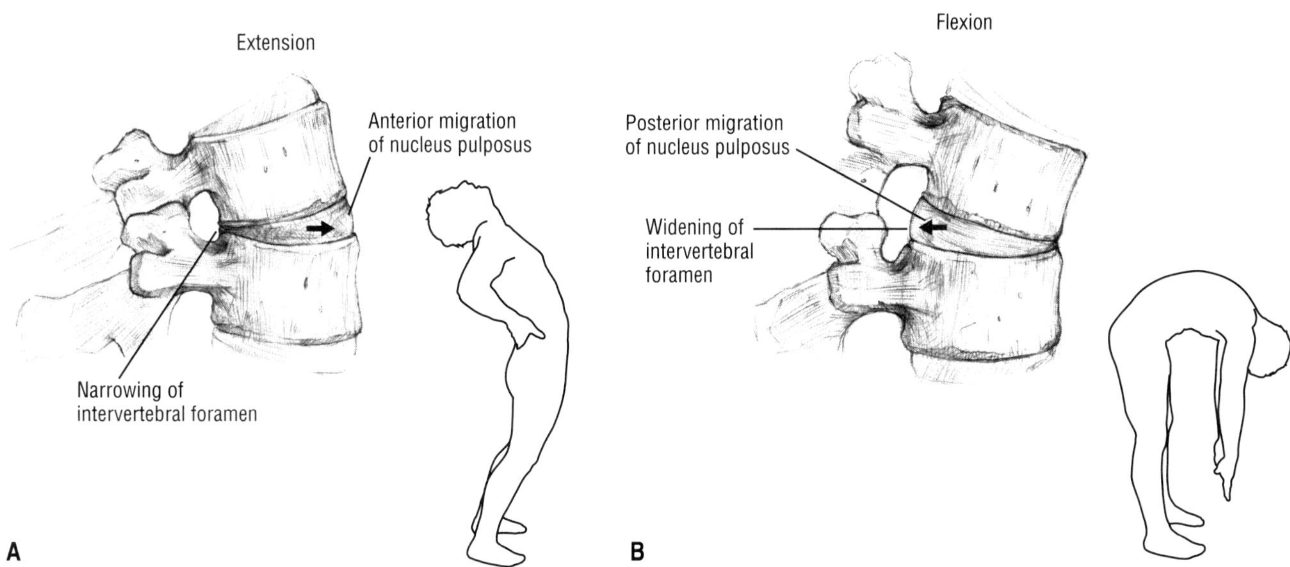

Figure 8-35 The effect of extension and flexion on the intervertebral disc. **A,** Lumbar extension producing a sight anterior migration of the nucleus pulposus and narrowing of the intervertebral foramen. **B,** Lumbar flexion producing a sight posterior migration of the nucleus pulposus and widening of the intervertebral foramen.

Many therapeutic techniques used for treatment of individuals with disc problems are based on the mechanics of spinal motion at the lumbar spine. For example, a patient with a posterior herniated nucleus pulposus in the lumbar spine is often treated with extension exercises. In theory, spinal extension exercises help push the nucleus pulposus anteriorly, back toward the center of the disc and away from the delicate spinal elements. Extreme care must be used, however, when attempting to exercise or move anyone with acute back pain. A major component of treatment involves educating patients in safer ways of lifting as well as explaining the benefits of proper sitting posture.

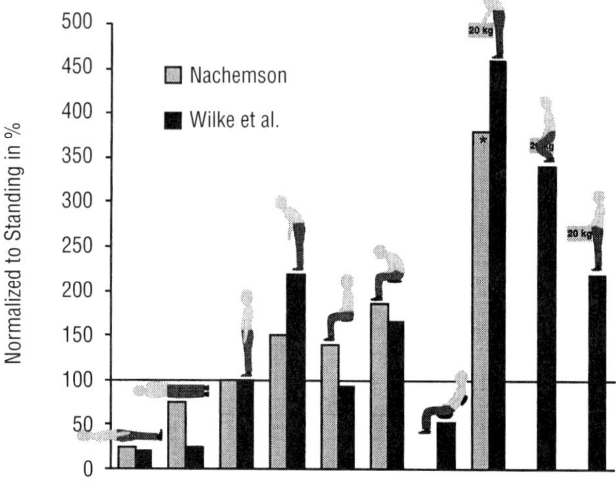

Figure 8-36 Comparison of pressure on the intervertebral disc in a variety of different postures. (Modified from Wilke H-J, Neef P, Caimi M et al: New in vivo measurements of pressures in the intervertebral discs in daily life, *Spine* 24:755-762, 1999. See Additional Readings on p. 225 for data sources.)

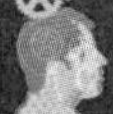

Consider this...

Scoliosis

Scoliosis (from the Greek, meaning "curvature") is a deformity of the vertebral column characterized primarily by abnormal frontal plane curvatures (lateral bends) within the thoracolumbar region. Because the motions of the spine are mechanically coupled, scoliosis typically also involves abnormal curvatures in the horizontal plane and, to a lesser extent, sagittal plane.

The most common pattern of scoliosis consists of a single lateral curve, with an apex in the T7-T9 region. Many other patterns involve a compensatory curve, most often in the lumbar region. For example, Figure 8-37 shows a posterior view of an adolescent girl with a right thoracic and left lumbar scoliosis. Note that the type of scoliosis is defined according to the apex or convex side of the curve. In cases of structural (fixed) scoliosis, a characteristic "rib hump" is often evident on forward flexion (see Figure 8-37, *B*) as a result of the ribs being forced to follow the unwanted rotation of the thoracic vertebrae.

Clinicians treat scoliosis through a variety of conservative methods including stretching of the tissues on the shortened—concave—side of each curve, strengthening of the muscles on the convex side, bracing, soft tissue mobilization, and postural education. Surgery may be required in severe cases or when conservative treatment does not arrest the progression of the deformity.

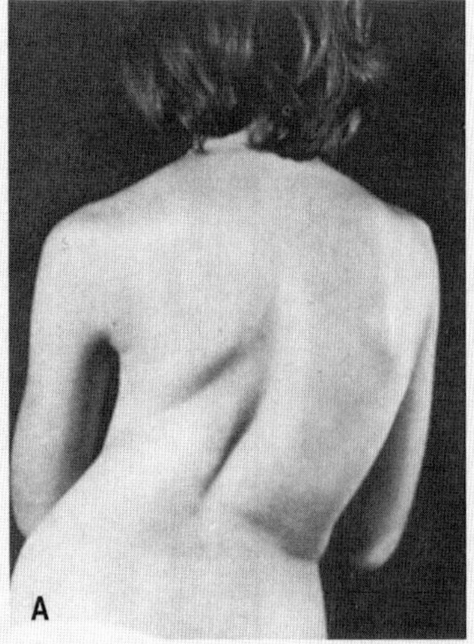

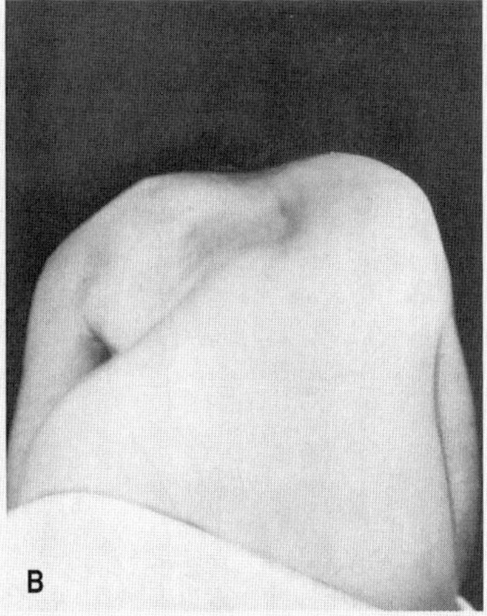

Figure 8-37 **A,** Posterior view of right thoracic and left lumbar scoliosis. **B,** "Rib hump" on the right is visible during forward flexion. (From Gartland JJ: *Fundamentals of orthopedics*, Philadelphia, 1979, Saunders.)

THERAPEUTIC IMPLICATIONS OF ANTERIOR AND POSTERIOR PELVIC TILTS

An **anterior pelvic tilt** is a short-arc anterior rotation of the pelvis about the hip joints, with the trunk held upright and stationary. As shown in Figure 8-38, *A*, an anterior pelvic tilt naturally extends the lumbar spine and increases the lumbar lordosis. A **posterior pelvic tilt,** on the contrary, is a short-arc posterior rotation of the pelvis. A posterior pelvic tilt (Figure 8-38, *B*) flexes the lumbar spine and therefore decreases the lumbar lordosis.

As described later, some physical therapy approaches to treating low back pain incorporate anterior and posterior tilting of the pelvis. These pelvic motions produce relatively small flexion or extension movements of the lumbar spine. Flexing or extending the lumbar region has many potential biomechanical consequences (Table 8-6). The specific reason for choosing flexion or extension depends on the underlying pathology and therapeutic goals established for the patient. For example, a patient with **stenosis** (narrowing) of the intervertebral foramen may be instructed in therapeutic exercises that promote a posterior pelvic tilt. Such a posture flexes the lumbar spine and thereby widens the intervertebral foramen (Figure 8-38, *D*). This may reduce painful symptoms caused by an impingement of an exiting nerve root. An individual suffering from a posterior disc herniation, in contrast, may be instructed to hold his or her pelvis in a more anteriorly tilted position, maintaining or increasing the lordosis of the lumbar spine. This posture may help prevent a posterior migration of the nucleus pulposus, limiting or preventing pressure on the nearby neural elements (Figure 8-38, *C*).

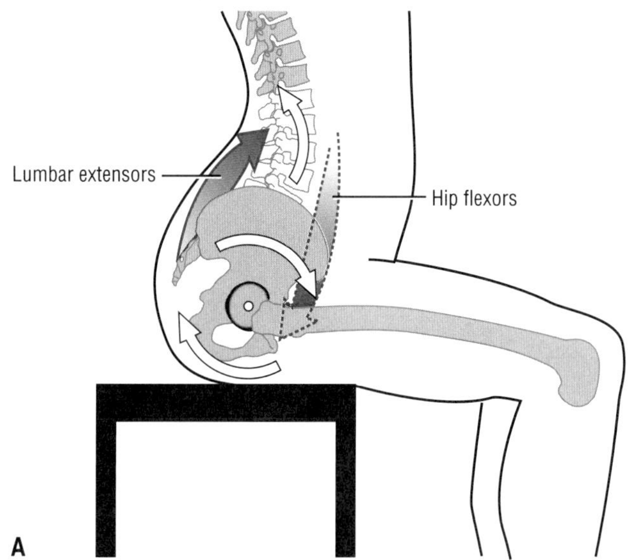

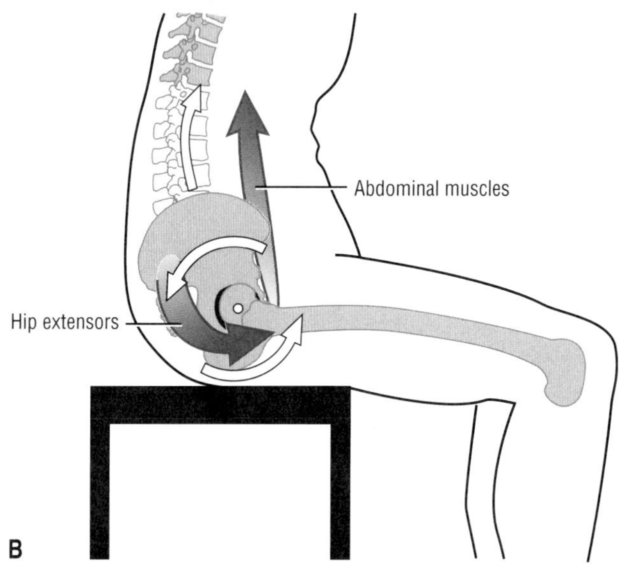

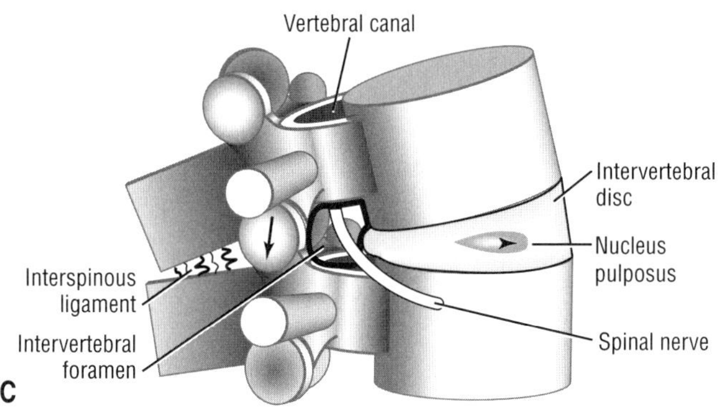

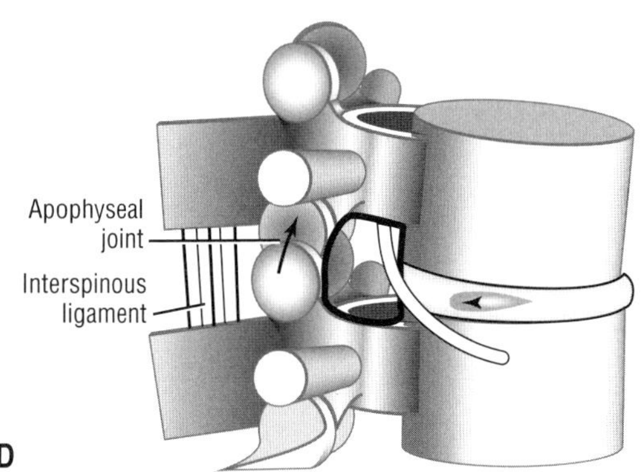

Figure 8-38 Anterior and posterior pelvic tilts of the pelvis and their effect on the lumbar spine. **A** and **C,** An anterior pelvic tilt increases the lordosis of the lumbar spine. This action tends to shift the nucleus pulposus anteriorly and decrease the diameter of the intervertebral foramina. **B** and **D,** Posterior pelvic tilt flexes the lumbar spine and decreases lumbar lordosis. This action tends to shift the nucleus pulposus posteriorly and increases the diameter of the intervertebral foramina. (From Neumann DA: *Kinesiology of the musculoskeletal system: foundations for physical rehabilitation,* St Louis, 2002, Mosby, Figure 9-68.)

Lumbosacral and Sacroiliac Joints

LUMBOSACRAL JUNCTION

The articulation between L5 and S1 is known as the lumbosacral junction (Figure 8-39). The weight of the entire trunk and upper body is transferred to the pelvis at this area. The L5-S1 junction has an interbody joint anteriorly and a pair of apophyseal joints posteriorly. Normally, the lumbosacral junction is aligned such that the base of the sacrum is inclined *forward* about 40 degrees from the horizontal plane. This alignment is referred to as the *sacrohorizontal angle* (Figure 8-40). The facet joints of the L5-S1 are typically oriented close to the frontal plane (see Figure 8-39), which helps prevent the lower spine from translating "downhill" in a forward direction relative to the sacrum. Excessive anterior translation of the lumbar spine relative to the base of the sacrum is called anterior spondylolisthesis, which is formed from the Greek words *spondylo* meaning "spine" and *listhesis* meaning "to slip."

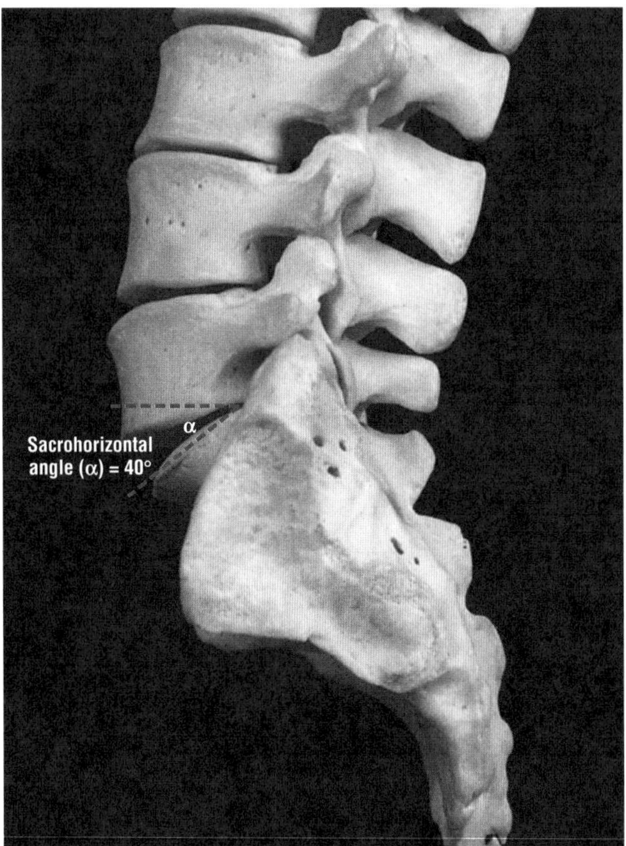

Figure 8-40 A lateral view of the lumbosacral junction, highlighting the sacrohorizontal angle. (Modified from Neumann DA: *Kinesiology of the musculoskeletal system: foundations for physical rehabilitation*, St Louis, 2002, Mosby, Figure 9-40. Created with the assistance of Guy Simoneau.)

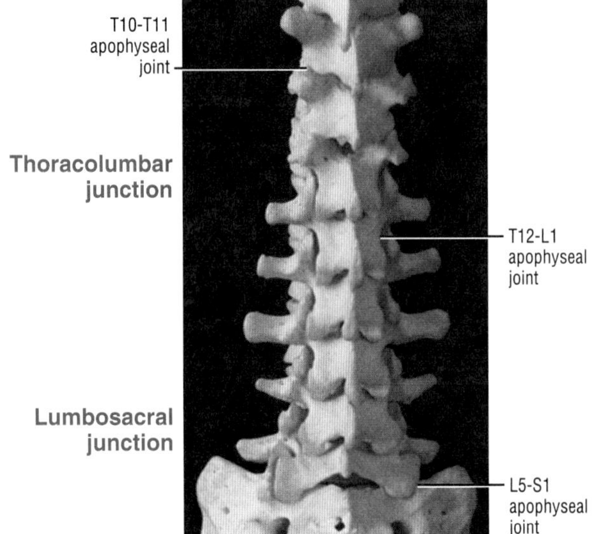

Figure 8-39 A posterior view of the thoracolumbar spine, highlighting the lumbosacral junction. (From Neumann DA: *Kinesiology of the musculoskeletal system: foundations for physical rehabilitation*, St Louis, 2002, Mosby, Figure 9-60.)

SACROILIAC JOINTS

The sacroiliac (SI) joints are formed by the articulation between the articular surfaces of the sacrum and both iliac bones. An important function of the SI joints is to allow the wedge-shaped sacrum to transfer forces of body weight to the pelvis and lower extremities. While standing in a weight-bearing position, these forces are redirected upward from the lower extremities to the sacrum and ultimately the vertebral column (Figure 8-42). In women, the SI joints become looser during childbirth, thereby helping to open the birth canal.

The SI joints typically allow little motion. The relative rigidity of these joints promotes stability between the ilium and sacrum, which is a requirement to adequately transfer large forces such as when walking or running. The SI joints are supported by many thick ligaments (Figure 8-43) and roughened articular surfaces. Further dynamic stability is created by muscles such as the piriformis, hamstrings, and abdominals—muscles that act either directly or indirectly across the SI joints.

Clinical **INSIGHT**

Anterior Spondylolisthesis

Anterior spondylolisthesis is a general term that describes the anterior displacement of one vertebra over another. This displacement often occurs at the L5-S1 junction (Figure 8-41). Most commonly this pathology results from a fracture of the pars interarticularis, a section of the vertebrae midway between the superior and inferior articular processes.

Severe anterior spondylolisthesis can injure the nerves within the cauda equina as they pass through the lumbosacral junction.

As a rule, exercises that promote full extension—or hyperlordosis—in the lumbar spine are contraindicated for a person with anterior spondylolisthesis. (This includes exercises that promote an extreme anterior pelvic tilt.) Such a movement or posture not only increases the sacrohorizontal angle, thereby increasing the likelihood of L5 sliding anteriorly over the base of the sacrum, but also decreases the space within the intervertebral foramen, further compromising the nerves that travel within that region.

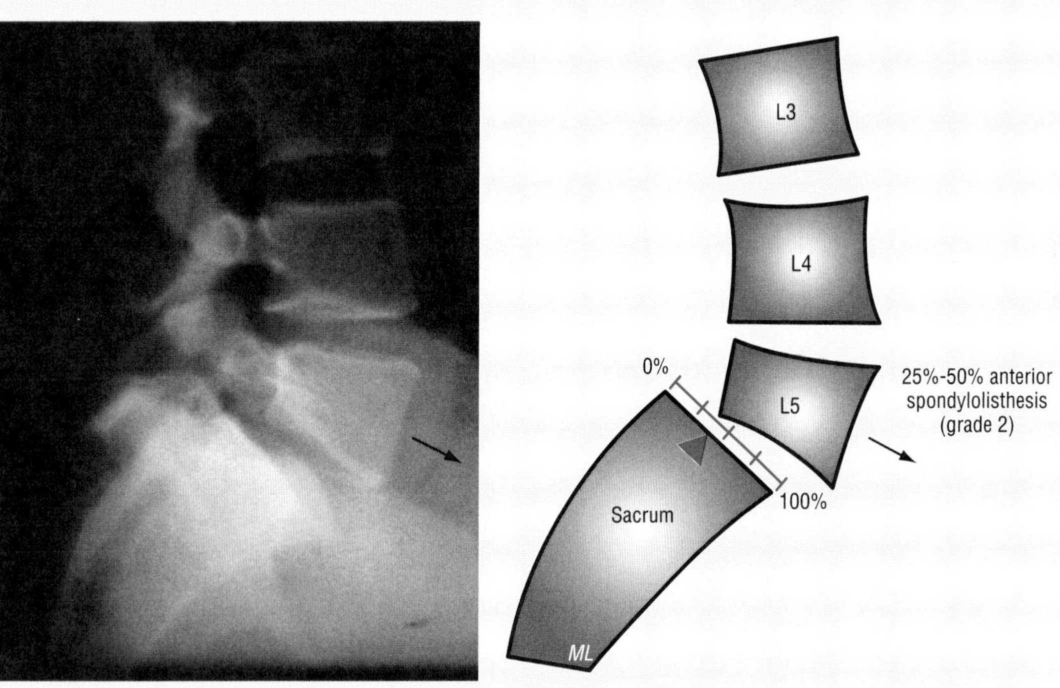

Figure 8-41 An illustration of an anterior spondylolisthesis. (From Marx J, Hockberger R, Walls R: *Rosen's emergency medicine: concepts and clinical practice*, ed 6, St Louis, 2006, Mosby, Figure 51-3.)

TABLE 8-6 BIOMECHANICAL CONSEQUENCES OF LUMBAR FLEXION AND EXTENSION

Movement	Biomechanical Consequences
Flexion	1. Tends to migrate the nucleus pulposus posteriorly, toward neural tissue 2. Increases the size of the opening of the intervertebral foramina 3. Transfers load from the apophyseal joints to the intervertebral discs 4. Increases tension in the posterior connective tissues (ligamentum flava, apophyseal joint capsules, interspinous and supraspinous ligaments, posterior longitudinal ligament) and posterior margin of the annulus fibrosus 5. Compresses the anterior side of the annulus fibrosus
Extension	1. Tends to migrate the nucleus pulposus anteriorly, away from neural tissue 2. Decreases the size of the opening of the intervertebral foramina 3. Transfers load from the intervertebral disc to the apophyseal joints 4. Decreases tension in the posterior connective tissues (see above) and posterior margin of the annulus fibrosus 5. Stretches the anterior side of the annulus fibrosus

From Neumann DA: *Kinesiology of the musculoskeletal system: foundations for physical rehabilitation*, St Louis, 2002, Mosby, Table 9-15.

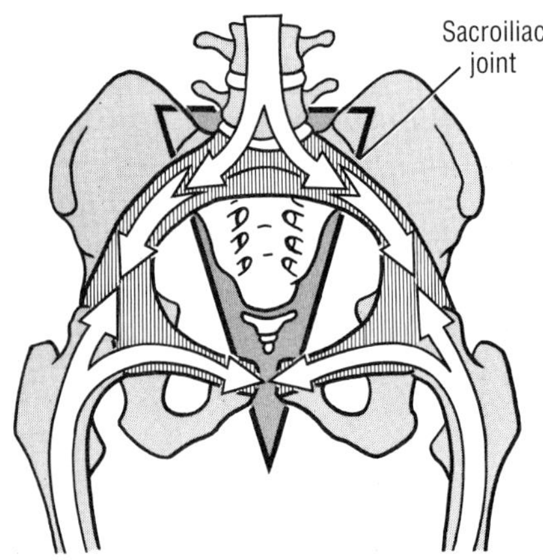

Figure 8-42 Anterior view of the pelvis, highlighting the transfer of body weight through the sacrum, eventually to the pelvic ring. (From Kapandji IA: *The physiology of joints*, vol 3, New York, 1974, Churchill Livingstone.)

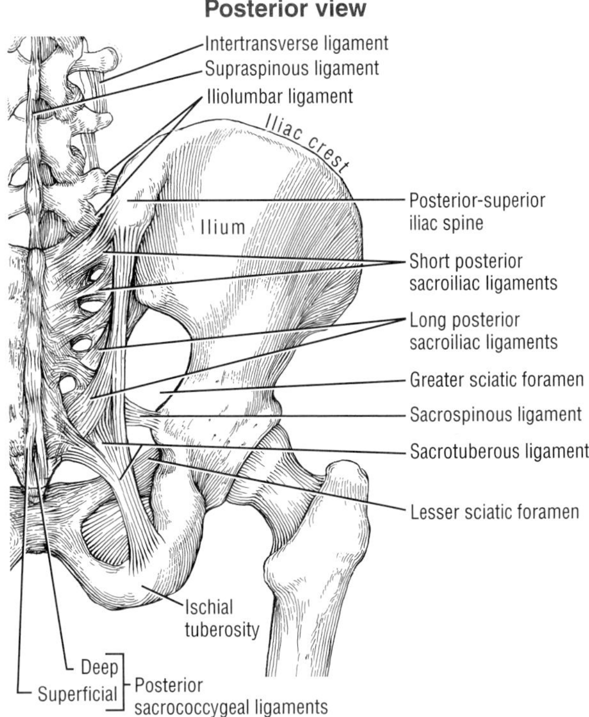

Figure 8-43 A posterior view of the right lumbosacral junction, showing the major ligaments that reinforce the sacroiliac joint. (From Neumann DA: *Kinesiology of the musculoskeletal system: foundations for physical rehabilitation*, St Louis, 2002, Mosby, Figure 9-75.)

The limited motion of the sacrum at the SI joints is usually not described as the result of specific muscle activation. Typical average reported rotations are 2 degrees or less. Small translations also occur but are usually less than

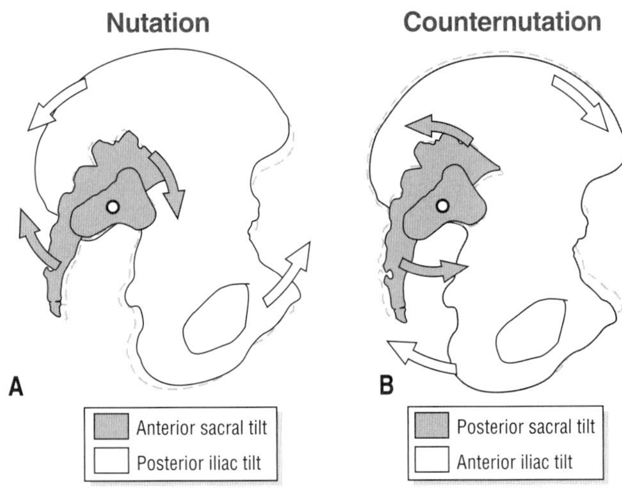

Figure 8-44 Kinematics of the sacroiliac joint. **A,** Nutation. **B,** Counternutation. (From Neumann DA: *Kinesiology of the musculoskeletal system: foundations for physical rehabilitation*, St Louis, 2002, Mosby, Figure 9-77.)

2 mm. Most kinematic descriptions of SI joint kinematics are complicated and beyond the scope of this text. The most basic terminology describes a short arc of rotations in the sagittal plane, called nutation and counternutation (Figure 8-44). **Nutation,** meaning "to nod," describes an anterior rotation of the sacrum relative to each ilium. **Counternutation** is a posterior rotation of the sacrum relative to each ilium. These movements are described by the movement of the anterior edge of the sacrum.

The SI joints are located at a stressful region of the body—the junction between the vertebral column and the pelvis and lower extremities. Despite an extensive network of ligaments, muscles, and fascia, the SI joints can become misaligned such as by falling on the hip or tailbone. This can quickly destabilize the pelvis and result in pain or significant postural compensations. Physical therapy may involve soft tissue mobilization, active exercise, and physical modalities to attempt to restore more natural alignment or at least reduce inflammation and pain.

Muscle and Joint Interaction

Innervation of the Craniocervical and Trunk Musculature

Once a spinal nerve exits an intervertebral foramen, it quickly divides into a ventral or a dorsal ramus (Figure 8-45). Dorsal rami form short nerves that innervate most muscles of the posterior neck and posterior trunk. Ventral rami not only form the cervical, brachial, and lumbosacral plexus, but also innervate most of the muscles of the anterior-lateral trunk and neck. Knowing this organization allows one to predict a craniocervical or trunk muscle's innervation. Although there are exceptions, muscle tissue, for example, found on the posterior aspect of the

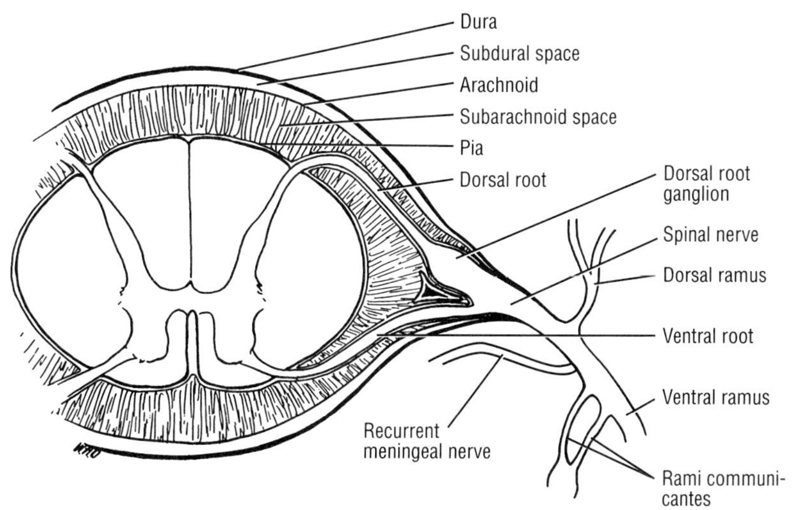

Figure 8-45 A cross section of the spinal cord shows the dorsal (sensory) and ventral (motor) roots forming a spinal nerve. The spinal nerve divides into a relatively small dorsal ramus and a much larger ventral ramus. (Modified from Jenkins DB: *Hollingshead's functional anatomy of the limbs and back,* ed 8, Philadelphia, 2002, Saunders.)

vertebral column that courses between the sixth and twelfth thoracic vertebrae is likely innervated by multiple dorsal rami from spinal nerves T6-T12. Muscle tissue of the anterior-lateral trunk spanning the same distance, on the other hand, would likely be innervated by nerves from the ventral rami of the T6-T12 region (called intercostal nerves). Box 8-1 defines some of the common functions of the various nerve components.

BOX 8-1

Common Functions of Nerve Components

- *Ventral nerve root:* contains primarily outgoing (efferent) axons that provide motor signals to muscle
- *Dorsal nerve root:* contains mostly incoming (afferent) dendrites that carry sensory information to the spinal cord from the periphery
- *Spinal nerve:* composed of dorsal and ventral nerve roots
- *Dorsal ramus:* posterior branches from the spinal nerve that innervate the deeper posterior musculature of the trunk and craniocervical regions
- *Ventral ramus:* anterior branches from the spinal nerve that innervate the anterior-lateral musculature of the trunk and craniocervical regions; also form the cervical, brachial, and lumbosacral plexus

Muscles of the Craniocervical Region

The numerous muscles within the craniocervical region can be divided into two groups: anterior and posterior. Anterior muscles flex the head or neck, whereas posterior muscles extend the head or neck. Nearly every muscle in this region also has some potential to also laterally flex or rotate the craniocervical regions in the horizontal plane.

ANTERIOR CRANIOCERVICAL MUSCLES

Superficial Muscles

The superficial muscles of the anterior craniocervical region include the sternocleidomastoid and the anterior, middle, and posterior scalenes. These muscles are typically much longer than the deeper muscles of the region. In addition to creating movement, these long, superficial muscles often function as "guy wires" to help stabilize the region.

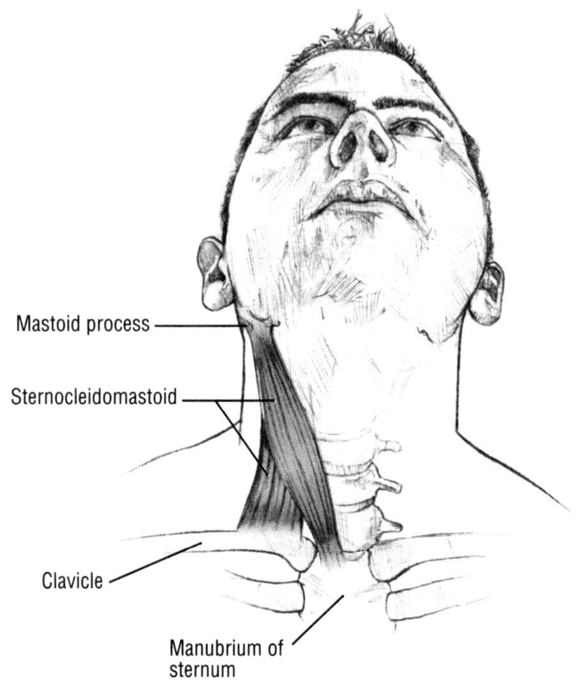

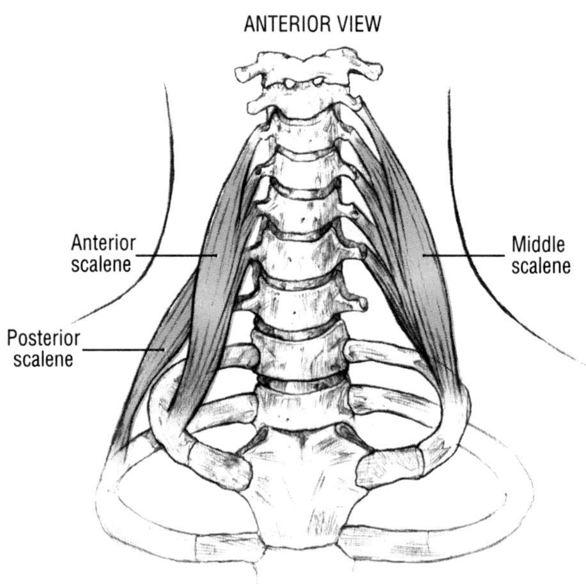

Sternocleidomastoid

Inferior Attachment: Sternal head: Superior aspect of the manubrium of the sternum
Clavicular head: Medial one third of the clavicle

Superior Attachment: Mastoid process of the temporal bone

Innervation: Spinal accessory nerve (cranial nerve XI)

Actions: Bilateral:
- Flexion of the head and neck

Unilateral:
- Contralateral rotation of the head and neck
- Lateral flexion of the head and neck

Comments: Tightness of one sternocleidomastoid results in a condition called torticollis (wryneck), which results in the head and neck becoming positioned into *all* of the actions of the sternocleidomastoid: flexion, lateral flexion, and rotation to the opposite side. This condition often occurs in young children and is typically treated conservatively with stretching of the muscle and mobilization of the surrounding soft tissues.

Scalenes

Anterior Scalene

Superior Attachment: Transverse processes of C3-C7

Inferior Attachment: First rib

Middle Scalene

Superior Attachment: Transverse processes of C2-C7

Inferior Attachment: First rib

Posterior Scalene

Superior Attachment: Transverse processes of C5-C7

Inferior Attachment: External surface of the second rib

Innervation of All Three Scalenes: Ventral rami (C3-C7)

Actions of all the scalene muscles:

Bilateral:
- Flexion of the neck (anterior and middle scalenes)
- Assist with inspiration via elevation of the first and second ribs

Unilateral:
- Lateral flexion

Comments: The (six total) scalenes provide a significant amount of stability to the craniocervical region, similar to the way cables are used to support large, free-standing antenna towers. The attachments of the scalenes to the ribs also allow these muscles to assist with inspiration by pulling upward on the ribs. Patients with chronic obstructive pulmonary disease may display prominent, hypertrophied scalenes resulting from long-term overuse of these muscles to assist with their labored breathing.

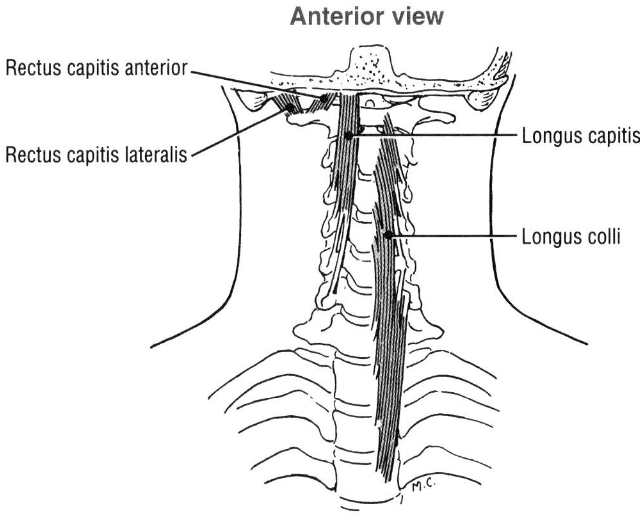

Figure 8-46 Anterior view of the deep anterior muscles of the neck. (From Luttgens K, Hamilton N: *Kinesiology: scientific basis of human motion*, ed 9, Madison, Wis, 1997, Brown and Benchmark/McGraw-Hill.)

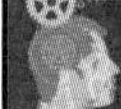

Consider this...

Thoracic Outlet Syndrome

Thoracic outlet syndrome is characterized by weakness, numbness, or tingling in the hand or arm, resulting from compression of the brachial plexus or subclavian artery.

The brachial plexus and the subclavian artery course between the anterior and middle scalenes. If either of these muscles is significantly tight or hypertrophied, the neurovascular bundle may become pinched, resulting in radicular signs and symptoms and diminished pulse.

Deep Anterior Muscles

The longus colli and longus capitis reside on the anterior aspect of the craniocervical region (Figure 8-46). These muscles flex the neck and head and also function as dynamic stabilizers of the craniocervical region.

The rectus capitis anterior and rectus capitis lateralis are short muscles that arise from the transverse processes of the atlas and insert on the occipital bone, near the foramen magnum (see Figures 8-6 and 8-46). These muscles function only at the atlanto-occipital joint. The rectus capitis anterior is a flexor, and the rectus capitis lateralis is a lateral flexor. The fine control afforded by these small muscles is important for visual and vestibular orientation. The specific anatomic attachments of these four muscles are listed in the table below.

POSTERIOR CRANIOCERVICAL MUSCLES

Suboccipital Muscles

The suboccipital muscles are a deep posterior group of four paired muscles that attach among the atlas, axis, and occipital bone (Figure 8-47). These short, relatively thick muscles provide fine control of movements in the atlanto-axial and atlanto-occipital joints. Such movements are important for positioning the head for vision, hearing, and vestibular function. Tightness and tenderness of these muscles is often associated with components of a "forward-head" posture. The specific anatomic attachments and functions of the suboccipital muscles are listed in the table on p. 211.

Superficial Cervical Extensors

The splenius capitis and splenius cervicis muscles are located just deep to the upper and middle trapezius. Although different anatomically, these muscles typically work together to extend, laterally flex, and rotate the head and neck to the same side. These muscles, along with the nearby levator scapula muscle, are pictured in the following sections.

DEEP ANTERIOR CRANIOCERVICAL MUSCLES

Muscle	Inferior Attachment	Superior Attachment	Actions	Innervation
Longus colli	Bodies and transverse processes of C3-T3	Transverse processes and bodies of C1-C6	Flexion of the neck	Ventral rami C2-C8
Longus capitis	Transverse processes of C3-C6	Anterior to the foramen magnum (occipital bone)	*Bilateral:* flexion of the head and neck	Ventral rami C1-C3
Rectus capitis anterior	Transverse processes of C1	Just anterior to the occipital condyles	Flexion of the head (AO joint only)	Ventral rami C1-C2
Rectus capitis lateralis	Transverse processes of C1	Just lateral to the occipital condyles	*Unilateral:* lateral flexion (AO joint only)	Ventral rami C1-C2

AO, Atlanto-occipital.

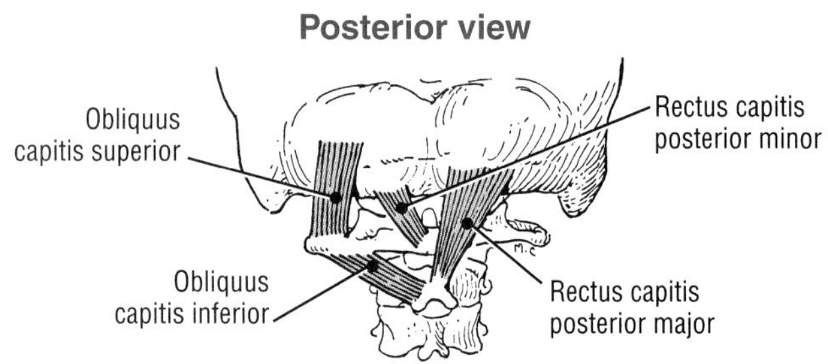

Figure 8-47 A posterior view of the suboccipital muscles. (From Luttgens K, Hamilton N: *Kinesiology: scientific basis of human motion*, ed 9, Madison, Wis, 1997, Brown and Benchmark/McGraw-Hill.)

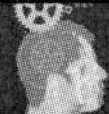

Consider this...

Muscular Trauma Associated with Whiplash

A common consequence of being in a car accident is whiplash of the head and neck. Whiplash is the result of uncontrolled acceleration of the head and neck into flexion or extension, or both (Figure 8-48).

Whiplash associated with cervical hyperextension generally creates greater strain on the muscles and soft tissues than whiplash associated with cervical flexion. This is explained, in part, because the maximum extent of cervical flexion is blocked by the chin striking the chest (see Figure 8-48, *B*). The longus colli and capitis are particularly vulnerable to injury from hyperextension-associated whiplash.

Clinically, a person with a hyperextension injury shows marked tenderness and protective spasm in the region of the longus colli and capitis (deep in the anterior neck). These impairments can lead to cervical instability, as well as difficulty shrugging the shoulders. Without adequate stabilization provided by the longus colli and other flexors, the upper trapezius loses its stable cranial attachment. Consequently, the upper trapezius loses its effectiveness at elevating the shoulder girdle.

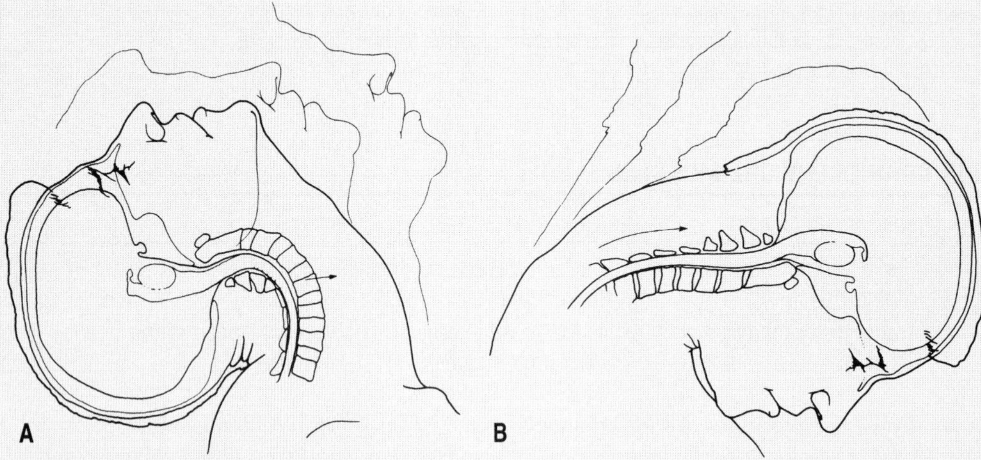

Figure 8-48 During acceleration (whiplash) injuries, cervical extension **(A)** typically exceeds cervical flexion **(B)**. As a result, the anterior structures of the cervical region are more vulnerable to injury. (From Porterfield JA, DeRosa C: *Mechanical neck pain: perspectives in functional anatomy*, Philadelphia, 1995, Saunders.)

SUBOCCIPITAL MUSCLES

Muscle	Inferior Attachment	Superior Attachment	Actions (Head and Neck)	Innervation
Rectus capitis posterior major	Spinous process of C2	Lateral aspect of inferior nuchal line	*Bilateral:* extension (AO and AA joints) *Unilateral:* lateral flexion (AO joint only); rotation to the same side (AA joint only)	Suboccipital nerve (dorsal ramus C1)
Rectus capitis posterior minor	Posterior tubercle of C1	Medial aspect of inferior nuchal line	*Bilateral:* extension (AO joint only)	Suboccipital nerve (dorsal ramus C1)
Obliquus capitis superior	Transverse process of C1	Between the inferior and superior nuchal lines—lateral aspect	*Bilateral:* extension (AO joint only) *Unilateral:* lateral flexion (AO joint only)	Suboccipital nerve (dorsal ramus C1)
Obliquus capitis inferior	Apex of the spinous process of C2	Inferior margin of the transverse process of C1	*Bilateral:* extension (AA joint only) *Unilateral:* rotation to the same side (AA joint only)	Suboccipital nerve (dorsal ramus C1)

AA, Atlanto-axial; AO, atlanto-occipital.

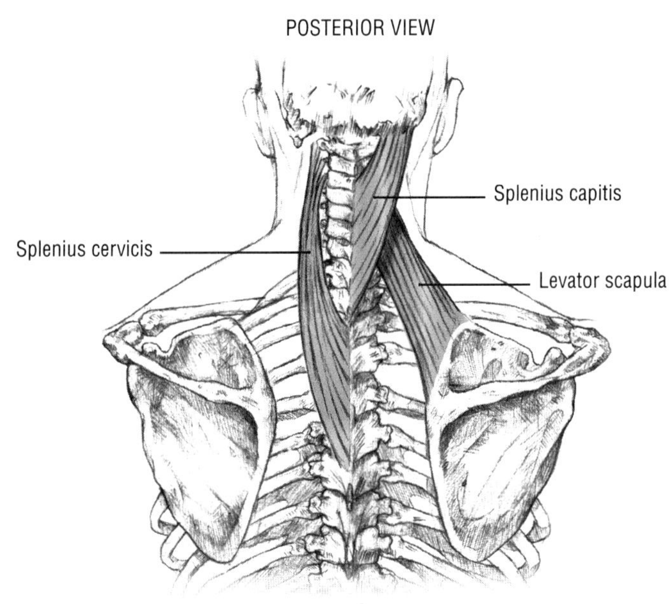

A posterior view of the left splenius cervicis and right splenius capitis. The levator scapula is pictured for reference.

Splenius Capitis

Inferior Attachment: Lower half of ligamentum nuchae and spinous processes of C7-T3

Superior Attachment: Mastoid process and lateral one third of the superior nuchal line

Innervation: Dorsal rami (C2-C8)

Actions: Bilateral:
- Extension of the head and neck

Unilateral:
- Lateral flexion of the head and neck
- Ipsilateral rotation of the head and neck

Splenius Cervicis

Inferior Attachment: Spinous processes of T3-T6

Superior Attachment: Transverse processes of C1-C3

Innervation: Dorsal rami (C2-C8)

Actions: Bilateral:
- Extension of the neck

Unilateral:
- Ipsilateral rotation of the neck
- Lateral flexion of the neck

Comments: The splenius capitis and cervicis are thin, bandage-like muscles that reinforce the (craniocervical) actions of the upper trapezius.

FUNCTIONAL CONSIDERATION: FINE-TUNING MOTIONS OF THE HEAD AND NECK

Optimal control over the movements and posture of the craniocervical region is an extremely important component of our everyday lives. Ample control of the head and neck is essential for coordinated alignment of the eyes and ears, such as when turning to locate and listen to someone speak. Neurologically, many of the muscles of the head and neck are closely linked to the visual and vestibular systems of the brain. To appreciate this, attempt this small experiment. Gaze forward, looking at an object directly in front of you, and then quickly look as far to the left as possible without rotating the head. Despite attempts to hold the head stationary, a small amount of craniocervical rotation toward the direction of gaze often occurs.

Although the head and neck can produce large range of motion in all three planes, a primary function of the numerous deeper craniocervical muscles is to fine-tune movements of the head and neck. As mentioned earlier in the chapter, motions of the spine are often mechanically coupled with other motions, depending on the orientation of the local facet joints. The deeper craniocervical muscles such as the suboccipital muscles are effective at neutralizing secondary (and often undesired) actions that are otherwise dictated by the plane of the facet joints. These neutralizing actions of these deep muscles are subtle yet important.

Muscles of the Trunk

ANTERIOR-LATERAL MUSCLES OF THE TRUNK

The anterior-lateral muscles of the trunk include matching pairs of the rectus abdominis, external oblique, internal oblique and transverse abdominis. These muscles, often referred to as the abdominals, provide an important source of mobility and stability to the trunk. The ability to maintain a stable trunk, or core, is an especially important function of the abdominals used during many physical activities. Contraction of the abdominal muscles increases intra-abdominal and intrathoracic pressures, which helps in many functions, including stabilizing the lumbar spine during lifting, coughing, defecation, and the process of childbirth.

When contracting bilaterally, the abdominal muscles decrease the distance between the xiphoid process of the sternum and pubic bone. This is expressed by either flexing the thoracic region (such as when performing "crunches"), posteriorly tilting the pelvis, or both actions simultaneously. The ability to posteriorly tilt the pelvis is an important and often poorly appreciated action of the abdominal muscles. This action is necessary to neutralize the strong anterior tilting potential caused by contraction of the hip flexor muscles. Clinicians therefore often promote abdominal activation prior to any strong activation of hip flexors (such as when performing straight leg raise) to prevent unwanted lumbar lordosis.

Acting unilaterally, the abdominal muscles are also able to rotate or laterally flex the trunk. Most often these muscles work bilaterally in a coordinated fashion to produce the appropriate combination of flexion, rotation, and lateral flexion. Consider, for example, the combined flexion, rotation, and lateral flexion of the trunk required to get in or out of a car.

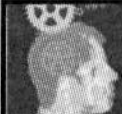

Consider this...

Thoracolumbar Fascia

Two of the four abdominal muscles attach directly into the thoracolumbar fascia. This fascia consists of an extensive, dense sheet of connective tissue that attaches to the spinous processes of all lumbar vertebrae, posterior sacrum, and the posterior ilium. This tissue tightly wraps around several muscles including the erector spinae, quadratus lumborum, and latissimus dorsi.

Contraction of the abdominal muscles increases the tension in the thoracolumbar fascia. The thoracolumbar fascia therefore allows a way for the abdominal muscles to transfer a force to mechanically support the lower back. People often strongly contract their abdominal muscles and temporally hold their breath just prior and during a lift. This may be a natural mechanism employed to engage this protective mechanism.

Slumped sitting with an overly flexed low back may, in time, over-stretch the thoracolumbar fascia. Reduced stiffness in this tissue may reduce the effectiveness of force transfer from the abdominal muscles and lower back. This is another reminder of why proper sitting posture is so important.

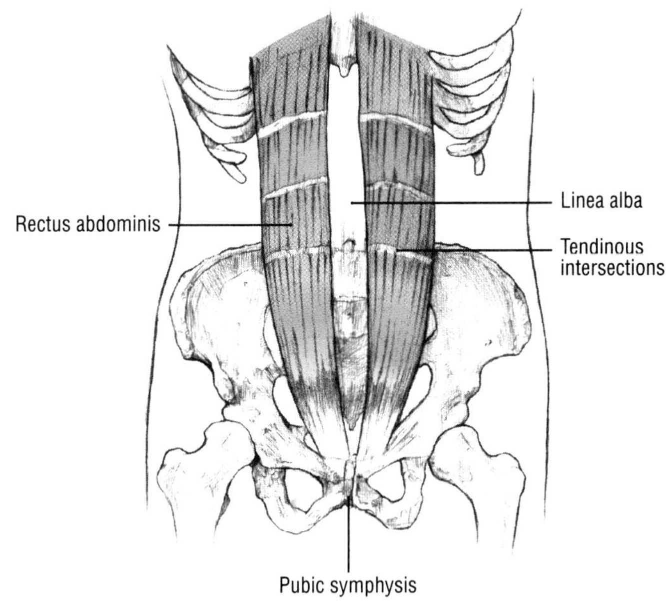

Rectus Abdominis

Inferior Attachment: Crest of the pubis

Superior Attachment: Xiphoid process and cartilages of ribs 5-7

Innervation: Intercostal nerves (T7-T12)

Actions:
- Flexion of the trunk
- Posterior pelvic tilt
- Increases intra-abdominal and intra-thoracic pressure

Comments: The two halves of the rectus abdominis are separated by a tendinous sheath known as the linea alba. This tissue (meaning "white line" in Latin) is a longitudinal strip of tough connective tissue that mechanically links the right and left sets of abdominal muscles. The rectus abdominis muscle is also intersected by three *tendinous intersections,* which can give a rippled look to the anterior abdominal region.

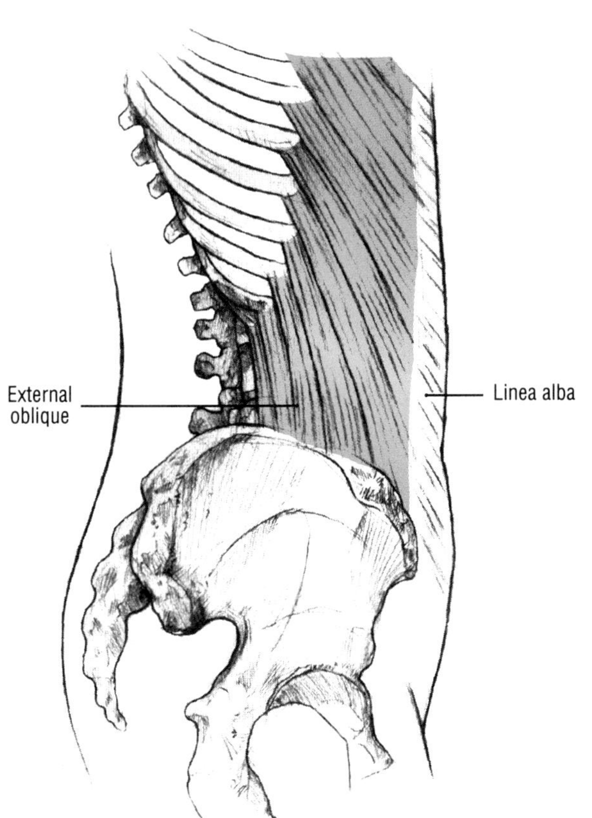

External Oblique

Lateral Attachment: Lateral side of ribs 4-12

Medial Attachment: Iliac crest and linea alba

Innervation: Intercostal nerves (T8-T12)

Actions: Bilateral:
- Flexion of the trunk
- Posterior pelvic tilt
- Increases intra-abdominal and intra-thoracic pressure

Unilateral:
- Rotation of the trunk to the contra-lateral side
- Lateral flexion of the trunk

Comments: The external oblique, formally named the obliquus externus abdominis, is the largest of the lateral abdominal muscles. The fibers of this muscle travel in an inferior-medial direction, similar to the direction of the fingers when placing one's hands in the front pockets. The external oblique is the primary contralateral (opposite side) rotator of the trunk.

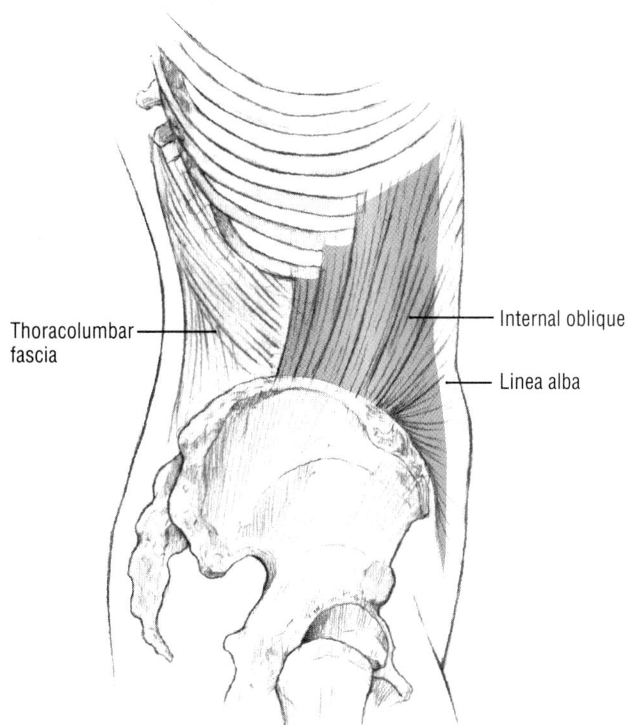

Internal Oblique

Lateral Attachment: Iliac crest, inguinal ligament, and thoracolumbar fascia

Medial Attachment: Ribs 9-12, linea alba

Innervation: Intercostal nerves (T8-T12)

Actions: Bilateral:

- Flexion of the trunk
- Posterior pelvic tilt
- Increases intra-abdominal and intra-thoracic pressure
- Increases tension in thoracolumbar fascia

Unilateral:

- Lateral flexion of the trunk
- Rotation of the trunk to the ipsilateral side

Comments: Formally called the obliquus internus abdominis, the internal oblique lies deep to the external oblique. This muscle courses in a superior-medial direction (from the iliac crest toward the sternum), nearly perpendicular to the deeper fibers of the external oblique. This muscle is the primary ipsilateral (same side) rotator of the trunk.

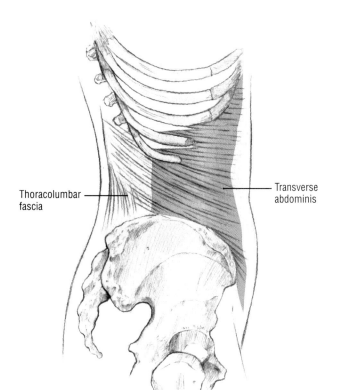

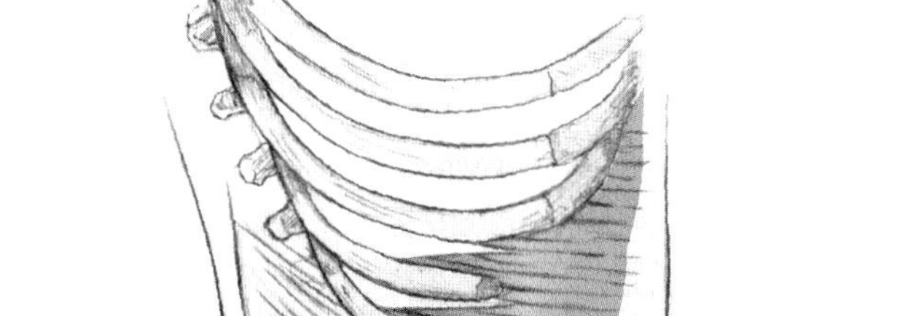

Transverse Abdominis

Lateral Attachment: Iliac crest, thoracolumbar fascia, cartilages of ribs 6-12, and inguinal ligament

Medial Attachment: Linea alba

Innervation: Intercostal nerves (T7-T12)

Actions:

- Increases intra-abdominal pressure
- Increases tension in thoracolumbar fascia

Comments: The transverse abdominis muscle is the deepest of the abdominal muscles. This muscle is also known as the "corset muscle," reflecting its primary function of increasing intra-abdominal pressure. As with the internal oblique, contraction of this muscle also pulls on the thoracolumbar fascia. The resulting increased tension in the thoracolumbar fascia helps stabilize the lumbar region when performing lifting activities.

Other Functionally Associated Muscles: Iliopsoas and the Quadratus Lumborum

Although the iliopsoas and quadratus lumborum are not actually considered muscles of the trunk, they are strongly associated with the movements and stability of the lumbar region.

The iliopsoas is a combination of two muscles: the iliacus and the psoas major. The muscle is a primary hip flexor and also plays a dominant role in other motions of the trunk and pelvis such as performing a sit-up or, if contracting without abdominal muscle support, creating a strong anterior pelvic tilt. The iliopsoas is covered in greater detail in Chapter 9, but some anatomic details are presented in this chapter to allow a complete analysis of the traditional sit-up maneuver.

The quadratus lumborum is anatomically considered a muscle of the posterior abdominal wall. This muscle attaches inferiorly to the iliac crest and superiorly to the twelfth rib and transverse processes of L1-L4. Unlike the abdominal muscles, bilateral activation of the quadratus lumborum results in extension of the lumbar spine.

The quadratus lumborum and the psoas major muscles run nearly vertical on either side of the lumbar vertebrae. A strong bilateral contraction of these muscles affords excellent vertical stability throughout the entire base of the spine including the L5-S1 junction.

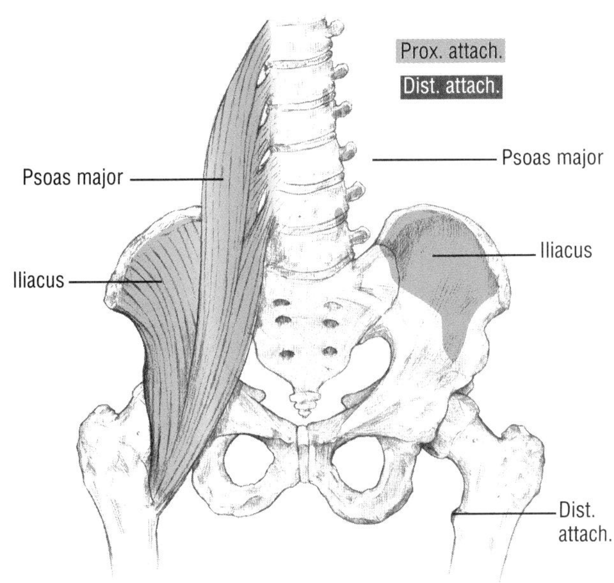

Iliopsoas

Psoas Major

Proximal Attachments:	Transverse processes of T12-L5

Iliacus

Proximal Attachment:	Iliac fossa
Distal Attachment:	Lesser trochanter of femur
Innervation:	Femoral nerve
Actions:	• Hip flexion • Trunk flexion • Anterior pelvic tilt
Comments:	The abdominal muscles produce a posterior pelvic tilt, whereas the iliopsoas produces an anterior pelvic tilt. These muscles can be activated together to firmly stabilize the pelvis within the sagittal plane.

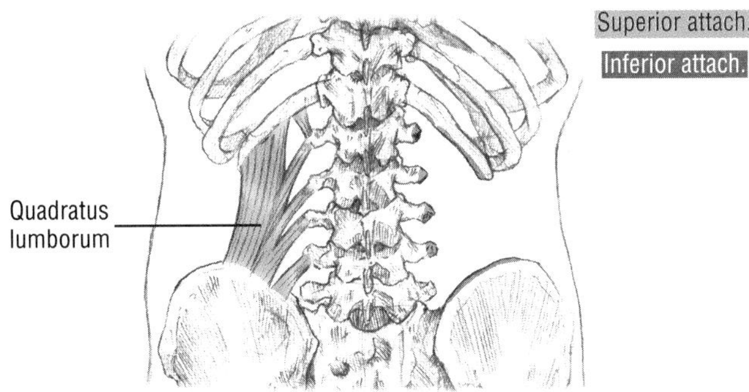

Quadratus Lumborum

Inferior Attachment:	Crest of the ilium
Superior Attachment:	Transverse processes of L1-L4 and twelfth rib
Innervation:	Ventral rami (T12-L3)
Actions:	Bilateral: • Extension of the lumbar region Unilateral: • Lateral flexion of the trunk
Comments:	Clinically, the quadratus lumborum is known as a "hip-hiker," describing its ability to elevate one side of the pelvis. Patients with weak or paralyzed hip flexors can be taught to contract their quadratus lumborum to elevate one side of the pelvis, helping to clear the foot from the ground as it is advanced forward during gait.

FUNCTIONAL CONSIDERATIONS

Analysis of a Sit-Up

The iliopsoas (and all other hip flexors) and the abdominal muscles share the responsibility of performing a basic sit-up. Although the sit-up is often discussed within the context of abdominal strengthening programs, this basic action is essential for the performance of many routine movements such as rising out of bed in the morning.

Figure 8-49 depicts the sit-up as occurring in two phases: a trunk flexion phase and a hip flexion phase. During the *trunk flexion phase*, the abdominal muscles (notably the rectus abdominis) are highly activated, bringing the xiphoid process toward the pubis and flattening the lordotic curve of the lumbar spine. This initial phase concludes as both scapulae clear the supporting surface. Although the

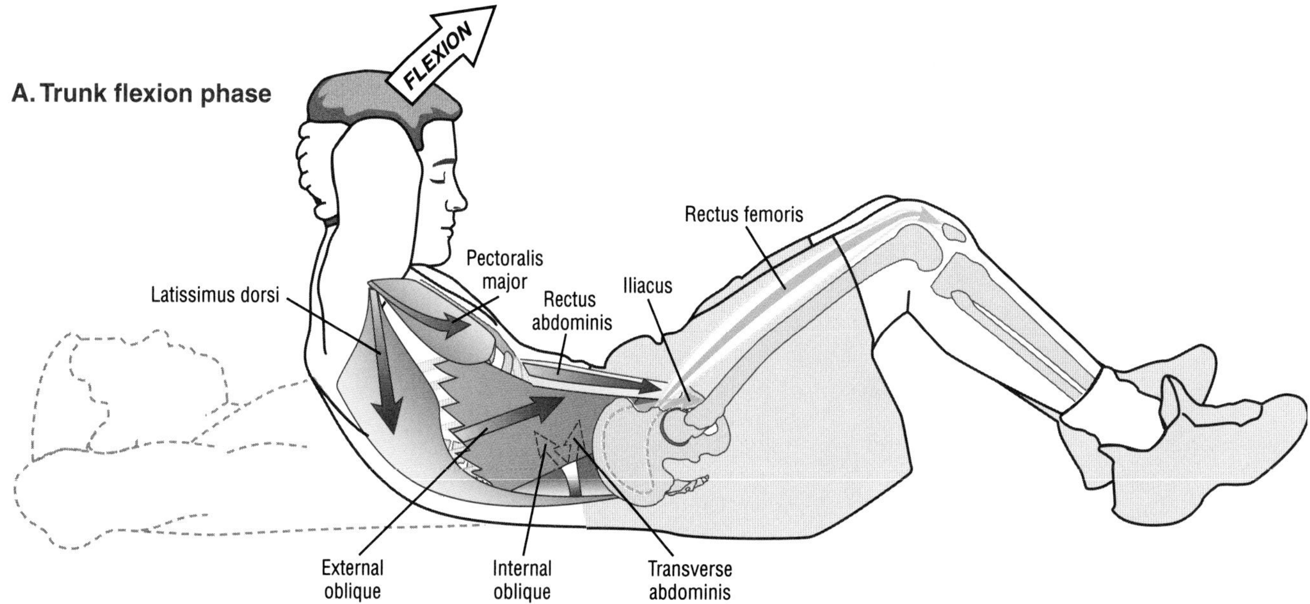

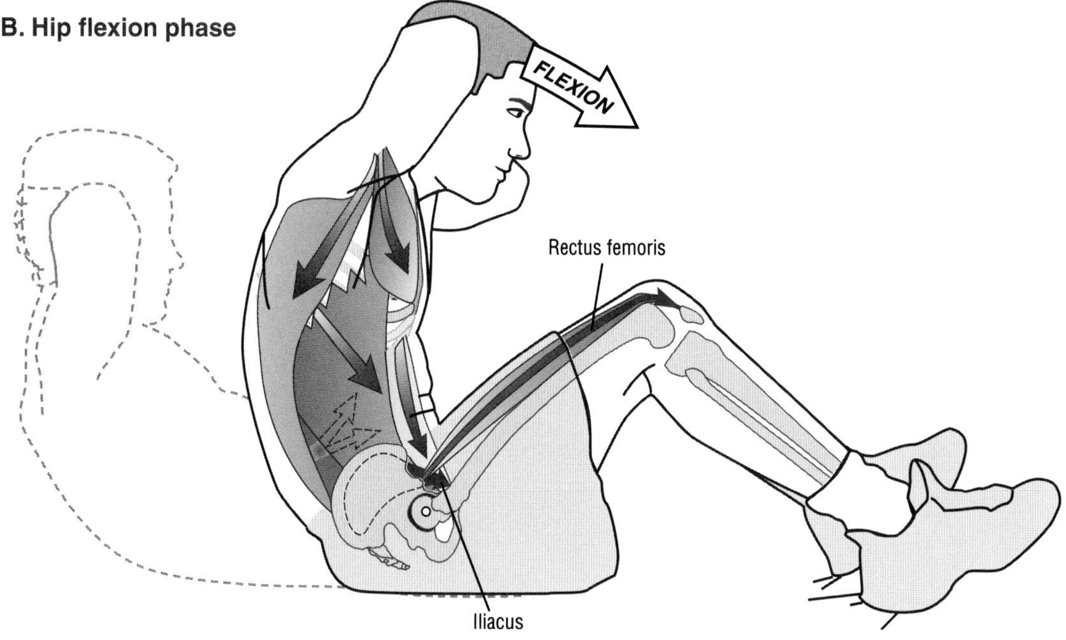

Figure 8-49 Typical activation pattern is shown during a traditional sit-up. **A,** The trunk flexion phase of the sit-up involves strong activation of the abdominal muscles. **B,** The hip flexion phase of the sit-up involves strong activation of the hip flexor muscles (and abdominals). (From Neumann DA: *Kinesiology of the musculoskeletal system: foundations for physical rehabilitation*, St Louis, 2002, Mosby, Figure 10-23.)

abdominal muscles remain active throughout the entire sit-up, strong activation of the hip flexor muscles (such as the iliopsoas and rectus femoris) defines the start of the *hip flexion phase* of the sit-up (see Figure 8-49, *B*). During this phase, the hip flexor muscles rotate the pelvis and attached trunk anteriorly, drawing the chest closer to the knees.

A person with weak abdominal muscles usually demonstrates a characteristic strategy when attempting to perform a sit-up, one that is dominated by strong contraction of the hip flexor muscles. Consequently, the hip flexors immediately take over the action—most notably by the exaggerated anterior pelvic tilt and increased lumbar lordosis—as the pelvis and trunk are rotated forward and upward.

Synergistic Action of the Oblique Abdominal Muscles

As a set, the abdominal muscles frequently contract to produce a combination of movements involving all three planes. Consider, as an example, the person depicted in Figure 8-50 performing a diagonal sit-up. This illustration shows the right and left oblique muscles working synergistically to control movement of the trunk. As depicted, trunk flexion with rotation to the left is controlled by contraction of the right external oblique and the left internal oblique muscles. Compare this movement with lateral flexion of the trunk such as a side sit-up (lateral flexion from a side-lying position). This motion is controlled by the internal and external oblique muscles on the *same* side. For example, a person performing lateral flexion to the left (from a side-lying position) must activate the left internal and left external oblique muscles. As described subsequently, the motions of lateral flexion and rotation are assisted by muscles of the posterior trunk.

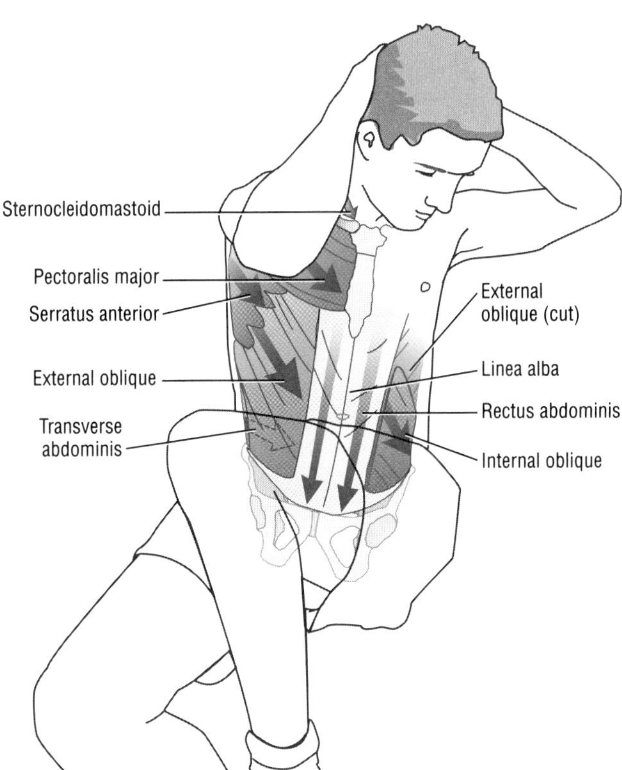

Figure 8-50 A diagonal sit-up to the left involves strong activation of the right external oblique and left external oblique, as well as the rectus abdominus. (From Neumann DA: *Kinesiology of the musculoskeletal system: foundations for physical rehabilitation*, St Louis, 2002, Mosby, Figure 10-16.)

POSTERIOR MUSCLES OF THE TRUNK

Erector Spinae Muscles

The erector spinae muscles are a large, disorganized group of muscles that run essentially vertically on either side of the spine, roughly one hand's width from the spinous processes. As a group, these muscles extend and stabilize the entire vertebral column and craniocervical region.

The erector spinae consist of three thin columns of muscles: spinalis, longissimus, and iliocostalis muscles

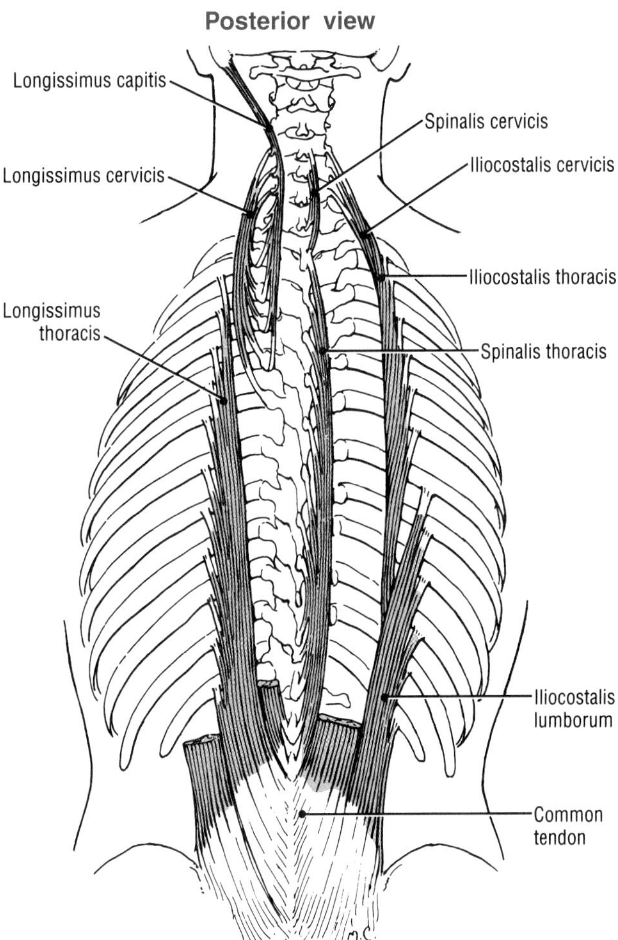

Figure 8-51 The muscles of the erector spinae group. (From Luttgens K, Hamilton N: *Kinesiology: scientific basis of human motion*, ed 9, Madison, Wis, 1997, Brown and Benchmark/McGraw-Hill.)

ERECTOR SPINAE MUSCLES

Muscle	Inferior Attachment	Superior Attachment	Actions	Innervation
Iliocostalis				
Lumborum	Common tendon	Angle of ribs 6-12	*Bilateral:* extension	Dorsal rami of adjacent spinal nerves
Thoracis	Angle of ribs 6-12	Angle of ribs 1-6	*Unilateral:* lateral flexion	
Cervicis	Angle of ribs 3-7	Transverse processes of C4-C6		
Longissimus				
Thoracis	Common tendon	Transverse processes of T1-T12	*Bilateral:* extension	Dorsal rami of adjacent spinal nerves
Cervicis	Transverse processes of T1-T4	Transverse processes of C2-C6	*Unilateral:* lateral flexion	
Capitis	Transverse processes of T1-T5 and near facet joints C3-C7	Mastoid process of temporal bone		
Spinalis				
Thoracis	Common tendon	Spinous processes of T1-T6	*Bilateral:* extension	Dorsal rami of adjacent spinal nerves
Cervicis	Ligamentum nuchae and spinous processes of C7-T1	Spinous process of C2		
Capitis	Blends with semispinalis capitis	Blends with semispinalis capitis		

(Figure 8-51). Each muscular column is further subdivided topographically into three regions. The inferior parts of the erector spinae share a common attachment to a broad thick tendon, just superficial to the sacrum. This thick *common tendon* blends with the more superficial part of the thoracolumbar fascia. The anatomic attachments and functions are listed in the table on this page.

Transversospinal Muscles

The transversospinal muscles include the semispinalis, multifidus, and rotators (Figures 8-53 and 8-54). The muscles lie deep to the erector spinae and course in an oblique direction, from the transverse processes of one vertebra to the spinous processes of more superior vertebrae. Most of the transversospinal muscles have a similar fiber direction, varying only in length and the number of vertebral segments they cross (see the table on p. 220). These muscles are particularly well developed at the lumbar and craniocervical regions, providing an extra element of stability to these regions of the vertebral column.

All transversospinal muscles extend the vertebral column. In addition, the oblique fiber direction of most of these muscles equips them with a favorable line of pull to produce contralateral (opposite side) rotation. The more horizontal (and shorter) the muscle, the greater its potential to produce horizontal plane rotation. For example, the multifidi are more effective rotators than the semispinales.

The transversospinal muscles work in conjunction with the oblique abdominal muscles during trunk rotation. Rotation to the left, for example, is driven primarily by the right external oblique and left internal oblique and reinforced by the right transversospinal muscles.

The table on p. 220 shows the various attachments, actions, and innervations.

Short Segmental Group

The short segmental group is composed of the intertransversarus and interspinales muscles (see Figure 8-54). The intertransversarus muscles attach between consecutive transverse processes. When activated unilaterally, the short segmental group assists with lateral flexion. Each interspinalis muscle attaches between consecutive spinous processes; these muscles extend the spine.

The paired, segmental nature of these muscles allows them to control movement at individual intervertebral junctions. Therefore these small muscles are most effective at furnishing fine control over the vertical stability of the vertebral column in both sagittal and frontal planes. This group also provides a rich source of sensory feedback, essential for subconscious control of postural alignment.

Functional Considerations

Segmental versus Gross Stabilization of the Vertebral Column. The muscles of the posterior trunk have an important function in vertically stabilizing the vertebral column. Each muscle group within the posterior trunk, however, provides vertical stability in a different manner.

The erector spinae muscles are the most superficial of the posterior trunk muscles, ascending vertically on either side of the vertebral column. Because of their parallel path, they are often referred to as the paraspinals. Each muscular column (within the erector spinae group) crosses many intervertebral segments and is therefore only capable of furnishing gross control over extension and lateral flexion of the vertebral column. Although lacking precise

Clinical INSIGHT

Hip and Low Back Regions Sharing the Flexibility Required for Forward Flexion

Bending the trunk forward toward the floor requires adequate flexibility in the muscles and other soft tissues in both the hip and low back regions (Figure 8-52, *A*). The woman in Figure 8-52, *B*, displays tightness of the hamstrings, which restricts flexion of the hip *(see red circle)*. Note that her functional range of motion into forward trunk flexion is only minimally limited because of the additional flexibility of the low back region. The opposite scenario is exhibited in Figure 8-52, *C*. In this common scenario the low back region is tight *(noted by red circle)*, but extra flexibility of the hip (such as the hamstrings) allows an adequate amount of forward flexion.

These two forward flexion compensations depicted in Figure 8-52, *B* and *C*, are quite common, and careful clinical observation can alert clinicians to the primary area of a particular limitation. Tightness in one region can place large demands on the other—possibly increasing the likelihood of stress-related pathology. These two scenarios also reinforce the importance of learning to visually isolate the components of a particular movement to help determine the origin of a particular limitation.

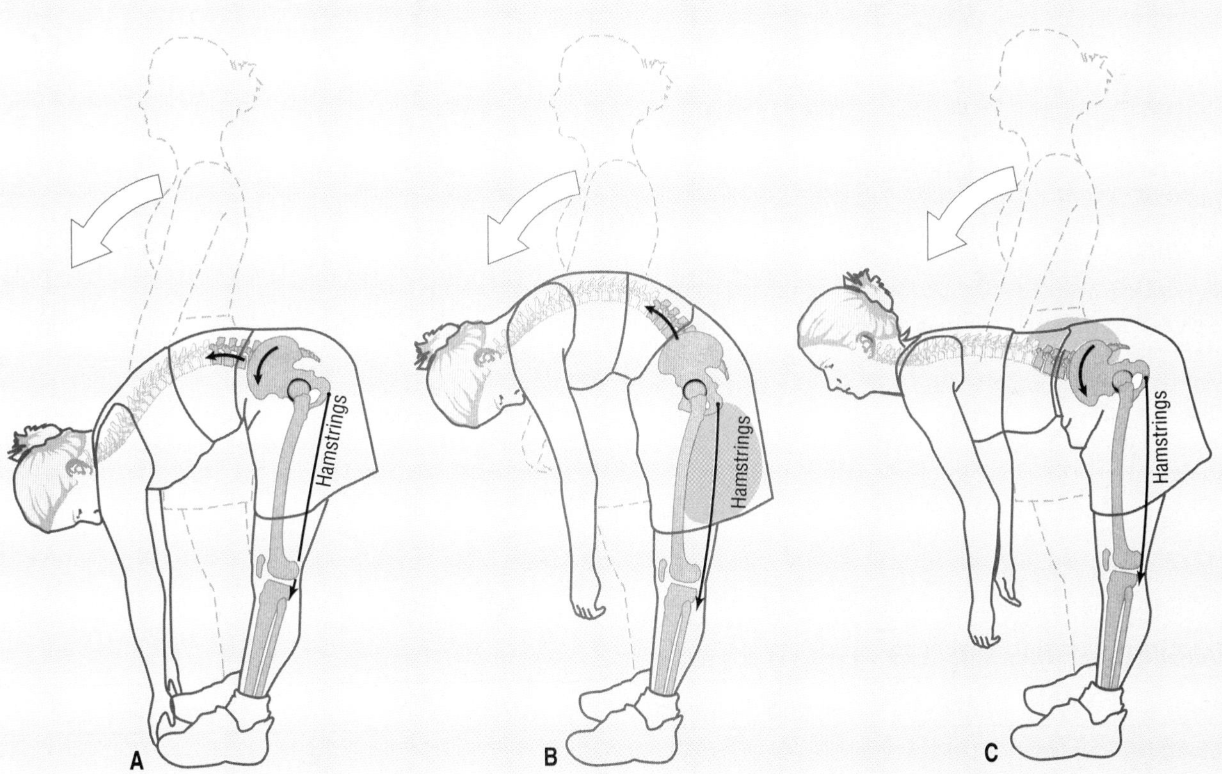

Figure 8-52 An illustration showing how the low back region and hip must both cooperate to allow full forward flexion. **A,** The hip (e.g., the hamstrings) and low back region display adequate flexibility to allow full forward flexion. **B,** Tightness of the hamstrings with excessive lumbar flexion. **C,** Tightness within the low back, but excessive flexibility of the hamstrings. The circles in B and C indicate the regions of tightness. (Modified from Neumann DA: *Kinesiology of the musculoskeletal system: foundations for physical rehabilitation,* St Louis, 2002, Mosby, Figure 9-66.)

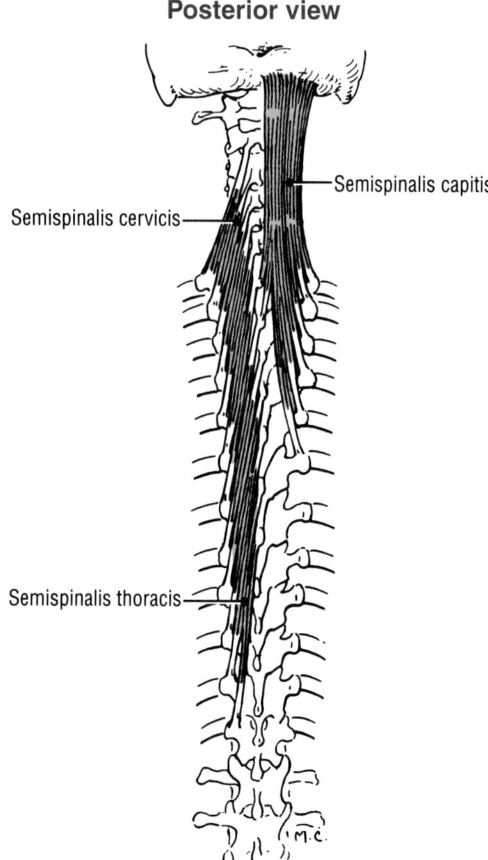

Figure 8-53 A posterior view of the semispinalis thoracis, semispinalis cervicis, and semispinalis capitis. (From Luttgens K, Hamilton N: *Kinesiology: scientific basis for human motion*, ed 9, Madison, Wis, 1997, Brown and Benchmark/ McGraw-Hill.)

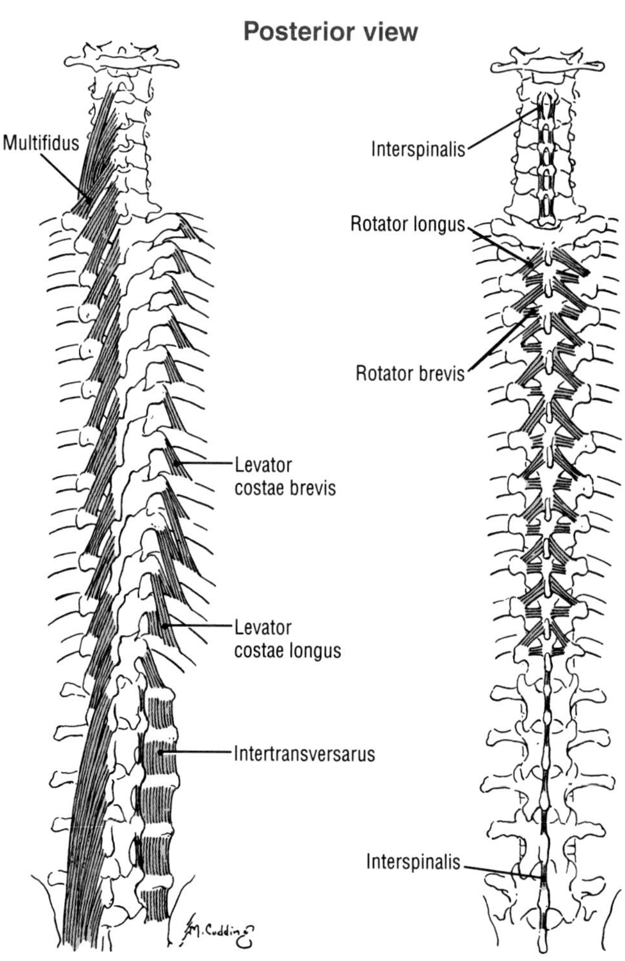

Figure 8-54 A posterior view of the transversospinal muscles (multifidi and rotators) and the muscles within the short segmental group (interspinalis and intertransversarus). (From Luttgens K, Hamilton N: *Kinesiology: scientific basis of human motion*, ed 9, Madison, Wis, 1997, Brown and Benchmark/ McGraw-Hill.)

TRANSVERSOSPINAL MUSCLES

Muscle	Inferior Attachment	Superior Attachment	Actions	Innervation
Semispinalis	Transverse processes of C4-T12	Spinous process located 6-8 vertebral segments above the inferior attachment Semispinalis capitis attaches just above the inferior nuchal line	*Bilateral:* extension *Unilateral:* rotation to the opposite side	Dorsal rami of adjacent nerves (C1-T12)
Multifidus	Transverse processes of T1-T12 Mamillary processes of L1-L5 Sacrum	Spinous processes located 2-4 vertebral segments above the inferior attachment	*Bilateral:* extension *Unilateral:* rotation to the opposite side	Dorsal rami of adjacent nerves (C4-S3)
Rotators	Transverse processes of all vertebrae	Spinous processes located 1-2 vertebral segments above the inferior attachment	*Bilateral:* extension *Unilateral:* rotation to the opposite side	Dorsal rami of adjacent nerves (C4-L4)

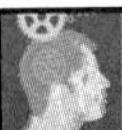

Consider this...

Getting to the Core of Spinal Stabilization

Active muscle force provides the primary form of stability to the vertebral column. Although ligaments and other connective tissues provide secondary sources of stability, only muscle can adjust the magnitude and timing of their forces. The forces produced by the abdominals and posterior trunk muscles provide much of the stability to the core of the body as a whole. Core stabilization exercises are often an integral component of back rehabilitation programs. These exercises focus on strengthening muscles that maintain the normal curvatures of the vertebral column. Such spinal alignment, often referred to as a **neutral spine**, is believed to disperse internal and external forces evenly throughout the region's supporting structures.

Core stabilization exercises are designed to challenge both intrinsic and extrinsic muscular stabilizers of the trunk. Intrinsic muscular stabilizers, attaching primarily within the vertebral column, include the transversospinal and short segmental groups of muscles. As mentioned previously, these muscles are particularly important for more precise segmental stabilization of the vertebral column. Extrinsic muscular stabilizers attach to points outside the vertebral column, including the head, sternum, ribs, or pelvis. These muscles include the abdominal muscles, erector spinae, quadratus lumborum, and psoas major. These muscles are responsible for generating large forces across a wide region of the body—from the spine, through the pelvis and lower extremities, and ultimately to the ground.

Increasing the strength and simultaneous control over both the intrinsic *and* extrinsic stabilizers is believed by many clinicians to limit the potentially destabilizing forces that may produce a back injury. A core stabilization program often involves holding a neutral or optimally positioned lumbar spine and pelvis while simultaneously performing a variety of movements or dynamic posturing. For example, after the desired posture of a patient's vertebral column (and trunk as a whole) is able to be maintained in a static position such as standing, dynamic movements such as mini-squats or lunges are performed.

intervertebral control, the erector spinae still provide an important source of extension torque for many common anti-gravity activities, ranging from maintaining upright posture to lifting objects from the floor.

The transversospinal muscles course obliquely (from nearly vertical to nearly horizontal) across relatively few intervertebral segments. This anatomic organization allows the muscles to exert a more refined, multidirectional control over the alignment of the vertebral column.

Finally, the deep segmental muscles cross only one intervertebral segment. As a set, these muscles afford the most precise control over vertical stability of the vertebral column.

Correct versus Incorrect Lifting. Lifting even moderately sized objects can generate large compression and shear forces throughout the body, most notably at the base of the spine. At some critical level, these forces may exceed the structural tolerance of the local muscles, ligaments, facet joints, and intervertebral disc within the lumbar region. Lifting is a leading risk factor associated with low-back injury in the workplace; therefore physical therapists and physical therapist assistants often educate patients on proper (and how to avoid improper) lifting techniques.

Ideally, optimal lifting technique allows the forces on the low back to be shared by muscles of the arms, legs, and trunk (Figure 8-55). Incorrect lifting, however, concentrates much of the force demands of the lift directly on the structures in the low back region. This not only taxes the muscles of the low back, but proportionally increases the compression forces on the discs and facet joints in the lumbar and lumbosacral regions. Lifting incorrectly with a flexed or rounded lumbar spine increases the stress on the muscles, joints, and intervertebral discs, thereby increasing the risk of injury. The primary factors that contribute to safe lifting are listed and explained in Table 8-7.

Summary

The vertebral column is involved with many functions that are essential to the normal kinesiology of the body. Its semirigid structure provides a stable axis for the entire trunk, head, and neck, and, indirectly, the upper extremities. In addition, the vertebral column provides the primary source of protection to the delicate spinal cord and exiting spinal nerves, from the atlas to the lower sacrum. Fractures or dislocations anywhere along the vertebral column can result in spinal cord injury and subsequent quadriplegia or paraplegia.

The joints and vertebrae of the cranial end of the vertebral column are highly specialized. The atlanto-occipital, atlanto-axial, and intracervical joints interact to provide extensive three-dimensional placement of the head and neck, essential for optimal spatial orientation of the special senses. In fact, range of motion of the craniocervical region exceeds that of any other region of the vertebral column. The highly specialized muscles that control the fine movements in the craniocervical region often become painful and inflamed when stressed due to poor posture, cervical arthritis, or compressed exiting spinal nerves.

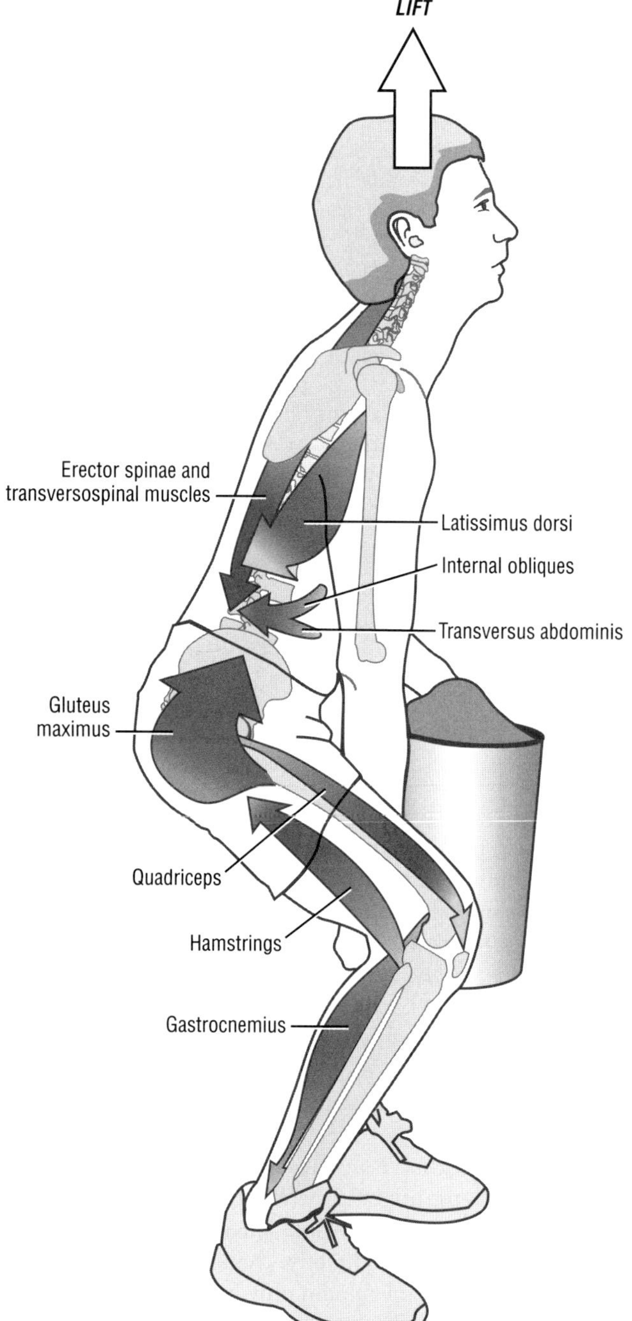

Figure 8-55 The typical activation pattern of selected muscles is shown as a healthy person lifts a load. (From Neumann DA: *Kinesiology of the musculoskeletal system: foundations for physical rehabilitation*, St Louis, 2002, Mosby, Figure 10-37.)

The thoracolumbar region has three major requirements. First, the thoracic region must protect the many important organs such as the heart and lungs. Second, the joints and muscles in the region must be sufficiently mobile and coordinated to function as a mechanical chamber for breathing, which includes coughing and forced exhalation. And third, the abdominal muscles, posterior trunk muscles, iliopsoas, and quadratus must provide core stability to the trunk and body as a whole. Controlling such core stability establishes a firm base of support for the extremities, as well as mechanical support for the vulnerable and naturally high-stressed lumbar and lumbosacral regions.

The most inferior (or caudal) end of the vertebral column is specialized for two important and interrelated functions. First, the lumbosacral junction and SI joints must transfer, at times, large forces from body weight and activated muscle through the pelvis and to the lower extremities. These large forces may exceed the physical tolerance of the region, causing impairments such as anterior spondylolisthesis or partial dislocation of the SI joints. Second, the more caudal end of the vertebral column must interact mechanically with the hip joints (pelvis or femurs) to maximize the movement of the trunk. The ability to reach and touch the floor while standing, for instance, requires ample forward bend in the lumbar region, as well as the pelvis relative to the femurs. A limitation in either region can increase the range of motion demands on the other, possibly leading to arthritis of the hip or disc herniation and inflamed facet joints in the lumbar spine.

Pain with limited mobility anywhere within the vertebral column can originate from many sources such as tight or weakened muscles; torn ligaments; herniated discs; bone spurs compressing nerve roots; inflamed joints; or, most likely, a combination of these pathologies. Regardless of the actual cause of the impairment, physical therapy is often the first line of conservative treatment for pain and dysfunction of the vertebral column. Understanding not only the medical diagnosis but also the rationale behind the many treatment approaches requires a sound understanding of the anatomy and kinesiology.

TABLE 8-7 FACTORS CONSIDERED TO CONTRIBUTE TO SAFE LIFTING TECHNIQUES

Consideration	Rationale	Comment
Maintain the external load as close to the body as possible.	Minimizes the external moment arm of the load, thereby reduces torque and force demands on back muscle.	Holding the load between the knees while lifting is ideal but not always possible.
Lift with the lumbar spine held as close to a neutral lordotic posture as possible. Avoid the extremes of flexion and extension. Exact position of the spine can vary based on comfort and practicality.	Concentrating on holding the lumbar spine in a neutral lordotic position may help prevent the spine from extremes of flexion and extension. Vigorous contraction of the back extensor muscles, with the lumbar spine maximally flexed, may produce damaging forces on the intervertebral discs. In contrast, vigorous contraction of the back extensor muscles with the lumbar spine maximally extended may damage the apophyseal joints.	Lifting with minimal-to-moderate flexion or extension in the lumbar spine may be acceptable for some persons, depending on the health and experience of the lifter and the situation. Minimal-to-moderate flexion or extension both have a biomechanical advantage: *Minimal-to-moderate flexion* increases the passive tension generated by the posterior ligamentous system, possibly reducing the force demands on extensor muscles. *Minimal-to-moderate extension* places the apophyseal joints nearer to their close-packed position, thereby providing greater stability to the region.
When lifting, fully utilize the hip and knee extensor muscles to minimize the force demands on the low-back muscles.	Very large forces produced by low-back extensor muscles can injure the muscles themselves, intervertebral discs, vertebral endplates, or apophyseal joints.	Persons with hip or knee arthritis may be unable to effectively use the muscles in the legs to assist the back muscles. The squat lift may encourage the use of the leg muscles but also increases the overall work demands on the body.
Minimize the vertical and horizontal distance that a load must be lifted.	Minimizing the distance that the load is moved reduces the total work of the lift, thereby reducing fatigue; minimizing the distance that the load is moved reduces the extremes of movement in the low back and lower extremities.	Using handles or an adjustable-height platform may be helpful.
Avoid twisting when lifting.	Torsional forces applied to vertebrae can predispose the person to intervertebral disc injury.	Properly designed work environment can reduce the need for twisting while lifting.
Lift as slowly and smoothly as conditions allow.	A slow and smooth lift reduces the large peak force generated in muscles and connective tissues.	
Lift with a moderately wide and slightly staggered base of support provided by the legs.	A relatively wide base of support affords greater overall stability of the body, thereby reducing the chance of a fall or slip.	
When possible, use the assistance of a mechanical device or additional people while lifting.	Using assistance while lifting can reduce the demand on the back of the primary lifter.	Using a mechanical hoist (Hoyer lift) or a "two-man" transfer may be prudent in many settings.

From Neumann DA: *Kinesiology of the musculoskeletal system: foundations for physical rehabilitation*, St Louis, 2002, Mosby, Table 10-15.

Study Questions

1. Which of the following statements is (are) true regarding the normal curvatures of the vertebral column?
   a. The cervical and lumbar regions are both normally lordotic
   b. The thoracic and lumbar regions are both normally kyphotic.
   c. The cervical and sacral areas are both normally kyphotic.
   d. The lumbar region is the only region of the spine that is normally lordotic.
2. The central fluid-filled portion of the intervertebral disc is called the:
   a. Vertebral end plate
   b. Nucleus pulposus
   c. Annulus fibrosis
   d. Pedicle
3. Which of the following vertebrae possess transverse foramina?
   a. Cervical
   b. Thoracic
   c. Lumbar
4. Which of the following terms is used to describe the second cervical vertebra?
   a. Cauda equina
   b. Pedicle
   c. Atlas
   d. Axis
5. The lumbar region allows the most motion in the:
   a. Frontal plane
   b. Sagittal plane
   c. Horizontal plane
6. The craniocervical region allows the most motion in the:
   a. Frontal plane
   b. Sagittal plane
   c. Horizontal plane
7. Which motion of the lumbar spine results in a posterior migration of the nucleus pulposus of an intervertebral disc?
   a. Lateral flexion
   b. Rotation
   c. Flexion
   d. Extension
8. An anterior pelvic tilt is naturally accompanied by:
   a. Increased lordosis of the lumbar spine
   b. Decreased lordosis of the lumbar spine
   c. Strong activation of the abdominals
   d. Near maximal elongation of the hip flexors
9. Which of the following motions decreases the diameter of the intervertebral foramen?
   a. Flexion
   b. Extension
10. Which of the following statements best describes an anterior spondylolisthesis?
    a. Reduced flexion of the cervical vertebrae
    b. Elongation of the ligamentum flavum
    c. Anterior slippage, or translation, of one vertebra relative to another
    d. Simultaneous elongation of the anterior longitudinal ligament and the rectus abdominis muscle.
11. Forward flexion of the lumbar spine involves:
    a. Elongation of the anterior longitudinal ligament
    b. Increased diameter of the intervertebral foramen
    c. Posterior migration of the nucleus pulposus
    d. B and C
    e. All of the above
12. Torticollis is typically caused by:
    a. Tightness of the lumbar erector spinae muscles
    b. Tightness of the sternocleidomastoid
    c. Excessive lateral flexion of the thoracic and lumbar spine
    d. Weakness of the quadratus lumborum
13. Which of the following statements is true regarding the external oblique muscle?
    a. Activation of the right external oblique produces rotation to the left.
    b. Activation of the right external oblique produces rotation to the right.
    c. Bilateral activation of the external obliques can produce a posterior pelvic tilt.
    d. A and C
    e. B and C
14. Which of the following muscles or muscle groups is involved with producing an anterior pelvic tilt?
    a. Erector spinae
    b. Hip flexors
    c. Rectus abdominis
    d. A and B
    e. B and C
15. Which of the following statements is (are) true regarding scoliosis?
    a. *Scoliosis* refers primarily to a frontal plane deviation in the thoracolumbar regions of the vertebral column.
    b. Scoliosis is named by the concave side of the spinal curve.
    c. Scoliosis is named by the convex side of the spinal curve.
    d. A and B
    e. A and C
16. Which muscle is part of the transversospinal muscle group?
    a. Multifidus
    b. Internal oblique
    c. Iliocostalis
    d. Transverse abdominis
17. Lateral flexion of the cervical spine occurs in the:
    a. Frontal plane
    b. Sagittal plane
    c. Horizontal plane
18. Performing a full sit-up requires strong activation of the:
    a. Quadratus lumborum and erector spinae

b. Iliocostalis and transversospinal muscles
c. Iliopsoas and rectus abdominis
d. Scalenes and suboccipital muscles

19. The right quadratus lumborum is able to:
    a. Rotate the lumbar spine to the left
    b. "Hike" the left side of the pelvis
    c. "Hike" the right side of the pelvis
    d. Laterally flex the trunk to the left
20. Thoracic outlet syndrome is often the result of tightness or excessive hypertrophy of the:
    a. Iliopsoas muscle
    b. Anterior and middle scalenes
    c. External obliques
    d. Foramen magnum
21. Which of the following muscles is referred to as the corset muscle owing to its primary function of increasing intra-abdominal pressure?
    a. Quadratus lumborum
    b. Erector spinae
    c. Transversus abdominis
    d. Splenius capitis and splenius cervicis
22. A posterior pelvic tilt involves activation of the abdominal muscles.
    a. True
    b. False
23. The dens is a bony projection found on the first cervical vertebrae.
    a. True
    b. False
24. The amount of lateral flexion that occurs in the thoracic region is largely limited by the articulation of the ribs with the thoracic vertebrae.
    a. True
    b. False
25. The cervical vertebrae have the widest, thickest bodies of all the vertebrae.
    a. True
    b. False
26. An individual with an anterior spondylolisthesis in the lumbar region would likely perform hyper-extension exercises as part of a therapeutic regimen.
    a. True
    b. False
27. About one half of the rotation available to the head and neck occurs from motion at the atlanto-axial joint.
    a. True
    b. False
28. The facet (apophyseal) joint surfaces of most lumbar vertebrae are oriented largely in the frontal plane.
    a. True
    b. False
29. A posterior pelvic tilt typically results in a decreased diameter of the lumbar intervertebral foramina.
    a. True
    b. False
30. The spinal nerves exit the vertebral column through the transverse foramina.
    a. True
    b. False
31. The craniocervical region typically allows 90 degrees of axial rotation to each side.
    a. True
    b. False

ADDITIONAL READINGS

Adams MA, Hutton WC: Prolapsed intervertebral disc: a hyperflexion injury. 1981 Volvo Award in Basic Science, *Spine* 7(3):184-191, 1982.

Albert TJ, Eichenbaum MD: Goals of cervical disc replacement, *Spine J* 4(6 Suppl):292S-293S, 2004.

Bogduk N: *Clinical anatomy of the lumbar spine*, ed 3, New York, 1997, Churchill Livingstone.

Bogduk N, Macintosh JE: The applied anatomy of the thoracolumbar fascia, *Spine* 9(2):164-170, 1984.

Bogduk N, Mercer S: Biomechanics of the cervical spine. I: Normal kinematics, *Clin Biomech* 15(9):633-648, 2000.

Calliet R: *Neck and arm pain*, Philadelphia, 1974, FA Davis.

Cholewicki J, Ivancic PC, Radebold A: Can increased intra-abdominal pressure in humans be decoupled from trunk muscle co-contraction during steady state isometric exertions? *Eur J Appl Physiol* 87(2):127-133, 2002.

De Troyer A, Estenne M, Ninane V et al: Transversus abdominis muscle function in humans, *J Appl Physiol* 68(3):1010-1016, 1990.

Ferreira PH, Ferreira ML, Maher CG et al: Specific stabilisation exercise for spinal and pelvic pain: a systematic review, *Aust J Physiother* 52(2):79-88, 2006.

Halpern AA, Bleck EE: Sit-up exercises: an electromyographic study, *Clin Orthop* November/December(145):172-178, 1979.

Harrison DE, Harrison DD, Troyanovich SJ: The sacroiliac joint: a review of anatomy and biomechanics with clinical implications, *J Manipulative Physiol Ther* 20(9):607-617, 1997.

Holmes A, Han ZH, Dang GT et al: Changes in cervical canal spinal volume during in vitro flexion-extension, *Spine* 21(11):1313-1319, 1996.

Ishii T, Mukai Y, Hosono N et al: Kinematics of the cervical spine in lateral bending: in vivo three-dimensional analysis, *Spine* 31(2):155-160, 2006.

Magnusson ML, Aleksiev AR, Spratt KF et al: Hyperextension and spine height changes, *Spine* 21(22):2670-2675, 1996.

McGill SM: Biomechanics of the thoracolumbar spine. In Dvir Z, editor: *Clinical biomechanics*, Philadelphia, 2000, Churchill Livingstone.

McKenzie RA: *The lumbar spine: mechanical diagnosis and therapy*, Waikanae, New Zealand, 1981, Spinal Publications.

Nachemson A: Lumbar intradiscal pressure. Experimental studies on post-mortem material, *Acta Orthop Scand Suppl* 43:1-104, 1960.

Neumann DA: Arthrokinesiologic considerations for the aged adult. In Guccione AA, editor: *Geriatric physical therapy*, Chicago, 2000, Mosby.

Salo PK, Ylinen JJ, Malkia EA et al: Isometric strength of the cervical flexor, extensor, and rotator muscles in 220 healthy females aged 20 to 59 years, *J Orthop Sports Phys Ther* 36(7):495-502, 2006.

Wilke HJ, Neef P, Caimi M et al: New in vivo measurements of pressures in the intervertebral disc in daily life, *Spine* 24(8):755-762, 1999.

Zhao F, Pollintine P, Hole BD et al: Discogenic origins of spinal instability, *Spine* 30(23):2621-2630, 2005.

CHAPTER 9

Structure and Function of the Hip

CHAPTER OUTLINE

OBJECTIVES

- Identify the bones and bony features of the hip and pelvis.
- Describe the supporting structures of the hip joint.
- Cite the normal ranges of motion for hip flexion and extension, abduction and adduction, and internal and external rotation.
- Describe the three kinematic strategies used to produce different functional motions at the hip.
- Describe the planes of motion and axes of rotation for all motions of the hip.
- Justify the actions of the hip muscles through knowledge of the muscle's proximal and distal attachments.
- Describe the force-couple involved in producing an anterior pelvic tilt and a posterior pelvic tilt.
- Explain the biomechanical consequences of a hip flexion contracture.
- Explain how the position of the hip and knee affect the length and ultimate function of the multi-articular muscles of the hip.
- Explain the function of the hip abductor muscles during the single-limb support phase of walking.
- Describe why a cane is most effective when used in the hand opposite the weakened or painful hip.

KEY TERMS

angle of inclination
anterior pelvic tilt
contracture
coxa valga
coxa vara
force-couple
hip drop
hip hiking
joint reaction force
normal anteversion
posterior pelvic tilt
Trendelenburg sign

The hip joint is the articulation between the large rounded head of the femur and the acetabulum, or socket, of the pelvis. Being the base of the lower extremity, the hip must provide a wide range of movement in all three planes. Generally speaking, hip movement can occur (1) by rotating the femur relative to a stationary or otherwise fixed pelvis, as when lifting the leg up a step or (2) by rotating the pelvis (and often trunk) relative to a fixed or stationary femur. The second situation occurs during many common activities such as walking, running, and transitioning

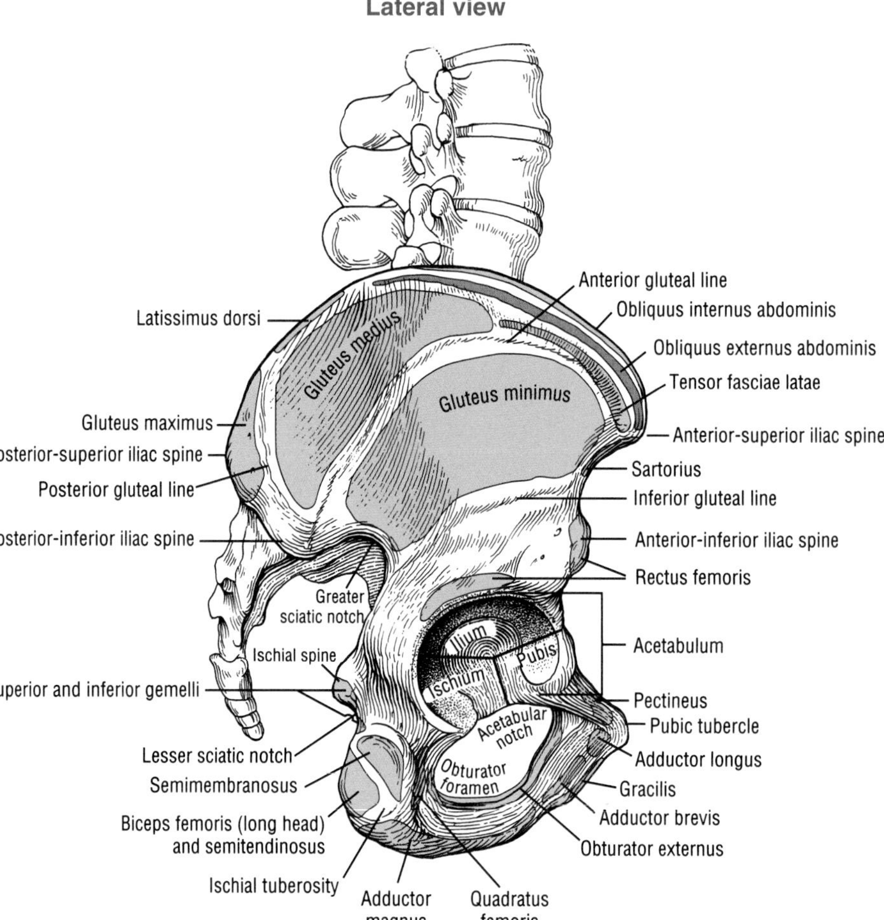

Figure 9-1 A lateral view of the right innominate bone. Proximal attachments of muscles are shown in red, distal attachments in gray. (From Neumann DA: *Kinesiology of the musculoskeletal system: foundations for physical rehabilitation*, St Louis, 2002, Mosby, Figure 12-1.)

from sitting to standing or picking up objects off the ground. Consider, for example, a golfer flexing forward on one leg to pick up a tee. One foot is securely planted on the ground, while the free leg and entire pelvis and trunk rotate around the femoral head. In this example, the primary pivot point for the rotation of the entire body is the hip joint of the supporting leg.

The hip has many anatomic features that provide stability during standing, bending, walking, and running. The femoral head is stabilized by a deep socket that is surrounded by an extensive set of capsular ligaments. Numerous muscles provide additional stability, while others supply the large forces required for a wide variety of functional activities. Weakness of these muscles, therefore, can have a profound impact on the functional mobility of the body as a whole.

This chapter discusses the structure, kinematics, and muscles of the hip joint with an emphasis on establishing a foundation for providing optimal treatment of hip dysfunction.

Osteology

The pelvis is also called the *innominate bone* (meaning "nameless" in Latin; Figure 9-1). Each right and left innominate bone is formed by the union of three bones: the *ilium*, *ischium*, and *pubis*. The wedge-shaped sacrum completes the posterior side of the pelvis. The junction of the two innominate bones with the sacrum forms the *sacroiliac joints* (Figures 9-2 and 9-3).

Ilium

The ilium is the wing-shaped superior portion of the innominate (see Figures 9-1, 9-2, and 9-3). The *iliac crest* is a long, palpable ridge of bone that marks the superior border of the ilium; clinicians often compare the heights of the right and left iliac crests to determine pelvic symmetry. The anterior tip of the iliac crest comes to a sharp point called the *anterior-superior iliac spine* (ASIS). Just inferior to the ASIS is the *anterior-inferior iliac spine* (AIIS), the proximal attachment for the rectus femoris muscle. The posterior tip of the iliac crest, called the *posterior-superior iliac spine* (PSIS), is more rounded than the ASIS but also readily palpable. Often, a small dimple located just superficial to each PSIS helps identify the general location of the nearby sacroiliac joints. The *posterior-inferior iliac spine* (PIIS) is the small bony prominence located inferior to the PSIS, marking the superior tip of the greater sciatic notch. The *greater sciatic notch*

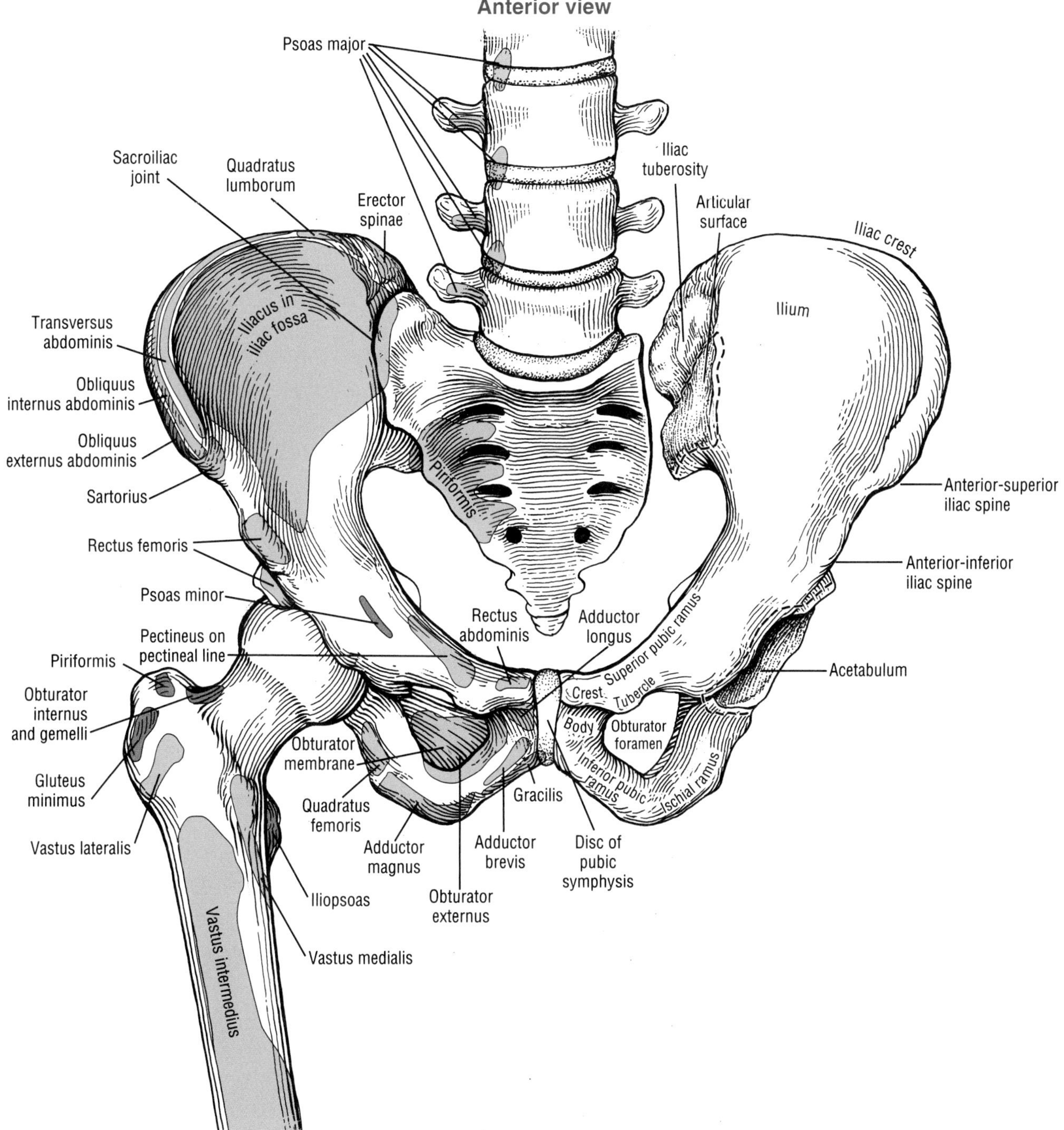

Figure 9-2 An anterior view of the pelvis, sacrum, and right proximal femur. Proximal attachments of muscles are shown in red, distal attachments in gray. A section of the left side of the sacrum is removed to expose the articular surface of the sacroiliac joint. (From Neumann DA: *Kinesiology of the musculoskeletal system: foundations for physical rehabilitation*, St Louis, 2002, Mosby, Figure 12-2.)

is a semicircular space between the PIIS and the ischial spine that provides space for the large sciatic nerve to exit the pelvis. The *sacrospinous* and *sacrotuberous ligaments* convert the greater sciatic notch to the greater *sciatic foramen*.

The *iliac fossa* is the smooth, concave, anterior surface of the ilium, which provides the proximal attachment of the *iliacus* muscle. The *articular surface* of each ilium articulates with the sacrum forming the *sacroiliac* joints.

Ischium

The ischium is located on the posterior-inferior aspect of the innominate (see Figures 9-1, 9-2, and 9-3). The *ischial*

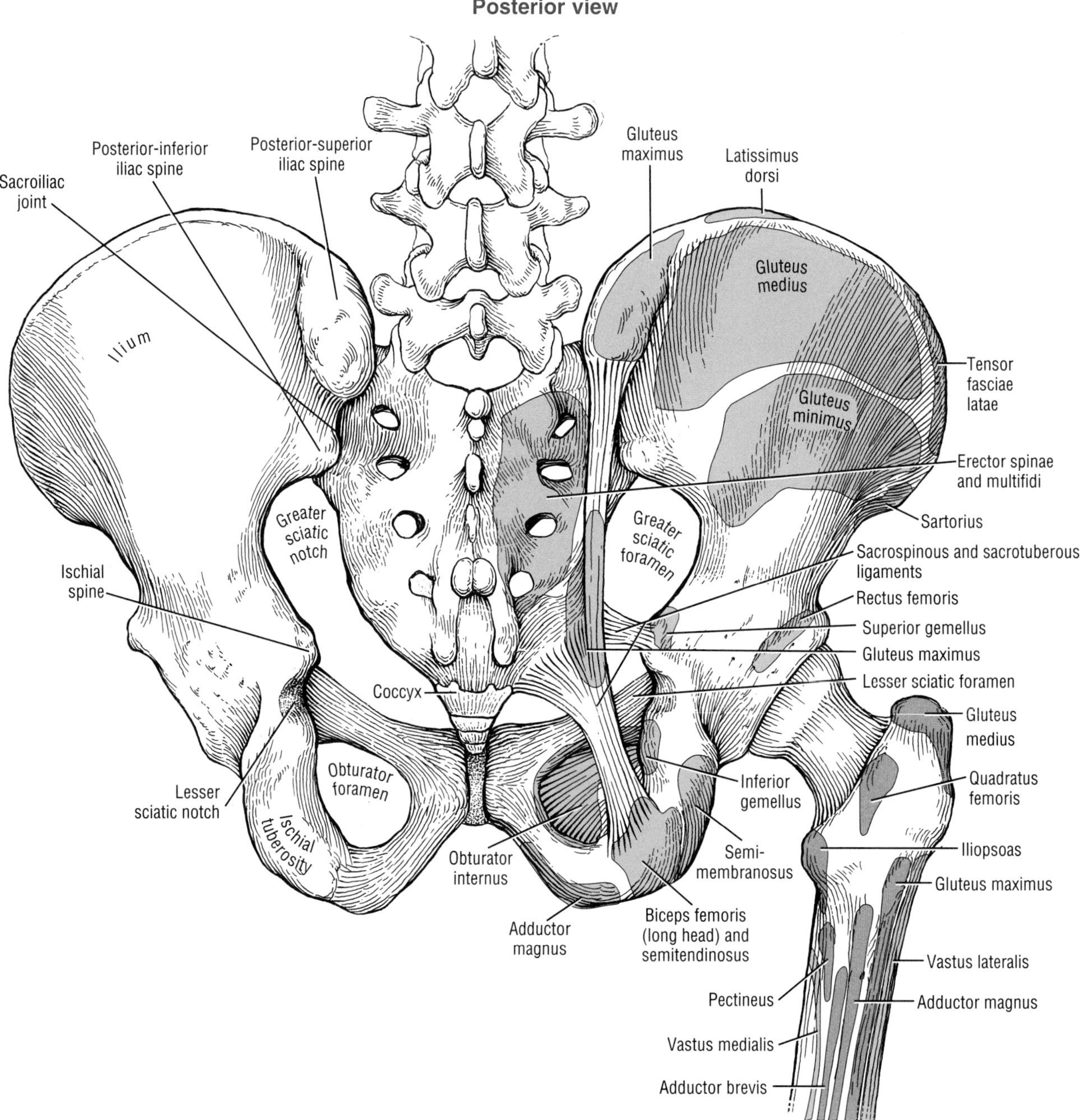

Figure 9-3 A posterior view of the pelvis, sacrum, and right proximal femur. Proximal attachments of muscles are shown in red, distal attachments in gray. (From Neumann DA: *Kinesiology of the musculoskeletal system: foundations for physical rehabilitation*, St Louis, 2002, Mosby, Figure 12-3.)

spine is a posterior projection of bone that marks the inferior aspect of the greater sciatic notch. The *ischial tuberosity* is a bumpy projection from the posterior-inferior aspect of the ischium that serves as the proximal attachment for three of the four hamstring muscles. In a seated position, people literally sit on their ischial tuberosities. These prominent structures are often the site of pressure sores, which may occur in persons who lack normal sensation and the ability to frequently alter their seated position. The *ischial ramus* extends anteriorly from the ischial tuberosity to join with the inferior pubic ramus.

Pubis

The pubis is composed primarily of two arms, or rami: (1) the *superior pubic ramus* and (2) the *inferior pubic ramus*, which coalesce anteriorly to form the *pubic crest*. The junction between the pubic crests of each innominate is called the pubic symphysis. This relatively immobile joint completes the anterior "ring" of the pelvis (see Figures 9-2 and 9-3).

The large circular opening formed by the pubic rami and the ischium forms the *obturator foramen*. This foramen is covered by the *obturator membrane*, which serves as the proximal attachment for the *obturator internus* and *obturator externus* muscles.

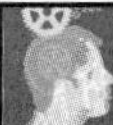

Consider this...

Implications of Pregnancy on Joint Laxity

During pregnancy, a woman's body receives an influx of a hormone called relaxin, which increases the flexibility of the pelvic ligaments in preparation for childbirth. Because of this, the bones of the pelvis are more likely to shift, possibly resulting in malalignment of the pelvic bones, particularly the sacroiliac joints and the pubic symphysis. Physical therapists often recommend strengthening exercises, which target the muscles that assist in stabilizing and supporting the pelvis.

Acetabulum

The *acetabulum* is the deep, cup-shaped structure that encloses the head of the femur at the hip joint (Figure 9-4). Interestingly, the acetabulum is formed by a combination of all three bones of the pelvis: the ilium, pubis, and ischium.

The *lunate surface* is the horseshoe-shaped articular superior surface of the acetabulum. Heavily lined with articular cartilage, it is the only part of the acetabulum that normally contacts the femoral head. The *acetabular fossa* is a depression deep within the floor of the acetabulum; normally the fossa does not contact the femoral head and is therefore not lined with articular cartilage.

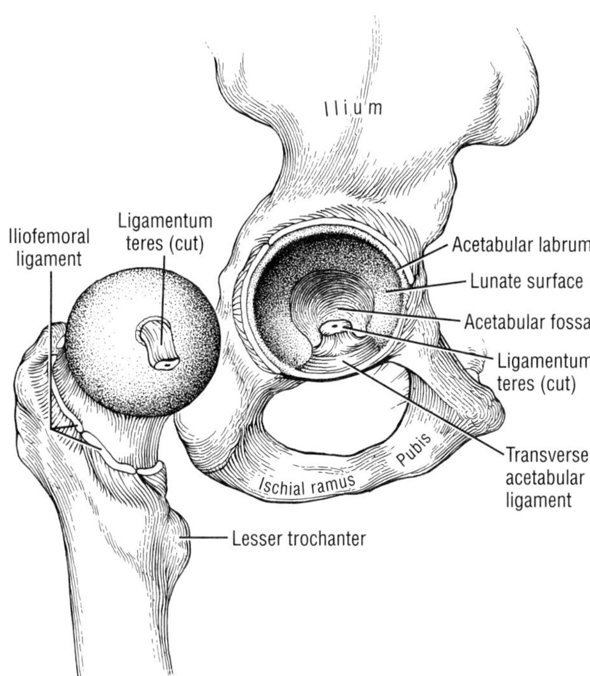

Figure 9-4 The right hip is opened to expose the internal components of the acetabulum. (Modified from Neumann DA: *Kinesiology of the musculoskeletal system: foundations for physical rehabilitation*, St Louis, 2002, Mosby, Figure 12-13.)

Femur

The femur is the longest bone in the body, which helps contribute to the extensive stride length of human gait (Figures 9-5 and 9-6). The proximal portion of each

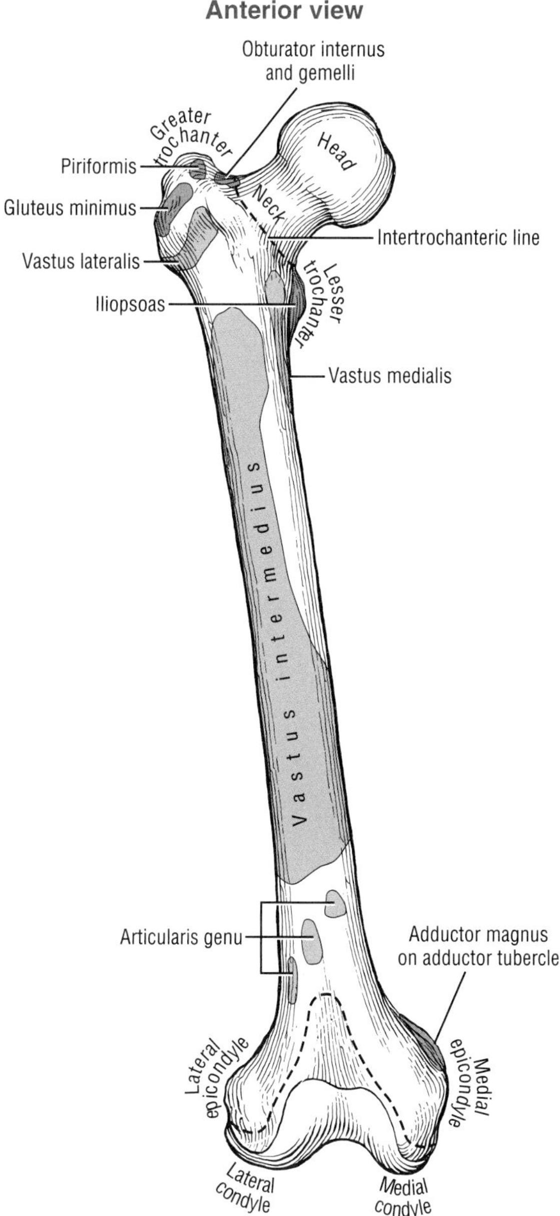

Figure 9-5 An anterior view of the right femur. Proximal attachments of muscles are shown in red, distal attachments in gray. Capsular attachments are shown as a dashed line. (From Neumann DA: *Kinesiology of the musculoskeletal system: foundations for physical rehabilitation*, St Louis, 2002, Mosby, Figure 12-4.)

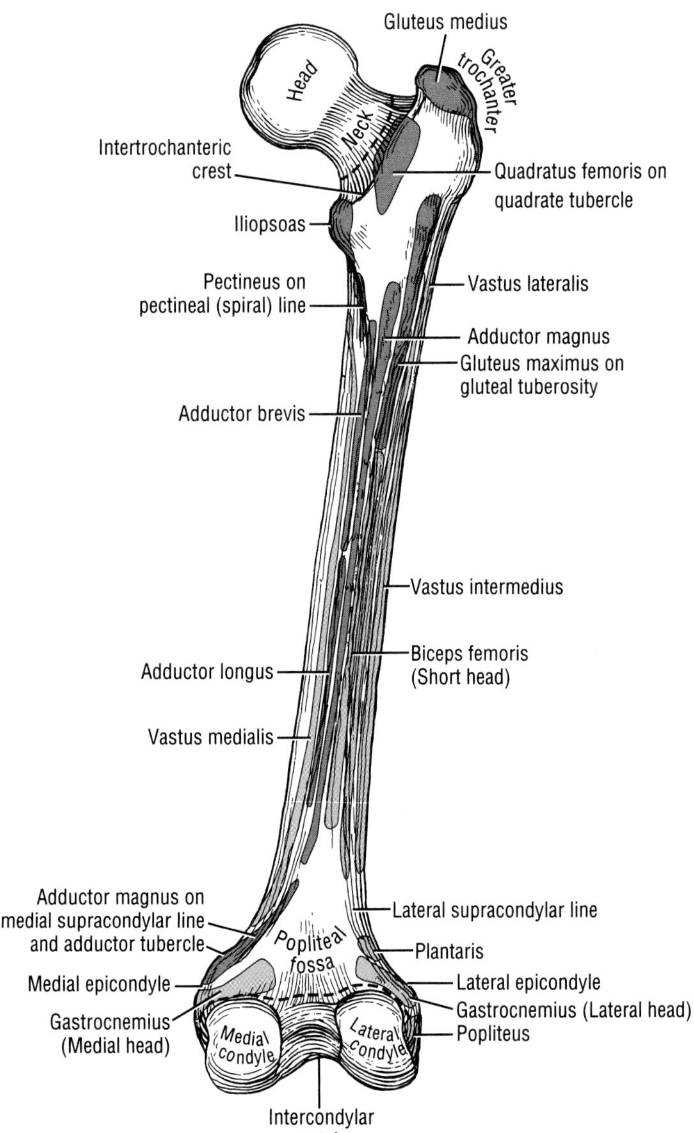

Figure 9-6 A posterior view of the right femur. Proximal attachments of muscles are shown in red, distal attachments in gray. Capsular attachments are shown as a dashed line. (From Neumann DA: *Kinesiology of the musculoskeletal system: foundations for physical rehabilitation*, St Louis, 2002, Mosby, Figure 12-6.)

femur is composed of a head, neck, and shaft. The *head* of the femur contains a small cup-like depression called the fovea, which accepts the ligamentum teres. The *neck* connects the head to the shaft of the femur, which is bordered superior-laterally by the greater trochanter.

The *greater trochanter* is the large, palpable projection of bone that extends laterally from near the junction of the femoral neck and shaft. It serves as an important distal attachment for numerous muscles of the hip. The *lesser trochanter* is a sharp posterior-medial projection of bone, which is the distal attachment for the iliopsoas muscle. The *intertrochanteric crest* is a ridge of bone that connects the posterior aspects of the greater and lesser trochanters. The *intertrochanteric line* courses anteriorly between the greater and lesser trochanters. This line marks the distal attachment for the anterior capsule of the hip. The trochanteric fossa is a small pit on the posterior-medial side of the greater trochanter. Many of the short external rotators of the hip attach near or on the trochanteric fossa.

More distally is the *linea aspera* (from Latin, meaning "rough line"), a line of slightly raised bone that courses along much of the posterior side of the femur. This bony ridge is the distal attachment for many of the adductor muscles and the proximal attachment for two of the quadriceps muscles. The *pectineal line*, which serves as the distal attachment for the *pectineus* muscle, is a small crest of bone that runs from the lesser trochanter to the superior aspect of the linea aspera. The *gluteal tuberosity* arises from the superior-lateral portion of the linea aspera and serves as a distal attachment for the *gluteus maximus*. The *adductor tubercle* is a palpable, raised portion of bone, located just proximally to the medial side of the knee, which

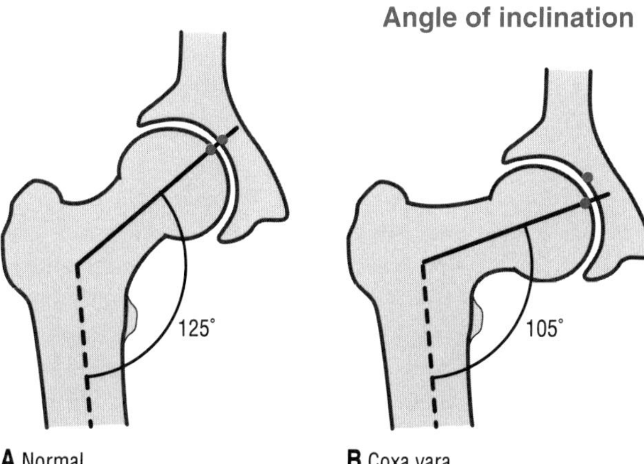

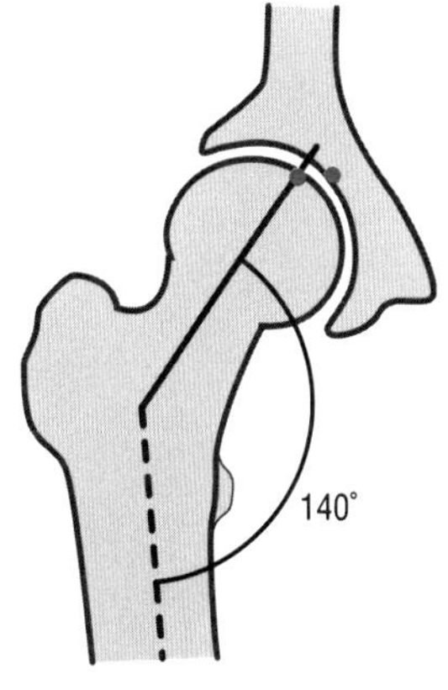

Figure 9-7 The proximal femur is shown: normal angle of inclination **(A)**, coxa vara **(B)**, and coxa valga **(C)**. The pair of red dots in each figure indicates the different alignments of the hip joint surfaces. Optimal alignment is shown in **A.** (From Neumann DA: *Kinesiology of the musculoskeletal system: foundations for physical rehabilitation*, St Louis, 2002, Mosby, Figure 12-8.)

marks the distal attachment of the *adductor magnus* muscle. The medial and lateral condyles and epicondyles, intercondylar notch, and intercondylar groove of the femur are important features more relevant to the *knee* and are therefore discussed in the next chapter.

Clinical INSIGHT

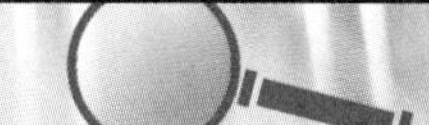

Relationship between Pressure Sores and Bony Anatomy

Pressure sores often occur when the skin and superficial tissues of the body are compressed over an extended period of time and are subsequently deprived of adequate blood flow. Bony areas around the hip such as the greater trochanter, sacrum, and ischial tuberosities are particularly at risk for developing pressure sores. These areas have a relatively small amount of soft tissue surrounding the underlying bone, so any prolonged pressure constricts the flow of blood and nutrients. Also, these bony areas are subject to high localized pressure while sitting or lying in bed. Pressure sores are often referred to as bed sores or "decubitus" ulcers (from Latin, meaning "lying down").

Individuals who have had a spinal cord injury are especially at a higher risk of developing a pressure sore because they often lack normal sensation and are unable to perceive the pain signals that normally accompany high pressure over a region of the body. Physical therapists and physical therapist assistants often play a large role in prevention of pressure sores by the following:

- Obtaining a proper pressure-relieving cushion: These are generally placed in wheelchairs and decrease the direct pressure over high-risk bony prominences.
- Educating patients on the following:
  - The importance of proper positioning (e.g., avoid lying on bony tuberosities for extended periods of time)
  - Performing pressure-relieving maneuvers such as "boosts" at regular intervals
  - Maintaining good hygiene, in particular keeping these at-risk areas clean and dry

ANGLE OF INCLINATION

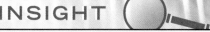

The **angle of inclination** refers to the frontal plane angle created between the femoral neck and the shaft of the femur (Figure 9-7, *A*). This angle, normally measuring about 125 degrees, directs the shaft of the femur toward the midline, thereby positioning the knee joint directly under the weight of the body. An angle of inclination of about 125 degrees is typically associated with the most optimal alignment of the hip joint, indicated in Figure 9-7, *A*, by the alignment of the red dots.

Deviations in the angle of inclination of the hip can occur from abnormal development in early childhood or from trauma. **Coxa valga** describes an angle of inclination that is significantly greater than 125 degrees (Figure 9-7, *C*). **Coxa vara**, in contrast, describes an angle of inclination that is significantly less than 125 degrees (Figure 9-7, *B*); note the offset alignment of the red dots in Figure 9-7, *B* and *C*. In severe cases of either abnormal deformity, the hip joint can become increasingly unstable or be subjected to high stress. In these cases a surgical correction may become necessary to realign the proximal femur or acetabulum. Without the correction, the abnormally high stress on the joint may cause degeneration of the joint, pain, and abnormal gait.

TORSION ANGLE

Although difficult to visualize, the femur is naturally twisted along its long axis. This twist is described as a *torsion* between the shaft and neck of the femur. The angle of the torsion can be appreciated by placing a femur flat on a tabletop. Relative to the femoral condyles (which are parallel with the tabletop), the femoral neck normally projects upward about 15 degrees. This 15-degree torsion angle is often referred to as **normal anteversion**, shown from above in Figure 9-8, *A*. Similar to the normal angle of inclination, normal anteversion is typically associated with the most optimal alignment between the femoral head and acetabulum, indicated by the close alignment of the red dots in Figure 9-8, *A*. Figure 9-8, *B*, shows a hip with *excessive anteversion*. When extreme, excessive anteversion may lead to anterior instability of the hip, especially when the hip is maximally externally rotated.

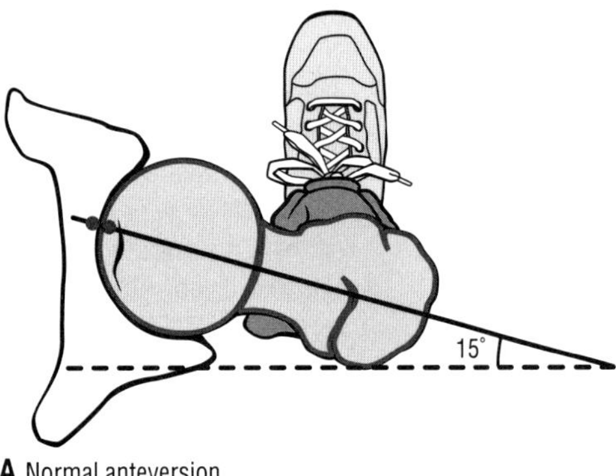

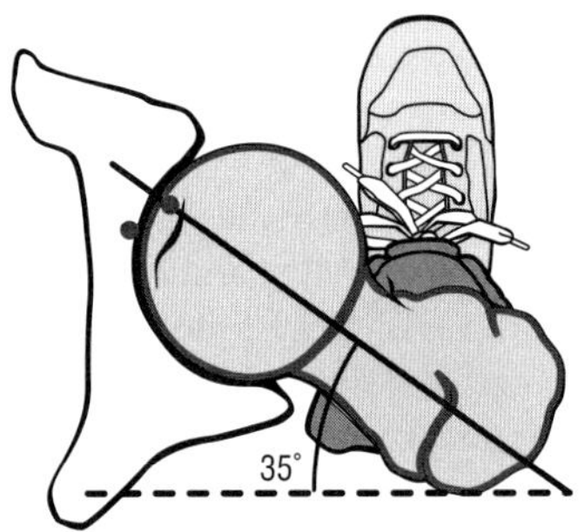

Figure 9-8 A superior view showing the angle of torsion of the right hip. **A,** The 15-degree anterior projection of the femoral head is considered normal anteversion of the hip. **B,** Excessive anteversion of the right hip. (From Neumann DA: *Kinesiology of the musculoskeletal system: foundations for physical rehabilitation*, St Louis, 2002, Mosby, Figure 12-9.)

Arthrology

General Features

The hip is anatomically designed to withstand the large and potentially dislocating forces that can routinely occur during walking and other more rigorous activities. An extensive ligamentous network maintains the femoral head securely within the deep acetabulum (described ahead). A thick layer of articular cartilage, muscle, and cancellous (spongy) bone in the proximal femur helps dampen the large forces that routinely cross the hip. Failure of any of these protective mechanisms, due to disease, injury, or even advanced age, may lead to deterioration and weakening of the joint structure.

Supporting Structures Located within the Hip Joint

Figure 9-4 illustrates the following supporting structures:

- *Transverse Acetabular Ligament:* Spans the acetabular notch, completing the "cup" of the acetabulum.
- *Ligamentum Teres:* A tubular sheath of connective tissue that runs from the transverse acetabular ligament to the fovea of the femoral head. A branch of the obturator artery travels through the ligamentum teres, providing the femoral head with a limited amount of its blood supply.
- *Acetabular Labrum:* A sharp ring or lip of fibrocartilage that surrounds the outer rim of the acetabulum. The labrum provides increased stability to the hip by deepening the socket and firmly gripping the femoral head. The labrum also helps "seal" the joint, thereby forming a partial vacuum that adds stability to the articulation.
- *Articular Cartilage:* Covers the lunate surface of the acetabulum and acts as a shock absorber within the joint. Thickest at the superior pole of the femoral head where the joint pressures are highest during the stance phase of gait.

Supporting Structures Located outside the Hip Joint

The external surface of the capsule of the hip is reinforced by a set of thick and important ligaments: the iliofemoral, ischiofemoral, and pubofemoral ligaments. Each ligament attaches proximally from the rim of the acetabulum and distally to the anterior aspect of the proximal femur. The following ligaments play an important role in stabilizing the hip:

- *Iliofemoral Ligament* or *"Y" Ligament* (Figure 9-9): A thick, strong ligament resembling an inverted Y. One of the thickest ligaments in the body, it attaches distally to the intertrochanteric line of the femur. Limits excessive extension of the hip.
- *Ischiofemoral Ligament* (Figure 9-10): Spirals around the femoral neck and attaches near the apex of the greater trochanter. Limits extension and internal rotation of the hip.
- *Pubofemoral Ligament* (see Figure 9-9): Attaches distally to the lower half of the intertrochanteric line of the femur. Limits abduction and extension of the hip.

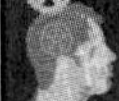

Consider this...

Gaining Strength by "Winding up" Passive Structures

Athletes such as field goal kickers and soccer players often enhance the power of their kicking by storing energy in the capsular ligaments of the hip. By "winding up," quickly extending the hip prior to the kick, the large ligaments are stretched and store energy in much the same way that a stretched rubber band stores energy. As the kick proceeds, these ligaments spring toward their normal length, providing the hip flexor muscles with an additional source of torque. Interestingly, stretched muscles also act as rubber bands, so the extended position of the pre-kick (or wind-up) allows the kicker to benefit from the elastic rebound of the ligaments *and* the muscles of the anterior hip.

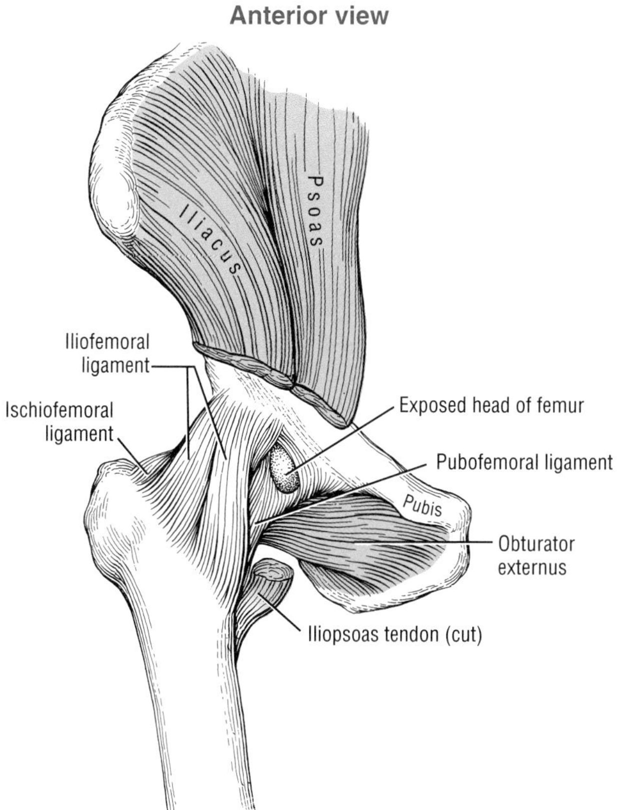

Figure 9-9 An anterior view of the right hip. The iliopsoas is cut to expose the iliofemoral and pubofemoral ligaments. (From Neumann DA: *Kinesiology of the musculoskeletal system: foundations for physical rehabilitation,* St Louis, 2002, Mosby, Figure 12-17.)

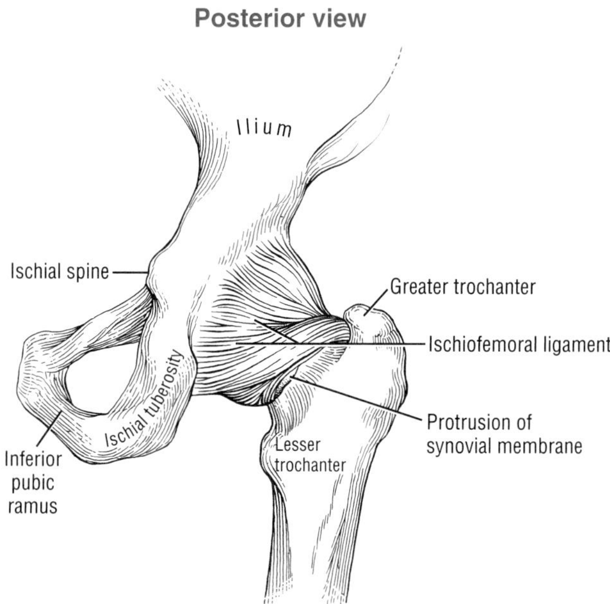

Figure 9-10 The posterior capsule and ischiofemoral ligament of the right hip. (From Neumann DA: *Kinesiology of the musculoskeletal system: foundations for physical rehabilitation,* St Louis, 2002, Mosby, Figure 12-18.)

Functional Importance of the Extendable Hip

MUSCULAR EFFICIENCY OF STANDING AT EASE

Most persons can stand for long periods of time using only minimal amounts of muscular energy about the hip. This near "free lunch" is attained primarily because of the relationship between the ligaments of the hip and the line of gravity. While standing in full upright posture, the line of gravity normally travels just *posterior* to the medial-lateral axis of rotation of the hips (Figure 9-11). Gravity, therefore, provides a passive extension torque at the hips, which, if not opposed, would cause a backward bending of the pelvis over the femurs. However, because all three ligaments of the hip are stretched in extension, they generate a passive rubber band–like flexion torque at the hips that offsets the extension torque caused by gravity. This balancing act, created between the tension in the stretched ligaments and the action of gravity, allows us to stand with

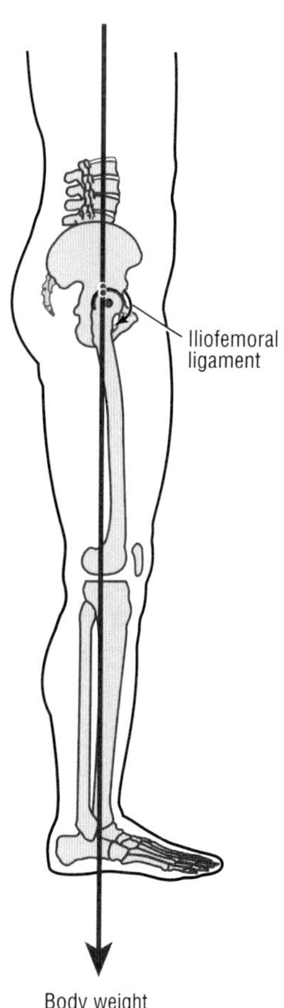

Figure 9-11 When standing fully extended, the line of gravity usually falls slightly posterior to the medial-lateral axis of rotation of the hip, which causes a passive extension torque at the hip. The anterior capsule and ligaments of the hip are pulled taut, limiting further extension of the hip. The red dots indicate optimal alignment of the hip. (From Neumann DA: *An arthritis home study course. The synovial joint: anatomy, function, and dysfunction.* The Orthopedic Section of the American Physical Therapy Association, 1998.)

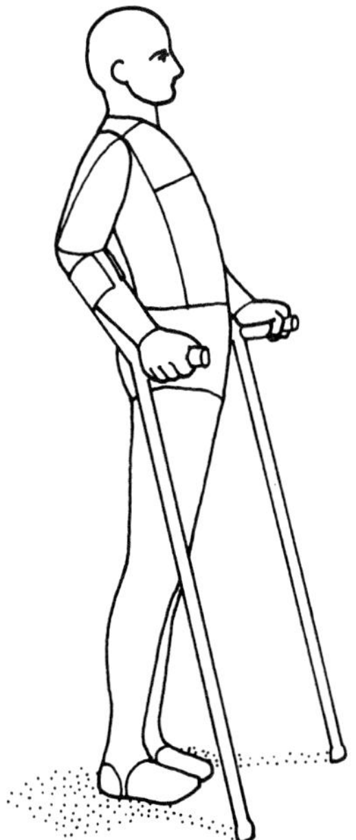

Figure 9-12 A person with paraplegia is shown standing with the aid of braces at the knees and ankles. Leaning of the pelvis and trunk posteriorly, relative to the hip joints, stretches structures such as the iliofemoral ligaments, providing a passive flexor torque that stabilizes the hip and pelvis. (From Somers MF: *Spinal cord injury: functional rehabilitation,* Norwalk, Conn, 1992, Appleton & Lange.)

surprisingly little muscular activation across the hips. In fact, this mechanism is so effective that it can enable standing by persons with paralysis of the lower extremities. For example, Figure 9-12 illustrates an individual with paralysis of the lower extremities following a lumbar spinal cord injury, standing with the aid of crutches and braces at the knees and ankles. By leaning the trunk and pelvis posteriorly relative to the hip joints, the large ligaments of the hip become stretched, stabilizing the trunk, hips, and pelvis without any muscular activation at the hip.

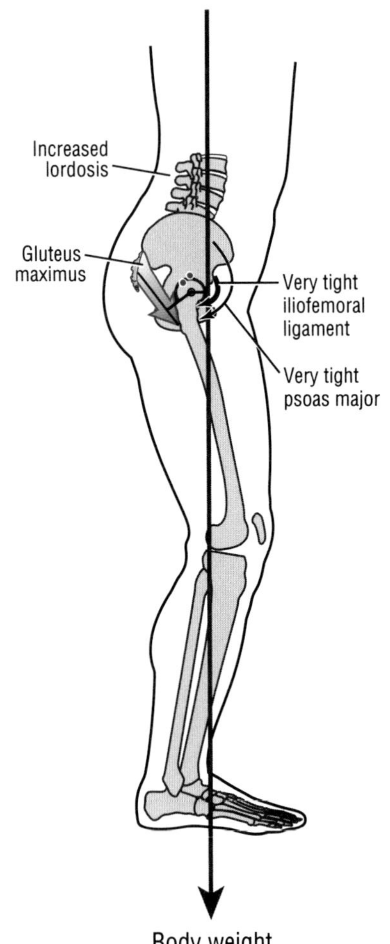

Figure 9-13 A lateral view of an individual with a hip flexion contracture illustrating some of the compensatory strategies: increased lordosis, flexion of the knees, and activation of the hip extensors (gluteus maximus). Offset red dots indicate malalignment of the hip. (From Neumann DA: *An arthritis home study course. The synovial joint: anatomy, function, and dysfunction.* The Orthopedic Section of the American Physical Therapy Association, 1998.)

HIP FLEXION CONTRACTURE

By definition, a hip flexion **contracture** is a limitation of passive hip extension caused by a lack of extensibility of the muscles or ligaments of the hip. Whether mild or severe, hip flexion contractures are relatively common impairments in persons with compromised mobility.

Persons most susceptible to a hip flexion contracture are those who spend a great deal of time in a sitting or otherwise hip-flexed position. Consider the flexed position of the hips in a person who is confined to a wheelchair or chronically assumes a fetal position in bed. Over time, a slackened ligament or muscle will adapt to its shortened position and remain shortened. Once shortened or contracted, the flexor muscles and ligaments of the hip are difficult to re-lengthen, even with aggressive stretching. The long-term effects of a hip flexion contracture can destabilize the hip and have a negative impact on many other regions and structures of the body.

When a person with a hip flexion contracture attempts to stand upright, the line of gravity shifts *anterior* to the medial-lateral axis of rotation (Figure 9-13). This disables the passive standing mechanism discussed earlier, resulting in the need for continuous activation of the hip and back extensor muscles to maintain an upright position. Often a person becomes fatigued and opts to sit, which places the hip flexor muscles and ligaments in a shortened position, thereby perpetuating the vicious cycle.

In order to "right" the trunk in the presence of a moderate to severe hip flexion contracture, the lower spine must be overly extended, resulting in increased lordosis of the lumbar spine (see Figure 9-13). If severe, this can eventually create tightness of the low back extensor muscles and increase the wear and tear on the lumbar facet joints.

This hip-flexed posture depicted in Figure 9-13 interferes with the body's ability to optimally dissipate the compression forces that naturally cross the hips. Normal standing, with the hips in extension, directs the compressive forces through the thicker regions of articular cartilage, more evenly dispersing the compressive loads. Standing with a hip flexion contracture directs the compressive forces from weight bearing through regions of the hip that are not anatomically designed to dissipate these large forces (indicated by the offset alignment of the red dots in Figure 9-13). Over time, this may generate abnormal wear and tear on the joint, increasing the chance of developing osteoarthritis. Standing with a severe hip flexion contracture usually involves the need to stand with the knees flexed. Such a posture requires continuous activation of the quadriceps muscles and increases the likelihood of developing knee flexion contractures.

Clinical **INSIGHT** 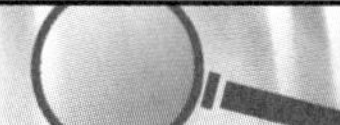

An Ounce of Prevention

Hip flexion contractures can have a number of potentially harmful effects that can spiral toward decreasing function. As mentioned earlier, once a hip flexion contracture has formed, it is extremely difficult to correct. Importantly, clinicians should identify at-risk individuals and prevent contractures before they occur.

Common Techniques for Preventing Hip Flexion Contractures

- *Lying prone:* This places the hips in a neutral or extended position. If tolerated, this activity can provide a prolonged low-intensity stretch of the capsular ligaments and hip flexor muscles.
- *Strengthening of the hip extensors:* This accomplishes the following two important elements:
  - The hips are actively moved out of the flexed position, into extension.
  - The muscular strength bias of the hips is shifted (slowly but surely) toward extension.
- *Patient education:* Moving out of the flexed position on a regular basis greatly reduces the likelihood of developing a contracture. Emphasize the following:
  - When tolerable, encourage standing versus sitting.
  - Lie flat (keep the head of the hospital bed in the down position).
  - Avoid sleeping with pillows under the knees.
- *Stretching of the hip flexors:* Encourage regular stretching through a home exercise program.

Kinematics

The hip allows six basic motions: (1) flexion, (2) extension, (3) abduction, (4) adduction, (5) internal rotation, and (6) external rotation. Because of the central and pivotal location of the hip relative to the entire body, movement between the femur and pelvis can be performed using three different kinematic strategies, as follows:

- Femoral-on-Pelvic Motion

  The femur rotates about a relatively fixed (stationary) pelvis (e.g., as you lift your leg to ascend a step). This open-chain motion is relatively easy to visualize.
- Long-Arc Pelvic-on-Femoral Motion

  The pelvis can rotate through a relatively long arc relative to fixed femurs. This closed-chain hip motion is often performed to maximize the range of motion of the trunk relative to the stationary femurs (e.g., bending forward or to the side to pick an object off the floor; Figure 9-14, *A*). Note that in order to maximize the displacement of the trunk, the lumbar spine moves in the *same* direction as the pelvis.
- Short-Arc Pelvic-on-Femoral Motion

  The pelvis can rotate relative to a fixed femur (or pair of femurs) as the trunk remains essentially stationary. Like the movement strategy described above, this is also considered a closed-chain hip motion. What is different about this kinematic strategy, however, is that the pelvis moves only through a short arc, as the trunk remains essentially upright (Figure 9-14, *B*). In order for the trunk to remain stationary, the lumbar spine must rotate in the *opposite* direction. A familiar example of this type of motion is an anterior or posterior pelvic tilt—movements described in Chapter 8.

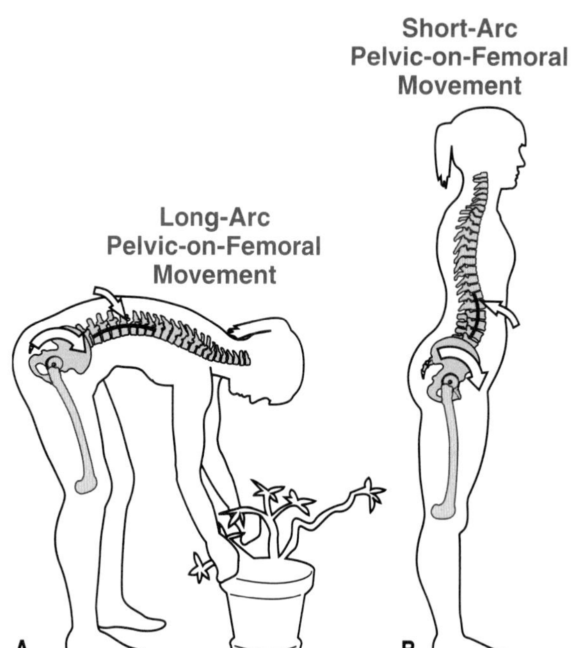

Figure 9-14 Closed-chain motions of the hip. **A,** Long-arc pelvic-on-femoral motion of the hip. Note that the trunk and pelvis move in the same direction. **B,** Short-arc pelvic-on-femoral motion of the hip. Note that the pelvis and lumbar spine move in opposite directions. (From Neumann DA: *Kinesiology of the musculoskeletal system: foundations for physical rehabilitation,* St Louis, 2002, Mosby, Figure 12-24.)

The following sections highlight the six motions allowed at the hip. Within each motion, these three aforementioned kinematic strategies are briefly described.

HIP FLEXION

Hip flexion involves a movement between the femur and the pelvis within the sagittal plane about a medial-lateral axis of rotation. Each kinematic strategy involving flexion reduces the distance between the anterior aspect of the pelvis and the anterior surfaces of the femurs, as follows:

- Femoral-on-Pelvic Motion

  Femoral-on-pelvic flexion of the hip occurs as the femur moves anteriorly about a fixed pelvis: This motion can be observed as the knee (or thigh) is brought toward the chest (Figure 9-15, A). The normal range of motion for hip flexion is about 0 to 120 degrees, with 0 degrees being the neutral, "straight" position of the hip.
- Long-Arc Pelvic-on-Femoral Motion

  Long-arc pelvic-on-femoral flexion of the hip is often performed to bend over and touch the toes or pick an object off the ground (Figure 9-15, B). The pelvis rotates anteriorly about the stationary femoral heads, while the lumbar spine flexes to exaggerate the forward bend of the entire trunk.
- Short-Arc Pelvic-on-Femoral Motion

  An **anterior pelvic tilt** occurs as a short-arc pelvic-on-femoral hip motion, with the trunk remaining upright (Figure 9-15, C): The pelvis rotates, or tilts, anteriorly around the medial-lateral axis of rotation of both hips. As introduced in Chapter 8, the term *tilt* implies a movement through a relatively short arc of motion. This action is easily understood by the following activity: While sitting or standing, tilt just the top of your pelvis anteriorly, keeping your trunk and chest upright. If performed correctly, the low back will have arched into greater extension (increased lordosis). Because the pelvis is rotating forward, the lumbar spine must extend—just as far—to keep the chest and trunk upright. In this way the lumbar spine allows the pelvis to rotate over the femoral heads, while allowing the trunk to remain upright. The range of motion of an anterior pelvic tilt is about 30 degrees, determined mostly by the available extension of the lumbar spine. This important relationship between the lumbar spine and the hip joints is discussed further as the chapter progresses.

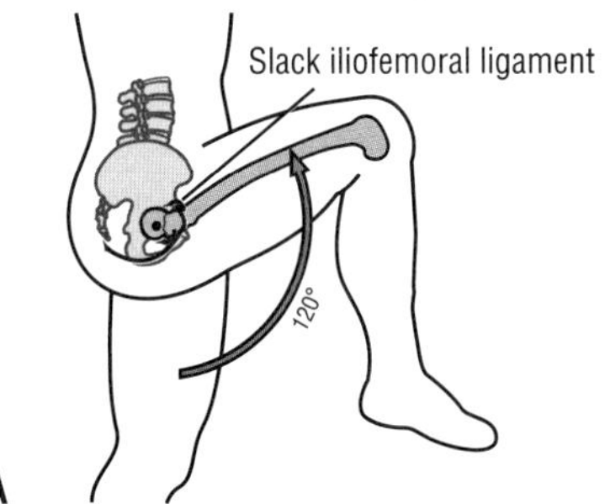

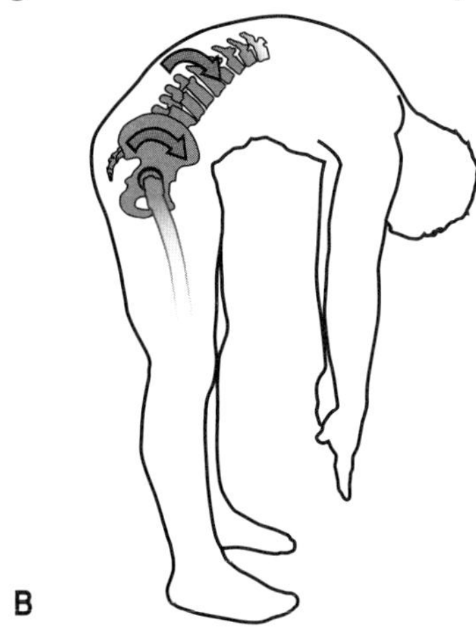

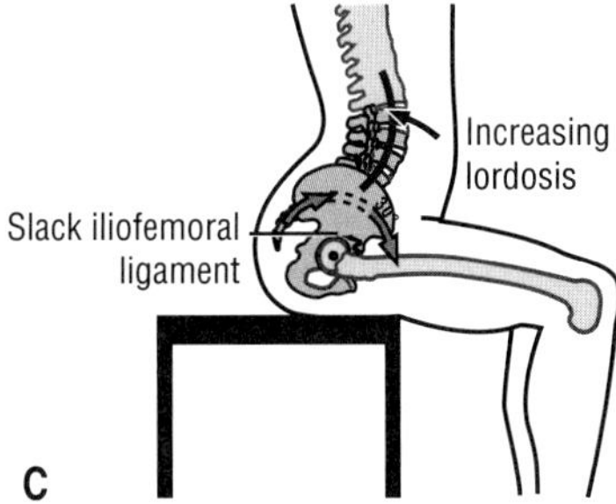

Figure 9-15 A, Femoral-on-pelvic (open-chain) flexion of the right hip. The thin black arrows represent stretched tissues. **B,** Long-arc pelvic-on-femoral flexion of the hips. **C,** Short-arc pelvic-on-femoral flexion of the hips—an anterior pelvic tilt. Note in **C** that flexion of the hips is coupled with extension of the lumbar spine. (Modified from Neumann DA: *Kinesiology of the musculoskeletal system: foundations for physical rehabilitation*, St Louis, 2002, Mosby, Figures 12-23, *A*; 9-8, *C*; and 12-25, *A*.)

HIP EXTENSION

Hip extension involves a movement between the femur and the pelvis within the sagittal plane about a medial-lateral axis of rotation. Each kinematic strategy for extension reduces the distance between the posterior aspect of the pelvis and the posterior surface of the femurs, as follows:

- Femoral-on-Pelvic Motion

  Femoral-on-pelvic extension of the hip occurs as the femur rotates posteriorly about a fixed pelvis (Figure 9-16, *A*). This motion can be observed as an individual extends the leg to walk backwards. The hip can normally be extended 20 degrees beyond the neutral position. As depicted in the illustration, this motion is typically limited by the tension in ligaments and muscles located on the anterior side of the joint.
- Long-Arc Pelvic-on-Femoral Motion

  Pelvic-on-femoral extension of the hips can occur with the lumbar spine and pelvis rotated in the same posterior direction. This action maximizes trunk displacement, as when arching the trunk backwards (as in Figure 9-16, *B*) or as one returns upright after touching the toes.
- Short-Arc Pelvic-on-Femoral Motion

  A **posterior pelvic tilt** is a short-arc, pelvic-on-femoral extension of the hip with the trunk remaining upright (Figure 9-16, C). This motion is the opposite of that described for the anterior pelvic tilt. During a posterior pelvic tilt, the lumbar spine must flex slightly (decreasing its lordosis) to maintain an upright position of the trunk.

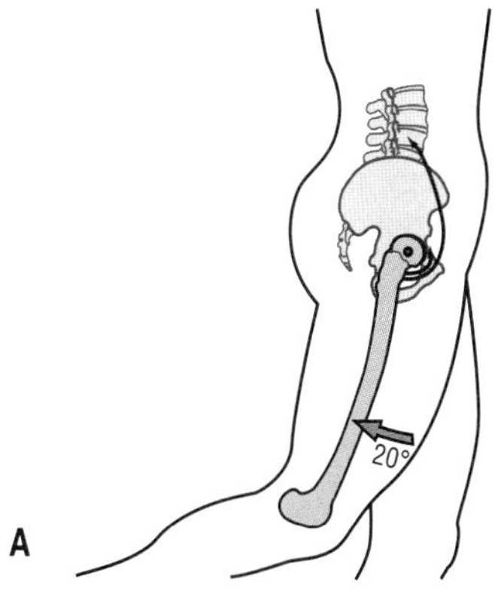

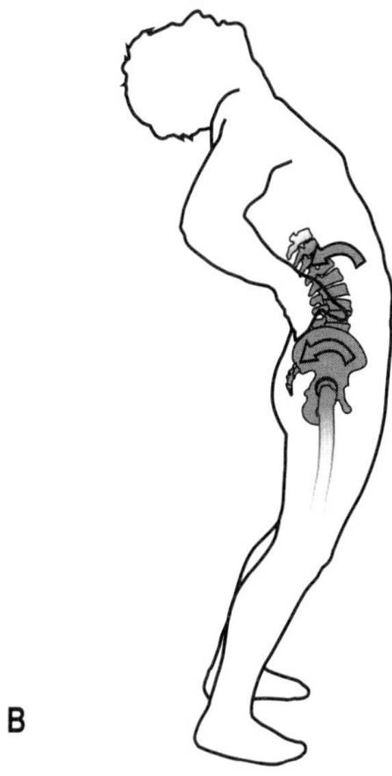

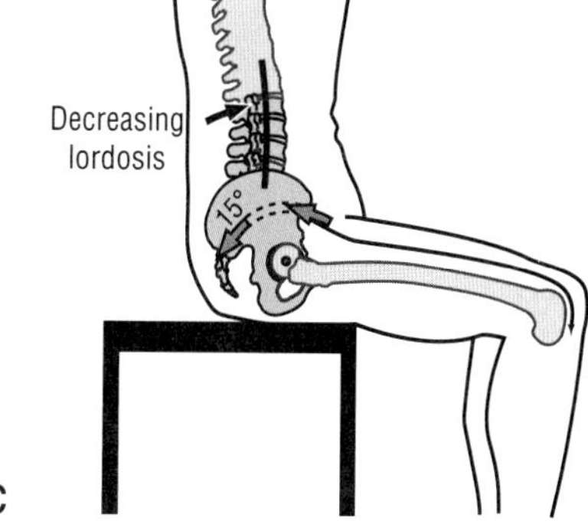

Figure 9-16 A, Femoral-on-pelvic (open-chain) extension of the right hip. **B,** Long-arc pelvic-on-femoral extension of the hips. Note the extension of the trunk to maximize backward bending. **C,** Short-arc pelvic-on-femoral extension of the hips—a posterior pelvic tilt. Thin black arrows indicate stretched tissues. (Modified from Neumann DA: *Kinesiology of the musculoskeletal system: foundations for physical rehabilitation,* St Louis, 2002, Mosby, Figures 12-23, *A*; 9-8, *B*; and 12-25, *A*.)

HIP ABDUCTION

Hip abduction involves a movement between the femur and the pelvis within the frontal plane about an anterior-posterior axis of rotation. Note that, regardless of which kinematic strategy is used, abduction reduces the distance between the iliac crest and the lateral aspect of the thigh, as follows:

- Femoral-on-Pelvic Motion

  Femoral-on-pelvic abduction of the hip occurs as the femur moves away from the midline relative to a fixed pelvis (Figure 9-17, A). The normal range of motion for this open-chain motion is about 0 to 40 degrees.

- Long-Arc Pelvic-on-Femoral Motion

  A long-arc pelvic-on-femoral abduction of the hip often occurs as the lumbar spine and pelvis move in the same frontal plane direction, relative to a stationary femur (Figure 9-17, B). This motion maximizes trunk displacement, as when one laterally flexes to the side to pick up a suitcase off the floor.

- Short-Arc Pelvic-on-Femoral Motion

  Hip hiking is a short-arc, pelvic-on-femoral abduction of the hip motion with the trunk remaining upright (Figure 9-17, C). Similar to anterior and posterior tilting of the pelvis, the lumbar spine rotates slightly in the opposite direction of the pelvis so that the trunk remains fixed and upright. As shown in Figure 9-17, C, hip hiking causes a rise in the contralateral side of the pelvis. This closed-chain movement is a common compensation used to clear the "swing leg" from the ground during ambulation, a gait pattern often used by patients requiring extra clearance to advance a leg, such as in those with marked weakness of the ankle or foot.

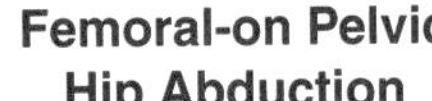

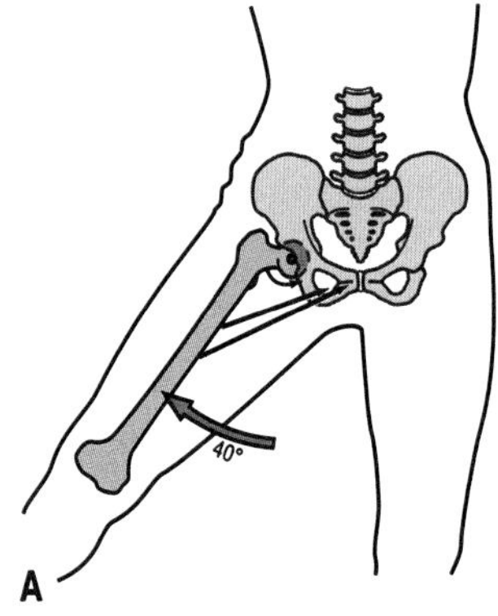

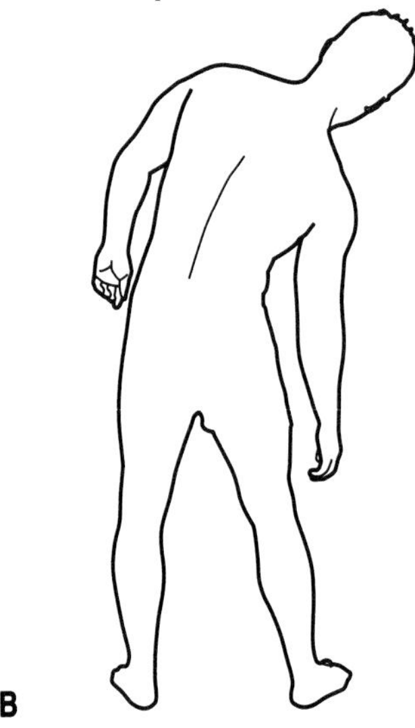

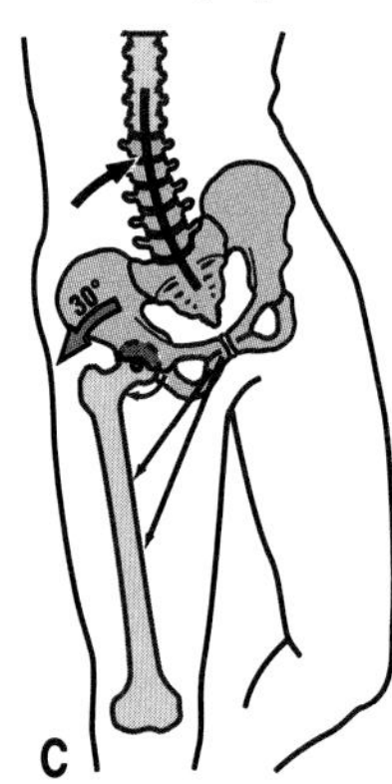

Figure 9-17 **A,** Femoral-on-pelvic (open-chain) abduction of the right hip. **B,** Long-arc pelvic-on-femoral abduction of the right hip. **C,** Short-arc pelvic-on-femoral abduction of the right hip—hip hiking. Thin black arrows indicate stretched tissues. (**A** and **C,** Modified from Neumann DA: *Kinesiology of the musculoskeletal, System: foundations for physical rehatilitation,* St Louis, 2002, Mosby, Figures 12-23, *B* and 12-25, *B*.)

HIP ADDUCTION

Hip adduction involves a movement between the femur and the pelvis within the frontal plane about an anterior-posterior axis of rotation. Regardless of which kinematic strategy is used, adduction results in a reduced distance between the midline of the pelvis and the medial aspect of the femur, as follows:

- Femoral-on-Pelvic Motion

  Femoral-on-pelvic hip adduction occurs as the femur moves toward, or across, the midline relative to a fixed pelvis (Figure 9-18, *A*). The normal range of motion for this open-chain action is 0 to 25 degrees.
- Long-Arc Pelvic-on-Femoral Motion

  Pelvic-on-femoral adduction of the hip can occur as the lumbar spine and pelvis both rotate in the frontal plane, away from fixed femur. This motion is relatively rare during normal activities but may be visualized by standing on the right leg and laterally flexing the body far to the left.
- Short-Arc Pelvic-on-Femoral Motion

  A **hip drop** is a short-arc pelvic-on-femoral motion that results in a slight drop of the contralateral side of the pelvis (Figure 9-18, *B*). For example, when standing on the right leg, the left side of the pelvis drops; to keep the trunk upright, the lumbar spine must laterally flex (just as far) to the right. This motion may be observed in individuals with weak hip abductor muscles who are unable to hold their pelvis level during the stance phase of gait.

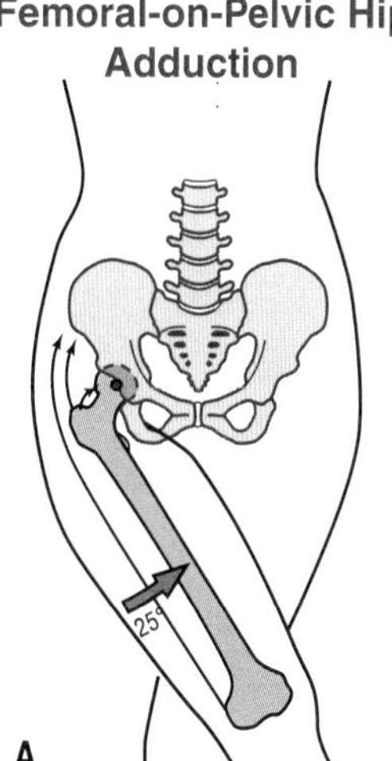

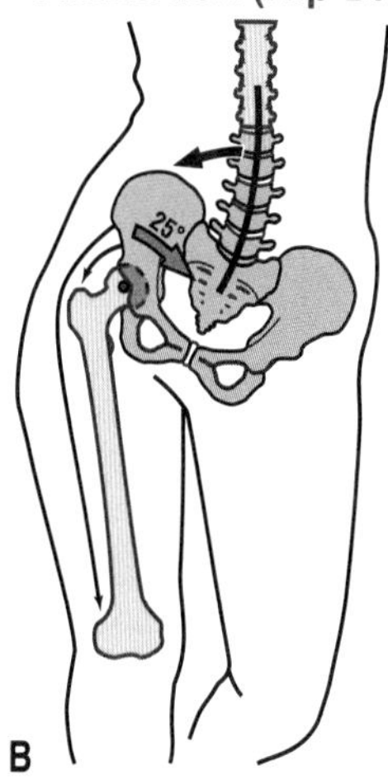

Figure 9-18 **A,** Femoral-on-pelvic (open-chain) adduction of the right hip. **B,** Short-arc pelvic-on-femoral adduction of the right hip—this may be referred to as a "hip drop" to the left. Thin black arrows indicate stretched tissues. (Modified from Neumann DA: *Kinesiology of the musculoskeletal system: foundations for physical rehabilitation*, St Louis, 2002, Mosby, Figures 12-23, *B*, and 12-25, *B*.)

Femoral-on-Pelvic
Hip External Rotation

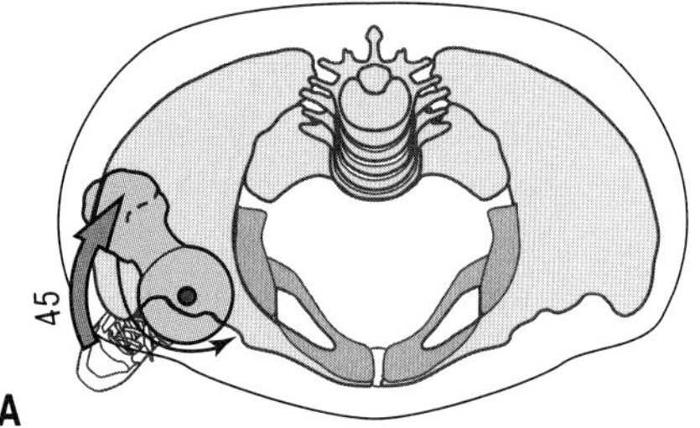

A

Long-Arc Pelvic-on-Femoral
Hip External Rotation

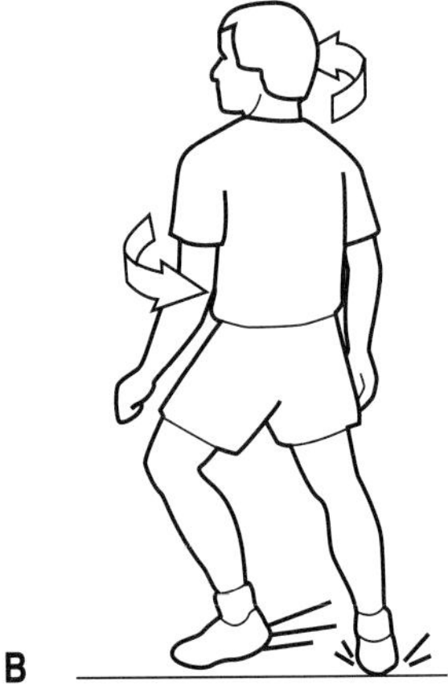

B

Short-Arc Pelvic-on-Femoral
Hip External Rotation

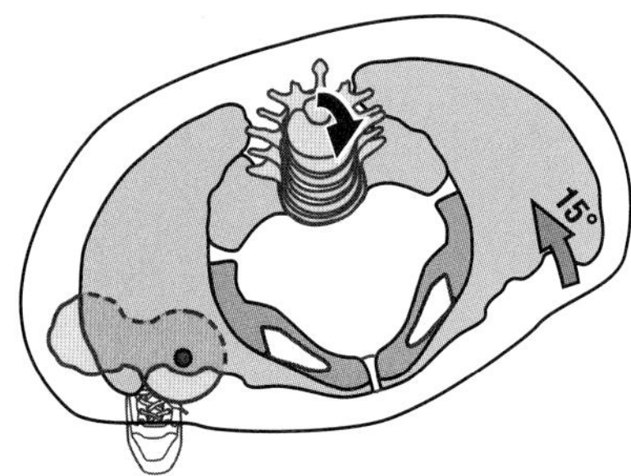

C

Figure 9-19 A, Femoral-on-pelvic (open-chain) external rotation of the right hip. **B,** Long-arc pelvic-on-femoral external rotation of the right hip. **C,** Short-arc pelvic-on-femoral external rotation of the right hip. Note the opposite direction rotation of the lumbar spine. (From Neumann DA: *Kinesiology of the musculoskeletal system: foundations for physical rehabilitation,* St Louis, 2002, Mosby, Figures 12-23, *C;* 12-47 [left]; and 12-25, *C.*)

INTERNAL AND EXTERNAL ROTATION OF THE HIP

Internal and external rotation of the hip occurs in the horizontal plane about a vertical or longitudinal axis of rotation. Due to their similarities, the kinematics of internal and external rotation are described together. As with other movements, three kinematic strategies are possible, as follows:

- Femoral-on-Pelvic Motion

  Femoral-on-pelvic internal and external rotation of the hip can be observed as an individual rotates an extended leg so that the foot and knee point inward (during internal rotation) and outward (during external rotation). Palpation of the greater trochanter can verify that these motions are the result of rotation of the femur. Normal range of motion is about 0 to 35 degrees for internal rotation, and 0 to 45 degrees for external rotation. Figure 9-19, *A*, *B*, and C, shows external rotation only.

- Long-Arc Pelvic-on-Femoral Motion

  With one limb off the ground, pelvic-on-femoral internal and external rotation of the supported hip occur relatively frequently throughout the day. This motion allows the trunk to follow the rotation direction of the pelvis. This strategy of rotation occurs as the pelvis, lumbar spine, and trunk all rotate in the same direction in the horizontal plane, relative to a fixed femur (see Figure 9-19, *B*). This type of movement maximizes the rotation of the entire body, as when planting the right foot and cutting sharply to the left (external rotation of right hip).

- Short-Arc Pelvic-on-Femoral Motion

  Pelvic-on-femoral internal and external rotation of the hip can also occur with the trunk remaining stationary (see Figure 9-19, C). These movements result in a short-arc rotation of the pelvis over the supporting limb as the lumbar spine rotates very slightly in the opposite direction as the pelvis. This motion is very subtle and difficult to observe, but nevertheless important in "decoupling" the motion of the pelvis from the trunk. This type of motion is used during walking or running, allowing the shoulders to remain square to the direction of progression. Note that the figure shows external rotation only.

TABLE 9-1 SUMMARY OF HIP KINEMATICS

Motion	Normal Range of Motion (Degrees)	Axis of Rotation	Plane
Flexion	0-120	Medial-lateral	Sagittal
Extension	0-20	Medial-lateral	Sagittal
Abduction	0-40	Anterior-posterior	Frontal
Adduction	0-25	Anterior-posterior	Frontal
Internal rotation	0-35	Vertical (longitudinal)	Horizontal
External rotation	0-45	Vertical (longitudinal)	Horizontal

ARTHROKINEMATICS

The arthrokinematics of the hip joint are usually described as a convex femoral head moving within the concave acetabulum of the pelvis. In this femoral-on-pelvic perspective, the arthrokinematics of abduction, adduction, and internal and external rotation involve a roll and slide in opposite directions. During flexion and extension of the hip, the femoral head spins in place about a medial-lateral axis of rotation. Normal ranges of motion for all the actions of the hip are listed in Table 9-1.

Muscle and Joint Interaction

Innervation of the Muscles of the Hip

The femoral and obturator nerves are the two largest nerves that exit the lumbar plexus (Figure 9-20). The femoral nerve innervates most of the hip flexors and all of the knee extensors. The obturator nerve innervates primarily the hip adductor muscles.

The sciatic nerve exits the sciatic plexus and is, in fact, the largest nerve in the body (Figure 9-21). Its large size reflects a bundle of two separate nerves, the tibial nerve and the common peroneal nerve. The tibial portion of the sciatic nerve innervates most of the hamstring muscles and the extensor head of the adductor magnus. The common peroneal portion of the sciatic nerve innervates the remaining hamstring—the short head of the biceps femoris—and a number of muscles of the ankle. Other nerves from the sacral plexus innervate the gluteal muscles, tensor fasciae latae, and five of the six short external rotator muscles. The table on p. 244 provides more specific details.

Clinical **INSIGHT**

Pelvic Tilts to Treat the Back

As described in Chapter 8, anterior and posterior pelvic tilts require simultaneous movement of the hips *and* lumbar spine. For this reason pelvic tilts are often a central component of rehabilitation programs designed to treat the lower back.

Some individuals have a natural postural bias that is expressed either as a swayback (hyperlordotic) lumbar or flatback (hypolordotic) lumbar posture. Over time, these postures may increase the likelihood of a herniated disc or damaged disc, over-compressed facet joints, or generalized lower back pain. Clinicians therefore often provide pelvic tilting exercises to reduce exaggerated postures in the lumbar spine. Anteriorly and posteriorly tilting the pelvis provides good visual clues as to the movements that are likely occurring at the lumbar spine. These clues can help guide the progress of an exercise program.

SUMMARY OF INNERVATION OF THE HIP MUSCLES

Nerve	Muscles Innervated	Region of Innervation
Femoral	Rectus femoris Sartorius Vastus lateralis Vastus medialis Vastus intermedius	Anterior thigh
Obturator	Gracilis Pectineus Adductor magnus—adductor head Adductor longus Adductor brevis Obturator externus	Medial thigh
Sciatic (tibial part)	Semimembranosus Semitendinosus Biceps femoris—long head Adductor magnus—extensor head	Posterior thigh
Superior gluteal	Gluteus medius Gluteus minimus Tensor fascia latae	Lateral gluteal region
Inferior gluteal	Gluteus maximus	Posterior gluteal region
Nerve to the piriformis Nerve to the obturator internus Nerve to the quadratus femoris	Piriformis Obturator internus and gemellus superior Quadratus femoris and gemellus inferior	Deep posterior gluteal region

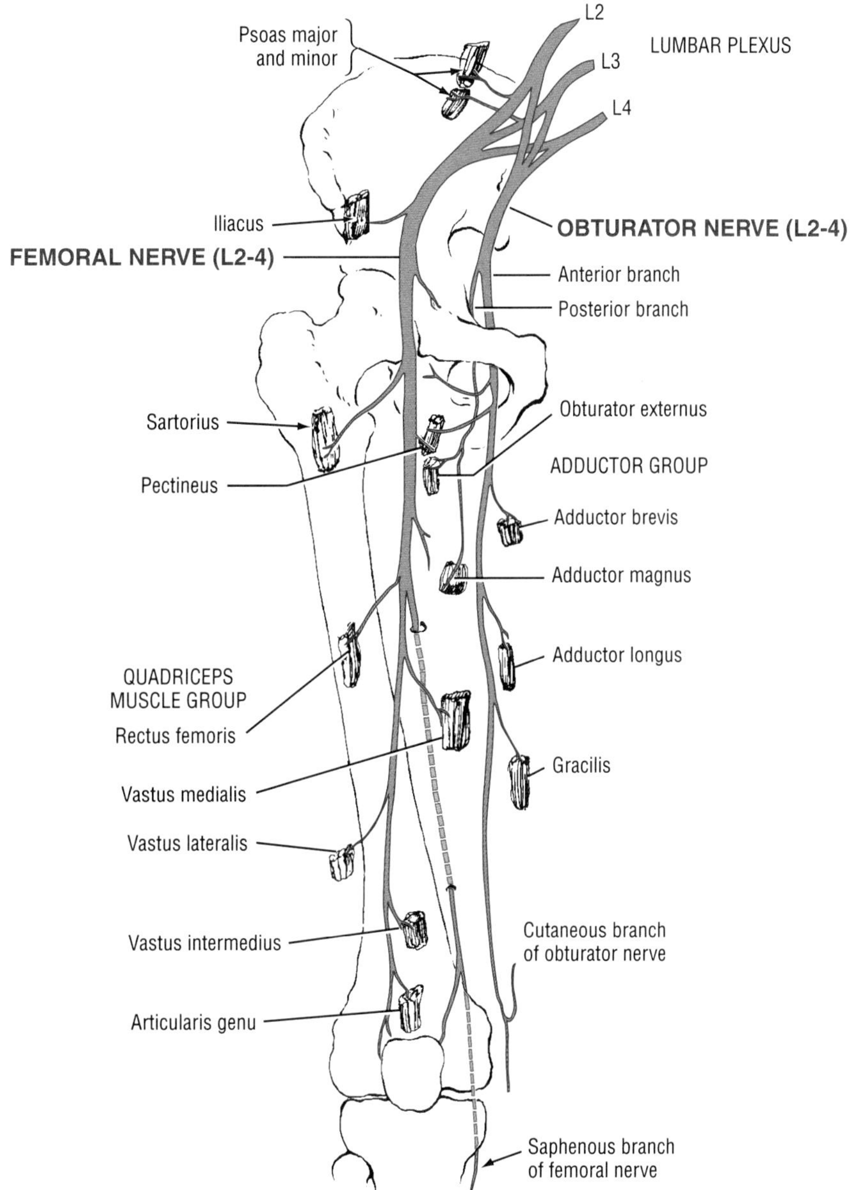

Figure 9-20 An anterior view of the right hip showing the general path of the femoral and obturator nerves. (Modified from Waxman S: *Correlative neuroanatomy,* ed 24, New York, 2000, Lange Medical Books/McGraw-Hill.)

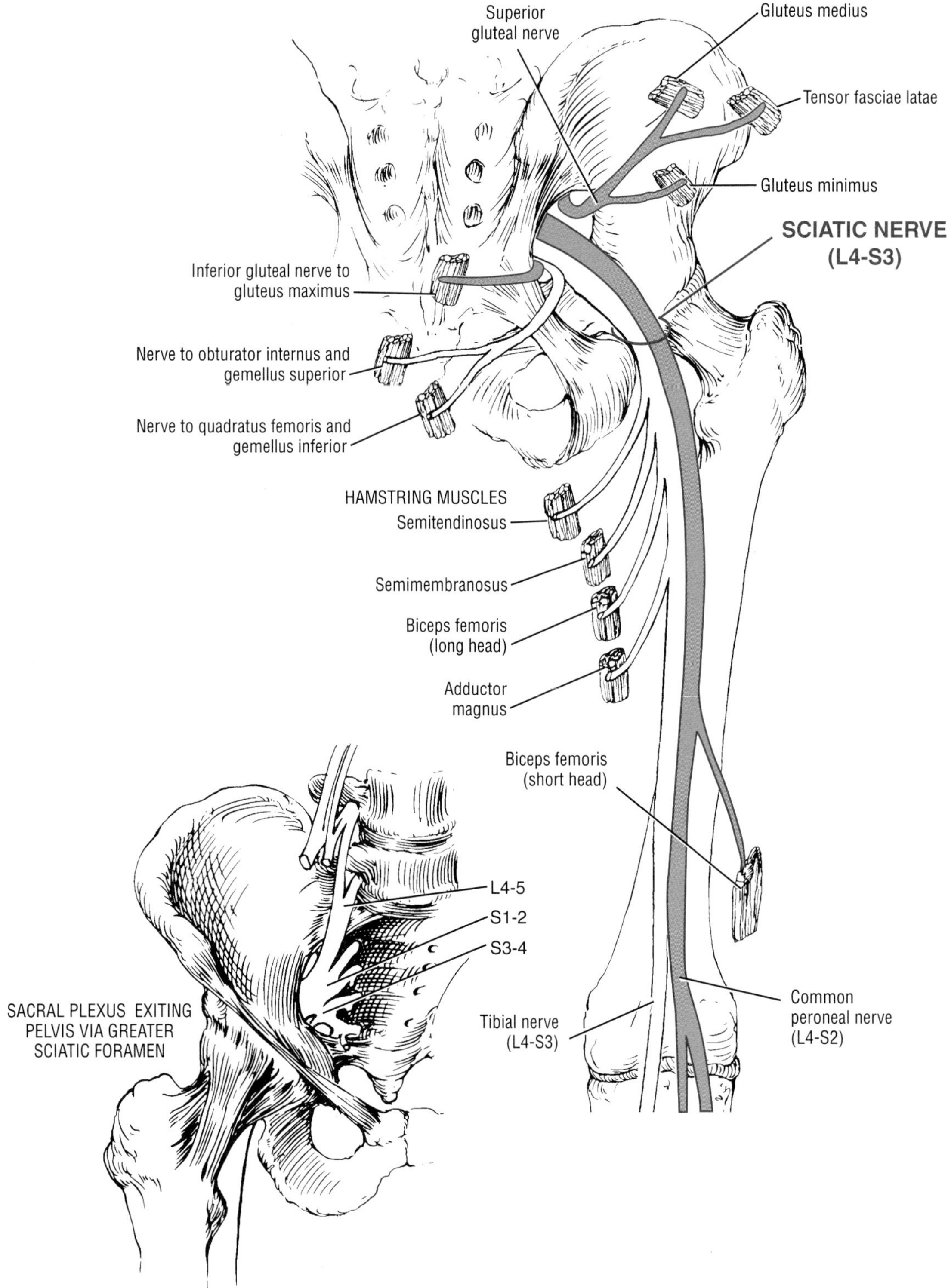

Figure 9-21 A posterior view of the right hip showing the sciatic nerve. Note that the sciatic nerve is composed of the tibial and common peroneal nerves. (Modified from Waxman S: *Correlative neuroanatomy,* ed 24, New York, 2000, Lange Medical Books/McGraw-Hill.)

Muscles of the Hip

Many large and powerful muscles surround the hip, producing the necessary forces to move the lower extremity through a variety of planes or propel the body in nearly any direction. Other relatively smaller muscles stabilize the hip and help fine-tune various actions of the lower extremity. Although these muscles are discussed individually, in reality, the ultimate function of the lower extremity is highly dependent on the interaction of all the surrounding musculature.

HIP FLEXORS

The primary hip flexors are the iliopsoas, rectus femoris, sartorius, and tensor fasciae latae. When analyzed from the anatomic position, most of the hip adductor muscles also flex the hip; these muscles will be described in detail in the hip adductor section. All hip flexor muscles have a line of pull that is anterior to the medial-lateral axis of rotation of the hip. Realize that *any* muscle with the potential to flex the hip has the same potential to anteriorly tilt the pelvis because, from a closed-chain perspective, an anterior pelvic tilt *is* hip flexion.

Primary Hip Flexors

- Iliopsoas
- Rectus femoris
- Sartorius
- Tensor fasciae latae

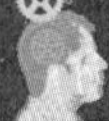

Consider this...

Iliopsoas: Built to Tilt

An anterior pelvic tilt by definition is a short-arc anterior rotation of the pelvis that occurs with the trunk held stationary. In order for the trunk to be held stationary, the lumbar spine must extend slightly (or increase its lordosis) to decouple the pelvic and trunk motions. The iliopsoas is perfectly suited for both of these tasks. With the femur held stationary, contraction of the iliacus muscle tilts the pelvis anteriorly, as the proximal attachment (iliac fossa) is drawn toward the lesser trochanter. At the same time, the psoas major pulls the lower part of the lumbar spine anteriorly, increasing the lumbar lordosis.

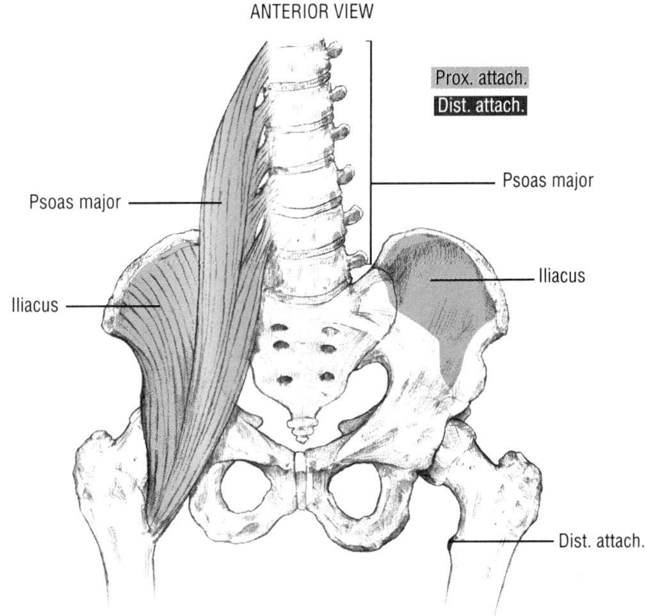

Iliopsoas

The iliopsoas consists of two muscles: the psoas major and the iliacus.

Psoas Major

Proximal Attachment: Transverse processes and lateral bodies of T12-L5 vertebrae including the intervertebral discs

Distal Attachment: Lesser trochanter of the femur

Iliacus

Proximal Attachment: Iliac fossa and inner lip of the iliac crest

Distal Attachment: Lesser trochanter of the femur

Innervation of the Iliacus and Psoas Major: Femoral nerve

Actions of the Iliacus and Psoas Major (Iliopsoas):

- Hip flexion
- Anterior pelvic tilt
- Flexion of the trunk relative to the lower extremity

Comments: The iliopsoas is the body's most powerful hip flexor and therefore equally well suited to flex the pelvis on the femurs—both from short- and long-arc perspectives. Tightness or weakness of the iliopsoas can lead to significant dysfunction within the trunk, lower back, pelvis, and hip.

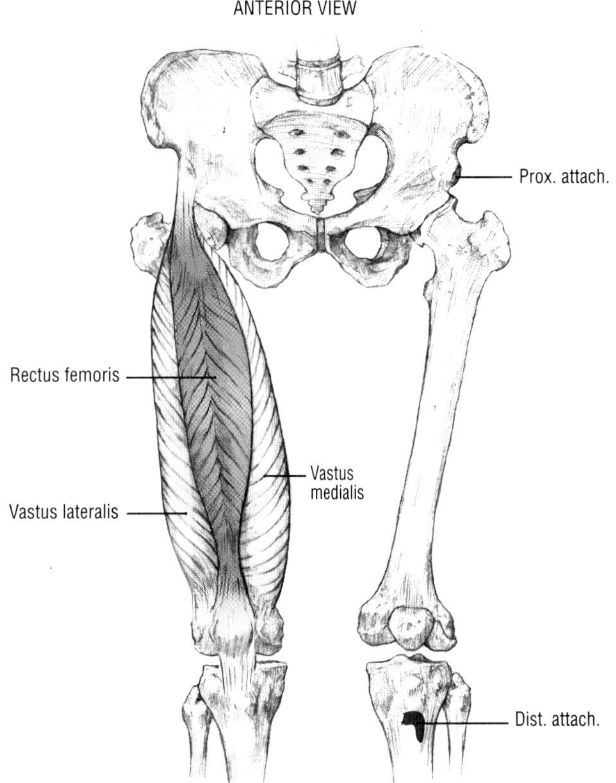

Rectus Femoris

Proximal Attachment: Anterior-inferior iliac spine
Distal Attachment: Tibial tuberosity
Innervation: Femoral nerve
Actions:
- Hip flexion
- Knee extension

Comments: The rectus femoris is the only muscle of the quadriceps group that crosses the hip and knee joints. This bi-articular muscle is both a flexor of the hip and extensor of the knee. Because the rectus femoris crosses both joints, the position of the knee influences the function of the rectus femoris at the hip and vice versa.

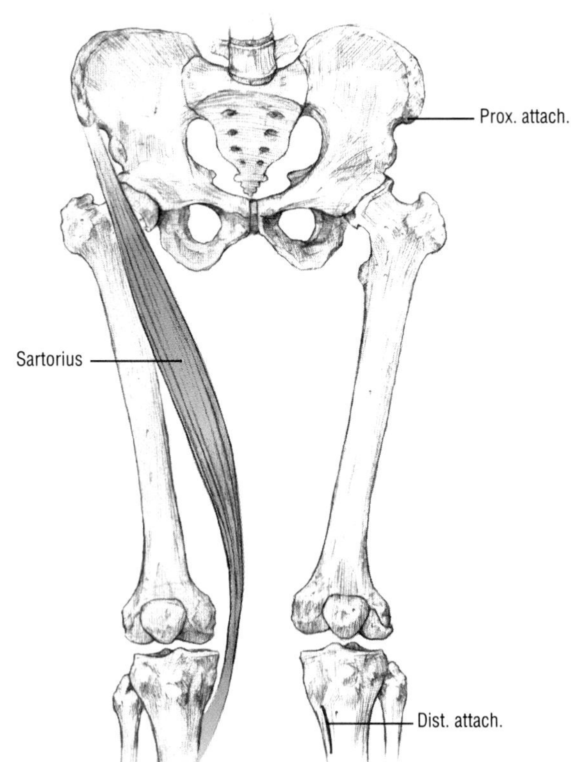

Sartorius

Proximal Attachment: Anterior-superior iliac spine
Distal Attachment: Proximal-medial surface of the tibia (via pes anserinus)

(The pes anserinus, meaning "goose's foot," refers to the three-pronged appearance of the sartorius, gracilis, and semitendinosus coalescing to insert on the proximal-medial tibia.)

Innervation: Femoral nerve
Actions:
- Hip flexion
- Hip abduction
- Hip external rotation
- Knee flexion
- Knee internal rotation

Comments: The sartorius is the longest muscle in the body. Wrapping diagonally across the anterior thigh, the sartorius crosses anterior to the medial-lateral axis of the hip and posterior to the medial-lateral axis of the knee, allowing this muscle to perform the opposite-direction actions of hip flexion and knee flexion. If you cannot remember all the actions of the sartorius, slide your heel up the opposite shin. The position of your leg, when your heel is at your knee, will tell you the answer: hip flexion, external rotation, and abduction, as well as flexion of the knee.

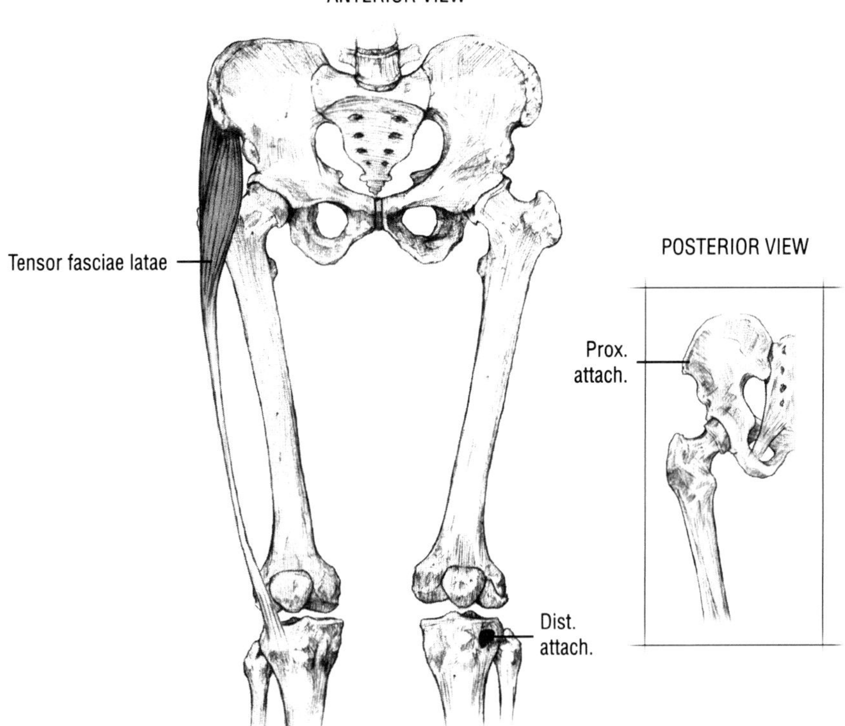

Tensor Fasciae Latae

Proximal Attachment: Outer surface of the iliac crest just posterior to the anterior-superior iliac spine

Distal Attachment: Proximal one third of the iliotibial band

Innervation: Superior gluteal nerve

Actions:
- Hip flexion
- Hip abduction
- Hip internal rotation

Comments: The iliotibial band is a thick band of connective tissue that runs from the iliac crest to the lateral tubercle of the tibia. One function of the tensor fasciae latae is to tighten the iliotibial band, providing increased stability across the lateral aspect of the hip and knee.

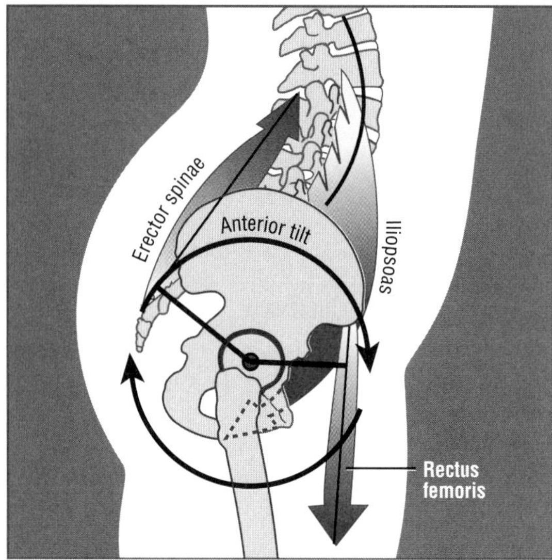

Figure 9-22 The force-couple is shown between the hip flexors and the erector spinae muscles, to anteriorly tilt the pelvis; note the increased lumbar lordosis. (From Neumann DA: *Kinesiology of the musculoskeletal system: foundations for physical rehabilitation*, St Louis, 2002, Mosby, Figure 12-30.)

Functional Considerations

Force-Couple for Performing an Anterior Tilt of the Pelvis. Actively anteriorly tilting the pelvis is created by a **force-couple** involving the hip flexor muscles and erector spinae (low back extensors) (Figure 9-22). The interaction between these two muscle groups is similar to the push and pull of one's hands when turning a steering wheel. The erector spinae muscles pull upward at the same time the hip flexors pull downward.

The close relationship between these muscles is often observed in cases of muscular tightness. For example, individuals who develop tightness of the hip flexor muscles are likely to develop tightness of the low back (erector spinae) muscles. This typically results in a swayback (excessive thoracic kyphosis with lumbar lordosis) in standing (see also Chapter 8, Figure 8-4). As outlined in Chapter 8, these postures—over time—can have a negative effect on the lumbosacral region. When addressing these faulty postures, clinicians must address tightness of the hip flexors *and* the musculature of the low back.

Abdominal Muscles as Proximal Stabilizers for the Hip Flexors. The hip flexor muscles are used for a variety of everyday functional activities such as advancing the lower extremity during gait, running, or lifting the leg when going up steps. Efficient execution of these hip flexion activities is highly dependent on the stabilizing forces provided by the abdominal muscles. This important point is nicely illustrated by analyzing the role of the rectus abdominis muscle while performing a straight leg raise. Figure 9-24, A, shows two primary hip flexor muscles generating a force to lift a fully extended lower extremity.

Clinical **INSIGHT**

Compensating for Tight Hip Flexors through Increased Lumbar Lordosis

Clinicians often use the Thomas test to check for tightness of the hip flexors. During a Thomas test, the patient is supine and holds the non-tested hip and knee fully flexed while the other leg is lowered toward the treatment table. If the leg does not lower to the level of the mat, the hip flexors are considered tight (Figure 9-23, *A*).

Note that the flexed position of the non-tested (left) leg stabilizes the pelvis in a neutral or slightly posteriorly tilted position. Without this stabilizing force, the test would be invalid because the tested (right) leg would likely drop to the level of the mat through increasing anterior pelvic tilt and lumbar lordosis, not through actual extension of the femur (Figure 9-23, *B*).

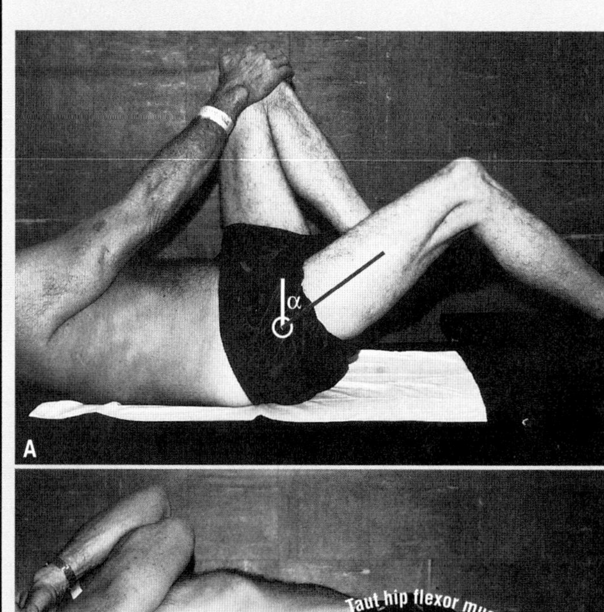

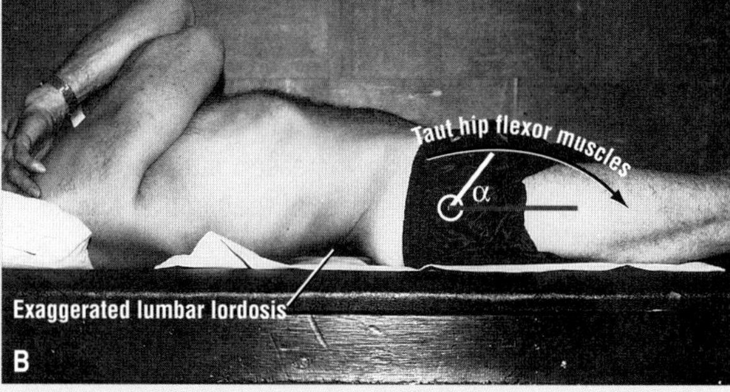

Figure 9-23 A, An individual performing a Thomas test, displaying tight hip flexors. With the pelvis and back stabilized, the tight hip flexors prevent the right leg from being lowered to the mat. **B,** The same individual is able to place the posterior thigh on the mat through an exaggerated lumbar lordosis—not the available extension of the hip. (From Neumann DA: *Kinesiology of the musculoskeletal system: foundations for physical rehabilitation*, St Louis, 2002, Mosby, Figure 9-69.)

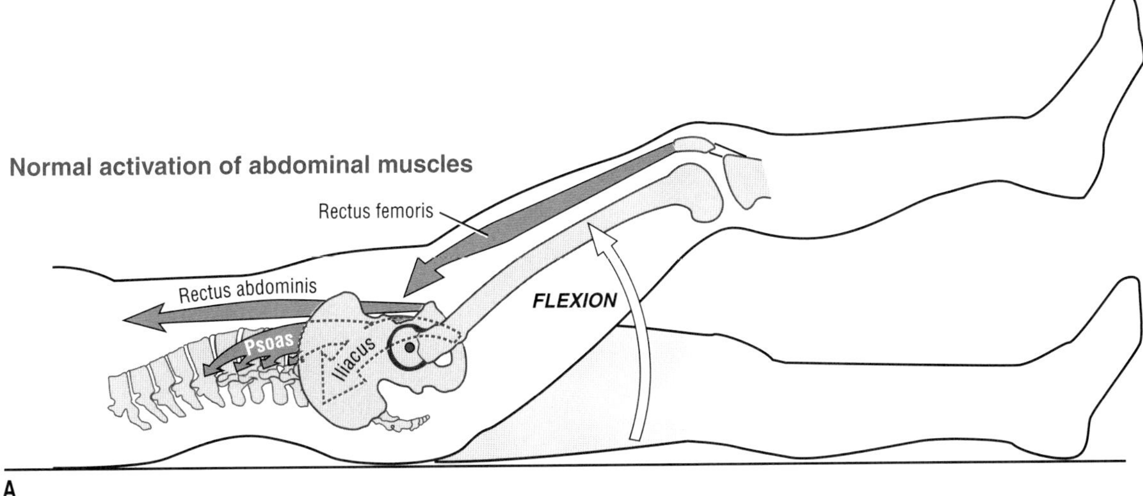

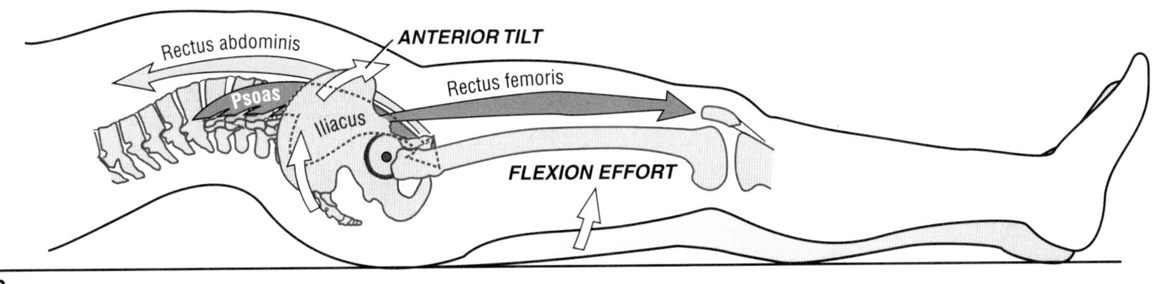

Figure 9-24 The stabilizing role of the abdominals is shown during a unilateral straight leg raise. **A,** With normal activation of the abdominals, the pelvis is stabilized, preventing an anterior tilt of the pelvis. **B,** With reduced activation or weakness of the abdominals, attempting a straight leg raise results in an anterior tilt of the pelvis. Note the increasing lordosis that accompanies an anterior pelvic tilt. (From Neumann DA: *Kinesiology of the musculoskeletal system: foundations for physical rehabilitation,* St Louis, 2002, Mosby, Figure 12-31.)

The relatively long extended leg places very large force demands on the hip flexor muscles. To successfully perform this action, the hip flexors must produce a force that likely exceeds 10 times the weight of the leg. With weakened abdominal muscles, attempts at flexing the leg often result in an unwanted anterior pelvic tilt and associated excessive lumbar lordosis (Figure 9-24, *B*). The unstable pelvis and lumbar spine are pulled *toward* the anterior femur—into an anterior pelvic tilt—because the pelvis and lumbar spine are more free to move than the leg. To prevent this, the abdominal muscles produce a posterior tilting force that stabilizes the pelvis (see Figure 9-24, *A*). As shown in Figure 9-24, *B*, the unwanted anterior tilt of the pelvis simultaneously increases the lordosis in the lumbar spine. For this reason, excessive lumbar lordosis is often a clinical sign of weak abdominal muscles.

HIP EXTENSORS

The primary hip extensors are the gluteus maximus and the hamstrings (i.e., the long head of the biceps femoris, the semitendinosus, and the semimembranosus). The extensor head of the adductor magnus (described later in this chapter) is also considered a primary hip extensor. This powerful group of hip extensors is used for functional activities involving upward and forward propulsion of the body such as for jumping, running, stair climbing, and transitioning from sitting to standing. With the femur well stabilized, activation of the hip extensors can also posteriorly tilt the pelvis.

Primary Hip Extensors

- Gluteus maximus
- Semitendinosus
- Semimembranosus
- Biceps femoris—long head
- Adductor magnus—extensor head

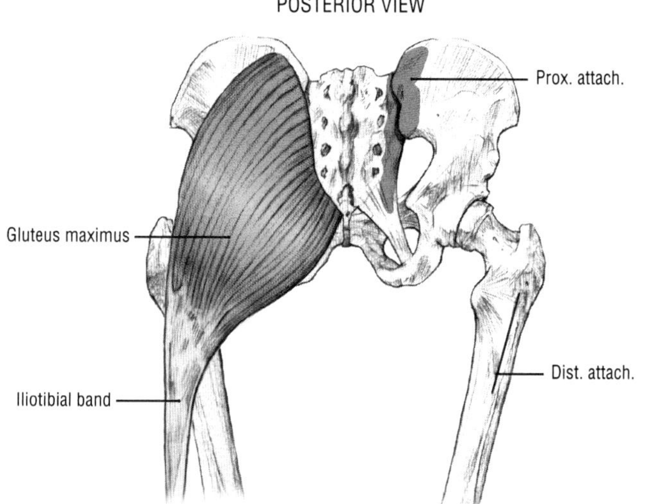

Gluteus Maximus

Proximal Attachment:	Posterior ilium, sacrum, coccyx, and sacrotuberous and sacroiliac ligaments
Distal Attachment:	Iliotibial band and the gluteal tuberosity of the femur
Innervation:	Inferior Gluteal Nerve
Actions:	• Hip extension • Hip external rotation • Posterior pelvic tilt • Extension of the trunk relative to the lower extremity
Comments:	The gluteus maximus is a strong hip extensor, often involved in high-powered, anti-gravity activities such as running uphill or quickly climbing steep steps.

Clinical INSIGHT

Using the Gluteus Maximus to Help Extend the Knee

The gluteus maximus is well known for its ability to extend the hip. This same muscle, however, can also perform the last 20 or 30 degrees of knee extension, provided the foot is in firm contact with the ground. The use of such proximal musculature to help extend the knee is a valuable substitution technique for those with knee extensor paralysis or a prosthetic leg who lack true knee extensors.

While standing over a slightly flexed knee, strong contraction of the gluteus maximus can pull the femur posteriorly. With the foot (or prosthesis) firmly in contact with the ground, the extending femur draws the attached tibia posteriorly, thereby extending the knee even without an active force from the knee extensor (quadriceps) muscles (Figure 9-25). The fully extended knee can then be mechanically locked by positioning body weight anterior to the medial-lateral axis of the knee. Some individuals become so effective at this technique that they are able to ascend steps or walk up moderately pitched inclines often, however, requiring the assistance of a hard rail. Effective use of this muscle substitution technique is only possible if the person has ample range of motion into hip extension. This explains, in part, why obtaining full hip extension (i.e., avoiding hip flexion contracture) is so emphasized in many lower-extremity amputation rehabilitation programs.

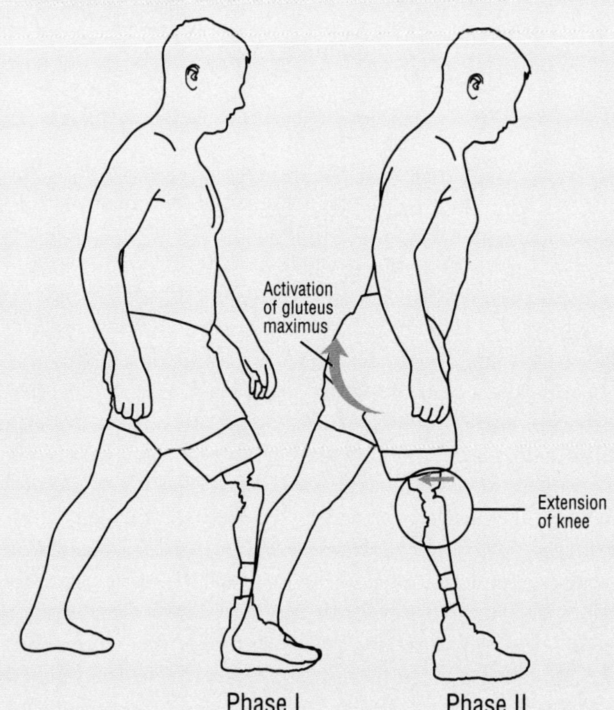

Figure 9-25 An individual is shown extending the prosthetic knee through activation of the hip extensor muscles.

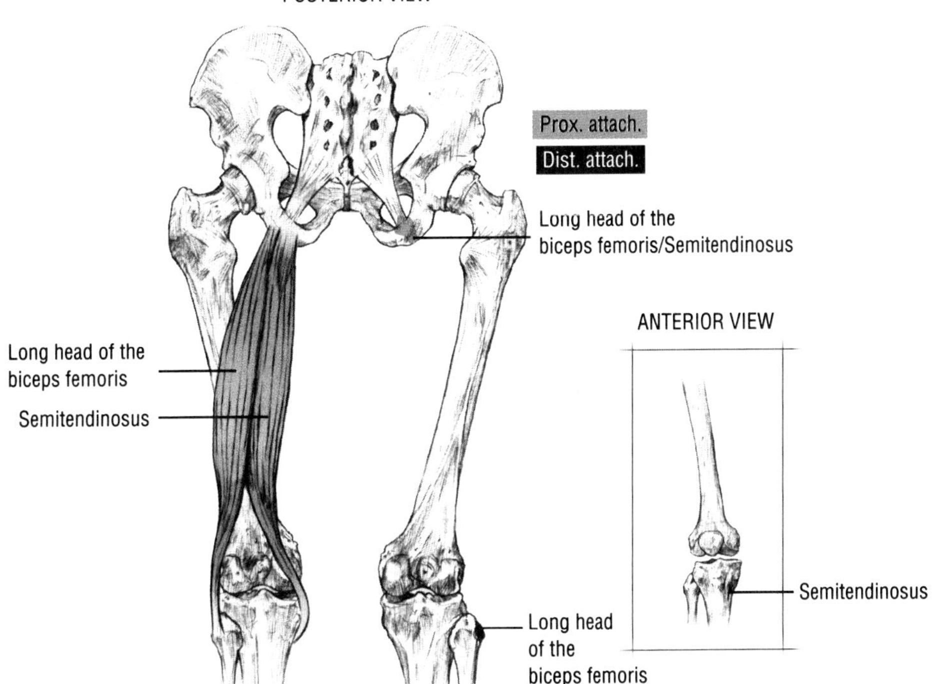

Semitendinosus

Proximal Attachment: Ischial tuberosity

Distal Attachment: Proximal-medial surface of the tibia (pes anserinus)

Innervation: Tibial portion of the sciatic nerve

Actions:

- Hip extension
- Posterior pelvic tilt
- Knee flexion
- Knee internal rotation

Comments: The cord-like tendon of this muscle is easily palpated as the most superficial structure on the posterior-medial aspect of the knee. Resisted knee flexion greatly enhances the ability to palpate this structure.

Biceps Femoris—Long Head

Proximal Attachment: Ischial tuberosity

Distal Attachment: Head of the fibula

Innervation: Tibial portion of the sciatic nerve

Actions:

- Hip extension
- Posterior pelvic tilt
- Knee flexion
- Knee external rotation

Comments: The biceps femoris is composed of a long head and a short head. The long head of the biceps femoris is a traditional hamstring muscle, crossing the posterior aspect of the hip and the knee, whereas the short head crosses only the knee. The distal tendon of the biceps femoris is easily palpated on the posterior-lateral aspect of the flexed knee during resisted knee flexion.

POSTERIOR VIEW

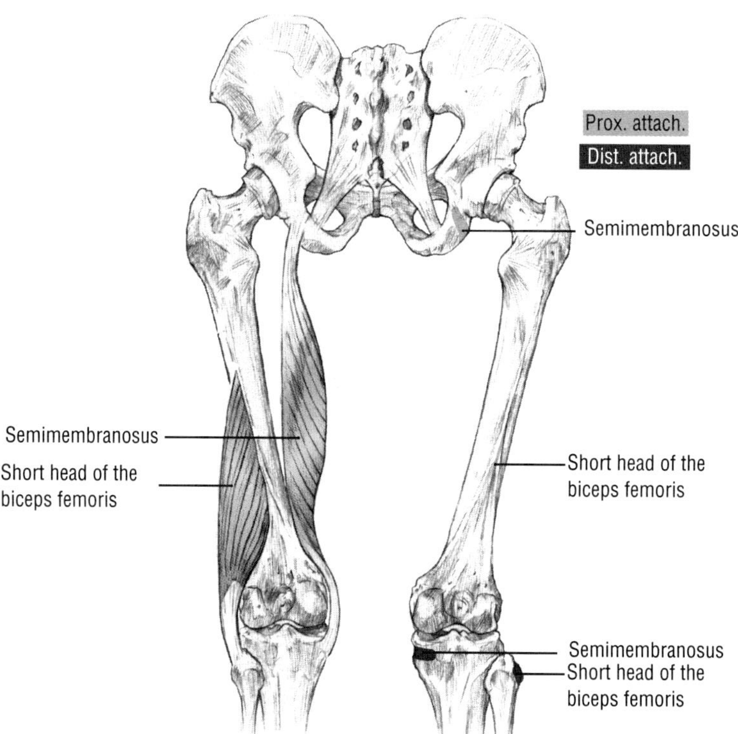

The semimembranosus is shown next to the short head of the biceps femoris. The semitendinosus and biceps femoris—long head have been removed to show this view. The anatomic details of the short head of the biceps femoris are provided in Chapter 10.

Semimembranosus

Proximal Attachment: Ischial tuberosity

Distal Attachment: Medial condyle of the tibia—posterior aspect

Innervation: Tibial portion of the sciatic nerve

Actions:

- Hip extension
- Posterior pelvic tilt
- Knee flexion
- Knee internal rotation

Comments: The semimembranosus and semitendinosus together are often referred to as the medial hamstrings. The semimembranosus is more flattened and membranous than the semitendinosus, hence its name.

Functional Considerations

Force-Couple for Performing a Posterior Pelvic Tilt. The motion of a posterior pelvic tilt is produced by a force-couple created by the abdominal muscles and the hip extensors (Figure 9-26). The interaction of these two groups of muscles provides enhanced control of the hip and pelvis in a wide variety of postures.

As mentioned in Chapter 8, a posterior pelvic tilt reduces the lordosis in the lumbar spine. For this reason, exercises that emphasize a posterior pelvic tilt are often used to address low-back problems. For example, a person with an anterior spondylolisthesis at L5/S1 is typically trained to hold his or her pelvis in a more posteriorly tilted position, which would minimize the lumbar lordosis and accompanying anterior shear at the base of the spine.

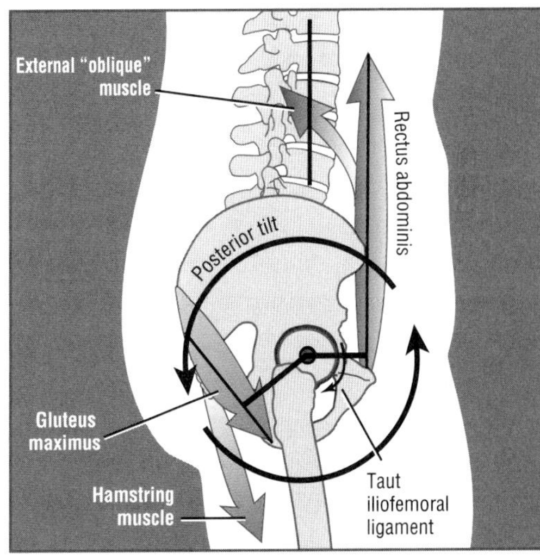

Figure 9-26 A posterior pelvic tilt produced by a force-couple between the hip extensors (gluteus maximus and hamstrings) and the abdominals. Note the decreased lordosis of the lumbar spine. (From Neumann DA: *Kinesiology of the musculoskeletal system: foundations for physical rehabilitation*, St Louis, 2002, Mosby, Figure 12-41.)

High-Powered Hip Extension. Activities such as running or jumping can require large hip extension torques, often generated very rapidly. These large hip extension torques are generally required just as the hip has cycled through full flexion. Likely not a coincidence, the position of hip flexion elongates the hip extensors, placing them at a more favorable length to produce large forces. Figure 9-27 illustrates the activation of three primary hip extensor muscles while climbing a steep hill with a heavy load. The hamstrings and gluteus maximus are both stretched across the hip, which helps maximize their force-generating ability. Also, the extensor head of the adductor magnus gains leverage as a hip extensor when the hip is fully flexed.

Interestingly, many of the hip adductor muscles, which can assist with hip flexion in the anatomic position, are converted to hip extensors when the hip is in a flexed position. Like switching gears in a car, the position of hip flexion strongly engages the available extension torque of numerous muscles of the hip.

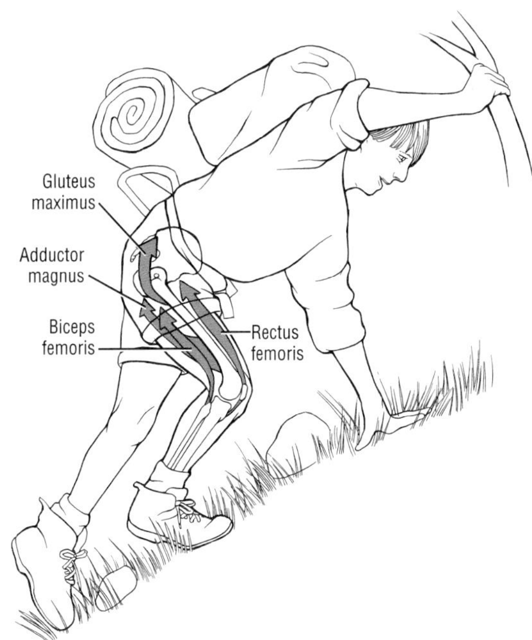

Figure 9-27 Relatively high demands are placed on the hip extensors when climbing up a mountain, requiring strong activation of the gluteus maximus, hamstrings, and adductors. (From Neumann DA: *Kinesiology of the musculoskeletal system: foundations for physical rehabilitation*, St Louis, 2002, Mosby, Figure 12-43.)

Consider this...

Hamstrings: Classic Bi-Articular Muscles in Action

The hamstrings are considered multi-articular muscles because they cross both the hip and the knee. This arrangement allows these muscles to contract a surprisingly short distance during many functional activities. As described in Chapter 3, minimizing the rate and amount of a muscle's contraction helps preserve its force-generating ability.

To explain further, consider the motion of standing up from a seated position. In the seated position, both the hip and knee are flexed. The hamstrings are therefore lengthened across the hip but relatively slackened across the knee (Figure 9-28, *A*). After coming to a full standing position, the hip and knee have extended; in this position the hamstrings are now relatively slackened across the hip but lengthened across the knee (Figure 9-28, *B*). The ability of the hamstrings to dynamically "trade" length across the hip and knee allows these muscles to operate while actually contracting a relatively short net distance. This ability helps keep the muscles strong throughout the entire range of motion.

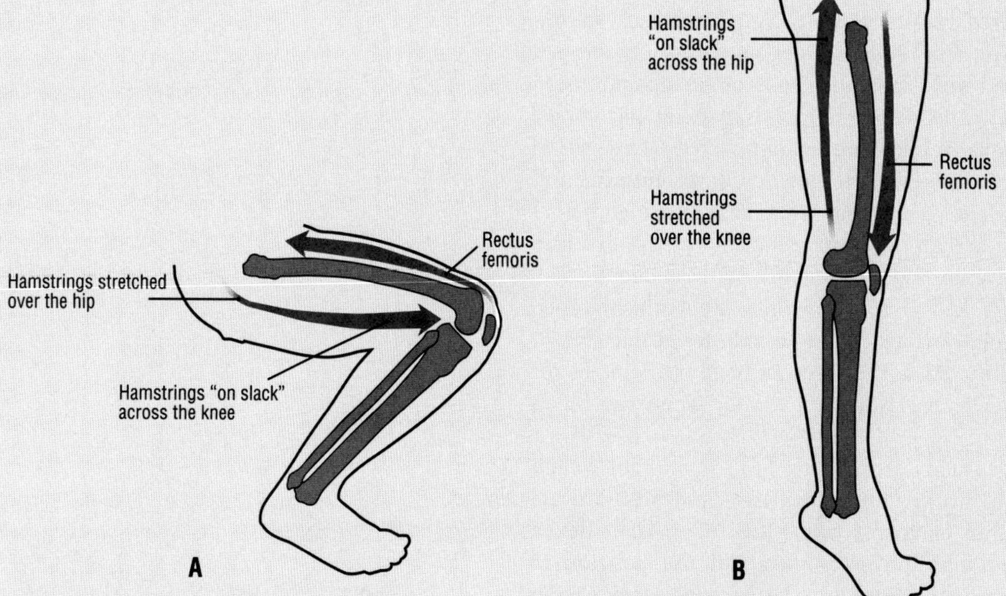

Figure 9-28 The hamstrings' ability to "trade length" when transitioning from a position of hip flexion and knee flexion to a position of hip extension and knee extension. **A,** In a squatting position the hamstrings are stretched over the hip but slackened at the knee. **B,** In standing, the hamstrings are slackened over the hip but stretched across the knee.

HIP ABDUCTORS

The primary hip abductor muscles include the gluteus medius, gluteus minimus, and tensor fasciae latae; the piriformis, sartorius, and superior fibers of the gluteus maximus are considered secondary hip abductors.

Primary Hip Abductors

- Gluteus medius
- Gluteus minimus
- Tensor fasciae latae

With the pelvis held fixed, contraction of the hip abductor muscles abducts the femur away from the midline. This action typically places a relatively low demand on these muscles. A more demanding (and common) activity imposed on these muscles occurs during closed-chain activities such as when the femur is fixed to the ground while standing on one leg (so-called single-limb support). Verify on yourself that while standing only on your right leg, "hiking" the left side of your pelvis is accomplished by a relatively strong contraction of your right hip abductors. (These muscles can be palpated midway between the greater trochanter and the iliac crest.) Similarly, eccentric activation of the right hip abductor muscles occurs while slowly lowering the left side of your pelvis. The axis of rotation for either pelvic action is in the anterior-posterior direction, through the center of the femoral head.

The most frequent demands placed on the hip abductors occur while walking. Consider, for example, the demands placed on the right abductor muscles when the right leg is in the single-limb support phase of gait, as the left limb is swinging forward (Figure 9-29). The right hip abductors must supply an adequate contraction force to keep the pelvis from "falling into the space" created by the advancing left leg. Weakness of these muscles results in an unstable pelvis while walking or while attempting to stand on one leg.

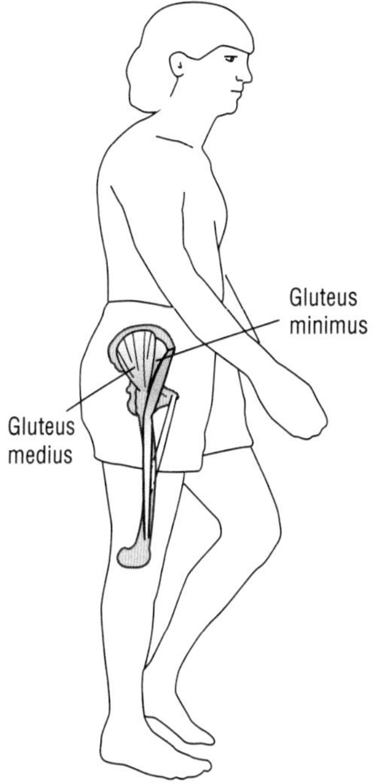

Figure 9-29 Activation of the hip abductor muscles (gluteus medius and gluteus minimus) during the stance phase of gait. (From Neumann DA: *Kinesiology of the musculoskeletal system: foundations for physical rehabilitation*, St Louis, 2002, Mosby, Figure 12-39 [*center*].)

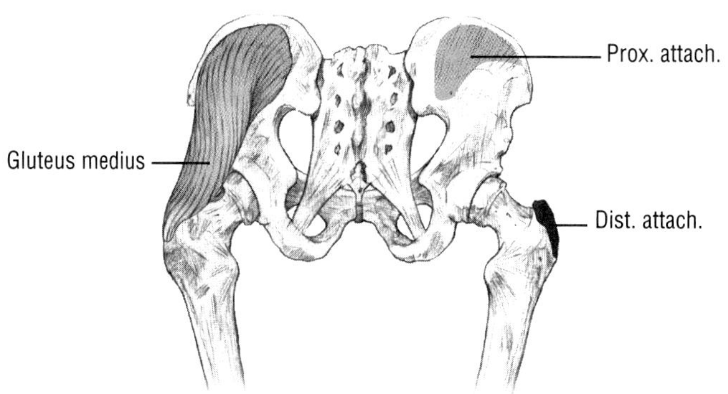

Gluteus Medius

Proximal Attachment: Outer surface of the ilium
Distal Attachment: Greater trochanter of the femur
Innervation: Superior gluteal nerve
Action: Hip abduction
Comments: The gluteus medius is the largest of the hip abductor muscles, occupying about 60% of the total abductor muscle cross-sectional area. The primary action of the gluteus medius is abduction. The muscle's anterior fibers can assist with flexion and internal rotation, whereas the posterior fibers can assist with extension and external rotation.

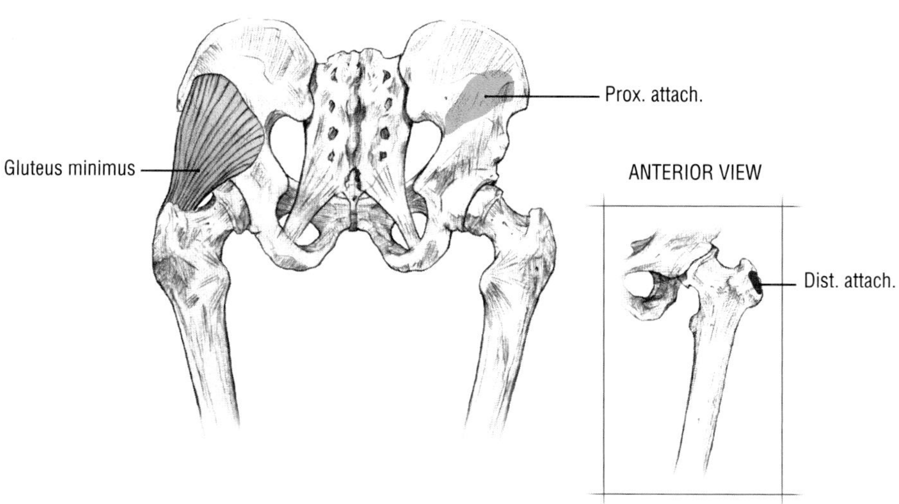

Gluteus Minimus

Proximal Attachment: Outer surface of the ilium, inferior to the gluteus medius
Distal Attachment: Greater trochanter
Innervation: Superior gluteal nerve
Actions:
- Hip abduction
- Hip internal rotation

Comments: The gluteus minimus has a similar shape to the gluteus medius, only slightly smaller. It is located deep and just anterior to the gluteus medius; this position provides the muscle with the ability to internally rotate and (with its anterior fibers) assist with flexion of the hip.

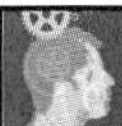

Consider this...

How the Greater Trochanter Helps Amplify Torque Production

The hip abductor muscles must generate considerable abduction torque during every single-limb support phase of gait. Recall that muscle torque is produced by the combination of a muscle's contraction force multiplied by its internal moment arm (see Chapter 1). The body often favors a design that limits the amount of force a muscle must produce for a given task—excessive force over a lifetime can damage the underlying joint. One way to minimize a muscle's force for a given task is to exaggerate the length of its internal moment arm. The gluteus medius and gluteus minimus do this by attaching to the prominent greater trochanter of the femur. This attachment significantly increases these muscles' internal moment arm for abduction. The abduction torque needed to hold the pelvis level during single-limb support can therefore be based more on moment arm length and less on muscle force. Orthopedic surgeons may purposely increase the lateral projection of the greater trochanter as a way to increase the gluteal muscles' moment arm for abduction. In theory, this alteration will reduce the force requirements on the hip abductor muscles for patients with either weak hip abductors or with a painful or unstable hip that is unable to tolerate large forces.

Functional Considerations

Important Function of the Hip Abductors: Holding the Pelvis Level While in the Single-Limb Support Phase of Walking. As introduced earlier, the hip abductor muscles play a critical role in controlling the pelvis within the frontal plane while walking. During the stance phase of gait (or while standing on one limb), the hip abductor muscles of the stance leg must hold the pelvis level, preventing it from dropping or sagging excessively to the opposite side. As the hip abductor muscles stabilize the pelvis, they also create significant forces within the hip. This fact has important clinical implications for treating someone with arthritis or an otherwise unstable or painful hip joint.

Figure 9-30 is designed to explain the force demands placed on the biomechanics of the hip abductor muscles (and hip joint) while standing on one limb. Figure 9-30 demonstrates the right hip abductor muscles (indicated by the black arrow pointing down) contracting to hold the pelvis level while standing only on the right leg. These muscles produce a pelvic-on-femoral hip abduction torque about the right hip: the product of hip abductor force *(HAF)* times the muscles' internal moment arm *(D)*. This abduction torque must counterbalance the pelvic-on-femoral adduction torque produced by body weight *(BW)* times its external moment arm (D_1). Both of these oppositely directed rotary torques are working against one another (compare dashed and solid circles). Once they are equal, the pelvis is considered to be in equilibrium: in other words, the pelvis is held level within the frontal plane.

Once in equilibrium, the compression forces produced between the femoral head and acetabulum reach several times body weight. The hip abductor muscles are responsible for most of the forces on the hip while standing on one limb—forces that can be much greater than body weight. These biomechanics exist because the hip abductors have an internal moment arm that is half the external moment used by body weight (compare D with D_1). This being the case, the hip abductors generate a force that is twice body weight—this is the only way the lever system will balance in the frontal plane.

The biomechanics of the hip abductors during single limb support (or standing on one limb) are similar to the mechanics of two persons sitting on a balanced but offset teeter-totter in the park (see D versus D_1 in the model on right). The only way the teeter-totter will remain balanced (i.e., for the pelvis to remain level and in equilibrium) is for the person on the short side of the teeter-totter (representing the hip abductors muscles) to weigh twice as much as the person on the long side (representing body weight). Every time a person stands on one limb, therefore, the hip abductors must produce a force that is at least two times body weight.

Clinical INSIGHT

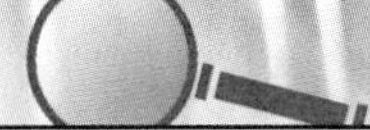

Trendelenburg Sign

Several medical conditions are associated with weakness of the hip abductor muscles. These conditions include muscular dystrophy, Guillain-Barré syndrome, and poliomyelitis. The hip abductors may also be weakened because of arthritis, instability, or surgery of the hip. The classic indicator of hip abductor weakness is a positive **Trendelenburg sign**. The Trendelenburg test is performed by having the patient assume a position of single-limb support over the affected leg. For example, if the right hip is suspected to be weak, the patient would be asked to lift the left leg and stand only on the right leg. If the patient's pelvis drops toward the unsupported leg, a positive Trendelenburg sign is registered.

Clinicians must use caution when observing this test, however, because patients often compensate by leaning their trunk to the side of the weakened stance leg. By leaning over the stance leg, the external moment arm (see D_1 in Figure 9-30) is brought closer to (or even directly over) the axis of rotation of the hip. This significantly reduces the hip abductor force needed to support the opposite side of the pelvis. When seen in gait, this compensatory lean to the side of the weakness is referred to as a gluteus medius limp or compensated Trendelenburg gait.

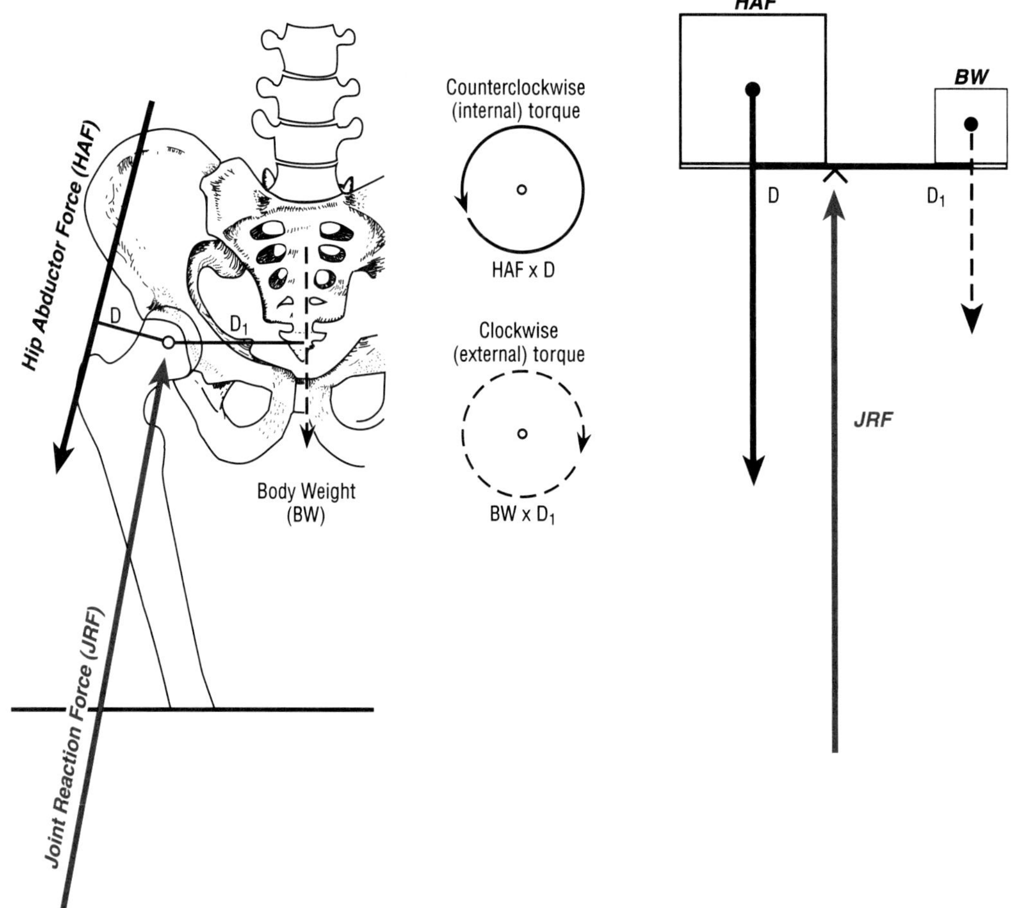

Figure 9-30 A frontal plane diagram of the right hip abductors holding the pelvis level. Note that the model *(left)* is showing a person standing only on the right leg. Hip abductor force *(HAF)* must be large because it is producing a torque about the relatively small internal moment arm of the hip *(D)*, whereas body weight *(BW)* is producing a torque in the opposite rotary direction about a much larger external moment arm (D_1). The counterclockwise torque *(solid circle)* is generated by HAF × D. The clockwise torque *(dashed circle)* is generated by BW × D_1. The combination of the hip abductor force and body weight force produces joint reaction forces *(JRF)* up to three times body weight *(red arrow)*. The analogy of the biomechanics of the hip abductor muscles is shown on right using a teeter-totter. The fulcrum of the teeter-totter is the axis of rotation of the hip joint. (From Neumann DA: Biomechanical analysis of selected principles of hip joint protection. *Arthritis Care Res* 2:146-155, 1989. Copyright American College of Rheumatology.)

Most studies indicate a total hip **joint reaction force** of three times body weight when standing on one limb. This total force is created by (1) the contraction force of the hip abductor muscles (which generates a force two times body weight) and (2) body weight itself. This total joint reaction force is indicated by the red arrows in Figure 9-30.

During the stance phase of walking, the large hip forces are well tolerated in the healthy hip. The forces actually help stabilize the hip and aid with the nutrition of the joint's articular cartilage. In a person with pain or osteoarthritis in the hip, however, these forces can aggravate the joint and can lead to further inflammation and degeneration. Clinicians often teach patients how to reduce these large forces on their hip, often referred to as principles of joint protection. Several principles, like using a cane in the hand opposite the painful hip, are based on the biomechanics of the hip abductors (Box 9-1).

Why Use a Cane in the Hand Opposite the Affected Hip? Several conditions may lead to a painful, unstable, and weak hip joint, such as osteoarthritis, fracture, loosened joint prosthesis, or many other inflammatory conditions. Therapeutic measures are often employed in physical therapy to reduce unnecessarily large forces that cross the painful or weakened hip. One easy and effective way to protect the hip from large forces is to use a cane—held in the hand opposite (contralateral to) the affected hip. Although this may sound counterintuitive, the following biomechanics will justify this premise.

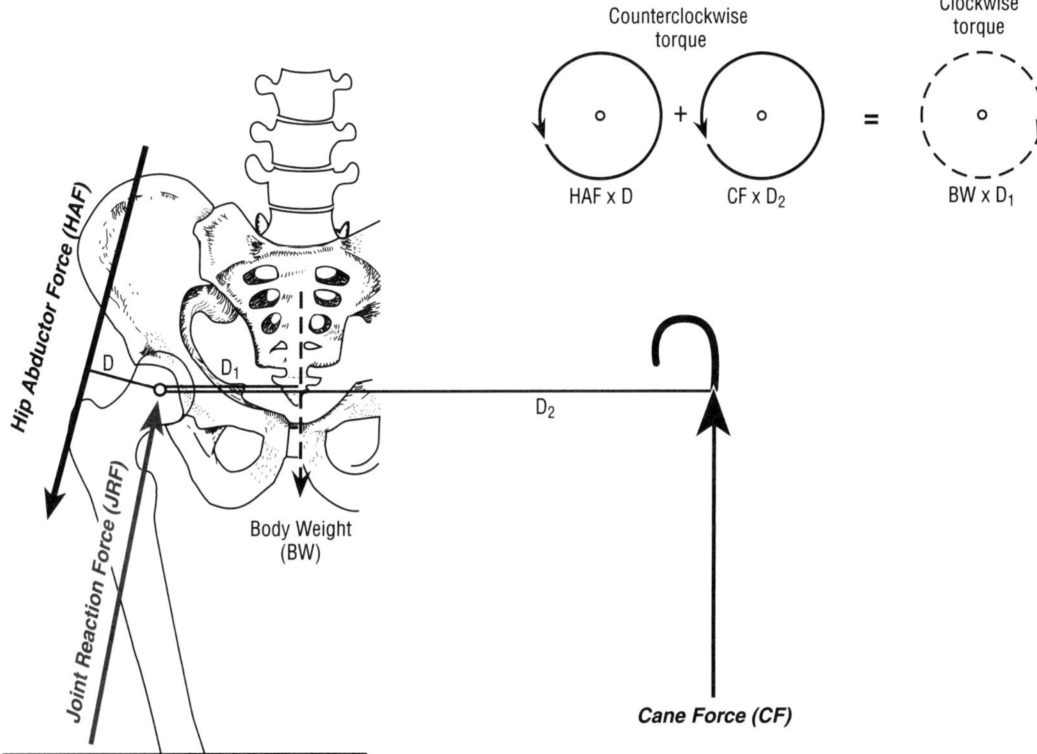

Figure 9-31 A frontal plane diagram shows how a cane used in the left hand reduces torque demands on the right hip abductor muscles. The model shows someone standing only on the right leg. Note by the direction of the small rotation circles that the torque produced by the cane force ($CF \times D_2$) acts in the *same* rotational direction as the torque produced by the hip abductors ($HAF \times D$). Less demand placed on the hip abductor muscles ultimately means less joint reaction force *(JRF)* on the hip. *D*, Internal moment arm of the hip abductors; D_1, external moment arm used by body weight (BW); D_2, external moment arm used by cane force; *HAF*, hip abductor force. (From Neumann DA: Hip abductor muscle activity in persons with a hip prosthesis while carrying load in one hand, *Phys Ther* 76:1320-1330, 1996. Copyright the American Physical Therapy Association.)

As explained previously, when in single-leg stance, the hip abductor muscles must produce large forces to hold the pelvis level. These large muscular forces (in combination with body weight) literally compress the acetabulum into the femoral head. One goal of using a cane is to reduce the demands on the hip abductor muscles and thereby reduce the compression forces on the diseased or unstable hip. Figure 9-31 shows a frontal plane model of the right hip while standing on only the right leg and applying a cane force with the left hand. The cane force acts upwards because the earth returns the same pushing force as applied downward by the hand. This cane force *(CF)*, acting with a very long moment arm (D_2), produces an abduction torque about the right hip. Note that this torque ($CF \times D_2$) tends to rotate the pelvis in the same rotation direction as the right-side hip abductor muscles ($HAF \times D$). The external torque ($BW \times D_1$) can now be balanced by $CF \times D_2$ *and* $HAF \times D$. In this way, the cane force acts as a very effective substitute for much of the torque that must be produced by the right hip abductors. The pelvis can therefore be kept level with less force demands on the hip abductor muscles and underlying hip joint. In theory, applying a modest cane force of only 10% of a person's body weight can reduce the hip joint force during the single limb support by about 50%.

BOX 9-1

Principles of Hip Joint Protection

Many solutions can help to protect a pathologic hip from further degeneration or inflammation, as follows:

- Use a cane in the hand opposite the affected hip.
- Lose excess body weight.
- Walk slowly.
- Correct faulty postures such as a hip flexion contracture.
- Maintain relative flexibility of muscles about the hip and lower back.
- Avoid carrying heavy loads, especially one-handed loads held on the side opposite the painful hip. Such a method of carrying a load produces large external torques on the hip abductors and underlying joint.
- Avoid excessive bending or standing on one limb.

HIP ADDUCTORS

The primary hip adductors are the pectineus, adductor longus, gracilis, adductor brevis, and adductor magnus. The primary function of this muscle group is, of course, to create adduction torque, bringing the lower extremity toward the midline. As explained later, this adduction torque can also bring the pubic symphysis region of the pelvis closer to the femur. From the anatomic position, the adductors are also considered hip flexor muscles.

Primary Hip Adductors

- Pectineus
- Adductor longus
- Gracilis
- Adductor brevis
- Adductor magnus—both heads

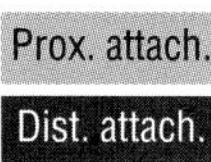

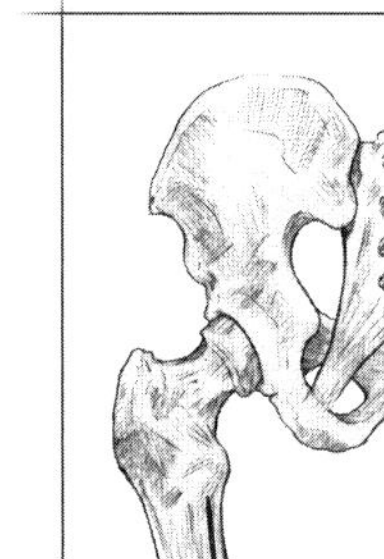

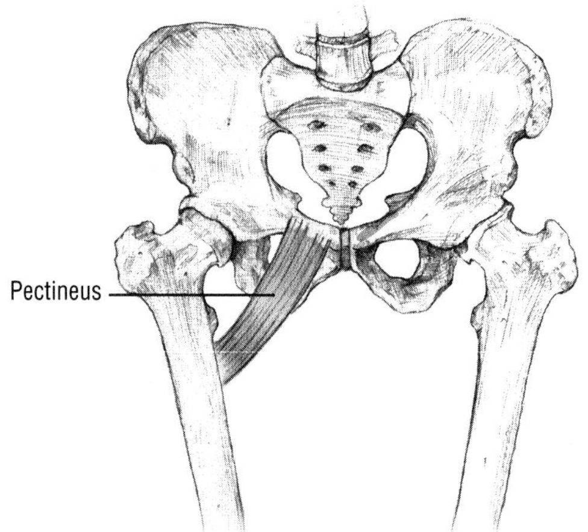

Pectineus

Proximal Attachment:	Pectineal line on superior pubic ramus
Distal Attachment:	Pectineal line on the posterior surface of the femur
Innervation:	Obturator nerve
Actions:	• Hip adduction • Hip flexion
Comments:	The short, rectangular pectineus muscle has the most proximal attachment to the femur of any hip adductor muscle.

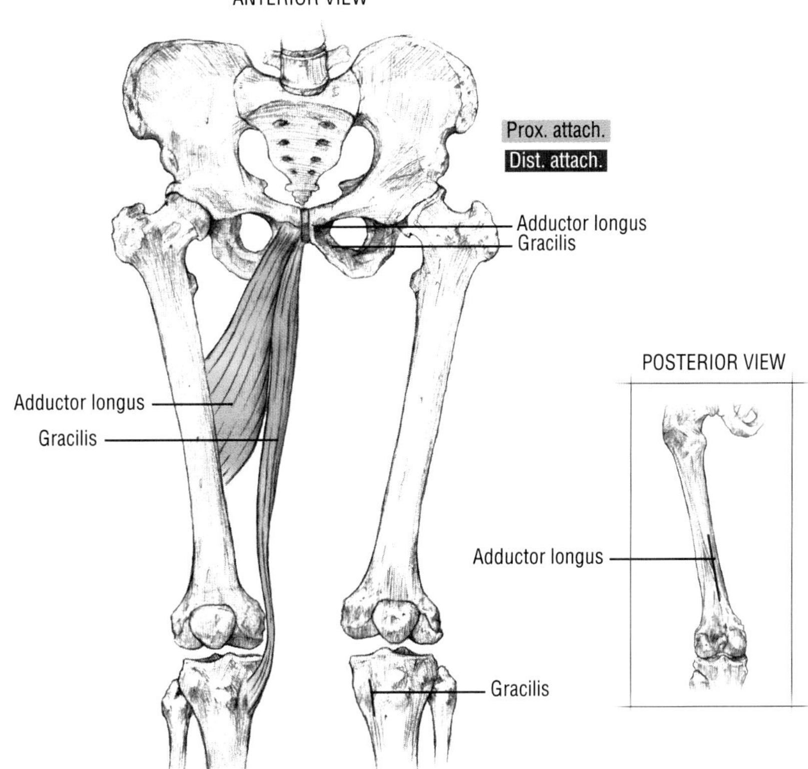

An anterior view of the hip showing the adductor longus and gracilis muscles.

Adductor Longus

Proximal Attachment: Anterior surface of the body of the pubis

Distal Attachment: Middle one third of the linea aspera of the femur

Innervation: Obturator nerve

Actions:
- Hip adduction
- Hip flexion

Comments: This is one of the most superficial adductor muscles.

Gracilis

Proximal Attachment: Body and inferior ramus of the pubis

Distal Attachment: Proximal-medial aspect of the tibia (pes anserinus)

Innervation: Obturator nerve

Actions:
- Hip adduction
- Hip flexion
- Knee flexion
- Knee internal rotation

Comments: The word *gracilis* is related to the word *gracile*, which means "gracefully slender." The tendinous insertion of the gracilis forms part of the pes anserinus, providing some medial support to the knee.

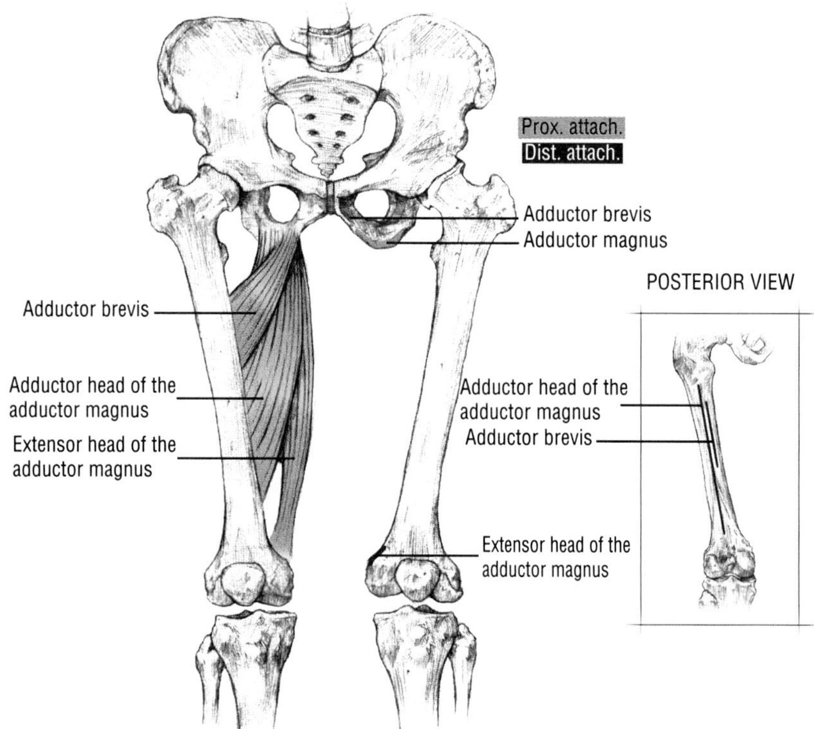

Adductor Brevis

Proximal Attachment: Anterior surface of the inferior pubic ramus

Distal Attachment: Proximal one third of the linea aspera of the femur

Innervation: Obturator nerve

Actions:
- Hip adduction
- Hip flexion

Comments: The adductor brevis occupies the middle layer of the adductors, just deep to the adductor longus.

Adductor Magnus

Extensor (Posterior) Head

Proximal Attachment: Ischial tuberosity

Distal Attachment: Adductor tubercle on distal femur

Innervation: Tibial portion of the sciatic nerve

Actions:
- Hip extension
- Hip adduction

Adductor (Anterior) Head

Proximal Attachment: Ischial ramus

Distal Attachment: Entire linea aspera of femur

Innervation: Obturator nerve

Actions:
- Hip adduction
- Hip flexion

Comments: The adductor magnus has two distinct heads: an adductor (anterior) head and an extensor (posterior) head. Both muscles are primary adductors of the hip. The extensor head, however, is similar to the hamstrings in its innervation (sciatic nerve), hip extension ability, and proximal attachments. The adductor head, in contrast, is similar to the adductor brevis in its innervation (obturator nerve), hip flexion ability, and proximal attachments.

Functional Considerations

Frontal Plane Function of the Adductor Muscles. The most obvious function of the adductor muscles is to adduct the femur (e.g., accelerating the lower extremity across the midline to kick a soccer ball). With the foot fixed to the ground, this muscle group can also rapidly lower the contralateral side of the pelvis. Figure 9-32 shows the adductor muscles contracting bilaterally to perform both these types of motions. In this figure, several of the right adductors are shown accelerating the lower extremity toward the ball. The left hip adductors add forcefulness to this action by actively lowering the right side of the pelvis.

Sagittal Plane Function of the Adductor Muscles. Regardless of the position of the hip, the extensor head of the adductor magnus is a powerful hip extensor. The remaining hip adductor muscles, however, can function as either hip flexors or hip extensors, depending on the position of the hip. At first, this may seem impossible for one muscle to have opposite actions. To explain, Figure 9-33 shows the adductor longus as a representative adductor muscle during a fast sprint. When the hip is flexed greater than about 50 to 60 degrees (see Figure 9-33, *A*), the line of pull of the adductor longus falls *posterior* to the medial-lateral axis of the hip,

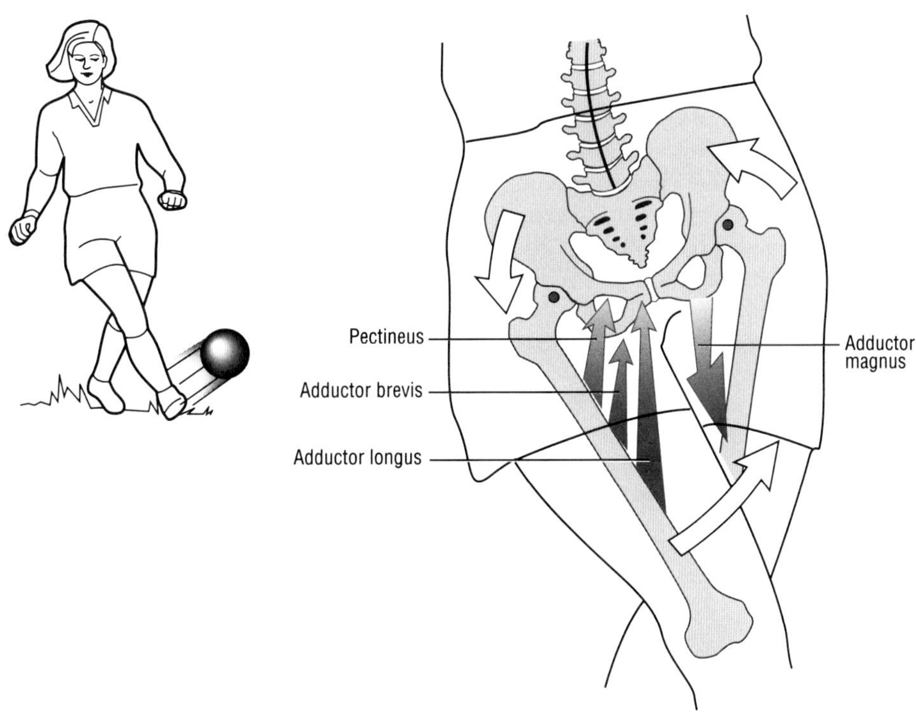

Figure 9-32 The bilateral cooperation of the adductor muscles while kicking a soccer ball. The left adductor magnus is shown actively producing pelvic-on-femoral adduction, lowering the right side of the pelvis. Several right adductors are shown producing femoral-on-pelvic adduction, accelerating the right lower extremity toward the midline. (From Neumann DA: *Kinesiology of the musculoskeletal system: foundations for physical rehabilitation*, St Louis, 2002, Mosby, Figure 12-35.)

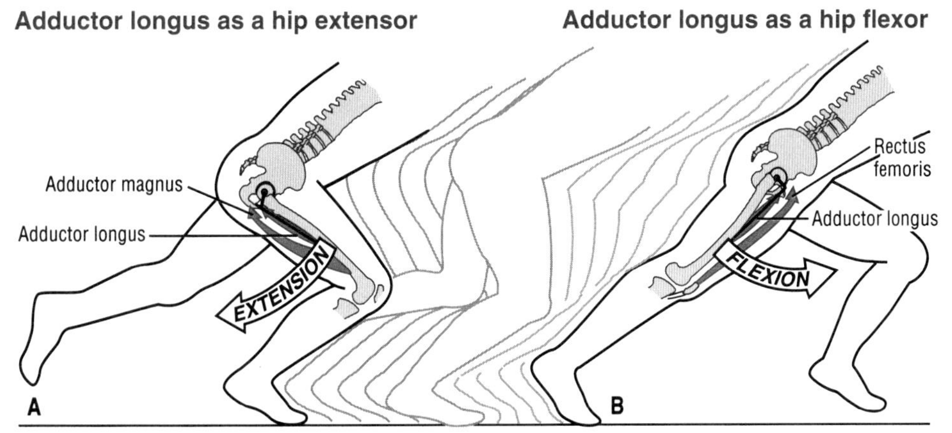

Figure 9-33 The adductor longus is shown as a representative adductor, displaying the ability to both flex and extend the hip. **A,** In a position of hip flexion, the adductors can produce hip extension torque. **B,** In a position of hip extension the adductors can produce hip flexion torque. (From Neumann DA: *Kinesiology of the musculoskeletal system: foundations for physical rehabilitation*, St Louis, 2002, Mosby, Figure 12-36.)

allowing it to function as a hip extensor, similar to the adductor magnus. In contrast, however, when the hip is in an extended position (see Figure 9-33, *B*), the line of pull of the adductor longus falls *anterior* to the medial-lateral axis of the hip, similar to that in the rectus femoris. The sagittal plane action of the adductors therefore shifts as the muscles shift their position relative to the axis of rotation. The adductors therefore provide a useful source of flexion and extension torque for the hip during activities such as sprinting and cycling or descending and rising from a deep squat. This task of switching from flexor to extensor may help explain the relatively high susceptibility of the adductors to muscle strain injuries while running.

EXTERNAL ROTATORS

The primary external rotators of the hip are the gluteus maximus, sartorius, and the six short external rotators: piriformis, gemellus superior, obturator internus, gemellus inferior, obturator externus, and quadratus femoris (Figure 9-34). The anatomy of the gluteus maximus and sartorius were discussed in previous sections. The attachments, innervation, and action of the six short external rotators are listed in the table on p. 267. The function of the short external rotators is described as a group, not individually.

Primary Hip External Rotators

- Gluteus maximus
- Sartorius
- Piriformis
- Gemellus superior
- Obturator internus
- Gemellus inferior
- Obturator externus
- Quadratus femoris

Functional Considerations: Driving the Cutting Motion in Many Sporting Activities

Like many of the muscles of the hip, the external rotators express their primary function when the lower limb is in contact with the ground. As a point of reference, horizontal plane rotation of the pelvis (relative to a stationary femur) is described by the rotational direction of a point on the *anterior side* of the pelvis, such as the pubic symphysis. For example, with the right femur securely fixed, contraction of the right external rotators will rotate the pelvis to the left (an action often referred to as contralateral pelvic rotation). Contralateral pelvic rotation occurs commonly during cutting motions while running (e.g., when a

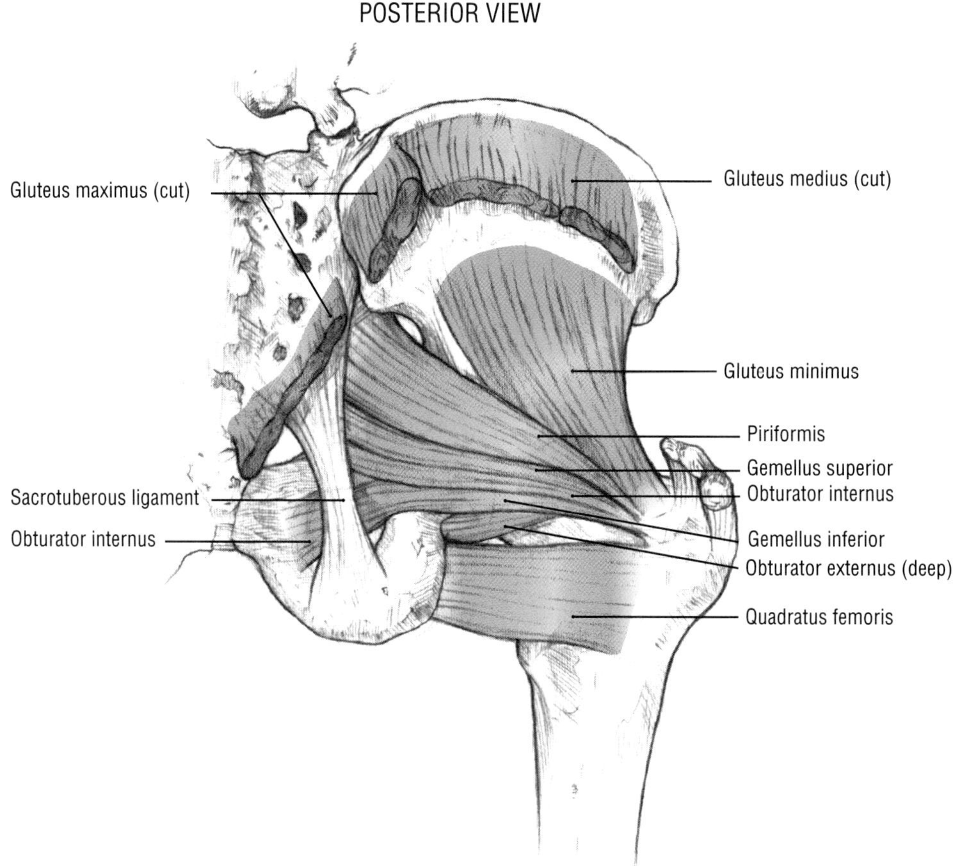

Figure 9-34 The short external rotators of the hip: piriformis, gemellus superior, obturator internus, gemellus inferior, obturator externus, and quadratus femoris.

SUMMARY OF THE SIX SHORT EXTERNAL ROTATOR MUSCLES

Muscle	Proximal Attachment	Distal Attachment	Action	Innervation
Piriformis	Anterior side of sacrum	Apex of the greater trochanter	External rotation	Nerve to the piriformis
Obturator internus	Internal side of the obturator membrane and surrounding structures	Greater trochanter	External rotation	Nerve to the obturator internus
Obturator externus	External surface of the obturator membrane and surrounding structures	Greater trochanter (at the trochanteric fossa)	External rotation	Obturator nerve
Gemellus superior	Dorsal surface of the ischial spine	Greater trochanter; blends with the tendon of the obturator internus	External rotation	Nerve to the obturator internus
Gemellus inferior	Tuberosity of the ischium	Greater trochanter; blends with the tendon of the obturator internus	External rotation	Nerve to the quadratus femoris
Quadratus femoris	Lateral surface of the ischial tuberosity	Quadrate tubercle	External rotation	Nerve to the quadratus femoris

sprinting football player plants his right foot and cuts sharply to the left). This action is driven by the right external rotator muscles (Figure 9-35).

The powerful gluteus maximus is near-perfectly designed to assist the other external rotators with this action. Recall that the gluteus maximus is a hip extensor *and* external rotator. Upon planting the right foot (with the left leg free), the right gluteus maximus can quickly and powerfully rotate the pelvis to the left (contralateral pelvic-on-femoral rotation). Once the pelvis has rotated, the gluteus maximus is immediately poised to provide the large hip extension torque needed to accelerate the athlete in the new direction.

The six external rotator muscles can assist the gluteus maximus with the cutting motion. In addition to generating fine control over the pelvic rotation, the short external rotators are also important dynamic stabilizers of the hip. Similar to the rotator cuff muscles of the shoulder, the short external rotators have a nearly horizontal line of pull, allowing them to efficiently compress the femoral head securely into the acetabulum.

INTERNAL ROTATORS

For any muscle to produce a strong internal rotation torque, it must have a significant portion of its fibers oriented in the horizontal plane. Such an orientation allows the muscle's line of pull to intersect the shaft of the femur at a 90-degree angle—this position would maximize a muscle's torque potential. This orientation is

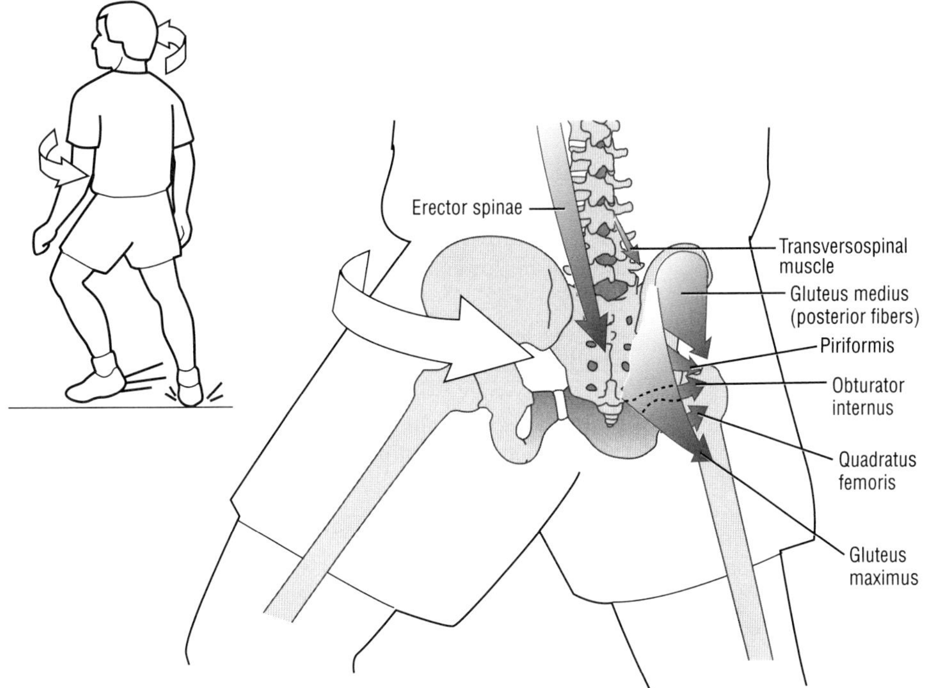

Figure 9-35 The right external rotators are shown performing pelvic-on-femoral (closed-chain) external rotation during a cutting motion to the left. (From Neumann DA: *Kinesiology of the musculoskeletal system: foundations for physical rehabilitation,* St Louis, 2002, Mosby, Figure 12-47.)

precisely why the external rotator muscles (discussed earlier) are so effective at active contralateral rotation of the pelvis relative to the stationary femur. Most internal rotator muscles, however, have a near-vertical orientation, at least from the anatomic position. For this reason no individual muscle is capable of generating a very strong internal rotation torque. The internal rotation torque that is generated occurs as a summation of forces from three muscles: the anterior fibers of the gluteus medius, the gluteus minimus, and the tensor fasciae latae. The anatomy of these muscles was described previously in this chapter. These muscles help change the direction of the advancing limb while walking and help balance the force of other flexor muscles that are also external rotators, such as the sartorius.

Primary Internal Rotators of the Hip

- Gluteus medius (anterior fibers)
- Gluteus minimus
- Tensor fasciae latae

Although the internal rotator muscles are oriented nearly parallel to the shaft of the femur when the hip is extended, their orientation approaches a 90-degree intersection with the femur when the hip is flexed. Consequently, internal rotation torque increases by 50% when the hip is shifted from extension to a flexed position. This fact should be kept in mind when performing a manual muscle test on a person's internal rotator muscles.

Clinical **INSIGHT**

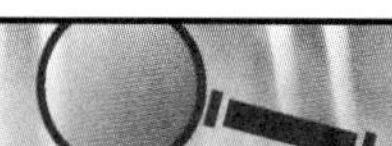

Unwanted Strength Dominance in the Internal Rotator Muscles

Many persons with cerebral palsy are able to ambulate, often with the assistance of a cane or crutches. A typical gait pattern often displayed by these individuals is called a crouched gait. The term *crouched* refers primarily to the flexed and internal rotated position of the hips while walking.

Weak hip extensors and overly strong (and often spastic) hip flexor muscles are largely responsible for the exaggerated hip flexion component of the crouched gait. Interestingly (and as described earlier), increased hip flexion significantly enhances the leverage and therefore strength of the internal rotator muscles. In fact, the internal rotator muscles often dominate the crouched appearance of the gait. One form of conservative treatment for the crouched gait is to stretch the hip flexor muscles and strengthen the hip extensor muscles. If successful, this approach will result in the ability of the person to stand and walk in greater hip extension. A posture of greater hip extension (and less hip flexion) will rob some of the excessive dominance of the internal rotator muscles. Often surgery is required to release some of the more dominating internal rotator muscles, as well as some of the adductor muscles.

Summary

Like all the joints of the body, the hip must satisfy the needs of stability and mobility. Functional activities such as walking, running, going up steps, and transitioning from sitting to standing all require large ranges of hip motion. At the same time, however, the hip must provide the stability needed to support the large weight-bearing, gravitational, and muscular forces that assault the hip in a nearly infinite number of directions. The hip joint solves both problems through its bony structure, ligamentous support, and the balance of the numerous surrounding muscles.

The ball-in-socket structure of the joint not only provides ample mobility in all three planes, but the deep cup of the acetabulum creates a stable bony structure to house the femoral head. In addition, strong ligaments exist that stabilize the hip. This ligamentous stability is strongly reinforced by a number of other strong muscles.

To truly understand the function of the hip, one must appreciate its relationship to the lumbar spine. The lumbar spine is directly linked to the pelvis (both anatomically and functionally) and is often called on to amplify pelvic-on-femoral motion (e.g., bending forward to pick an object off the ground requires simultaneous flexion of the hip and spine). Conversely, the lumbar spine may be required to compensate for certain pelvic-on-femoral motions, such as increasing its lordosis during an anterior pelvic tilt.

Because of its central location, dysfunction of the hip can generate a number of problems up and down the kinematic chain. In fact, many problems of the lower back and lower limb are thought to originate at the hip. Facilitating proper alignment and function of the hip is often the basis for treating dysfunction in the low-back region and the more distal lower limb.

Study Questions

1. *Coxa valga* describes:
   a. The position of the hip when standing with an anterior pelvic tilt
   b. An angle of inclination significantly greater than 125 degrees
   c. The position of the hip when standing with a posterior pelvic tilt
   d. An angle of inclination significantly less than 125 degrees

2. The anterior superior iliac spine is a bony landmark found on the:
   a. Ischium
   b. Proximal femur
   c. Ilium
   d. Pubis
3. The iliofemoral, ischiofemoral, and pubofemoral ligaments all limit:
   a. Extension of the hip
   b. Flexion of the hip
   c. Abduction of the hip
   d. Internal rotation of the hip
4. Standing with a hip flexion contracture is likely to:
   a. Involve a hyperlordotic posture of the lumbar spine
   b. Involve a posterior pelvic tilt
   c. Over-stretch the iliofemoral ligament
   d. A and C
   e. B and C
5. Which of the following best describes an anterior pelvic tilt?
   a. Short-arc, pelvic-on-femoral hip extension with the trunk remaining essentially upright
   b. Short-arc, pelvic-on-femoral hip flexion with the trunk remaining essentially upright
   c. An open-chain hip extension motion
   d. Long-arc hip flexion with the trunk moving the same direction as the pelvis
6. The normal range of motion for hip flexion is:
   a. 0 to 90 degrees
   b. 0 to 50 degrees
   c. 0 to 30 degrees
   d. 0 to 120 degrees
7. Which of the following statements is true regarding an individual hiking the right side of the pelvis?
   a. This motion is produced by active contraction of the right hip abductors
   b. This motion involves closed-chain abduction of the left hip
   c. This motion involves activation of the left gluteus medius
   d. A and C
   e. B and C
8. Which group of muscles is largely innervated by the obturator nerve?
   a. Hip extensors
   b. Hip abductors
   c. Hip adductors
   d. Hip external rotators
9. Which of the following actions occurs in the horizontal plane?
   a. Hip flexion
   b. Hip internal rotation
   c. Hip abduction
   d. Hip extension
10. Which of the following muscles is a primary hip flexor?
    a. Iliopsoas
    b. Semitendinosus
    c. Piriformis
    d. Gluteus maximus
11. Which of the following muscles is involved with the force-couple that produces a posterior pelvic tilt?
    a. Iliopsoas
    b. Gluteus maximus
    c. Rectus abdominis
    d. A and B
    e. B and C
12. An anterior pelvic tilt involves:
    a. A force-couple between the gluteus maximus and the erector spinae
    b. Increasing lordosis of the lumbar spine
    c. Decreasing lordosis of the lumbar spine
    d. Strong activation of the hamstring muscles
13. If the abdominal muscles are weak, resisted hip flexion will likely result in:
    a. Increased lordosis of the lumbar spine
    b. Decreased lordosis of the lumbar spine
    c. Co-activation of the gluteus maximus
    d. Rupture of the pubofemoral ligament
14. Which of the following statements is true regarding a posterior pelvic tilt?
    a. Involves increasing lordosis of the lumbar spine
    b. Is performed by a force-couple involving the iliopsoas and the erector spinae
    c. Involves decreasing lordosis of the lumbar spine
    d. A and B
    e. B and C
15. When the hip is flexed to 70 degrees:
    a. The gluteus maximus is slackened.
    b. Many of the adductors have a favorable line of pull to perform hip extension.
    c. The iliofemoral ligament becomes taut.
    d. The psoas major is maximally elongated.
16. When standing only on the right leg, the primary muscles involved in keeping the left side of the pelvis from dropping are the:
    a. Left hip abductors
    b. Right hip abductors
    c. Left hip adductors
    d. Right hip adductors
17. If a patient's left hip is arthritic or painful, a clinician would most likely recommend:
    a. The patient perform heavy resistive exercises with the left leg
    b. The patient use a cane in the left hand
    c. The patient perform deep squatting exercises
    d. The patient use a cane in the right hand
18. The right external rotators of the hip are highly involved in which of the following activities?
    a. Planting the right foot and cutting sharply to the left
    b. Planting the left foot and cutting sharply to the right
    c. Strongly adducting the hip across the midline
    d. Flexing the hip past 100 degrees

19. Which of the following is *not* an action of the gluteus maximus?
    a. Hip extension
    b. Hip external rotation
    c. Posterior pelvic tilt
    d. Hip internal rotation
20. Which of the following statements is true?
    a. Normal range of motion for hip external rotation is 0 to 15 degrees
    b. Normal range of motion for hip extension is 0 to 90 degrees
    c. Normal range of motion for hip abduction is 0 to 40 degrees
    d. Normal range of motion for hip flexion is 0 to 100 degrees
21. When stretching the iliopsoas muscle, the pelvis must be stabilized to prevent:
    a. Unwanted lordosis of the lumbar spine
    b. Unwanted stretching of the hamstrings
    c. Excessive flattening of the lumbar spine
    d. Activation of the quadriceps muscles
22. An anterior pelvic tilt is a type of hip flexion.
    a. True
    b. False
23. During standing at ease, the line of gravity (from body weight) normally travels anterior to the medial-lateral axis of the hip.
    a. True
    b. False
24. A posterior pelvic tilt is accompanied by decreasing lordosis of the lumbar spine.
    a. True
    b. False
25. If a man with osteoarthritis of the right hip must carry a load such as a suitcase, he should carry it on the right side.
    a. True
    b. False
26. The rectus femoris is maximally elongated in a position of hip flexion and knee flexion.
    a. True
    b. False
27. Three of the four hamstring muscles attach proximally to the ischial tuberosity.
    a. True
    b. False
28. The hip joint is a condyloid joint allowing 2 degrees of freedom.
    a. True
    b. False
29. Abduction of the hip occurs about a medial-lateral axis of rotation.
    a. True
    b. False
30. A positive Trendelenburg sign indicates weakness of the hip adductors.
    a. True
    b. False

ADDITIONAL READINGS

Andersson E, Oddsson L, Grundstrom H et al: The role of the psoas and iliacus muscles for stability and movement of the lumbar spine, pelvis and hip, *Scand J Med Sci Sports* 5:10-16, 1995.

Arnold AS, Asakawa DJ, Delp SL: Do the hamstrings and adductors contribute to excessive internal rotation of the hip in persons with cerebral palsy? *Gait Posture* 11:181-190, 2000.

Bergmann G, Graichen F, Rohlmann A: Hip joint loading during walking and running, measured in two patients, *J Biomech* 26:969-990, 1993.

Broadhurst NA, Simmons DN, Bond MJ: Piriformis syndrome: correlation of muscle morphology with symptoms and signs, *Arch Phys Med Rehabil* 85:2036-2039, 2004.

Cahalan TD, Johnson ME, Liu S et al: Quantitative measurements of hip strength in different age groups, *Clin Orthop* September (246):136-145, 1989.

Crawford JR, Villar RN: Current concepts in the management of femoroacetabular impingement, *J Bone Joint Surg Br* 87:1459-1462, 2005.

Dewberry MJ, Bohannon RW, Tiberio D et al: Pelvic and femoral contributions to bilateral hip flexion by subjects suspended from a bar, *Clin Biomech (Bristol, Avon)* 18:494-499, 2003.

Dostal WF, Andrews JG: A three-dimensional biomechanical model of hip musculature, *J Biomech* 14:803-812, 1981.

Eckstein F, von Eisenhart-Rothe R, Landgraf J et al: Quantitative analysis of incongruity, contact areas and cartilage thickness in the human hip joint, *Acta Anatomica* 58:192-204, 1997.

Fuss FK, Bacher A: New aspects of the morphology and function of the human hip joint ligaments, *Am J Anat* 192:1-13, 1991.

Kendall FP, McCreary AK, Provance PG: *Muscles testing and function*, ed 4, Baltimore, 1993, Williams & Wilkins.

Krebs DE, Elbaum L, Riley PO et al: Exercise and gait effects on in vivo hip contact pressures, *Phys Ther* 71:301-309, 1991.

Kurrat HJ, Oberlander W: The thickness of the cartilage in the hip joint, *J Anat* 126:145-155, 1978.

Lengsfeld M, Pressel T, Stammberger U: Lengths and lever arms of hip joint muscles: geometrical analyses using a human multibody model, *Gait Posture* 6:18-26, 1997.

Lewis CL, Sahrmann SA: Acetabular labral tears, *Phys Ther* 86:110-121, 2006.

Moore KL, Persaud TVN: *The developing human: clinically oriented embryology*, ed 7, St Louis, 2003, Saunders.

Neumann DA: Hip abductor muscle activity in persons with a hip prosthesis while carrying loads in one hand, *Phys Ther* 76:1320-1330, 1996.

Neumann DA: Hip abductor muscle activity as subjects with hip prostheses walk with different methods of using a cane, *Phys Ther* 78:490-501, 1998.

Neumann DA: An electromyographic study of the hip abductor muscles as subjects with a hip prosthesis walked with different methods of using a cane and carrying a load, *Phys Ther* 79:1163-1173, 1999.

Neumann DA: Biomechanical analysis of selected principles of hip joint protection, *Arthritis Care Res* 2:146-155, 1989.

Neumann DA, Soderberg GL, Cook TM: Comparison of maximal isometric hip abductor muscle torques between hip sides, *Phys Ther* 68:496-502, 1988.

Roach KE, Miles TP: Normal hip and knee active range of motion: the relationship to age, *Phys Ther* 71:656-665, 1991.

Soderberg GL, Dostal WF: Electromyographic study of three parts of the gluteus medius muscle during functional activities, *Phys Ther* 58:691-696, 1978.

Standring S: *Gray's anatomy: the anatomical basis of clinical practice*, ed 39, New York, 2005, Churchill Livingstone.

Wingstrand H, Wingstrand A, Krantz P: Intracapsular and atmospheric pressure in the dynamics and stability of the hip: a biomechanical study, *Acta Orthop Scand* 61:231-235, 1990.

CHAPTER 10

Structure and Function of the Knee

CHAPTER OUTLINE

OBJECTIVES

- Identify the bones and primary bony features of the knee.
- Describe the primary supporting structures of the knee.
- Describe the planes of motion and axes of rotation for the motions of the knee.
- Cite the proximal and distal attachments of the muscles of the knee.
- List the innervation of the muscles of the knee.
- Justify the primary actions of the muscles of the knee.
- Describe the factors that contribute to excessive lateral tracking of the patella.
- Explain how patellofemoral joint compression force is increased or decreased relative to the depth of a squatting position.
- Describe one biomechanical consequence associated with hamstring tightness.
- Explain the principles of active and passive insufficiency in regard to the multi-articular muscles of the knee.
- Describe the combined movements at the hip and knee that promote the most effective force production in the hamstrings and rectus femoris.

KEY TERMS

compression forces
excessive genu valgum
extensor lag
genu recurvatum
genu valgum
genu varum
lateral tracking of the patella
pes anserinus
Q-angle
screw-home mechanism

The knee consists of the tibiofemoral joint and the patellofemoral joint. As illustrated in Figure 10-1, the tibiofemoral joint is formed between the large condyles of the distal femur and the relatively flat proximal tibia. The patellofemoral joint is formed between the patella and the distal femur. Both joints are considered anatomic components of the knee.

Motion at the knee occurs in two planes: flexion and extension in the sagittal plane and internal and external rotation in the horizontal plane. Most activities, however, require that the knee move simultaneously in both planes such as while running and quickly changing directions. Also, because the knee functions as the middle joint of the lower extremity, most everyday motions such as

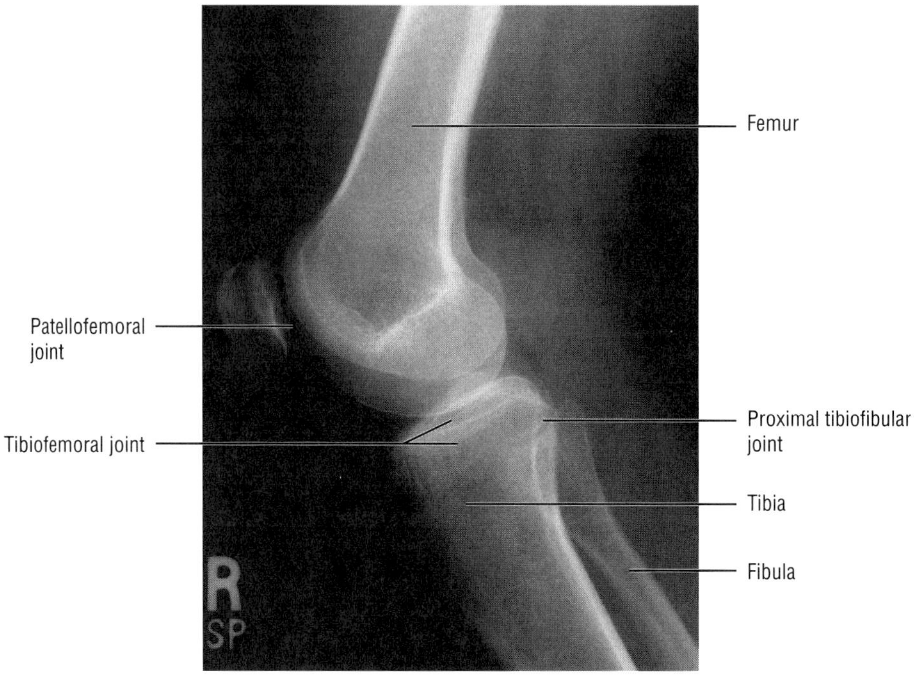

Femur
Patellofemoral joint
Proximal tibiofibular joint
Tibiofemoral joint
Tibia
Fibula

Figure 10-1 A radiograph showing the bones and associated articulations of the knee. (From Neumann DA: *Kinesiology of the musculoskeletal system: foundations for physical rehabilitation,* St Louis, 2002, Mosby, Figure 13-1.)

standing up from a seated position require simultaneous movement at the hip and ankle. This kinematic interdependence is evident by the many multi-articular muscles of the lower extremity such as the hamstrings, rectus femoris, and gastrocnemius. The anatomic and kinesiologic relationships among the knee, hip, and ankle provide the foundation for many treatment strategies used in the rehabilitation of the knee.

Unlike the hip joint, the tibiofemoral joints of the knee lack a deep concave socket. From the perspective of bony fit, therefore, the knee is relatively unstable. Many strong ligaments and muscles are therefore required for stabilization. These soft tissues are very vulnerable to injury. Many principles of rehabilitation and assessment of the knee require a firm working knowledge of the anatomy of these soft tissues. The anatomy and function of these tissues is an important theme of this chapter.

Osteology

Distal Femur

The *medial* and *lateral condyles* (from the Greek *kondylos,* meaning "knuckle") are the large rounded projections of the distal femur that articulate with the medial and lateral condyles of the tibia. The *intercondylar groove* is the smooth rounded area between the femoral condyles that articulates with the posterior surface of the patella (Figure 10-2). The *intercondylar notch* is located on the posterior-inferior aspect of the distal femur, separating the medial and lateral condyles. This notch forms a passageway for the anterior and posterior cruciate ligaments. The *medial* and *lateral epicondyles* (Figure 10-3) are palpable bony projections on the medial and lateral femoral condyles, respectively; these projections serve as attachments for the medial and lateral collateral ligaments of the knee.

Proximal Tibia

The *medial* and *lateral condyles* of the *tibia* are smooth and shallow for articulation with the condyles of the femur (Figure 10-4). The flattened superior surfaces of the condyles are often called the tibial plateau. The *intercondylar eminence* is a double-pointed projection of bone separating the medial and lateral condyles of the tibia. This structure serves as an attachment for the anterior and posterior cruciate ligaments, as well as the medial and lateral meniscus. The *tibial tuberosity* is a protrusion of bone located on the anterior aspect of the proximal tibia, which serves as the distal attachment for the quadriceps muscle.

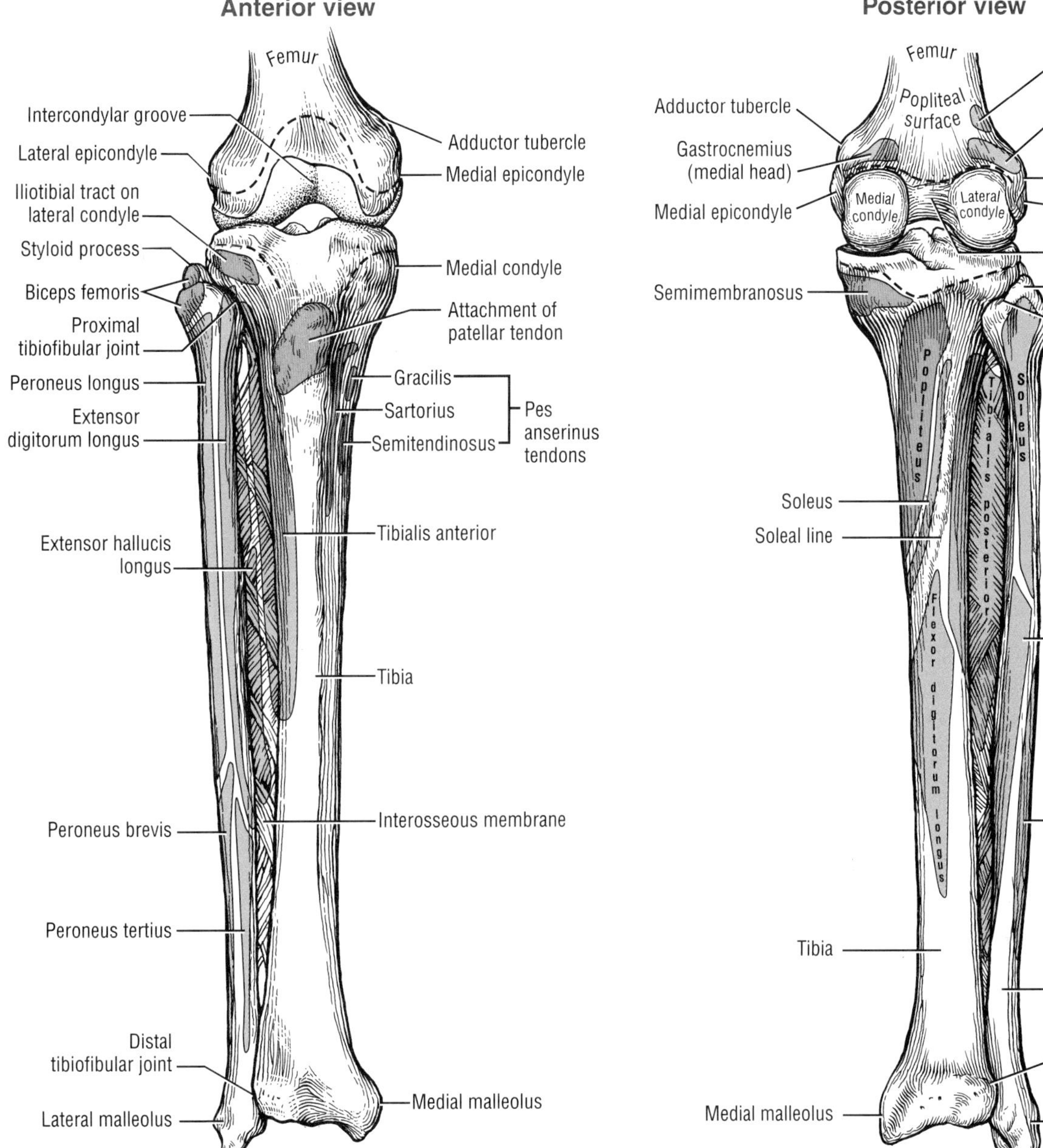

Figure 10-2 Anterior view of the right distal femur, tibia, and fibula. Proximal attachments of muscles are shown in red, distal attachments in gray. (From Neumann DA: *Kinesiology of the musculoskeletal system: foundations for physical rehabilitation*, St Louis, 2002, Mosby, Figure 13-2.)

Figure 10-3 Posterior view of the right distal femur, tibia, and fibula. Proximal attachments of muscles are shown in red, distal attachments in gray. (From Neumann DA: *Kinesiology of the musculoskeletal system: foundations for physical rehabilitation*, St Louis, 2002, Mosby, Figure 13-3.)

Figure 10-4 An anterior view of the tibia showing the tibial condyles, intercondylar eminence, and tibial tuberosity.

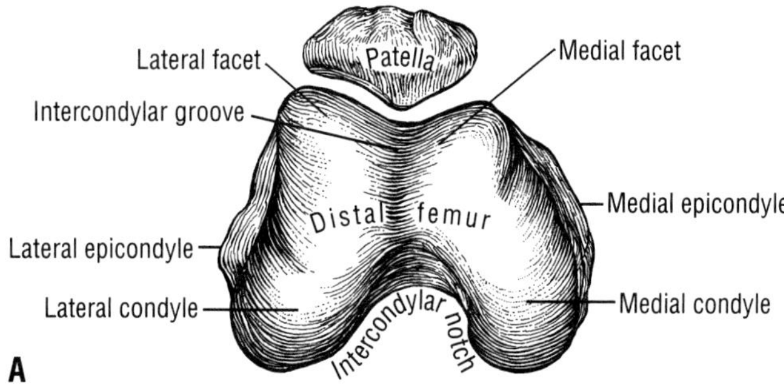

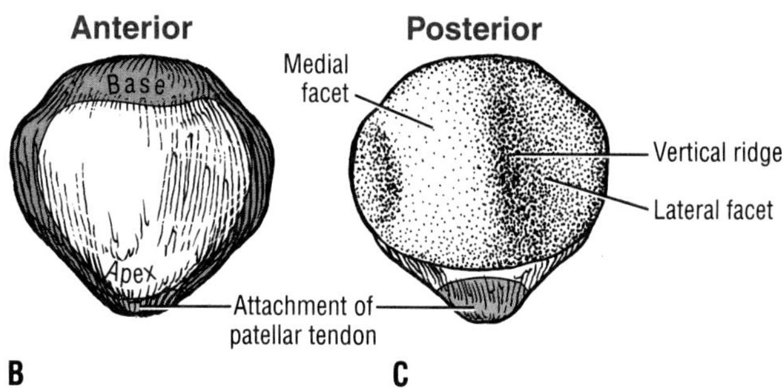

Figure 10-5 Three different views of the patella: **A**, inferior view, showing the matching articular surfaces of the posterior patella and intercondylar groove of the femur; **B**, anterior view of the patella; and **C**, posterior view of the patella. The attachment of the quadriceps muscle is shown in gray; the proximal attachment of the patellar tendon is shown in red. (Modified from Neumann DA: *Kinesiology of the musculoskeletal system: foundations for physical rehabilitation*, St Louis, 2002, Mosby, Figures 13-4 and 13-6.)

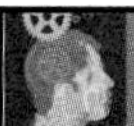

Consider this...

Osgood-Schlatter's Disease

Activities such as running and jumping require the quadriceps to generate large knee extension forces. The force generated from these muscles pulls strongly on the tibial tuberosity via the patellar tendon. During adolescence, excessively large and frequent quadriceps contractions may overwhelm the structural integrity of the immature bone of the tibia. As a result, fragments of immature bone are pulled from the tibial tuberosity. This condition, known as Osgood-Schlatter's disease, is often accompanied by pain and enlargement of the tibial tuberosity.

Proximal Fibula

The fibula (see Figure 10-4) is a long, slender bone that courses along the lateral shaft of the tibia. The *fibular head* is the rounded superior portion of the fibula that articulates with the superior-lateral aspect of the tibia. This articulation forms the firm *proximal tibiofibular joint*. The head of the fibula is the distal attachment of the lateral collateral ligament and biceps femoris muscle.

Patella

The patella, or knee cap, is a small, plate-like bone embedded within the quadriceps tendon. Because the patella exists within the quadriceps tendon, it is highly mobile and at risk for abnormal gliding or subluxation. A portion of the stability provided to the patellofemoral joint comes from the fit of posterior patella within the intercondylar groove of the femur (Figure 10-5, A). The *base*, or superior pole, of the patella accepts the quadriceps tendon; the *apex*, or inferior pole, accepts the proximal side of the patellar tendon (Figure 10-5, B). The *posterior articular surface of the patella* articulates with the intercondylar groove of the femur through *medial* and *lateral facets*. The lateral facet is steeper than the medial facet, matching the general shape of the intercondylar groove of the femur (Figure 10-5, C).

Arthrology

General Features

The tibiofemoral and patellofemoral joints each provide a unique contribution to the overall kinesiology of the knee. Consider walking, for example, in which the motion of the

Consider this...

Patellar Motion and Stability

The patella plays an integral part in the normal kinematics of the knee by:

- Acting as a transmitter of quadriceps force across the knee
- Enhancing the leverage (internal moment arm) of the quadriceps muscle

During normal patellofemoral joint motion, the patella glides distally as the knee is flexed and proximally as the knee is extended (Figure 10-6, *A-C*). As the patella glides proximally and distally, it must remain stable within the intercondylar groove of the femur. The anatomic design of the patella is normally well suited for this function. The jigsaw fit of the convex posterior patella fits snugly against the matching concavity of the intercondylar groove of the femur (Figure 10-6, *D*). Strong activation of the quadriceps naturally produces a net lateral pull on the patella. The steep slope of the lateral facet of the femur—and matching patellar surface—normally help prevent a lateral subluxation (dislocation) of the patella. Persons with a flattened lateral intercondylar groove are more likely to experience lateral subluxation of their patellofemoral joint.

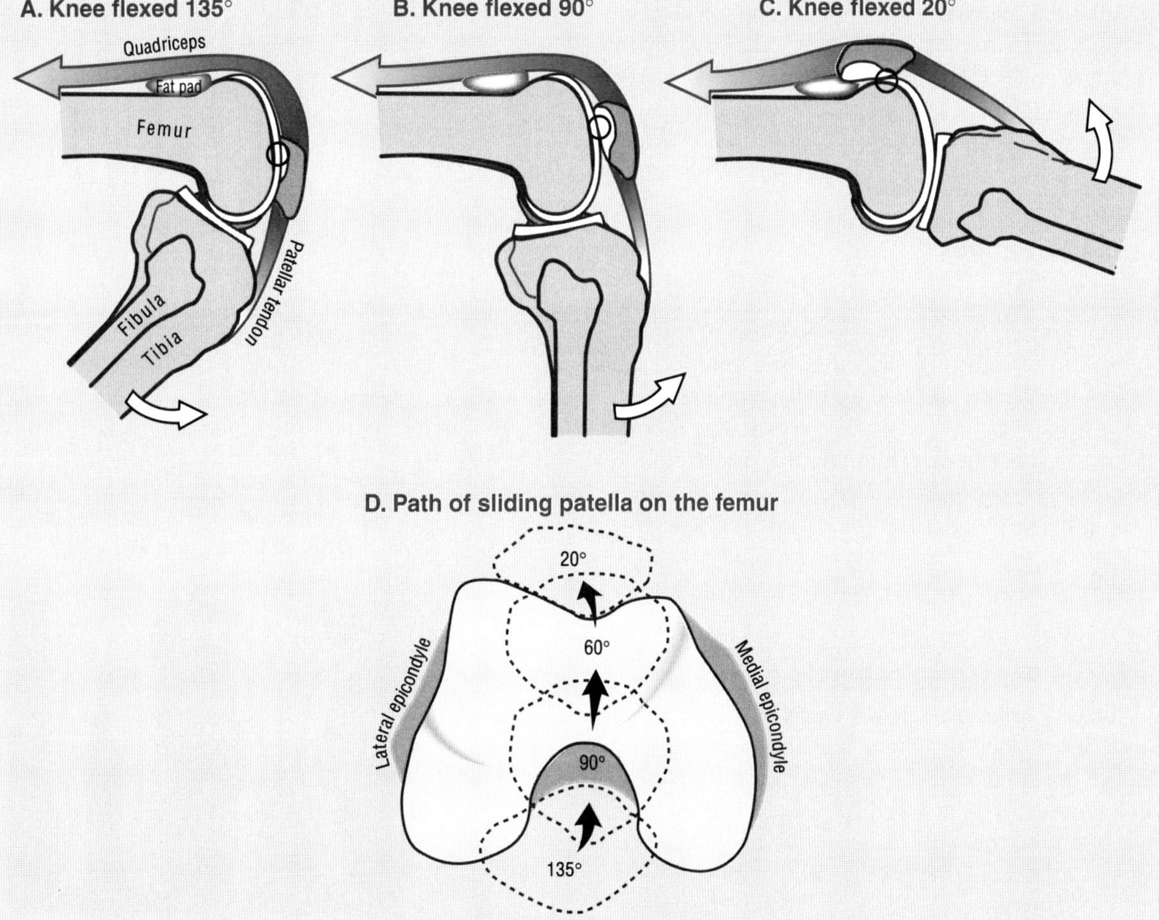

Figure 10-6 Kinematics of the patellofemoral joint as the knee is extending. Note the superior migration of the patella as the knee moves from 135 degrees of flexion **(A)** to 90 degrees of flexion **(B)** to 20 degrees short of full extension **(C)**. **D** shows a front view of the path and contact area of the patella as the knee moves from 135 degrees of flexion to 20 degrees short of full extension. (From Neumann DA: *Kinesiology of the musculoskeletal system: foundations for physical rehabilitation,* St Louis, 2002, Mosby, Figure 13-19, *A-D*.)

tibiofemoral joint is essential to the natural forward progression of the leg. Connective tissues surrounding the tibiofemoral joint not only guide these movements but also stabilize the articulation, as well as absorb and transmit forces. The surrounding musculature adds another critical element of stability and shock absorption across the knee.

The *patellofemoral joint* protects the delicate structures within the knee and improves the moment arm for the quadriceps, thereby improving the extensor torque-producing potential of this muscle group. Strong activation of the quadriceps produces proportionally large **compression forces** between the patella and femur. These large compressive forces are important to consider when designing quadriceps strengthening exercises or giving advice to patients on how to protect painful or arthritic knees from damaging forces.

Normal Alignment

As illustrated in Figure 10-7, *A* (and studied in Chapter 9), the 125-degree angle of inclination of the proximal femur directs the shaft of this bone toward the midline, for eventual articulation with the tibia at the knee. Because the tibia is oriented essentially vertically while standing, the articulation between the femur and the tibia does not typically form a straight line. As shown in Figure 10-7, *A*, the femur usually meets the tibia to form a lateral angle of 170 to 175 degrees. This alignment is referred to as normal **genu valgum**. Variations of this angle are not uncommon because the knee must adjust to malalignment at either the hip or ankle. A lateral angle of less than 170 degrees is considered **excessive genu valgum**, or knock-kneed (Figure 10-7, *B*). A lateral angle greater than 180 degrees is called **genu varum**, giving a bowlegged appearance (Figure 10-7, *C*).

Supporting Structures

The knee joint must remain stable even while subjected to large internal and external forces. In addition to muscle, the stability of the knee is provided by the anterior and posterior cruciate ligaments, medial and lateral collateral ligaments, posterior capsule, and the menisci. The following sections will describe the structure and basic function of these important connective tissues. Table 10-1 summarizes the primary functions of these structures and lists common mechanisms of their injury.

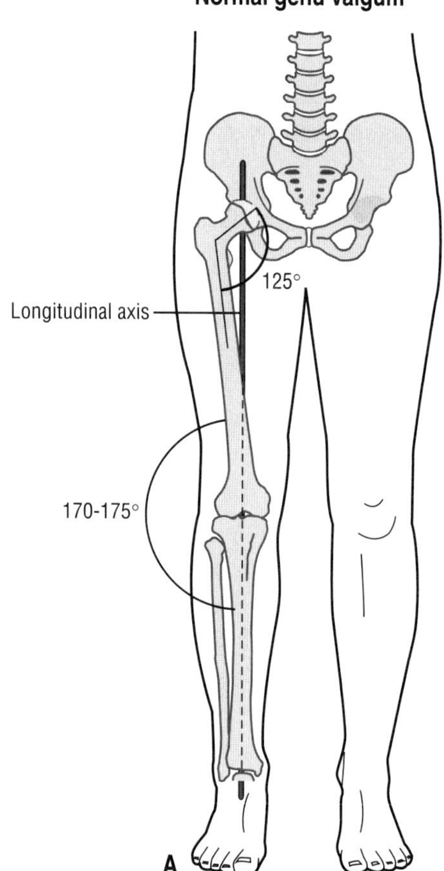

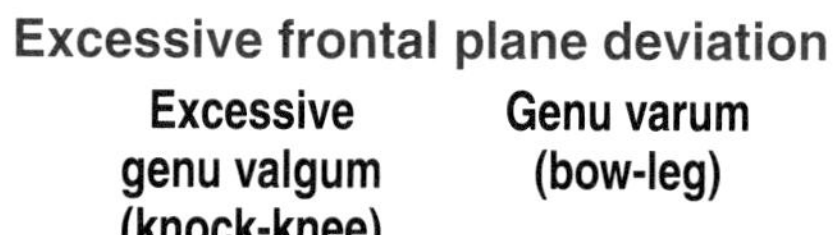

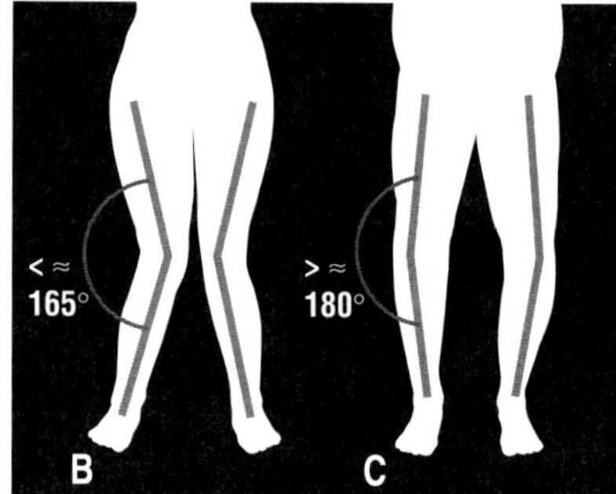

Figure 10-7 Frontal plane deviations of the knee. **A,** Normal genu valgum. **B,** Excessive genu valgum. **C,** Genu varum. (From Neumann DA: *Kinesiology of the musculoskeletal system: foundations for physical rehabilitation*, St Louis, 2002, Mosby, Figure 13-8.)

ANTERIOR AND POSTERIOR CRUCIATE LIGAMENTS

Cruciate, literally meaning "cross," describes the X shape of the anterior and posterior cruciate ligaments as they interconnect the tibia with the femur (Figure 10-8). The predominant anterior-posterior direction of the cruciate ligaments stabilizes the knee against the large anterior-posterior shear forces that occur while walking and running. The anterior and posterior cruciate ligaments, therefore, are the most important stabilizers of the knee in the sagittal plane.

The anterior cruciate ligament (ACL) is frequently injured during sporting events such as soccer, football, or skiing—activities that generate a combination of large rotational, side-to-side, and hyperextension forces through the knee. The posterior cruciate ligament (PCL) is injured less frequently but may be ruptured along with the ACL. Surgery is generally required to repair a ruptured cruciate ligament by replacing the torn ligament with a tendon from another muscle (autograft) or one harvested from a cadaver (allograft). Regardless of the type of surgical reconstruction, knowledge of the anatomy and function of the ACL and PCL is required for proper post-surgical rehabilitation and protection of the reconstructed ligaments.

The box on p. 280 summarizes the primary functions of the ACL and PCL, which are illustrated in Figures 10-9 and 10-10, respectively.

TABLE 10-1 FUNCTIONS AND MECHANISMS OF INJURY OF THE SUPPORTING STRUCTURES OF THE KNEE

Structure	Function	Most Common Mechanisms of Injury
Anterior cruciate ligament	(1) Resists anterior translation of the tibia relative to a fixed femur or posterior translation of the femur relative to a fixed tibia (2) Resists the extremes of knee extension (3) Resists valgus and varus deformations and excessive horizontal plane rotations	(1) Hyperextension (2) Large valgus- or varus-producing forces with foot planted (3) Either of the above combined with large torsional (rotational) force at the knee
Posterior cruciate ligament	(1) Resists posterior translation of the tibia relative to a fixed femur or anterior translation of the femur relative to a fixed tibia (2) Resists the extremes of knee flexion (3) Resists valgus and varus deformations and excessive horizontal plane rotations	(1) Hyperflexion of the knee (2) "Dashboard injuries" (i.e., the tibia being forcefully driven posteriorly relative to the femur) (3) Severe hyperextension (with a large gapping of the posterior side of the joint) (4) Large valgus- or varus-producing forces with foot planted (5) Any of the above combined with large torsional force at the knee
Medial collateral ligament	(1) Resists valgus deformation of the knee (2) Resists excessive knee extension	(1) Valgus-producing force with foot planted (2) Severe hyperextension of the knee
Lateral collateral ligament	(1) Resists varus deformation of the knee (2) Resists excessive knee extension	(1) Varus-producing force with foot planted (2) Severe hyperextension of the knee
Posterior capsule	(1) Resists excessive knee extension	(1) Severe hyperextension
Medial and lateral menisci	(1) Improve the overall congruency (fit) of the tibiofemoral joint (2) Dissipate compression and shear forces across the knee	(1) Extreme valgus- or varus-producing forces at the knee (2) Extreme rotations of the knee, especially under large compression forces

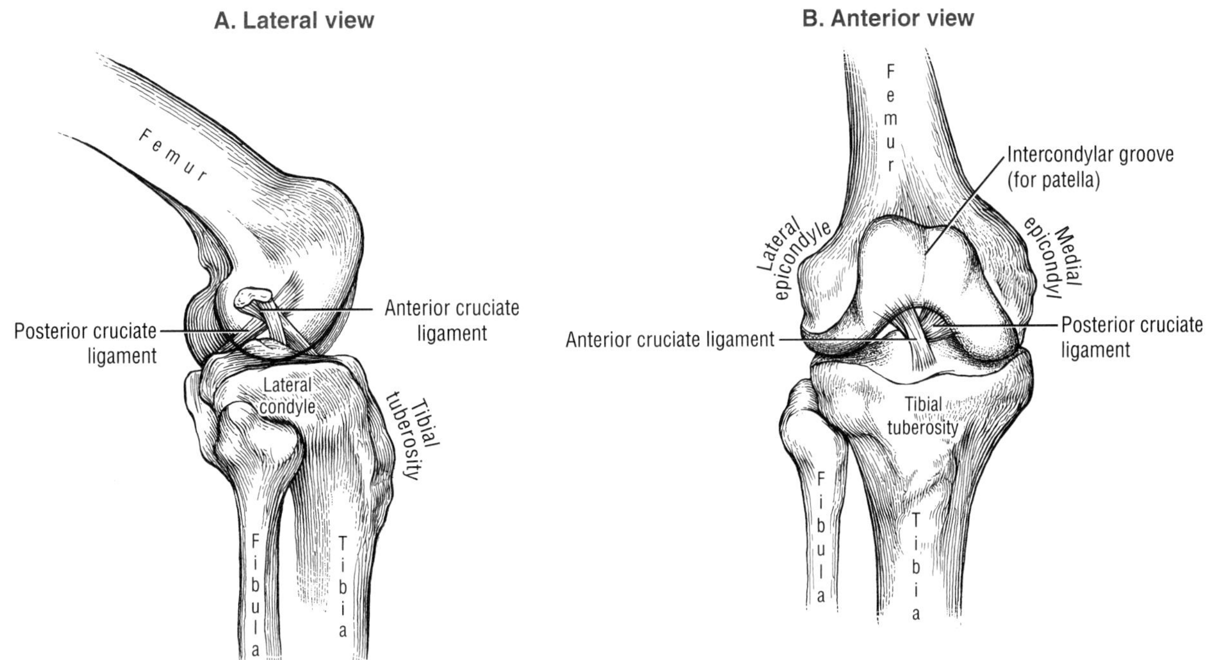

Figure 10-8 The anterior and posterior cruciate ligaments. **A,** Lateral view. **B,** Anterior view. (From Neumann DA: *Kinesiology of the musculoskeletal system: foundations for physical rehabilitation,* St Louis, 2002, Mosby, Figure 13-21.)

Clinical INSIGHT

Why Full Active Knee Extension Is Often Avoided after Anterior Cruciate Ligament (ACL) Reconstruction

Many post-surgical ACL rehabilitation protocols limit active or forceful knee extension from 40 degrees of flexion through full extension. Activation of the quadriceps at these ranges produces anterior shear forces that pull the tibia anterior relative to the femur. One of the primary functions of the ACL is to resist the anterior shear of the tibia relative to the femur. As a measure of protection, therefore, motions that maximally challenge the integrity of the new graft, such as heavily resisted, end-range (open-chain) knee extension exercises, are often avoided in the early stages of post-ACL reconstruction rehabilitation. During this time, therapists often design knee extension exercises that promote co-contraction of the muscles about the knee, such as supervised, relatively shallow, short-arc squats. Assuming the patient is progressing well, the later stage of rehabilitation may incorporate a safe balance between open- and closed-chain knee extension exercises. Therapists must always monitor the patient for complications following ACL reconstruction, such as increased pain, swelling, and instability, as well as prolonged atrophy within the quadriceps muscle.

Primary Functions of the Anterior and Posterior Cruciate Ligaments

Anterior Cruciate Ligament

- Resists anterior translation of the tibia relative to a fixed femur—open-chain perspective (see Figure 10-9, *A*)
- Resists posterior translation of the femur relative to a fixed tibia—closed chain perspective (see Figure 10-9, *B*)

Posterior Cruciate Ligament

- Resists posterior translation of the tibia relative to a fixed femur—open-chain perspective (see Figure 10-10, *A*)
- Resists anterior translation of the femur over a relatively fixed tibia—closed-chain perspective (see Figure 10-10, *B*)

MEDIAL AND LATERAL COLLATERAL LIGAMENTS

The medial and lateral collateral ligaments strengthen the medial and lateral sides of the capsule of the knee (Figure 10-11, A). These ligaments are the primary frontal plane stabilizers of the knee, protecting against forces that produce excessive genu valgus.

The wide, flat medial collateral ligament (MCL) spans the medial side of the knee between the medial epicondyle of the femur and the proximal medial tibia. The primary function of the MCL is to resist valgus-producing forces (Figure 10-11, *B*). Some fibers of the MCL attach to the medial meniscus of the

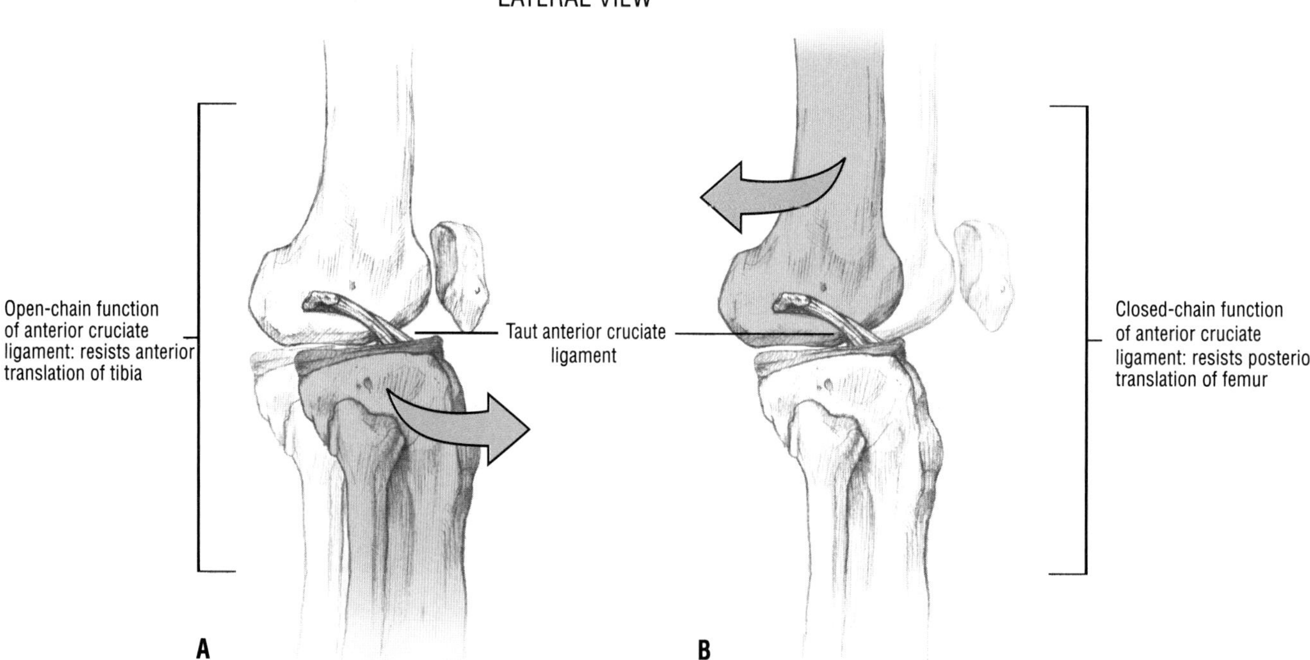

Figure 10-9 The primary sagittal plane functions of the anterior cruciate ligament. **A,** Resisting anterior translation of the tibia relative to the femur. **B,** Resisting posterior translation of the femur relative to the tibia.

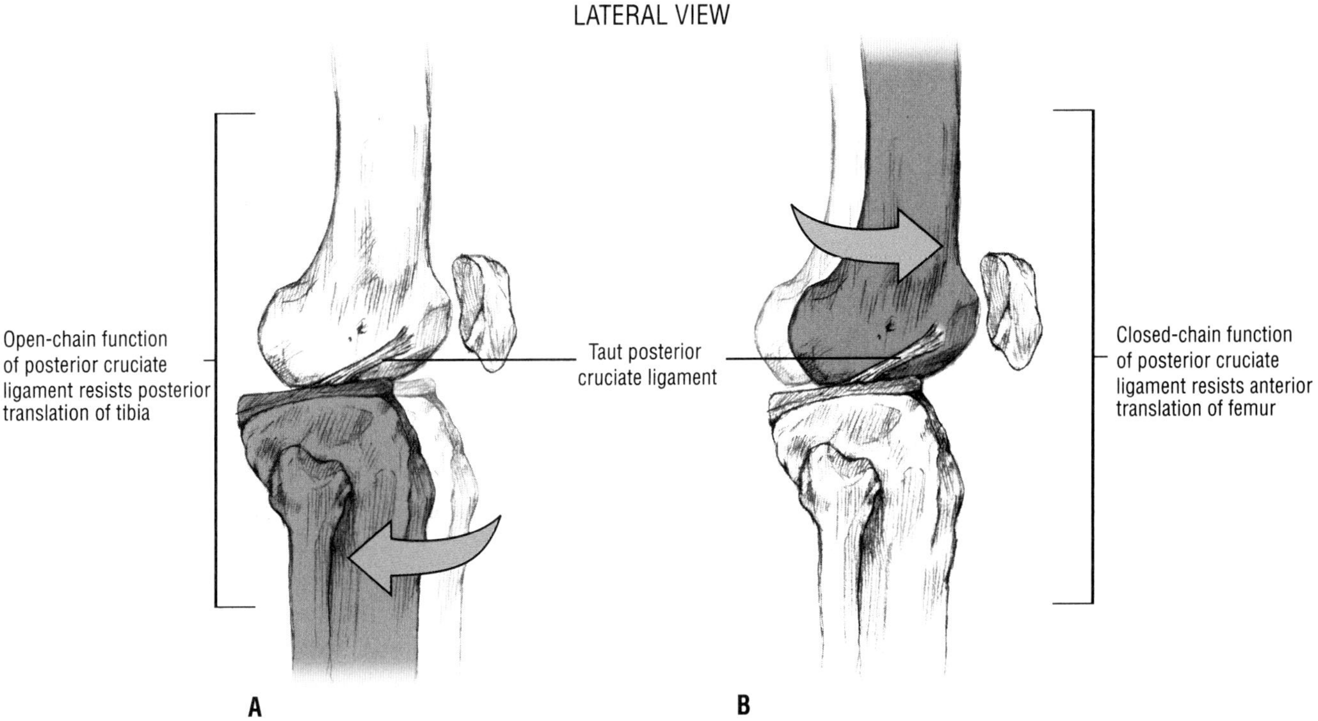

LATERAL VIEW

Open-chain function of posterior cruciate ligament resists posterior translation of tibia

Taut posterior cruciate ligament

Closed-chain function of posterior cruciate ligament resists anterior translation of femur

A

B

Figure 10-10 The primary sagittal plane functions of the posterior cruciate ligament. **A,** Resisting posterior translation of the tibia relative to the femur. **B,** Resisting anterior translation of the femur relative to the tibia.

knee; therefore injury to the MCL may involve injury to the medial meniscus as well.

The lateral collateral ligament (LCL) is a round, cord-like ligament that crosses the lateral side of the knee, attaching to the lateral epicondyle of the femur and the head of the fibula. The primary function of the LCL is to protect the knee from varus-producing forces (Figure 10-11, C).

Although the knee is stressed only minimally in the frontal plane while walking or running, rapid changes in direction or a large impact of external forces frequently injure the collateral ligaments, especially the MCL. Consider, for example, a football player who is tackled from the side (Figure 10-12). With the foot in firm contact with the ground, the medially directed force on the lateral side of the knee creates a forceful genu valgus, often tearing the MCL.

In addition to providing most of the medial-lateral stability to the knee, the collateral ligaments also become taut at full extension. This increased tension in the stretched

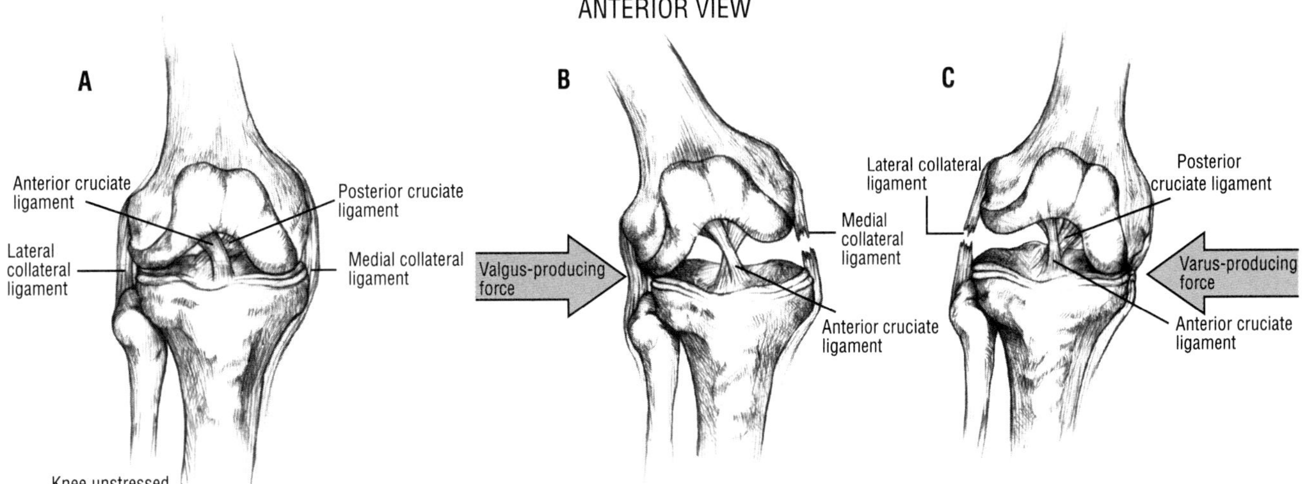

Figure 10-11 **A,** Anterior view of the right knee showing the medial and lateral collateral ligaments, anterior cruciate ligament, and posterior cruciate ligament. **B,** Valgus-producing force rupturing the medial collateral ligament. **C,** Varus-producing force rupturing the lateral collateral ligament.

ligaments is useful for locking the extended knee while standing—a mechanism that allows a person to periodically rest the quadriceps. The increased tension in the ligaments does, however, increase the likeliness of injury. The pre-stretched MCL of a fully extended knee places it much closer to its rupture point at the time of impact.

Primary Functions of the Collateral Ligaments

- *Medial collateral ligament:* Resists valgus-producing forces at the knee
- *Lateral collateral ligament:* Resists varus-producing forces at the knee
- Both ligaments are taut in full extension; assist with locking the knee

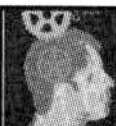

Consider this...

The "Terrible Triad"

The "terrible triad" describes the simultaneous injury of the anterior cruciate ligament, medial collateral ligament, and medial meniscus. Most often this injury occurs as a result of large rotational and valgus-producing forces to the nearly or fully extended knee, when the foot is firmly planted on the ground.

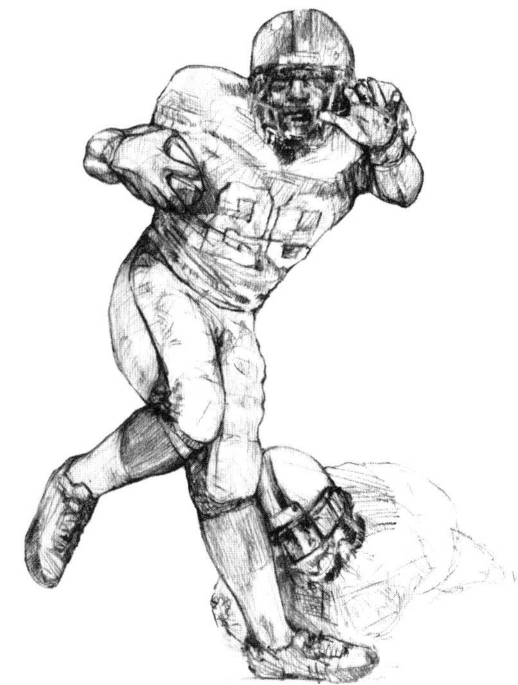

Figure 10-12 A large valgus-producing force at the knee resulting from a tackle against the lateral aspect of the extended knee.

MEDIAL AND LATERAL MENISCI

The medial and lateral menisci are crescent-shaped fibrocartilaginous discs located at the top of the medial and lateral condyles of the tibia (Figure 10-13). These structures play an important role in absorbing the compressive forces across the knee caused by muscular contraction and body weight. While walking, compressive forces at the knee routinely reach two to three times body weight. By nearly tripling the area of joint contact and expanding outward on weight bearing, the menisci significantly reduce the pressure across the knee. Also, the cup-shaped menisci "deepen" the articular surface of the knee, facilitating the arthrokinematics and further stabilizing the joint.

Part of the medial meniscus attaches to the MCL. For this reason, excessive stress or deformation of the MCL may also damage the medial meniscus.

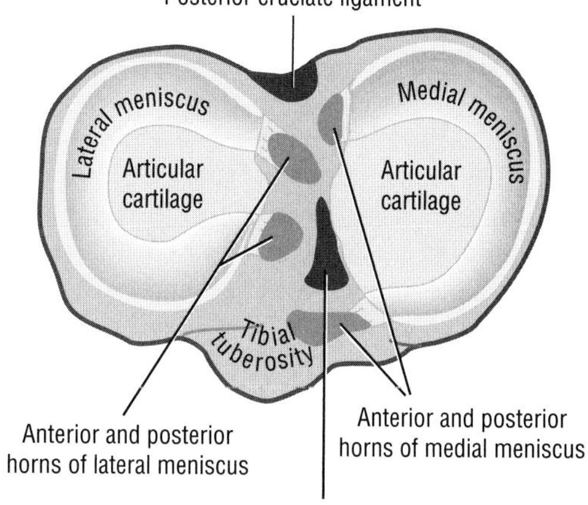

Figure 10-13 A superior view of the tibia showing the shapes of the medial and lateral meniscus. (From Neumann DA: *Kinesiology of the musculoskeletal system: foundations for physical rehabilitation,* St Louis, 2002, Mosby, Figure 13-12, *B.*)

Primary Functions of the Menisci

- Act as shock absorbers for the knee; reduce friction and dissipate compressive forces
- Increase surface area of joint contact, therefore reducing joint pressure
- Improve joint congruency
- Facilitate normal joint arthrokinematics

POSTERIOR CAPSULE

The primary role of the posterior capsule is to prevent hyperextension of the knee. Two major ligaments or thickenings of the posterior capsule exist: the arcuate popliteal ligament and the oblique popliteal ligament (Figure 10-15).

A variety of musculoskeletal disorders can create marked hyperextension at the knee due to an imbalance of forces.

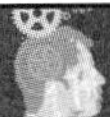

Consider this...

Injury and Healing of the Menisci

The primary role of the menisci is to absorb and disperse the large compressive forces transferred through the knee joint. These fibrocartilaginous structures, however, are susceptible to injury from torsion or "grinding" of the femoral condyles against the tibia. Once injured, the menisci may not heal well. This is especially true with the inner one third of the structure due to its poor blood supply (Figure 10-14).

- *Inner one third:* essentially avascular
- *Middle one third:* poor blood supply
- *Outer one third:* good blood supply

Injury to the outer one third of the meniscus may heal without surgery because of its relatively good blood supply.

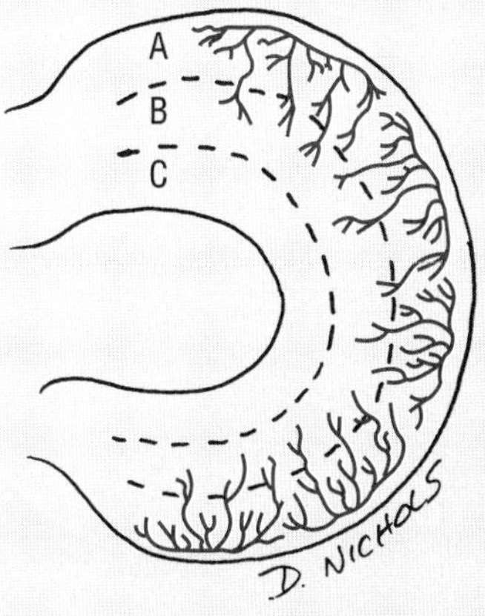

Figure 10-14 The blood supply to the meniscus. The outer regions *(A)* have good blood supply, the middle portion *(B)* has moderate blood supply, and the inner portion *(C)* has little to no blood supply. (Modified from Shankman G: *Fundamental orthopedic management for the physical therapist assistant*, ed 2, St Louis, 2004, Mosby, Figure 19-25.)

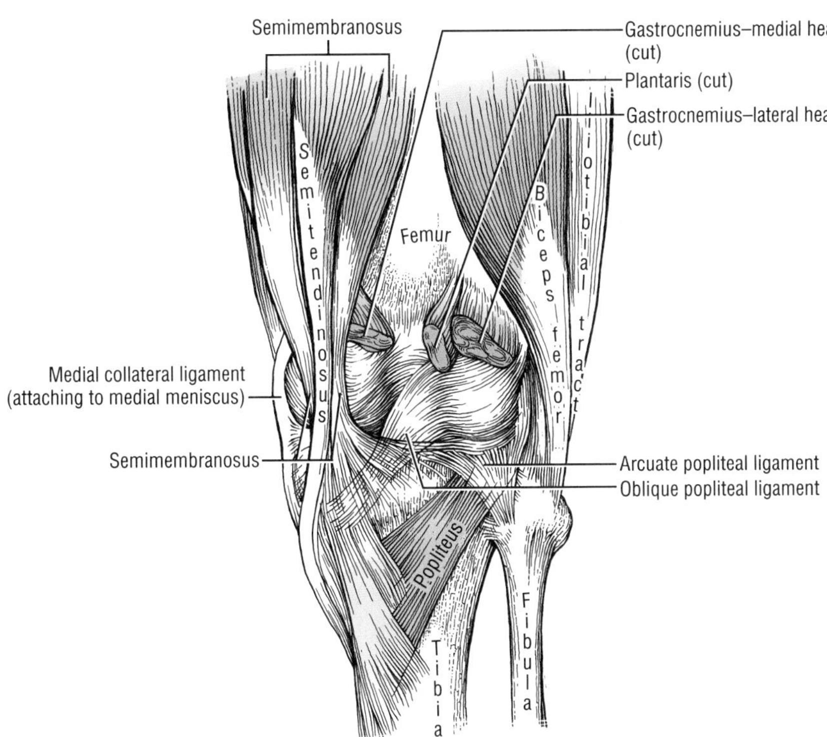

Figure 10-15 Posterior view of the right knee showing the posterior capsule, including the oblique popliteal and arcuate popliteal ligaments. (Modified from Neumann DA: *Kinesiology of the musculoskeletal system: foundations for physical rehabilitation*, St Louis, 2002, Mosby, Figure 13-10.)

Unlike the elbow, the knee joint has no bony block to resist full extension. As a result of prolonged hyperextension forces, the posterior capsule may become over-stretched. A knee that demonstrates marked hyperextension is referred to as **genu recurvatum**, a condition that strains the posterior capsule and many other structures of the knee.

Kinematics

OSTEOKINEMATICS OF THE TIBIOFEMORAL JOINT

The tibiofemoral (knee) joint allows 2 degrees of freedom, flexion and extension, as well as internal and external rotation.

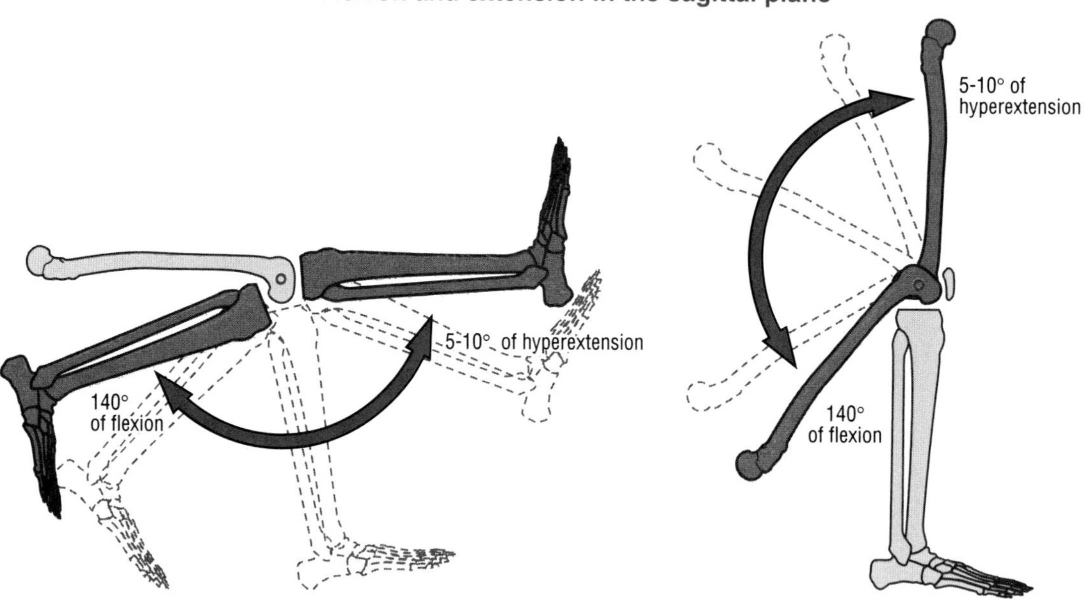

Figure 10-16 Sagittal plane motion of the knee. **A,** Tibial-on-femoral perspective. **B,** Femoral-on-tibial perspective. (From Neumann DA: *Kinesiology of the musculoskeletal system: foundations for physical rehabilitation,* St Louis, 2002, Mosby, Figure 13-14.)

TABLE 10-2 OSTEOKINEMATICS OF THE KNEE

Motion	Axis of Rotation	Plane of Motion	Normal Range of Motion
Flexion Extension	Medial-lateral through the femoral condyles	Sagittal	0-140 degrees 0-5 degrees of hyperextension
Internal rotation External rotation	Vertical (longitudinal)	Horizontal	0-15 degrees (with knee flexed) 0-30 degrees (with knee flexed)

Flexion and extension occur in the sagittal plane about a medial-lateral axis of rotation. Motion occurs from about 5 degrees of knee hyperextension to about 130 to 140 degrees of flexion. As illustrated in Figure 10-16, the range of motion at the knee is the same whether viewed from an open-chain (tibial-on-femoral) or closed-chain (femoral-on-tibial) perspective. The only difference is which bone is fixed and which is moving.

Internal and external rotation of the knee occurs within the horizontal plane about a vertical or longitudinal axis of rotation. This motion, also called axial rotation, refers to the rotation between the tibia and the femur. With the knee flexed, the knee joint permits 40 to 50 degrees of total rotation (Table 10-2); however, with the knee fully extended, essentially no rotation occurs between the two bones.

Closed-chain (femoral-on-tibial) axial rotation of the knee is an important but often overlooked motion. Consider, for example, a sharp 90-degree cutting motion while running. With the foot and attached tibia fixed to the ground, the rotating femur creates a critical horizontal plane pivot point for the entire trunk and upper body. Large force demands are placed on the muscles and ligaments of the knee as the femur (and rest of the upper body) accelerates or decelerates relative to the fixed tibia. This large demand partially explains the relatively high incidence of injury to the knee resulting from cutting motions associated with high-speed sporting events.

ARTHROKINEMATICS AT THE TIBIOFEMORAL JOINT

Figure 10-18, A, illustrates knee extension with an arthrokinematic pattern of rolling and sliding in the *same* direction. These open-chain arthrokinematics are based on the concave tibial condyles rotating around the convex condyles of the femur. Closed-chain extension, however, is based on the arthrokinematics of a roll-and-slide pattern occurring in *opposite* directions (Figure 10-18, *B*). The anterior roll of the femoral condyles must be accompanied by a posterior slide; otherwise, the femur would (theoretically) roll off the front of the tibial plateau. Although not

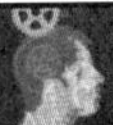

Consider this...

The Migrating Axis of Rotation at the Knee

Flexion and extension range of motion of the knee is typically measured by placing the axis of the goniometer directly over the medial-lateral axis of rotation of the knee—assumed to lie over the lateral epicondyle of the femur. In actuality, the axis of rotation of the knee is not fixed but moves (or migrates) slightly with knee movement (Figure 10-17).

Knee braces are often recommended after knee surgery or injury as a way to protect the region. Because a knee brace has a fixed axis and the knee joint does not, the brace may "piston" slightly as the knee flexes and extends. Therapists must be aware of this possible problem and monitor the patient's skin for abrasions or other signs of discomfort.

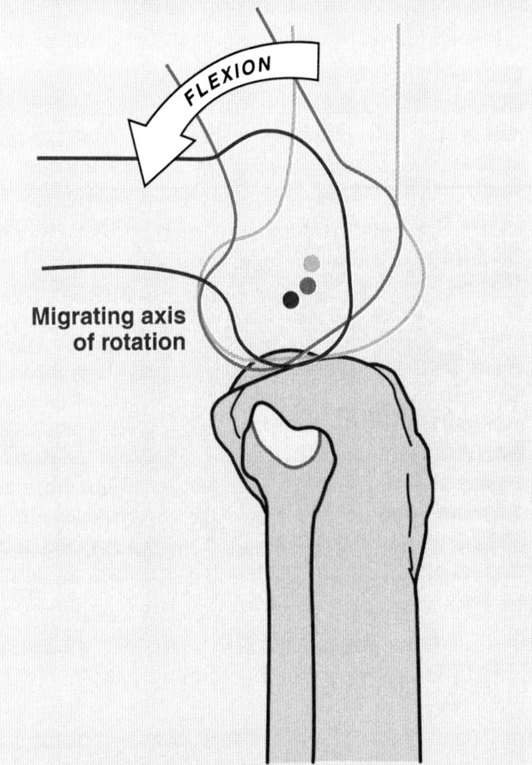

Figure 10-17 The flexing knee generates a migrating medial-lateral axis of rotation. (From Neumann DA: *Kinesiology of the musculoskeletal system: foundations for physical rehabilitation*, St Louis, 2002, Mosby, Figure 13-16.)

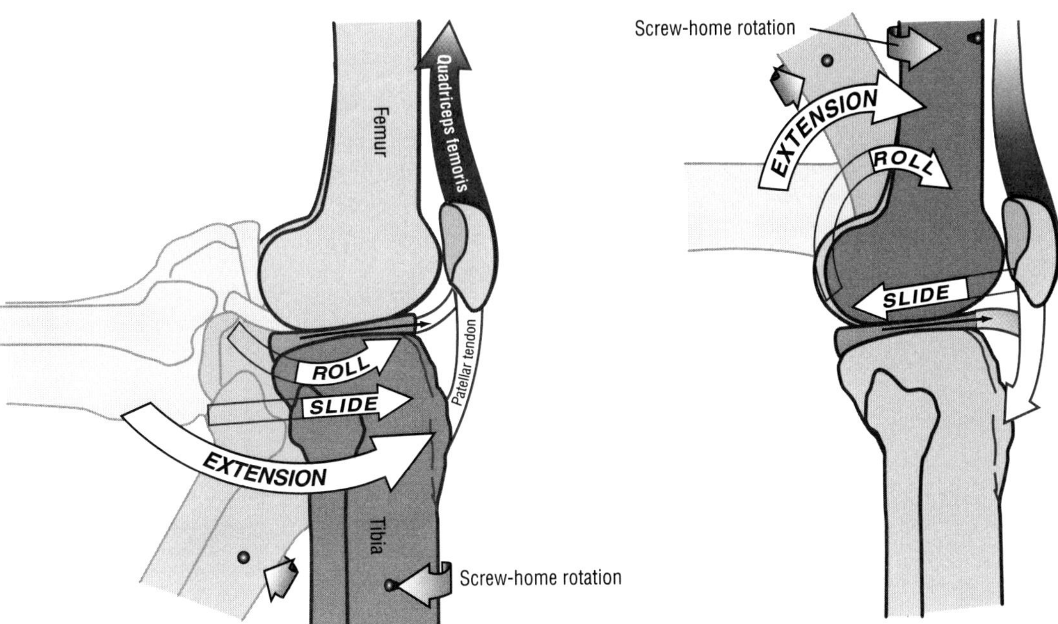

Figure 10-18 The active arthrokinematics of knee extension. **A,** Tibial-on-femoral perspective. **B,** Femoral-on-tibial perspective. (From Neumann DA: *Kinesiology of the musculoskeletal system: foundations for physical rehabilitation*, St Louis, 2002, Mosby, Figure 13-17.)

illustrated, the arthrokinematics for knee flexion are essentially the same as for knee extension, except that the movements occur in reverse directions.

The shape of the articular surfaces of the tibiofemoral joint necessitates that flexion and extension are accompanied by slight automatic rotational movements. As the knee nears full extension, the knee rotates externally about 10 to 15 degrees. This automatic rotation—defined by the position of the tibia relative to the femur—assists in locking the knee, the so-called **screw-home mechanism.** This locking mechanism can occur by rotation of the tibia on the femur or by rotation of the femur over a fixed tibia. In either case the rotation of the knee helps lock the knee into extension (see Figure 10-18).

PATELLOFEMORAL JOINT

The patellofemoral joint is the articulation between the smooth, posterior surface of the patella and the intercondylar groove of the femur. Many everyday activities such as ascending steps or standing up from a seated position require large active knee-extension torques generated by the quadriceps. These large torques are enhanced by the patella and are often used to swiftly accelerate the femur (and entire body) upward during activities such as running, jumping, or climbing.

An intact patella increases the internal moment arm for the quadriceps to about 2 inches (Figure 10-19, *A*). For the sake of discussion, assume that the quadriceps can produce a maximum force of 250 lb. With the moment arm provided by the patella, the quadriceps force is converted to a knee extension torque of 500 in-lbs (250 lb × 2 inches). Figure 10-19, *B*, shows a knee following a patellectomy, a surgical procedure that removes the patella, often following severe fracture. Without the patella, the internal moment arm available to the quadriceps is reduced to about 1½ inches. Given the same muscular effort and quadriceps force of 250 lb, the knee extensor torque is now reduced to 375 in-lbs (250 lb × 1.5 inches = 375 in-lbs). This (125 in-lb) *loss* of maximal knee extension torque may be significant, depending on the daily activity demands required of the patient.

In summary, the patella enhances the torque-producing capability of the quadriceps by about 25%. Alternatively stated, following a patellectomy, the quadriceps must produce 25% more force to produce an equivalent preoperative torque. Over time, the increased muscle force may cause fatigue or damage the patellofemoral or tibiofemoral joints.

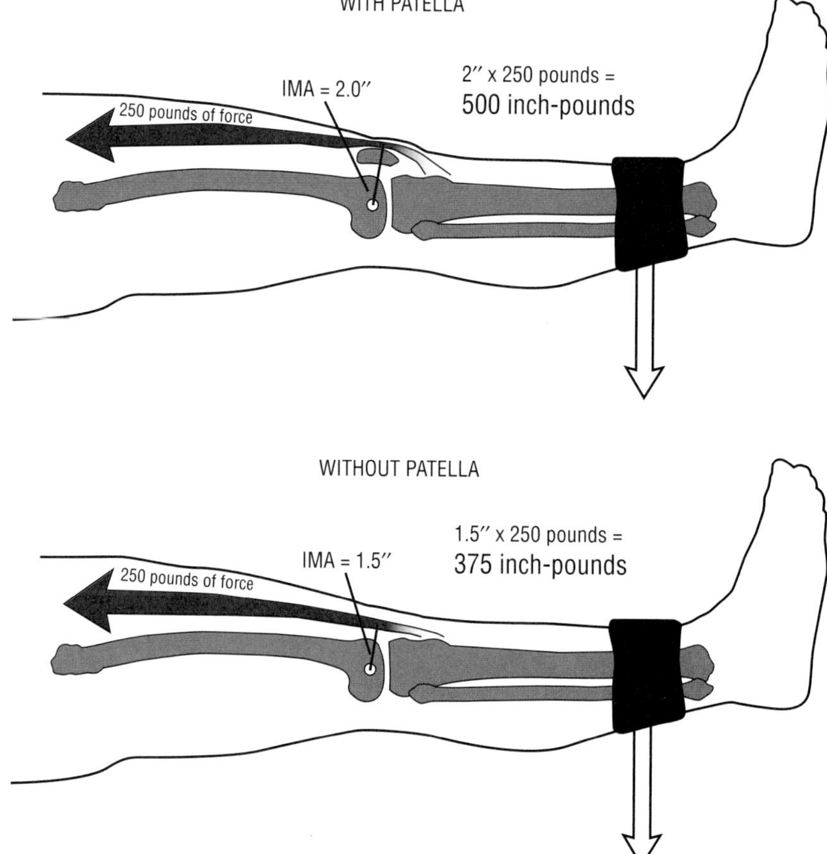

Figure 10-19 An illustration of two different knees supporting a weight. **A,** Normal knee with a patella shows the quadriceps generating 500 inch-pounds of torque. **B,** Knee without a patella. With the same amount of muscular force, the quadriceps are able to generate only 375 inch-pounds of torque. *IMA,* Internal moment arm.

Clinical INSIGHT

Positioning the Ankle to Change the Biomechanics of the Knee

While standing, the position of the ankle helps determine the position of the leg and ultimately the position of the knee. These closely related kinematics can be verified by assuming a shallow squat position and noting how the forward movement of the leg (tibia relative to the ankle) causes flexion of the knee. Rotating the leg posterior (at the ankle) causes the knee to extend. These relationships often have important clinical consequences. One such example is subsequently described.

Figure 10-20, *A*, shows an individual with the left ankle surgically fused in 25 degrees of plantar flexion. Because the subject has complete flaccid paralysis of the muscles of the left ankle, the ankle was fused to improve its stability. The resulting posterior position (tilt) of the lower leg shifts the line of body weight well *anterior* to the medial-lateral axis of rotation of the knee. This causes gravity to act with a long external moment arm (see *EMA* in figure), thereby producing a strong extension torque at the knee. Over many years, the extension torque has led to an over-stretched posterior capsule and subsequent genu recurvatum (see Figure 10-20, *A*). To help correct this stressful posture, the individual has been given a shoe with an elevated heel that tilts the tibia anteriorly (Figure 10-20, *B*). On weight bearing, the tibia is now better aligned with the femur, resulting in a relatively straight knee. The corrected position improves lower extremity function and removes the strain on the posterior structures of the knee.

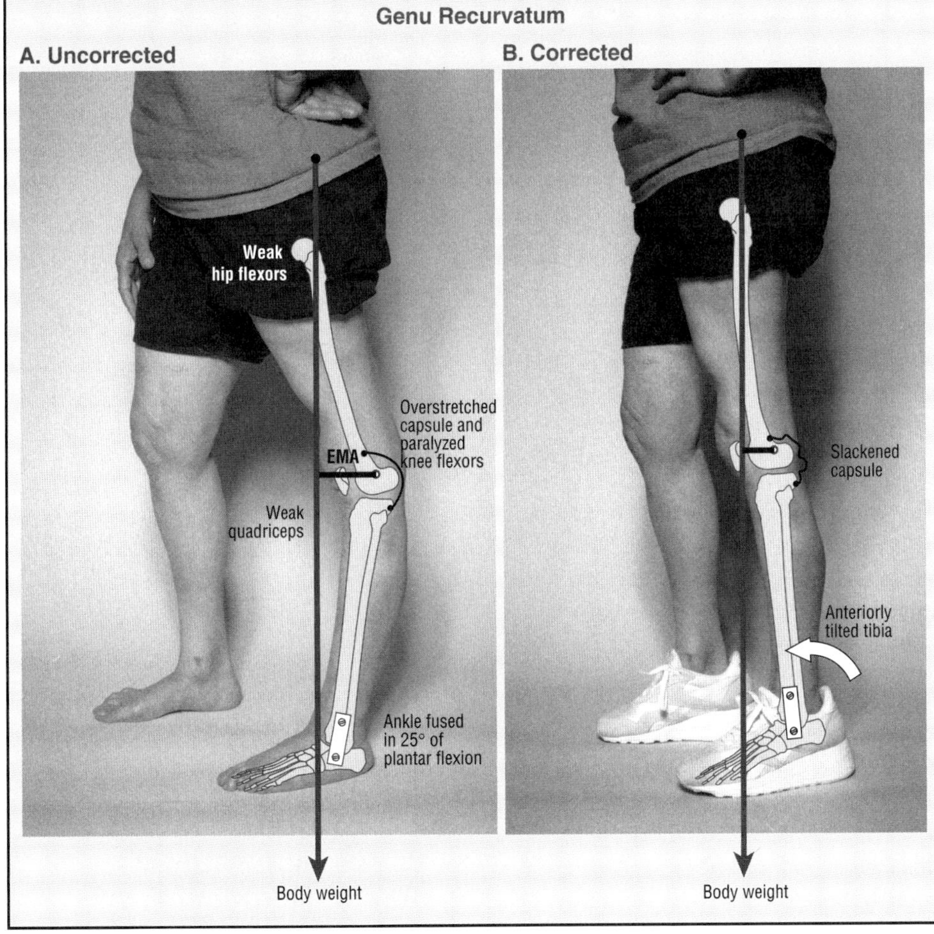

Figure 10-20 **A**, An individual with marked genu recurvatum of the left knee secondary to the ankle being fused in 25 degrees of plantar flexion producing a large extension torque on the knee. **B**, Subject is able to reduce the severity of the genu recurvatum by wearing a tennis shoe with a built-up heel. *EMA*, External moment arm. (From Neumann DA: *Kinesiology of the musculoskeletal system: foundations for physical rehabilitation*, St Louis, 2002, Mosby, Figure 13-42.)

Muscle and Joint Interaction

Innervation of the Muscles of the Knee

The muscles of the knee are innervated by three different nerves (Table 10-3): (1) femoral, (2) sciatic, and (3) obturator (see Chapter 9, Figures 9-20 and 9-21). The femoral nerve supplies the sole source of innervation to the quadriceps, so laceration or other damage to this one nerve can result in complete paralysis of the knee extensor muscles. The sciatic nerve has two branches: (1) tibial and (2) peroneal. The tibial portion of the sciatic nerve innervates most of the hamstrings: the semitendinosus, semimembranosus, and the long head of the biceps femoris. The

TABLE 10-3 INNERVATION OF THE MUSCLES OF THE KNEE

Innervation	Muscle
Femoral nerve	Rectus femoris Vastus medialis Vastus lateralis Vastus intermedius Sartorius
Sciatic nerve—tibial portion	Hamstrings: Semitendinosus Semimembranosus Biceps femoris—long head
Sciatic nerve—peroneal portion	Biceps femoris—short head
Obturator nerve	Gracilis
Tibial nerve	Gastrocnemius Popliteus Plantaris

peroneal portion of the sciatic nerve innervates the short head of the biceps femoris. The obturator nerve courses down the medial thigh and innervates the gracilis.

Muscles of the Knee

Knee muscles can be divided into two major groups: the knee extensors and the knee flexors. Although these muscles have important individual actions, most often they work in teams to maximize their control over movements of the knee. Consider, for example, that isolated contraction of the knee extensor muscles exerts minimal if any control of rotation at the knee but plays a major role in guiding the path (tracking) of the patella within the intercondylar groove of the femur. Conversely, isolated contraction of the knee flexor muscles exerts major control of knee flexion, as well as rotational movements at the knee, but has minimal effect on patellar tracking. Yet a common action like standing up from a seated position requires simultaneous activation of both the quadriceps and the hamstrings. Many of these muscular interactions are described later in this chapter.

KNEE EXTENSORS: QUADRICEPS

The term *quadriceps* is used to describe a group of four knee extensor muscles. This group includes the rectus femoris, vastus lateralis, vastus medialis, and vastus intermedius. Although all four muscles originate from a different area of the femur or pelvis, they join together and attach distally—as a group—to the tibial tuberosity via the patellar tendon. When active isometrically, the quadriceps may help to stabilize and protect the knee. When active eccentrically, the quadriceps may control the rate of descent of the body, such as when slowly transitioning from standing to sitting. When active concentrically, the quadriceps accelerate the knee into extension, often in association with hip extension such as when jumping.

Each of the four members of the quadriceps has a different line of pull to produce knee extension (Figure 10-21). Interestingly, however, each muscle transmits its unique force across the knee using the same patellar tendon and patella. As described later, the individual force produced by each member of the quadriceps must be balanced with the others in order for the patella to track naturally. Optimal tracking places as little stress as possible on the patella and associated cartilage as it migrates up and down the intercondylar groove of the femur.

Knee Extensor Muscles

- Rectus femoris
- Vastus lateralis
- Vastus medialis
- Vastus intermedius

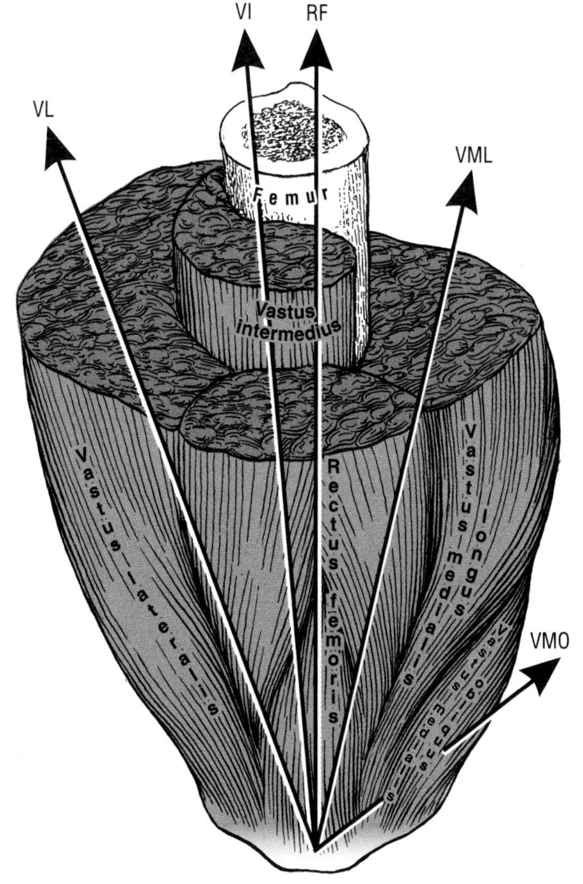

Figure 10-21 A cross section through the right quadriceps muscle. The arrows depict the approximate line of pull for each muscle of the quadriceps: vastus lateralis *(VL)*, vastus intermedius *(VI)*, rectus femoris *(RF)*, vastus medialis longus *(VML)*, and vastus medialis obliquus *(VMO)*. (From Neumann DA: *Kinesiology of the musculoskeletal system: foundations for physical rehabilitation*, St Louis, 2002, Mosby, Figure 13-23.)

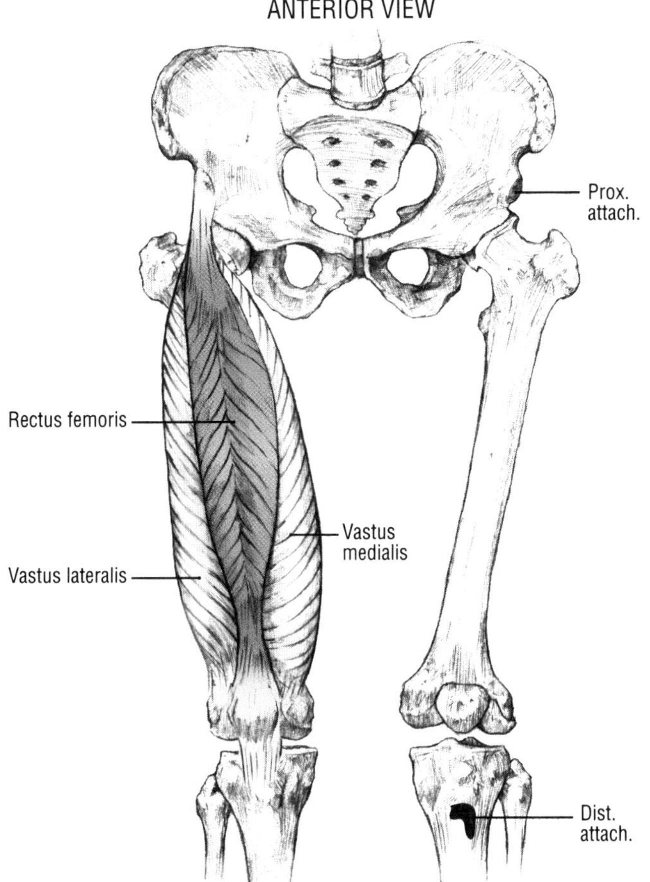

Rectus Femoris

Proximal Attachment: Anterior-inferior iliac spine

Distal Attachment: Tibial tuberosity

Innervation: Femoral nerve

Actions:
- Knee extension
- Hip flexion

Comments: Because this muscle crosses anterior to the hip and the knee, it functions as a hip flexor *and* a knee extensor. This long bipennate muscle is the only true antagonist to the hamstrings—muscles that extend the hip and flex the knee.

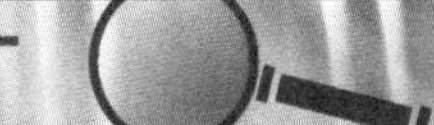

Clinical **INSIGHT**

Stretching the Rectus Femoris

As described, contraction of the rectus femoris can extend the knee and flex the hip. Therefore, maximally stretching this muscle requires that it be placed in a position opposite of *both* its actions. The rectus femoris, therefore, is stretched by extending the hip and flexing the knee.

In order to maximize the stretch of the rectus femoris, clinicians must pay close attention to any associated anterior tilting of the pelvis. For example, Figure 10-22, *A*, shows an individual attempting to stretch the rectus femoris with the pelvis poorly stabilized. In this scenario, as the femur is pulled posteriorly to extend the hip, the pelvis simultaneously tilts anteriorly. The anterior tilt of the pelvis (which is essentially a hip flexion motion) offsets any real stretch of the rectus femoris. This stretch is corrected in Figure 10-22, *B*, which shows strong activation of the abdominals to "hold" the pelvis in a posterior pelvic tilt. With the pelvis well stabilized, extension of the femur results in a more effective stretch on the rectus femoris.

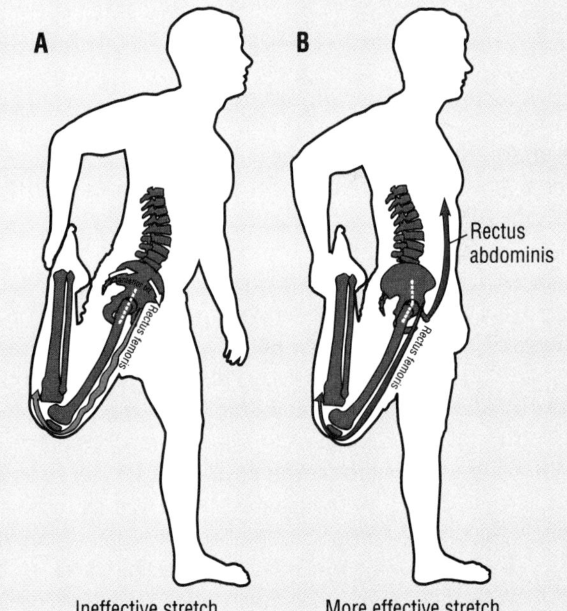

Figure 10-22 A, An ineffective stretch of the rectus femoris because minimal amounts of hip extension actually occur. **B,** A more effective stretch of the rectus femoris. The pelvis is well stabilized by the rectus abdominis as the hip is extended.

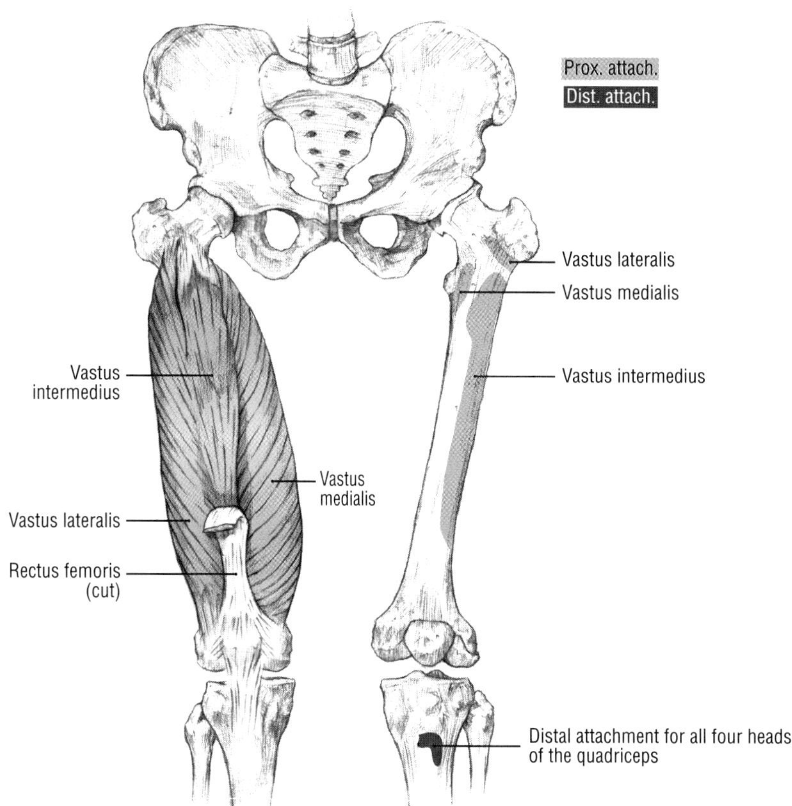

The vastus lateralis, vastus intermedius, and vastus medialis are shown with the rectus femoris cut for viewing.

Vastus Medialis

Proximal Attachment: Medial lip of the linea aspera and the intertrochanteric line of the femur

Distal Attachment: Tibial tuberosity

Innervation: Femoral nerve

Action: Knee extension

Comments: As this muscle courses distally toward the patella, it divides into two distinct fiber groups: the vastus medialis longus (VML) and the vastus medialis obliquus (VMO) (see Figure 10-21). The fibers of the vastus medialis longus are oriented longitudinally about 18 degrees from the midline, thereby directing most of its knee extension force in a line nearly parallel with the femur. The fibers of the vastus medialis obliquus, however, approach the patella at about a 50- to 55-degree angle to the midline. The more oblique orientation of the VMO provides a medially directed pull on the patella that counteracts the strong lateral pull of the larger, stronger vastus lateralis. Ideally, these two forces are balanced across the knee, resulting in optimal tracking of the patella.

Vastus Lateralis

Proximal Attachment: Lateral lip of the linea aspera, intertrochanteric line, and lateral region of the gluteal tuberosity

Distal Attachment: Tibial tuberosity

Innervation: Femoral nerve

Action: Knee extension

Comments: The vastus lateralis is the largest and hence the strongest of the quadriceps muscles. A significant portion of this muscle's force is directed laterally, which partially explains why abnormal tracking or dislocation of the patella occurs most frequently in a lateral direction.

Vastus Intermedius

Proximal Attachment: Upper two thirds of the anterior femoral shaft

Distal Attachment: Tibial tuberosity

Innervation: Femoral nerve

Action: Knee extension

Comments: The vastus intermedius is the deepest of the quadriceps muscles, located just deep to the rectus femoris.

Clinical INSIGHT

Q-Angle

The **Q-angle** describes the overall line of force of the quadriceps. This angle can provide clues to the causes of abnormal kinematics (or tracking) of the patellofemoral joint. This frontal plane angle is measured goniometrically as follows:

- *Axis:* Midpoint of the patella
- *Stationary arm:* Pointed toward the anterior-superior iliac spine
- *Movable arm:* Pointed toward the tibial tuberosity

The Q-angle (formally quadriceps angle) is normally 10 to 20 degrees (Figure 10-23), which reflects the normal genu valgus posture of the knee. The Q-angle indicates the relative lateral force that is applied to the patella during a quadriceps contraction. As illustrated in Figure 10-24, *A*, activation of the quadriceps naturally produces a lateral "bowstringing force" on the patella that is proportional to the strength of the quadriceps and the valgus alignment of the knee. *The larger the Q-angle (or genu valgum), the larger the lateral pull on the patella.* Larger lateral forces applied to the patella increase the chance of patellofemoral joint degeneration, abnormal lateral tracking, or even lateral patellar dislocation.

Interestingly, females have a slightly greater Q-angle than males. The proportionately larger Q-angle (and associated genu valgus) may account for the fact that women have a greater incidence of lateral dislocation of the patella and a higher frequency of patellofemoral joint pain.

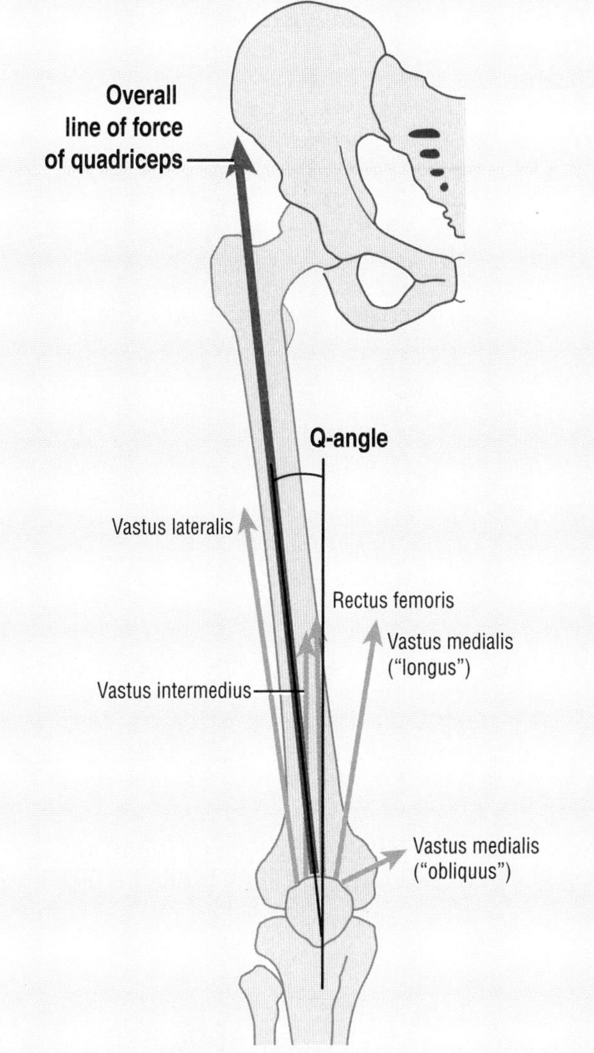

Figure 10-23 The overall line of force of the quadriceps as depicted by the Q-angle. (From Neumann DA: *Kinesiology of the musculoskeletal system: foundations for physical rehabilitation*, St Louis, 2002, Mosby, Figure 13-32.)

Functional Considerations

Excessive Lateral Tracking of the Patella. Normally, the patella tracks within the intercondylar groove without excessive deviation in either a medial or lateral direction. Normal tracking affords maximal contact area and minimal stress between the patella and the femur. Abnormal tracking of the patella is relatively common, however, and typically occurs in a lateral direction.

Excessive **lateral tracking of the patella** increases pressure and friction within the patellofemoral joint. This may result in pain, inflammation, and joint degeneration; in severe cases the patella may dislocate laterally. It is often helpful clinically to classify the factors that may contribute to an excessive lateral tracking of the patella as either *intrinsic*, originating at the knee, or *extrinsic*, originating proximally or distally to the knee (Box 10-1). Knowledge of these factors can help determine more effective treatment strategies.

Increased Compression within the Patellofemoral Joint during a Deep Squat. Patellofemoral joint pain is one of the most common clinical conditions of the knee. A common feature of this impairment is the inability of the patellofemoral joint to tolerate large compression forces. Often, clinicians recommend that patients with patellofemoral joint pain avoid or limit squatting as a way to reduce excessive compression and subsequent wear and tear of the

BOX 10-1

Factors That Can Cause Excessive Lateral Tracking of the Patella

Intrinsic Factors

- *Imbalance of forces between the vastus medialis obliquus (VMO) and the vastus lateralis (Figure 10-24, A)*
  Normally these two opposing heads of the quadriceps work together to track the patella "straight" within the intercondylar groove. Weakness of the VMO or hypertrophy of the vastus lateralis can create a force imbalance, likely resulting in an excessive lateral pull and subsequent lateral tracking of the patella.
- *Tight iliotibial band or lateral patellar retinaculum (see Figure 10-24, A)*
  The iliotibial band and lateral retinaculum (net-like connective tissue associated with distal attachments of the quadriceps) are firmly attached to the lateral aspect of the patella; therefore tightness of these structures can draw the patella laterally.
- *Decreased slope of the lateral facet on the intercondylar groove of the femur*
  The lateral facet of the femur is normally sloped at a relatively steep angle (see Figure 10-5, *A*). This slope naturally blocks the patella from gliding too far laterally. The slope of the lateral facet may be abnormally decreased, allowing the patella to glide laterally or dislocate out of the intercondylar groove of the femur.

Extrinsic Factors

- *Large Q-angle (Figure 10-24, B)*
  A large Q-angle resulting from malalignment of the hip or ankle creates a bowstringing force that naturally pulls the patella laterally on activation of the quadriceps.
- *Weak external rotators or abductors of the hip (see Figure 10-24, B)*
  During gait or weight-bearing activities, a person with weak hip external rotators and abductors may have difficulty preventing the femur from drifting into adduction and internal rotation. (This is often apparent while a person sits slowly from a standing position or slowly descends a step.) With the foot securely planted, excessive internal rotation and adduction of the femur (hip) increases the genu valgum of the knee. As a result, the patella is forced laterally.
- *Excessive pronation of the foot (see Figure 10-24, B)*
  Pronation of the foot can force the tibia medially, therefore creating increased valgus of the knee. The greater the valgus, the greater the potential for lateral tracking of the patella.

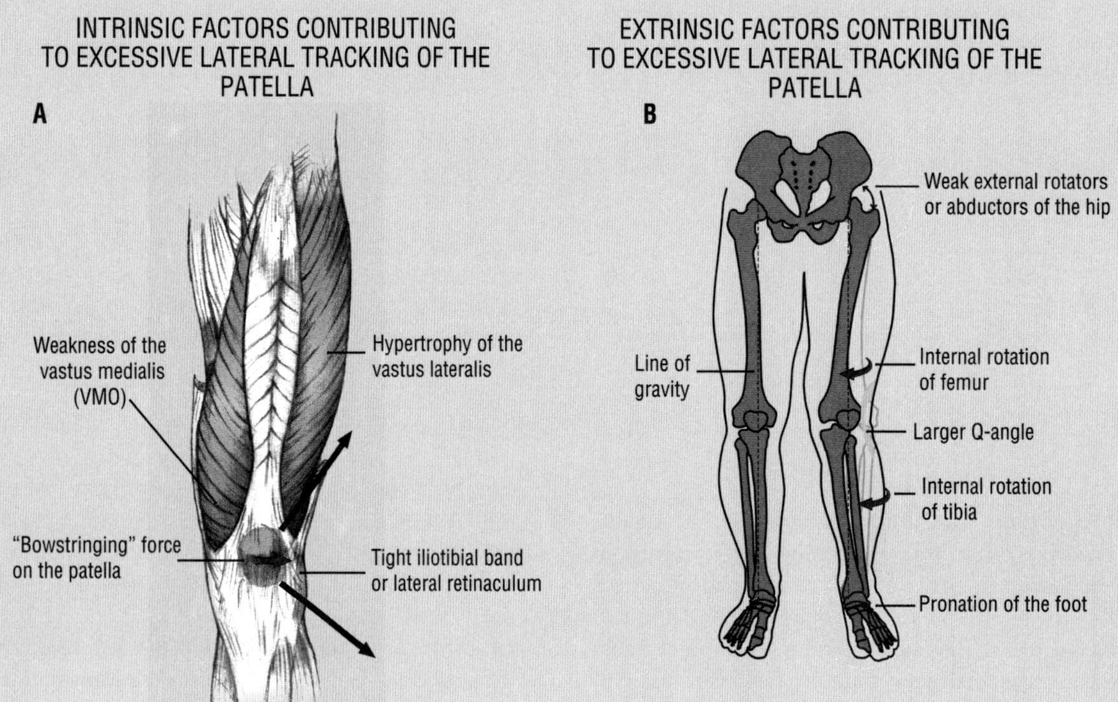

Figure 10-24 Factors that contribute to excessive lateral tracking of the patella. **A,** Intrinsic factors. **B,** Extrinsic factors.

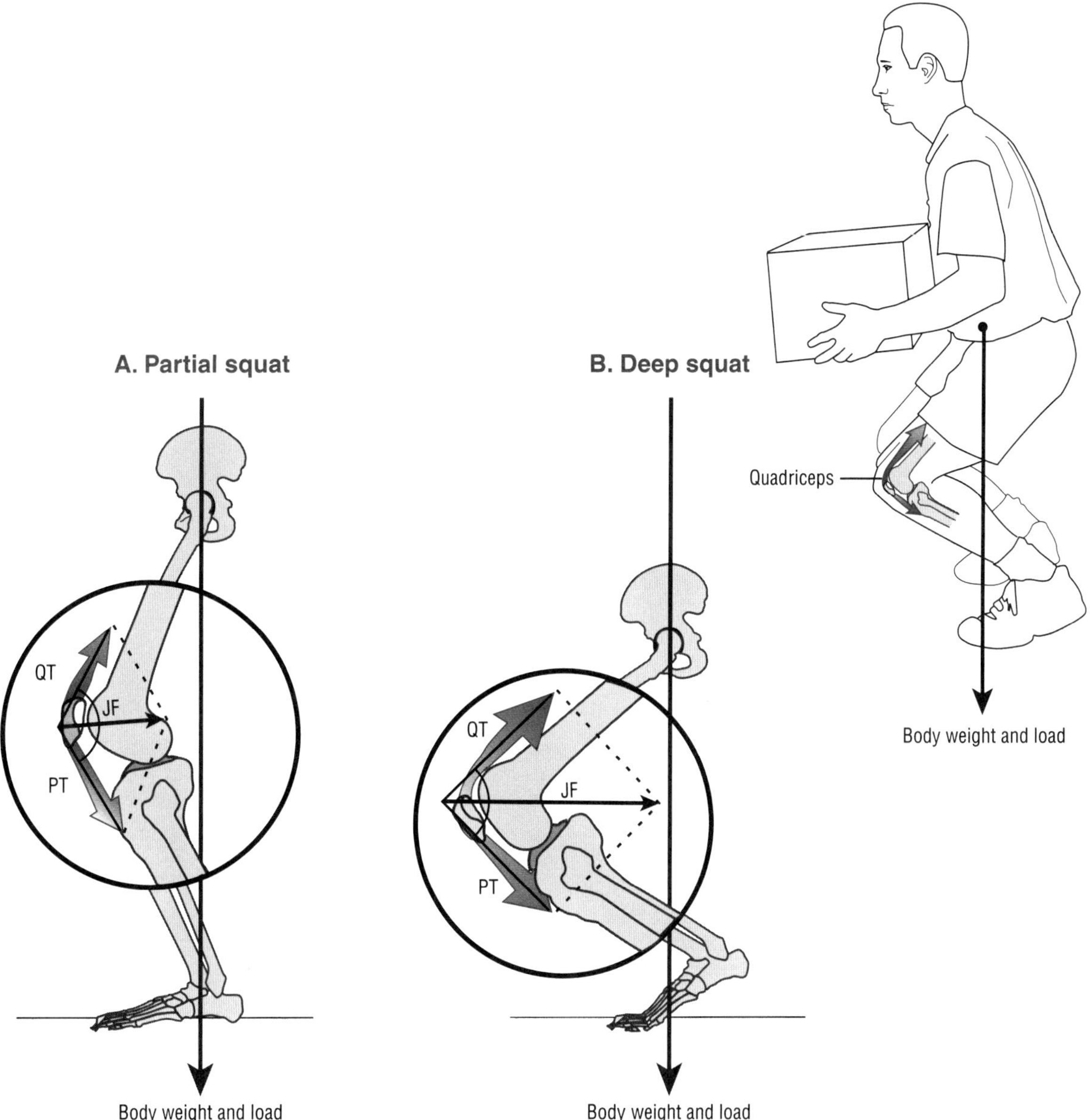

Figure 10-25 The relationship between the depth of a squat position and the compression force within the patellofemoral joint. **A,** Maintaining a partial squat requires that the quadriceps transmit a force through the quadriceps tendon *(QT)* and the patellar tendon *(PT)*. The vector addition of QT and PT provides an estimation of the patellofemoral joint force *(JF)*. **B,** The deeper squat not only requires greater quadriceps force because of the larger flexion torque at the knee, but the more acute angle increases the resultant joint force. (Modified from Neumann DA: *Kinesiology of the musculoskeletal system: foundations for physical rehabilitation*, St Louis, 2002, Mosby, Figure 13-29.)

posterior side of the patella. As illustrated in Figure 10-25, *A*, a squatting position places the line of body weight far posterior to the medial-lateral axis of the knee. In order to control the squat, the quadriceps must be strongly activated; this produces a compression force that strongly presses the patella into the intercondylar groove of the femur. Figure 10-25, *B*, illustrates the same individual performing a deeper squat. As indicated, the deeper squat places the line-of-body weight much farther posterior to the medial-lateral axis of the knee, which generates a proportionally greater demand on the quadriceps muscles. The increased knee extensor force results in a proportionally large increase in the compression force through the patellofemoral joint (see Figure 10-25, *B*). Also, by comparing Figure 10-25, *A* and *B*, it should be apparent that increased flexion of the knee results in a much larger resultant joint force (*JF* in Figure 10-25) than that of the more extended knee. The larger the resultant force produces a proportionately large increase in the patellofemoral compression force. These large forces may contribute to increased patellofemoral joint pain and inflammation, especially if the joint has a pre-existing condition, such as osteoarthritis of the knee.

Clinical INSIGHT

Extensor Lag

Many times after surgery or injury to the knee, the quadriceps show considerable difficulty in performing the last 15 to 20 degrees of active knee extension. Clinically, this impairment is referred to as an **extensor lag,** which can adversely affect lower extremity function.

Interestingly, the difficulty in completing full active knee extension is often attributed to effusion (swelling) within the knee. Swelling increases intra-articular pressure, which can physically impede full knee extension. This is especially true in the final degrees of extension where intra-articular pressure is naturally the greatest. Also, increased intra-articular pressure can cause neural inhibition of the quadriceps, preventing full activation of this muscle. Methods that reduce swelling of the knee therefore have an important role in rehabilitation of the knee.

KNEE FLEXOR MUSCLES

The knee flexors include the set of hamstrings, gracilis, sartorius, gastrocnemius, plantaris, and popliteus. Interestingly, most of these knee flexors also internally or externally rotate the knee. This important set of motions will be discussed in an upcoming section.

Knee Flexor Muscles

- Semimembransous
- Semitendinosus
- Biceps femoris—long and short heads
- Gracilis and sartorius
- Gastrocnemius and plantaris
- Popliteus

Hamstrings

The semitendinosus, semimembranosus, and biceps femoris (long and short heads) make up the hamstring group (Figure 10-26).

Spanning the posterior thigh, the hamstring muscles are the primary knee flexors. With the exception of the short head of the biceps femoris, the hamstrings also perform hip extension. Because three of the four hamstrings cross the hip, as well as the knee, the position of the hip (and knee) can significantly affect the operational length of these muscles. For this reason, both the extensibility and maximal force generated by the hamstrings are highly dependent on the position of the hip. This important point is revisited later in this chapter. The specific anatomy of the hamstrings is covered in the previous chapter, but a brief review is provided in the following table.

HAMSTRINGS

Muscle	Proximal Attachment	Distal Attachment	Actions	Innervation
Semitendinosus	Ischial tuberosity	Proximal-medial aspect of the tibia (via pes anserinus)	Hip extension Knee flexion Knee internal rotation	Tibial branch of the sciatic nerve
Semimembranosus	Ischial tuberosity	Posterior surface of the medial condyle of the tibia	Hip extension Knee flexion Knee internal rotation	Tibial branch of the sciatic nerve
Biceps femoris—long head	Ischial tuberosity	Head of the fibula	Hip extension Knee flexion Knee external rotation	Tibial branch of the sciatic nerve
Biceps femoris—short head	Lateral lip of the linea aspera	Head of the fibula	Knee flexion Knee external rotation	Peroneal branch of the sciatic nerve

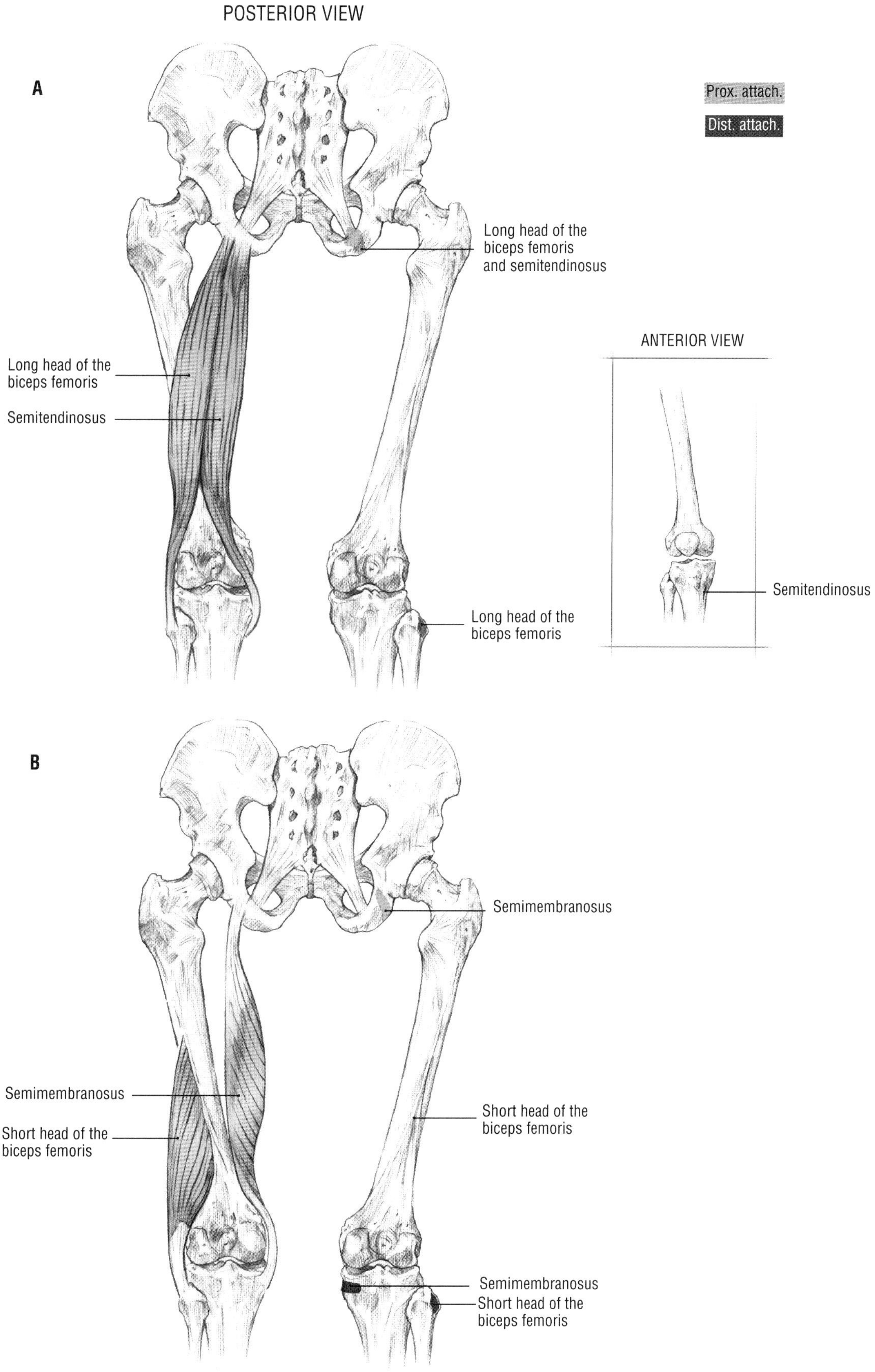

Figure 10-26 The hamstring muscles. **A,** The semitendinosus and long head of the biceps femoris. **B,** The semimembranosus and short head of the biceps femoris.

GRACILIS AND SARTORIUS

Muscle	Proximal Attachment	Distal Attachment	Actions	Innervation
Gracilis	Inferior pubic ramus	Proximal-medial tibia (via pes anserinus)	Hip adduction Hip flexion Knee flexion Knee internal rotation	Obturator nerve
Sartorius	Anterior-superior Iliac spine	Proximal-medial tibia (via pes anserinus)	Hip flexion Hip external rotation Hip abduction Knee flexion Knee internal rotation	Femoral nerve

Gracilis and Sartorius

The gracilis and sartorius are described in the previous chapter in reference to their functions at the hip (see pp. 263 and 248). These muscles also flex and internally rotate the knee and play an important role in providing stability to the medial side of the knee.

Both of these muscles attach proximally to the pelvis—the sartorius to the anterior-superior iliac spine (ASIS) and the gracilis to the inferior pubic ramus. Distally, these muscles travel side by side as they course posterior to the medial-lateral axis of rotation of the knee. The tendons of the gracilis and sartorius join the tendon of the semitendinosus for a collective insertion on the proximal-medial tibia. The three tendons conjoin to form one common tendon, commonly referred to as the **pes anserinus,** meaning "goose's foot" in Latin.

Consider this...

Pes Anserinus

The semitendinosus, sartorius, and gracilis all attach to the proximal-medial tibia through a broad sheet of connective tissue known as the pes anserinus. The pes anserinus, meaning "goose's foot," gets its name from the three-pronged appearance of the tendons of these three muscles as they course toward their common insertion.

Although all three of these muscles originate from a different bone of the pelvis, perform different actions at the hip, and are innervated by different nerves, they all perform three common functions at the knee, as follows:

- Flexion of the knee
- Internal rotation of the knee
- Dynamic support of the medial collateral ligament, providing medial stability to the knee

Gastrocnemius and Plantaris

The gastrocnemius is a powerful two-headed muscle, well known for its ability to produce large plantar flexion torques across the ankle. Because this muscle crosses the posterior aspect of the knee, it is also a knee flexor. This muscle, along with the relatively small plantaris, which also crosses the posterior knee, is described in greater detail in the next chapter.

Popliteus

As described previously in this chapter, the knee is locked into extension by the screw home mechanism (i.e., external rotation of the knee). The popliteus muscle, a very effective *internal* rotator muscle, provides the torque that unlocks the knee. As one transitions from a knee-extended position to a partial squat, for example, the popliteus externally rotates the femur slightly and, in a relative sense, internally rotates the knee. This action is essential to unlock the knee, thereby allowing it to flex.

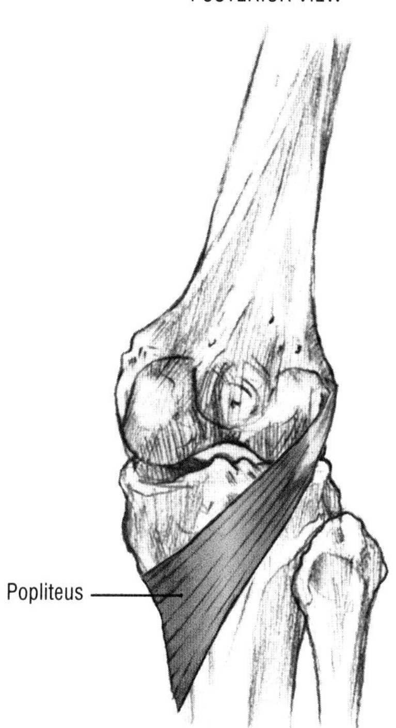

Popliteus

Proximal Attachment:	Posterior aspect of the lateral femoral condyle
Distal Attachment:	Posterior surface of the proximal tibia
Innervation:	Tibial nerve
Actions:	• Knee internal rotation • Knee flexion
Comments:	Based on this muscle's ability to unlock the knee, it is often referred to as the "key to the knee."

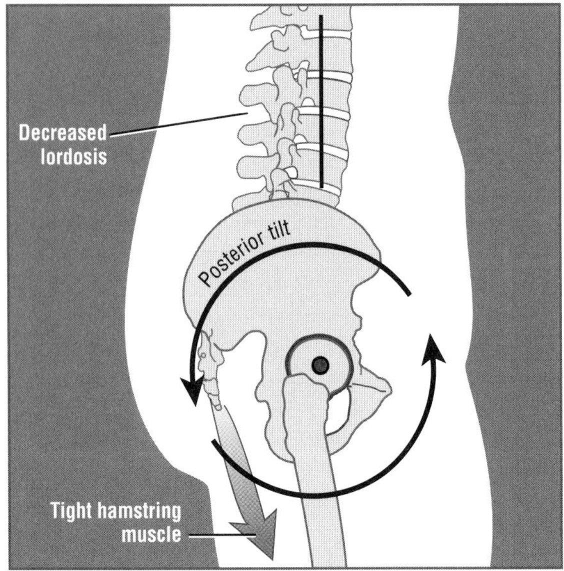

Figure 10-27 Passive tension from the already tight hamstrings pulls the pelvis into a posterior pelvic tilt as the knee is attempted to be extended. (Modified from Neumann DA: *Kinesiology of the musculoskeletal system: foundations for physical rehabilitation,* St Louis, 2002, Mosby, Figure 12-41.)

Functional Considerations

Consequences of Tight Hamstrings. Tightness of the hamstrings is a relatively common impairment, often due to spasticity, muscle irritability, or spending extended periods of time in a flexed-knee position such as sitting. When non–weight bearing, as when lying in bed, extreme tightness of the hamstring muscles is often observed as a knee flexion contracture. However, when attempting to stand upright, the additional stretch placed on the tight hamstrings is transferred proximally and can be expressed as an extreme posterior pelvic tilt and flattened lumbar spine (Figure 10-27). As described in Chapter 8, a flattened lumbar spine may over-stretch the connective tissues in the lumbar region, thereby increasing the likelihood of a posterior herniated intervertebral disc. It is interesting that a knee flexion contracture can have such negative kinesiologic consequences as far proximal as the lumbar spine.

When stretching the hamstrings, a clinician must be aware of the potential for passive tension in these muscles to posteriorly tilt the pelvis. Therefore it is important that the therapist (or patient) stabilize the pelvis as the stretch is being performed. Without adequate pelvic stabilization, attempts to stretch the hamstrings may result in an undesired posterior pelvic tilt, which would reduce the effectiveness of the hamstring stretch. Excessive posterior tilting may produce an unwanted over-stretching of the connective tissues within the lumbar region.

Synergy between the Rectus Femoris and Hamstrings. Most functional activities of the lower extremity combine the motions of (1) hip flexion and knee flexion or (2) hip extension and knee extension. Consider these motions while jumping or climbing up a steep hill, for example. These movements are not random but occur naturally to help the rectus femoris and hamstrings remain close to their optimal length for producing effective forces.

To explain further, consider the simultaneous action of hip extension *and* knee extension, a natural motion used during running (Figure 10-28). The semitendinosus, for example, actively shortens to extend the hip; however, at the same time, this muscle is passively stretched as the knee is actively extended by the quadriceps. As the active rectus femoris extends the knee, it is also simultaneously stretched across the extending hip. Therefore, during combined hip and knee extension, both the rectus femoris and semitendinosus muscle avoid over-contracting (shortening) across the hip and knee. If this were to happen, the muscles would rapidly become actively insufficient and unable to generate effective forces. Consider, for example, the consequence of trying to combine

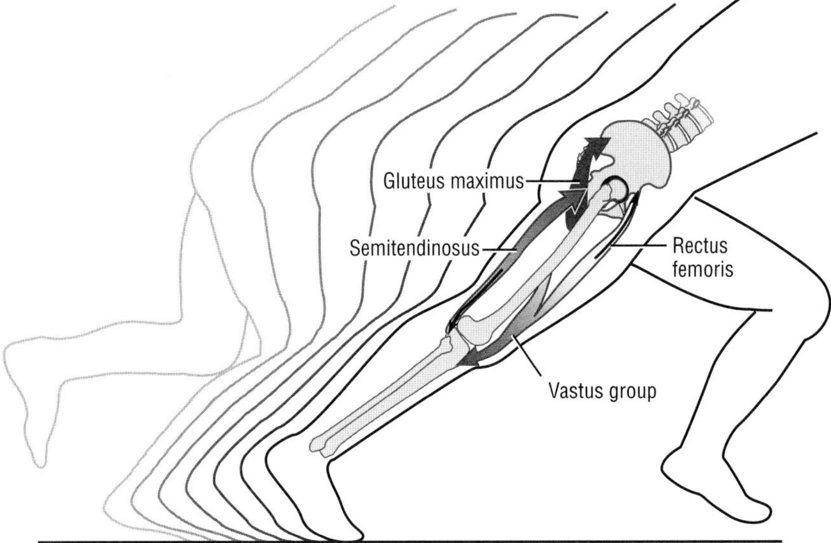

Figure 10-28 The muscular interaction of the right leg during the push-off phase of running. Note the relationship between the multi-articular rectus femoris and the semitendinosus. The position of hip extension and knee extension allows each muscle to "borrow length" from the hip *(semitendinosus)* or the knee *(rectus femoris).* The black arrows indicate the region of "stretch" within each muscle. (From Neumann DA: *Kinesiology of the musculoskeletal system: foundations for physical rehabilitation,* St Louis, 2002, Mosby, Figure 13-36.)

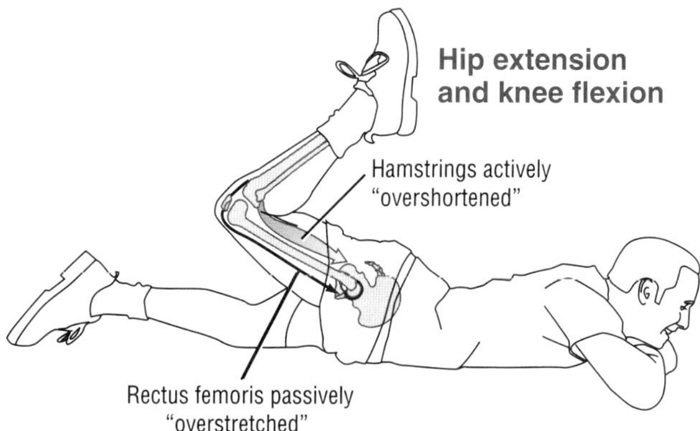

Figure 10-29 The combined motions of hip extension and knee flexion produce active insufficiency of the hamstring muscles and passive insufficiency of the rectus femoris, indicated by the thin black line. (From Neumann DA: *Kinesiology of the musculoskeletal system: foundations for physical rehabilitation*, St Louis, 2002, Mosby, Figure 13-37, *B*.)

active hip extension with knee flexion (Figure 10-29). During this seemingly unnatural motion, the hamstring muscles actively and quickly over-shorten across the hip and knee at once, a situation that significantly reduces their force-producing potential. Furthermore, the over-stretched rectus femoris becomes passively insufficient, thereby further limiting the ability of the hamstrings to flex the knee and extend the hip. Table 10-4 lists the various movement combinations that usually promote either effective or ineffective force production from the rectus femoris and hamstrings.

Internal and External Rotators of the Knee

All of the hamstrings muscles, as well as the gracilis, popliteus, and sartorius, control active rotation of the knee within the horizontal plane. The medial hamstrings (semitendinosus and semimembranosus), gracilis, and sartorius internally rotate the knee, whereas the lateral hamstrings (both heads of biceps femoris) externally rotate the knee.

Interestingly, the ability to perform rotation of the knee for either group is almost negligible when the knee is near full extension but maximal when the knee is flexed to 90 degrees. This reinforces the concept that a muscle has the best leverage when it approaches the shaft of the bone at a 90-degree angle.

The internal rotator muscles of the knee far outweigh the strength of the external rotator muscles. This should be no surprise considering that there are many more internal rotators than external rotators of the knee. Such a disparity favoring the internal rotator muscles likely reflects the functional need at the knee to either accelerate the knee into internal rotation (by concentric contraction) or decelerate external rotation of the knee (by eccentric

Internal and External Rotators of the Knee

Internal Rotators
- Semimembranosus
- Semitendinosus
- Gracilis
- Sartorius
- Popliteus

External Rotators
- Biceps femoris—long head
- Biceps femoris—short head

TABLE 10-4 MOVEMENT COMBINATIONS THAT PROMOTE EFFECTIVE AND INEFFECTIVE FORCE PRODUCTION

Position of Hip or Knee	Description
Effective Force Production	
Hip flexion *and* knee flexion	Hamstrings and rectus femoris are able to work synergistically, thereby maintaining optimal length-tension relationship
Hip extension *and* knee extension	As above, the hamstrings and rectus femoris are able to work synergistically, thereby maintaining optimal length-tension relationship
Ineffective Force Production	
Hip flexion and knee extension	Rectus femoris becomes *actively insufficient*—shortened over both joints, significantly reducing its force-producing ability
	Hamstrings become *passively insufficient*—stretched across both joints, creating passive resistance to the motion
Hip extension and knee flexion	Rectus femoris becomes *passively insufficient*—stretched across both joints, creating passive resistance to the motion
	Hamstrings become *actively insufficient*—shortened over both joints, significantly reducing their force-producing capability

Clinical INSIGHT

Manual Muscle Testing to Isolate the Gluteus Maximus

Clinically, it is important that the therapist be able to determine which individual muscle within a larger muscle group is exhibiting weakness. This situation may be necessary when evaluating the strength of the hip extensor muscles. Through an understanding of the form and function of these muscles, a procedure known as a manual muscle test (MMT) can help identify the specific muscle or muscles involved, as follows:

- MMT of *all* hip extensors (Figure 10-30, *A*): The subject lies prone and performs maximal-effort hip extension with the knee extended. The therapist resists this action and assigns the appropriate strength grade to the contracting muscle.
  A weak grade by the therapist indicates only that there is reduced strength within the hip extensor group as a whole.
- MMT of the gluteus maximus (Figure 10-30, *B*): The subject lies prone with the knee flexed, and then performs maximal-effort hip extension. The therapist once again resists this action to determine the muscle's strength grade.

The position of knee flexion and hip extension purposively over-shortens the hamstrings across both the hip and knee, thereby reducing the muscle's active force potential. This procedure is believed to "isolate" the gluteus maximus from the contracting hamstrings. Weakness demonstrated from this test strongly suggests reduced strength of the gluteus maximus.

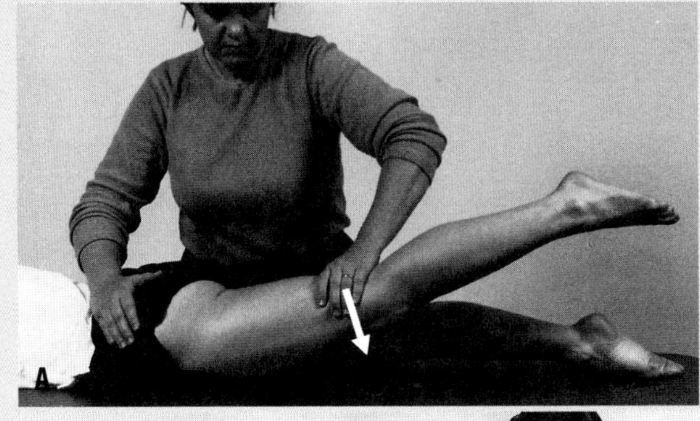

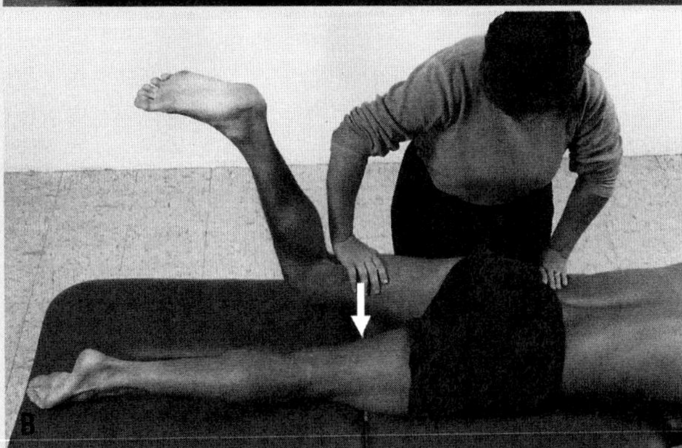

Figure 10-30 Two different manual muscle tests for the hip extensors. **A,** Manual muscle test for all the hip extensors (gluteus maximus and hamstrings). **B,** Manual muscle test that isolates the gluteus maximus. (From Reese NB: *Muscle and sensory testing*, ed 2, Philadelphia, 2005, Saunders, Figures 4-16, *A*, and 4-23, *B*.)

activation). An analysis of the "cutting" motion often performed in sports reinforces the importance of the eccentric activity of the internal rotators at the knee. For example, sharply cutting to the left normally involves firmly planting the right foot and pushing off to the left. As illustrated in Figure 10-31, this motion involves internal rotation of the right femur relative to the planted tibia; remember, this is actually external rotation of the *knee* (tibia relative to femur). Such a motion creates a valgus strain on the knee, which is easy to verify on one's self. Through eccentric activation, the internal rotators not only decelerate the external rotation of the knee, but dynamically support the medial collateral ligament, protecting the knee from excessive valgus strain.

Summary

The stability of the knee is maintained largely by the ligaments and surrounding musculature, as the bony containment provides little protective support. The combination of large forces and lack of bony constraint may account for the relatively high incidence of knee injuries. Because the knee is located between the hip and ankle, it is subjected to many large stresses that can originate at either end of the lower extremity.

From a therapeutic perspective, the knee must be considered within the functional context of the entire lower extremity. Rehabilitation approaches usually involve the knee itself, as well as surrounding joints and muscles. Therapeutic concerns that focus directly on the knee include stretching or strengthening of the muscles that cross the joint, the application of braces, and instructions on how to protect injured tissues. The prudent clinician, however, often addresses weakness or malalignment of the hip or ankle as part of a knee rehabilitation regimen.

Study Questions

1. Which of the following describes the primary sagittal plane function of the anterior cruciate ligament?
   a. Resists posterior translation of the femur relative to a fixed tibia

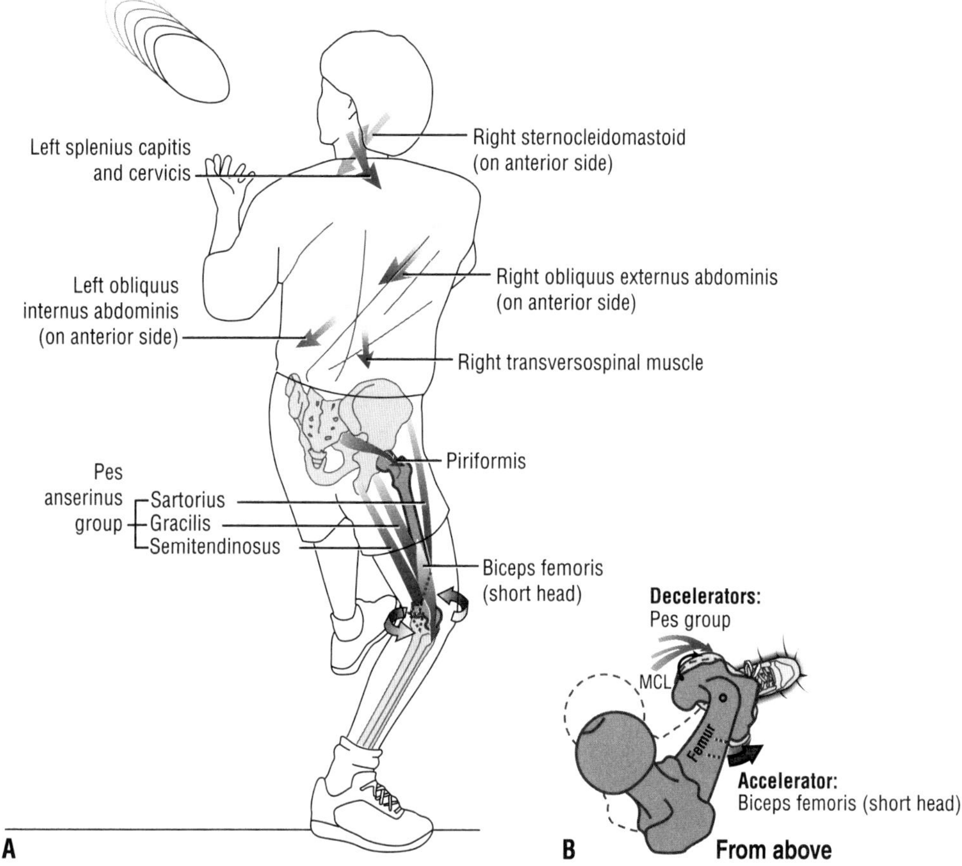

Figure 10-31 With the right foot fixed to the ground, the right knee becomes an important pivot point for controlling horizontal plane rotation **(A).** The short head of the biceps is shown accelerating the femur into internal rotation, while the medial hamstrings and the pes anserinus group are eccentrically activated to help decelerate and limit the amount of external rotation at the knee **(B).** (From Neumann DA: *Kinesiology of the musculoskeletal system: foundations for physical rehabilitation*, St Louis, 2002, Mosby, Figure 13-33.)

  b. Resists anterior translation of the femur relative to a fixed tibia
  c. Resists anterior translation of the tibia relative to a fixed femur
  d. A and C
  e. B and C
2. Which of the following structures is the distal attachment for all heads of the quadriceps?
  a. Tibial plateau
  b. Tibial tuberosity
  c. Pes anserinus
  d. Lateral epicondyle of the femur
3. Measured on the lateral side of the knee, normal genu valgum of the knee is typically:
  a. 30 degrees
  b. 100 degrees
  c. 120 to 140 degrees
  d. 170 to 175 degrees
4. The primary ligament involved in resisting large valgus-producing forces at the knee is the:
  a. Medial collateral ligament
  b. Posterior cruciate ligament
  c. Lateral collateral ligament
  d. Arcuate popliteal ligament
5. The "terrible triad" describes:
  a. Three primary muscles involved in a hamstring strain
  b. Triangular forces produced during a deep squat
  c. Simultaneous injury of the medial collateral ligament, anterior cruciate ligament, and medial meniscus
  d. Simultaneous activation of the quadriceps, hamstring, and gastrocnemius muscles
6. Which of the following statements best describes the function of the medial and lateral menisci of the knee?
  a. Absorb compressive forces between the patella and the femur
  b. Absorb and disperse the compressive forces between the tibia and the femur
  c. Prevent friction between the hamstring muscles and the epicondyles of the femur
  d. Significantly reduce the area of joint contact between the femur and the tibia

7. Which of the following best describes the screw-home mechanism of the knee?
   a. Active extension of the knee causes a superior migration of the patella
   b. Passive flexion of the knee results in an inferior migration of the patella
   c. An automatic rotation that assists in locking the knee into extension
   d. Simultaneous activation of the medial and lateral hamstring muscles
8. Which of the following muscles is innervated by the femoral nerve?
   a. Biceps femoris—long head
   b. Semitendinosus
   c. Rectus femoris
   d. A and C
   e. B and C
9. Which of the following muscles is able to perform hip extension and knee flexion?
   a. Semitendinosus
   b. Biceps femoris—long head
   c. Biceps femoris—short head
   d. A and B
   e. All of the above
10. Which of the following muscles is *not* associated with the pes anserinus?
   a. Sartorius
   b. Rectus femoris
   c. Gracilis
   d. Semitendinosus
11. Which of the following muscles is *not* innervated by the tibial branch of the sciatic nerve?
   a. Semitendinosus
   b. Biceps femoris—long head
   c. Semimembranosus
   d. Biceps femoris—short head
12. A muscle that courses anterior to the medial-lateral axis of rotation of the knee is able to perform:
   a. Knee flexion
   b. Knee extension
   c. Knee internal rotation
   d. Knee external rotation
13. Which of the following statements best describes genu recurvatum?
   a. Internal rotation of the tibia relative to a fixed femur
   b. A knee that displays marked hyperextension
   c. A knee that consistently displays a knock-kneed or valgus appearance
   d. A knee that consistently displays a bow-legged or varus appearance
14. Which of the following statements best describes a function of the patella?
   a. Prevents excessive hyperextension of the knee
   b. Assists the medial hamstrings with internal rotation of the patella
   c. Increases the internal moment arm of the quadriceps, enhancing knee extension torque
   d. Prevents excessive flexion of the knee
   e. B and D
15. Which of the following factors are likely to contribute to excessive lateral tracking of the patella?
   a. Tight iliotibial band or lateral retinaculum
   b. Excessive pronation of the ankle and foot
   c. Weakness of the hip abductors and hip external rotators
   d. B and C
   e. All of the above
16. An "extensor lag" is best described as:
   a. Activation of the vastus medialis and vastus lateralis occurring after activation of the rectus femoris
   b. Activation of the quadriceps that occurs after activation of the hamstrings
   c. Inability to complete the final few degrees of knee extension possibly due to swelling within the knee
   d. Extension of the knee occurring after extension of the hip
17. The hamstrings are maximally elongated in a position of:
   a. Hip flexion and knee flexion
   b. Hip extension and knee flexion
   c. Hip flexion and knee extension
   d. Hip extension and knee extension
18. On standing with the knees fully extended, an individual with tight hamstrings is most likely to display:
   a. A relative anterior pelvic tilt
   b. A relative posterior pelvic tilt
   c. Genu varum
   d. Genu valgum
19. The rectus femoris remains strong throughout a motion that combines hip flexion with knee flexion because:
   a. The rectus femoris becomes maximally elongated
   b. The hamstrings are able to assist with flexing the hip
   c. The rectus femoris is shortened across the hip but elongated across the knee—maintaining a near-optimal length for producing force
   d. The vastus medialis and vastus lateralis assist with flexing the hip, whereas the one-joint gluteus maximus assists with flexing the knee.
20. Which of the following muscles is *not* multi-articular?
   a. Vastus lateralis
   b. Vastus medialis
   c. Rectus femoris
   d. A and B
   e. All of the above are multi-articular muscles.
21. Which of the following muscles is *not* considered a quadriceps muscle?
   a. Semimembranosus
   b. Vastus intermedius
   c. Rectus femoris

d. Vastus lateralis
e. A and C

22. If the quadriceps are active eccentrically:
a. The knee is moving into extension.
b. The hip is moving into flexion.
c. The knee is moving into flexion.
d. The patella is migrating superiorly.

23. A large Q-angle can contribute to excessive lateral tracking of the patella.
a. True
b. False

24. The gastrocnemius muscles have the potential to perform knee extension.
a. True
b. False

25. Active extension of the knee involves a superior migration of the patella.
a. True
b. False

26. One of the primary functions of the popliteus muscle is to assist in locking the knee.
a. True
b. False

27. A deep squat produces more patellofemoral compression force than a shallow squat.
a. True
b. False

28. The rectus femoris becomes actively insufficient when performing the combined motions of hip flexion and knee extension.
a. True
b. False

29. One of the primary functions of the posterior cruciate ligament is to resist a posterior translation of the tibia relative to a fixed femur.
a. True
b. False

30. The medial and lateral collateral ligaments are at less risk of injury with the knee fully extended because they are slackened in knee extension.
a. True
b. False

ADDITIONAL READINGS

Adachi N, Ochi M, Uchio Y et al: Mechanoreceptors in the anterior cruciate ligament contribute to the joint position sense, *Acta Orthop Scand* 73(3):330-334, 2002.

Akima H, Furukawa T: Atrophy of thigh muscles after meniscal lesions and arthroscopic partial meniscectomy, *Knee Surg Sports Traumatol Arthrosc* 13(8):632-637, 2005.

Baker MM, Juhn MS: Patellofemoral pain syndrome in the female athlete, *Clin Sports Med* 19(2):315-329, 2000.

Besier TF, Lloyd DG, Ackland TR: Muscle activation strategies at the knee during running and cutting maneuvers, *Med Sci Sports Exerc* 35(1):119-127, 2003.

Beynnon BD, Johnson RJ, Abate JA et al: Treatment of anterior cruciate ligament injuries, part 1, *Am J Sports Med* 33(10): 1579-1602, 2005.

Beynnon BD, Johnson RJ, Abate JA et al: Treatment of anterior cruciate ligament injuries, part 2, *Am J Sports Med* 33(11):1751-1767, 2005.

Bodor M: Quadriceps protects the anterior cruciate ligament, *J Orthop Res* 19(4):629-633, 2001.

Christoforakis J, Bull AM, Strachan RK et al: Effects of lateral retinacular release on the lateral stability of the patella, *Knee Surg Sports Traumatol Arthrosc* 14(3):273-277, 2006.

Christou EA: Patellar taping increases vastus medialis oblique activity in the presence of patellofemoral pain, *J Electromyogr Kinesiol* 14(4):495-504, 2004.

Cibulka MT, Threlkeld-Watkins J: Patellofemoral pain and asymmetrical hip rotation, *Phys Ther* 85(11):1201-1207, 2005.

Fithian DC, Paxton EW, Stone ML et al: Epidemiology and natural history of acute patellar dislocation, *Am J Sports Med* 32(5):1114-1121, 2004.

Fleming BC, Oksendahl H, Beynnon BD: Open- or closed-kinetic chain exercises after anterior cruciate ligament reconstruction? *Exerc Sport Sci Rev* 33(3):134-140, 2005.

Gigante A, Pasquinelli FM, Paladini P et al: The effects of patellar taping on patellofemoral incongruence: a computed tomography study, *Am J Sports Med* 29(1):88-92, 2001.

Hewett TE, Myer GD, Ford KR: Anterior cruciate ligament injuries in female athletes. Part 1: Mechanisms and risk factors, *Am J Sports Med* 34(2):299-311, 2006.

Hewett TE, Ford KR, Myer GD: Anterior cruciate ligament injuries in female athletes. Part 2: A meta-analysis of neuromuscular interventions aimed at injury prevention, *Am J Sports Med* 34(3):490-498, 2006.

Lutz GE, Palmitier RA, An KN et al: Comparison of tibiofemoral joint forces during open-kinetic-chain and closed-kinetic-chain exercises, *J Bone Joint Surg Am* 75(5):732-739, 1993.

Mizuno Y, Kumagai M, Mattessich SM et al: Q-angle influences tibiofemoral and patellofemoral kinematics, *J Orthop Res* 19(5):834-840, 2001.

Mohtadi N: Rehabilitation of anterior cruciate ligament injuries: a review, *Clin J Sport Med* 15(4):287-288, 2005.

Powers CM: The influence of altered lower-extremity kinematics on patellofemoral joint dysfunction: a theoretical perspective, *J Orthop Sports Phys Ther* 33(11):639-646, 2003.

Powers CM: Patellar kinematics. Part I: The influence of vastus muscle activity in subjects with and without patellofemoral pain, *Phys Ther* 80(10):956-964, 2000.

Powers CM: Patellar kinematics. Part II: The influence of the depth of the trochlear groove in subjects with and without patellofemoral pain, *Phys Ther* 80(10):965-978, 2000.

Powers CM: Rehabilitation of patellofemoral joint disorders: a critical review, *J Orthop Sports Phys Ther* 28(5):345-354, 1998.

Powers CM, Chen PY, Reischl SF et al: Comparison of foot pronation and lower extremity rotation in persons with and without patellofemoral pain, *Foot Ankle Int* 23(7):634-640, 2002.

Powers CM, Chen YJ, Scher I et al: The influence of patellofemoral joint contact geometry on the modeling of three dimensional patellofemoral joint forces, *J Biomech* 39(15):2783-2791, 2006.

Powers CM, Ward SR, Fredericson M et al: Patellofemoral kinematics during weight-bearing and non–weight-bearing knee extension in persons with lateral subluxation of the patella: a preliminary study, *J Orthop Sports Phys Ther* 33(11):677-685, 2003.

Salsich GB, Brechter JH, Farwell D et al: The effects of patellar taping on knee kinetics, kinematics, and vastus lateralis muscle activity during stair ambulation in individuals with patellofemoral pain, *J Orthop Sports Phys Ther* 32(1):3-10, 2002.

Sendur OF, Gurer G, Yildirim T et al: Relationship of Q angle and joint hypermobility and Q angle values in different positions, *Clin Rheumatol* 25(3):304-308, 2006.

Takahashi M, Doi M, Abe M et al: Anatomical study of the femoral and tibial insertions of the anteromedial and posterolateral bundles of human anterior cruciate ligament, *Am J Sports Med* 34(5):787-792, 2006.

Witvrouw E, Danneels L, Van TD et al: Open versus closed kinetic chain exercises in patellofemoral pain: a 5-year prospective randomized study, *Am J Sports Med* 32(5):1122-1130, 2004.

CHAPTER 11

Structure and Function of the Ankle and Foot

CHAPTER OUTLINE

OBJECTIVES

- Identify the primary bones and bony features of the ankle and foot.
- Describe the connective tissues of the ankle and foot.
- Describe the primary motions that occur at the talocrural, subtalar, and transverse tarsal joints.
- Describe the most stable position of the talocrural joint.
- Describe the planes of motion and axes of rotation for dorsiflexion/plantar flexion, inversion/eversion, and adduction/abduction of the ankle and foot.
- Cite the components of the motions of pronation and supination.
- Explain the function of the medial longitudinal arch.
- Explain why the lateral ligaments of the ankle are injured far more often than the medial ligaments.
- Justify the actions of the muscles of the ankle and foot through knowledge of their proximal and distal attachments.
- Cite the innervation of the muscles of the ankle and foot.
- Explain the primary muscular interactions involved with rising up on tip-toes.
- Describe the common abnormal gait patterns involved with weakness of the dorsiflexor muscles.
- Explain how the interaction among the talocrural, subtalar, and transverse tarsal joints allows the foot to adapt to uneven ground while standing and walking.

KEY TERMS

abduction
adduction
dorsal
dorsiflexion
eversion
foot drop
gait cycle
inversion
mortise
pes cavus
pes planus
plantar
plantar flexion
pronation
stance phase
supination
swing phase
triceps surae

The bones, joints, and muscles of the ankle and foot cooperate to provide amazing adaptability to the distal end of the lower extremity. Consider, for example, an individual walking up a rocky embankment. The joints of the ankle and foot must be pliable enough to adapt to the changing shapes of the terrain while, at the same time, provide a solid foundation to support the weight of the body and the forces of strong muscular contraction. In many ways the structure of the ankle and foot resembles a functional three-dimensional puzzle that can be modified, when necessary, to promote either mobility or stability. This chapter provides an overview of the muscles and joints that make up this three-dimensional structure.

Terminology

The unique structure of the ankle and foot requires special terminology. The **plantar** aspect of the foot refers to the sole or its bottom, whereas the **dorsal** aspect refers to the top or its superior portion. Rearfoot, midfoot, and forefoot are commonly used clinical terms that indicate specific areas of the foot (Figure 11-1).

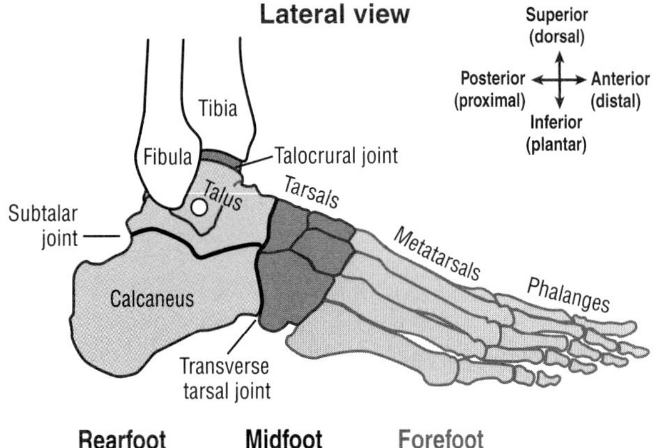

Figure 11-1 Lateral view of the right ankle and foot. (From Neumann DA: *Kinesiology of the musculoskeletal system: foundations for physical rehabilitation*, St Louis, 2002, Mosby, Figure 14-1.)

Brief Overview of the Gait Cycle

Some of the most important functions of the ankle and foot occur during walking, also referred to as *gait*. The kinesiologic events that occur during walking are usually referenced within a gait cycle (Figure 11-2). The **gait cycle** describes the events that occur (while walking) within two successive heel contacts of the *same* leg. Each gait cycle is divided into a stance phase and a swing phase. The **stance phase** refers to the events that occur when the foot is in contact with the ground, whereas the **swing phase** describes the events that occur when the foot is swinging through the air, advancing the lower extremity to the next step. The stance phase is typically subdivided into five events: (1) *heel contact*, (2) *foot flat*, (3) *mid stance*, (4) *heel off*, and (5) *toe off*. The swing phase is typically subdivided into (1) *early swing*, (2) *mid swing*, and (3) *late swing* (see Figure 11-2). The kinesiology of each event within these phases is described in Chapter 12.

Osteology

Distal Tibia and Fibula

The *medial malleolus* is the medial projection of bone from the distal tibia. The *lateral malleolus* projects laterally from the distal fibula (Figure 11-3). Both malleoli serve as the proximal attachments for the collateral ligaments of the ankle.

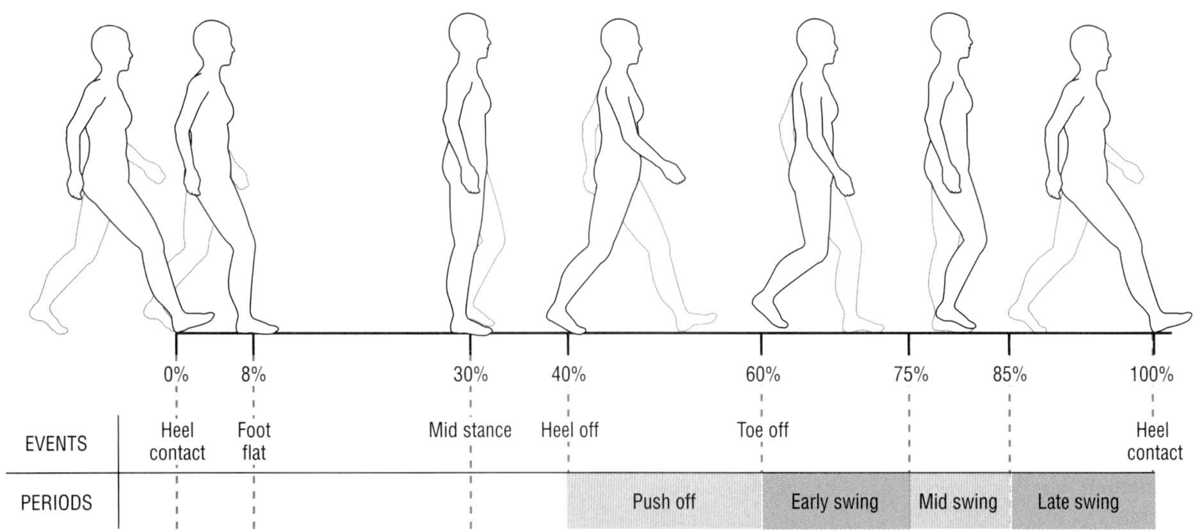

Figure 11-2 Traditional subdivisions of the gait cycle. (From Neumann DA: *Kinesiology of the musculoskeletal system: foundations for physical rehabilitation,* St Louis, 2002, Mosby, Figure 15-11.)

The *fibular notch* is a concave portion of the distal tibia that articulates with the fibula, forming the *distal tibiofibular joint* (see Figure 11-3). This firm articulation allows very little gliding motion between the tibia and fibula. The joint's primary function is to serve as a stable rectangular concavity (socket) that accepts the talus—forming the *talocrural (ankle) joint.*

Bones of the Foot

The osteology of the foot includes three sets of bones: (1) tarsals, (2) metatarsals, and (3) phalanges. Figure 11-4 displays the arrangement of these bones; the following text highlights the important features.

TARSAL BONES

The tarsal bones include the *talus, calcaneus, navicular, cuboid,* and the *medial, intermediate,* and *lateral cuneiforms.* The important features of these bones are outlined in Table 11-1 and Figures 11-4 to 11-6.

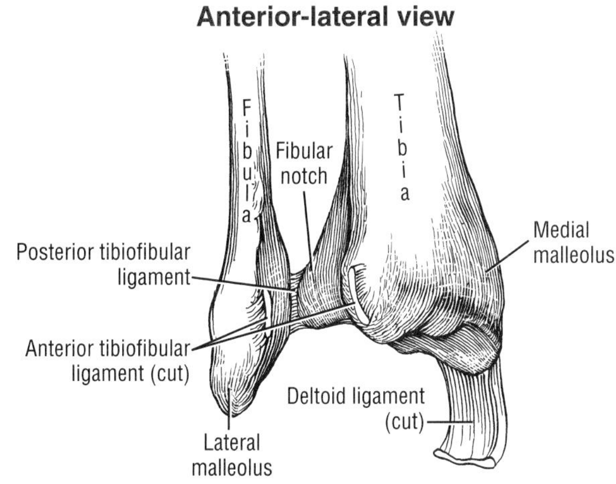

Figure 11-3 Anterior-lateral view of the distal tibiofibular joint. The fibula has been reflected to show the articular surfaces. (From Neumann DA: *Kinesiology of the musculoskeletal system: foundations for physical rehabilitation,* St Louis, 2002, Mosby, Figure 14-10.)

TABLE 11-1 TARSAL BONES

Bone	Important Features	Figure
Rearfoot		
Talus	*Trochlea:* dome-shaped superior portion of the talus	11-5 11-6
	Three facets on plantar aspect for articulation with calcaneus	
	Head: articulates with the navicular bone	
Calcaneus	*Calcaneal tuberosity:* attachment of the Achilles tendon	11-5 11-6
	Three facets on the superior (dorsal) aspect for articulation with the talus	
	Sustentaculum talus: medial projection of bone that serves as a shelf to support the medial side of the talus	
Midfoot		
Navicular	*Navicular tuberosity:* prominent medial projection of bone; site of distal attachment for the spring ligament and tibialis posterior muscle	11-5 11-6
Medial, Intermediate, and Lateral Cuneiforms	Form the medial half of the *transverse arch* of the foot	11-5
Cuboid	Forms the lateral half of the *transverse arch* of the foot	11-5 11-4
Forefoot		
Metatarsals	All 5 metatarsals consist of a: • Base (proximal aspect) • Shaft • Convex head (distal aspect)	11-5 11-4
Phalanges	Each of the 14 phalanges is composed of a: • Concave base • Shaft • Convex head	11-5 11-4

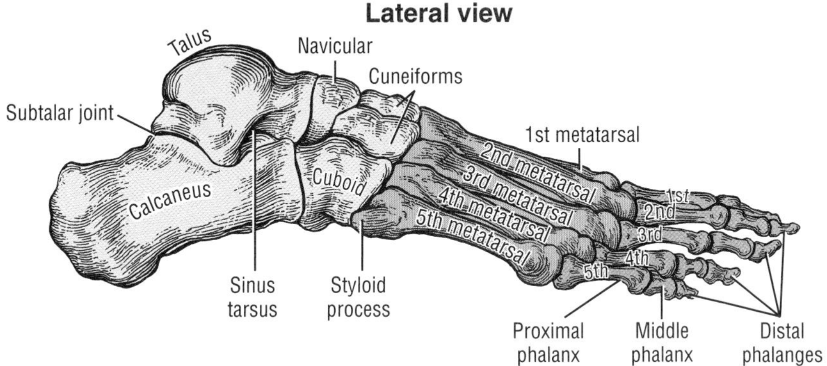

Figure 11-4 Lateral view of the bones of the right ankle and foot. The tarsal bones are in pink, the metatarsals are in gray, and the phalanges are in red. (Modified from Neumann DA: *Kinesiology of the musculoskeletal system: foundations for physical rehabilitation,* St Louis, 2002, Mosby, Figure 14-7.)

Arthrology of the Ankle and Foot

General Features

The ankle and foot consist of numerous joints. For organizational purposes, the joints will be portioned into proximal and distal sets (Table 11-2). The proximal joints, which occupy most of the kinesiologic discussion within this chapter, consist of the talocrural, subtalar, and transverse tarsal joints (see Figure 11-1). The distal joints include the tarsometatarsal, metatarsophalangeal, and interphalangeal joints. Although other smaller joints exist, they are not covered in this text.

Kinematics of the Ankle and Foot

The kinematics of the ankle and foot may be the most complex in the human body. Many irregularly shaped joints are capable of producing unique motions not yet introduced in this text. Two sets of terminology are therefore necessary to fully describe the complex kinematics at the ankle and foot: fundamental and applied.

Fundamental movements are those that occur within a plane that is perpendicular to the three classic axes of rotation: medial-lateral, anterior-posterior, and vertical. Unfortunately, these relatively familiar concepts do not adequately describe the kinematics across all the joints of the ankle and foot. Joints such as the subtalar and transverse tarsal, for instance, produce a more oblique movement that is best described with the *applied* terms of *pronation* or *supination*. The significance of these two sets of definitions becomes more apparent as the chapter evolves.

FUNDAMENTAL MOVEMENT TERMINOLOGY

Dorsiflexion and Plantar Flexion

Dorsiflexion and plantar flexion occur in the sagittal plane about a medial-lateral axis of rotation (Figure 11-7, A). **Dorsiflexion** describes the motion of bringing the dorsal part (top) of any region of the foot toward the anterior aspect of the tibia. **Plantar flexion**, in contrast, most often describes the motion of pushing the foot downward or, more correctly, moving the dorsal part of any region of the foot *away* from the anterior aspect of the tibia. Plantar flexion of the ankle, for example, occurs as one pushes down on the accelerator of a car.

Inversion and Eversion

Inversion and eversion occur in the frontal plane about an anterior-posterior axis of rotation (Figure 11-7, B). **Inversion** turns a point anywhere on the plantar aspect

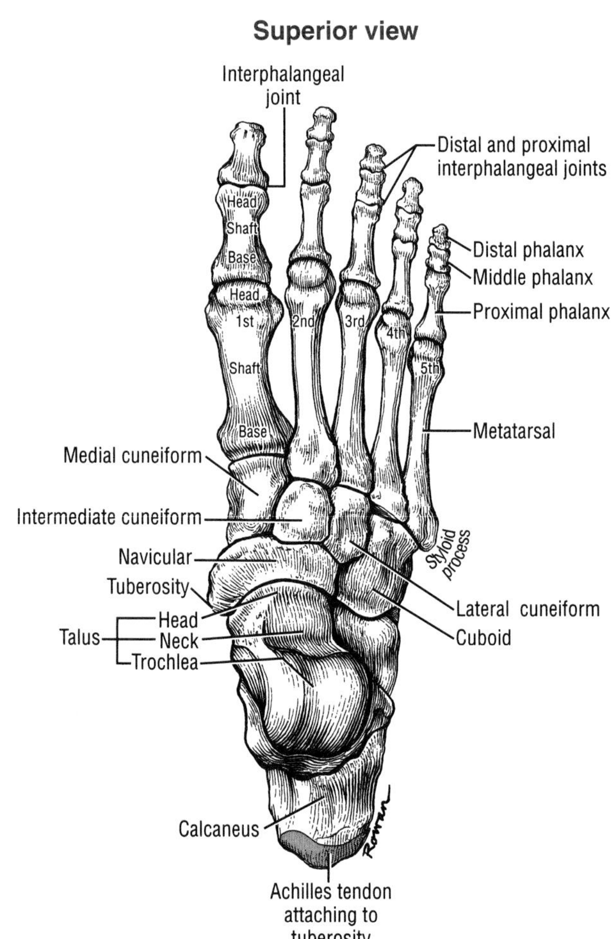

Figure 11-5 Superior view of the bones of the right ankle and foot. (From Neumann DA: *Kinesiology of the musculoskeletal system: foundations for physical rehabilitation,* St Louis, 2002, Mosby, Figure 14-4.)

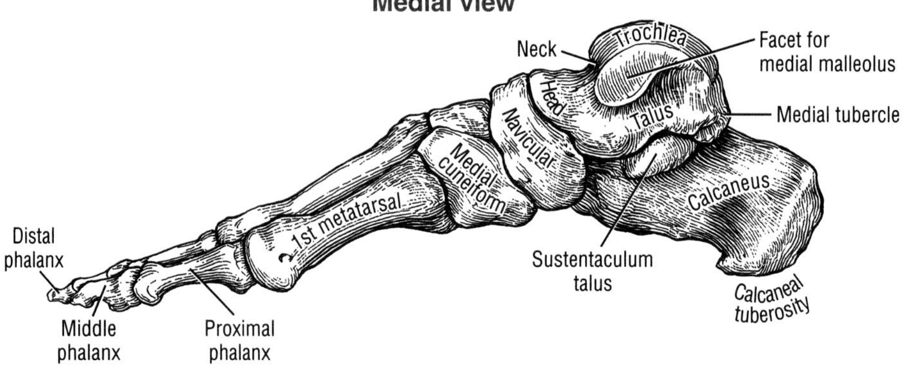

Figure 11-6 Medial view of the bones of the right ankle and foot. (From Neumann DA: *Kinesiology of the musculoskeletal system: foundations for physical rehabilitation,* St Louis, 2002, Mosby, Figure 14-6.)

TABLE 11-2 JOINTS OF THE ANKLE AND FOOT: ARTICULATIONS AND IMPORTANT FEATURES

Joint	Articulation	Important Features	Comments
Proximal Joints			
Talocrural	Trochlea of the talus articulates with the rigid concavity formed by the distal tibia and fibula	Designed primarily for dorsiflexion and plantar flexion The primary joint of the distal leg that allows a forward progression of the body while walking	Joint resembles a carpenter's mortise See Figure 11-9
Subtalar	Composed of the articulation between the three inferior facets of the talus and the matching superior facets of the calcaneus	Designed primarily to permit an arc of motion that combines inversion/adduction and eversion/abduction During the stance phase of walking, this joint allows the lower leg to rotate slightly within frontal and horizontal planes, independent of the fixed calcaneus (heel)	Effective subtalar joint motion requires that the trochlea (dome) of the talus remains mechanically stable within the mortise shape of the talocrural joint
Transverse tarsal	Consists of 2 articulations: talonavicular joint and calcaneocuboid joint	Designed to allow motions that cut through all three planes (i.e., allows the most pure form of pronation and supination)	Greatly enhances the overall kinematic versatility of the foot
Distal Joints			
Tarsometatarsal	Formed by the articulation between the distal surfaces of the three cuneiforms and cuboid with the base of all 5 metatarsals	The relatively flattened joint surfaces allow a variety of adaptive motions	The second ray functions as a stable central longitudinal pillar throughout the foot
Metatarsophalangeal	Formed by the articulation between the convex metatarsal head and the concave base of each corresponding phalanx	Designed to allow 2 degrees of freedom: flexion-extension and abduction-adduction	About 60-65 degrees of hyperextension are required at the first metatarsophalangeal joint during the push-off phase of walking
Interphalangeal	Formed by articulations between the convex head of the more proximal phalanx and concave base of the more distal phalanx	Designed to allow extension and flexion only	The first toe has only one interphalangeal joint; the other 4 digits each have a proximal and distal interphalangeal joint

of the foot toward the midline. **Eversion** turns a point on the plantar aspect of the foot laterally, or away from the midline.

Abduction and Adduction

These motions occur in the horizontal plane about a vertical axis of rotation (Figure 11-7, *C*). **Adduction** describes a horizontal plane rotation of the foot as a point on its anterior surface moves *toward* the midline. **Abduction** describes the opposite movement, in which a point on its anterior surface rotates *away from* the midline.

APPLIED MOVEMENT TERMINOLOGY

Pronation and Supination

These specialized *applied* motions are based on a combination of the fundamental movements described above. **Pronation** (Figure 11-8, *A*) is a combined movement that includes eversion, abduction, and dorsiflexion of any region of the ankle and foot. **Supination**, in contrast, is a combined movement of inversion, adduction, and plantar flexion of any region of the ankle and foot (Figure 11-8, *B*). As indicated in this figure, these specialized movements occur most regularly at the subtalar and transverse tarsal joints. This concept will be reinforced again later in the chapter.

Proximal Joints of the Ankle and Foot

The talocrural, subtalar, and transverse tarsal joints are large and extremely important joints, each belonging within the *proximal* set of joints of the ankle and foot. The *talocrural joint* allows motion in the sagittal

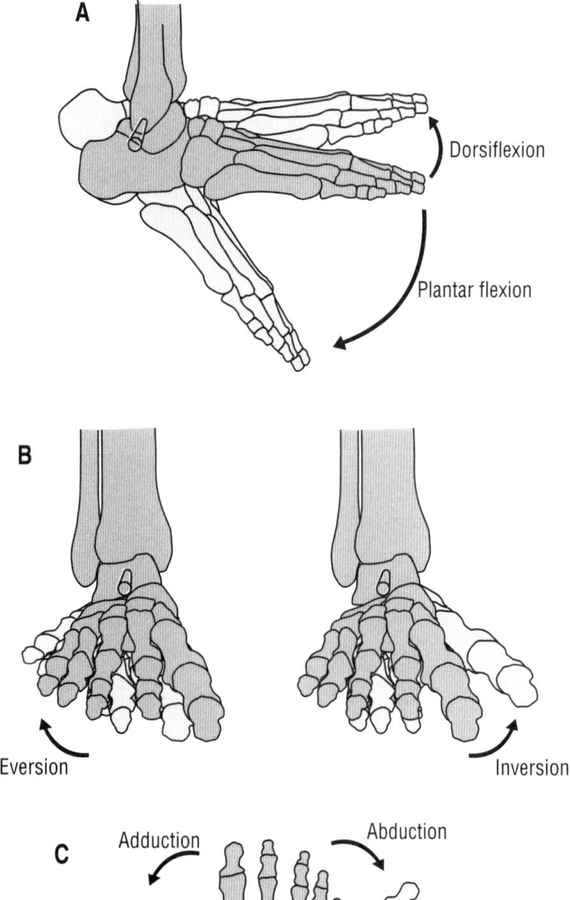

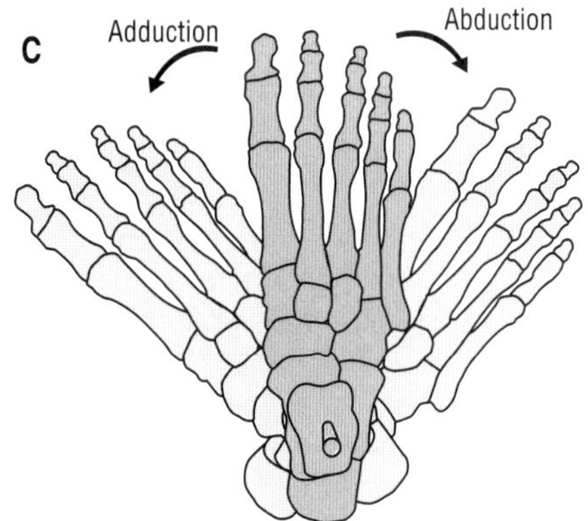

Figure 11-7 Fundamental movements of the ankle and foot defined about the traditional axes of rotation. **A,** Dorsiflexion and plantar flexion. **B,** Eversion and inversion. **C,** Adduction and abduction. The axis of rotation for each movement is indicated by the red cylinder.

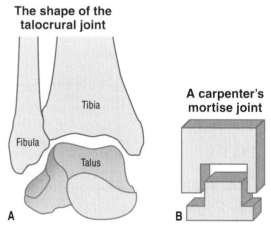

plane: dorsiflexion and plantar flexion. The *subtalar joint* allows an oblique arc of motion that results primarily in the combined motions of inversion and adduction, or eversion and abduction; two of the three components of supination and pronation, respectively. The *transverse tarsal joint* permits the most oblique motion, one that cuts through all three planes of motion. The transverse tarsal joint, therefore, allows the purest form of pronation and supination.

TALOCRURAL JOINT

General Features

The talocrural joint, commonly called the ankle joint, is created by the articulation between the trochlea of the talus and the concavity formed by the distal tibia and fibula. This concave part of the joint is often referred to as the **mortise** because of its resemblance to a mortise joint used by carpenters (Figure 11-9).

Several factors contribute to the stability of this joint: the tight rectangular fit of the talus in the mortise, the support of numerous collateral ligaments and muscles, and the strength of the distal tibiofibular joint.

The shape of the talocrural joint
Tibia
Fibula
Talus
A
A carpenter's mortise joint
B

Figure 11-9 Similarity in shape of the talocrural joint **(A)** to that of a carpenter's mortise joint **(B)**. (From Neumann DA: *Kinesiology of the musculoskeletal system: foundations for physical rehabilitation,* St Louis, 2002, Mosby, Figure 14-12.)

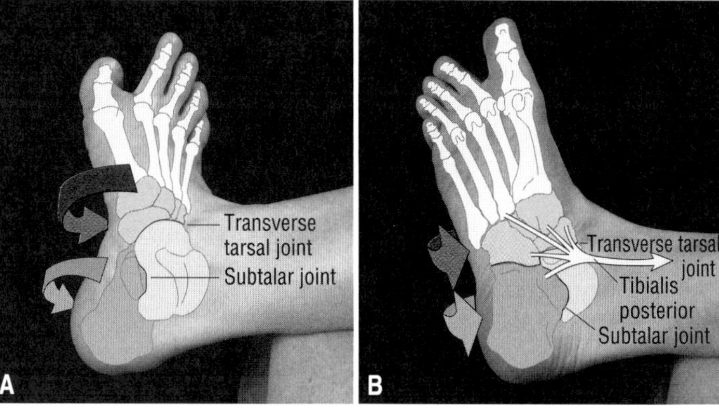

Figure 11-8 As described in the text, pronation **(A)** includes the combined movements of eversion, abduction, and dorsiflexion. Supination **(B),** on the other hand, combines inversion, adduction, and plantar flexion. Note that these oblique movements occur predominately across the subtalar and transverse joints. (From Neumann DA: *Kinesiology of the musculoskeletal system: foundations for physical rehabilitation,* St. Louis, 2002, Mosby, Figure 14-24, *B* and *D.*)

Supporting Structures

The following structures support the talocrural joint:

- Interosseous membrane
- Anterior and posterior tibiofibular ligaments (Figure 11-10, A)
- Deltoid ligament (Figure 11-10, B)
- Lateral collateral ligaments (see Figure 11-10, A)
  - Anterior talofibular
  - Calcaneofibular
  - Posterior talofibular

These structures and their functions are summarized in the table on the next page.

Kinematics

The talocrural joint possesses 1 degree of freedom, permitting dorsiflexion and plantar flexion of the ankle. This sagittal plane motion is essential to the forward progression of movement while walking. Dorsiflexion and plantar flexion are also important in permitting squatting motions, such as when transitioning between sitting and standing. Note that in this type of motion, the tibia moves relative to the foot; consider, for example, the dorsiflexed position of the ankle when holding a deep squat.

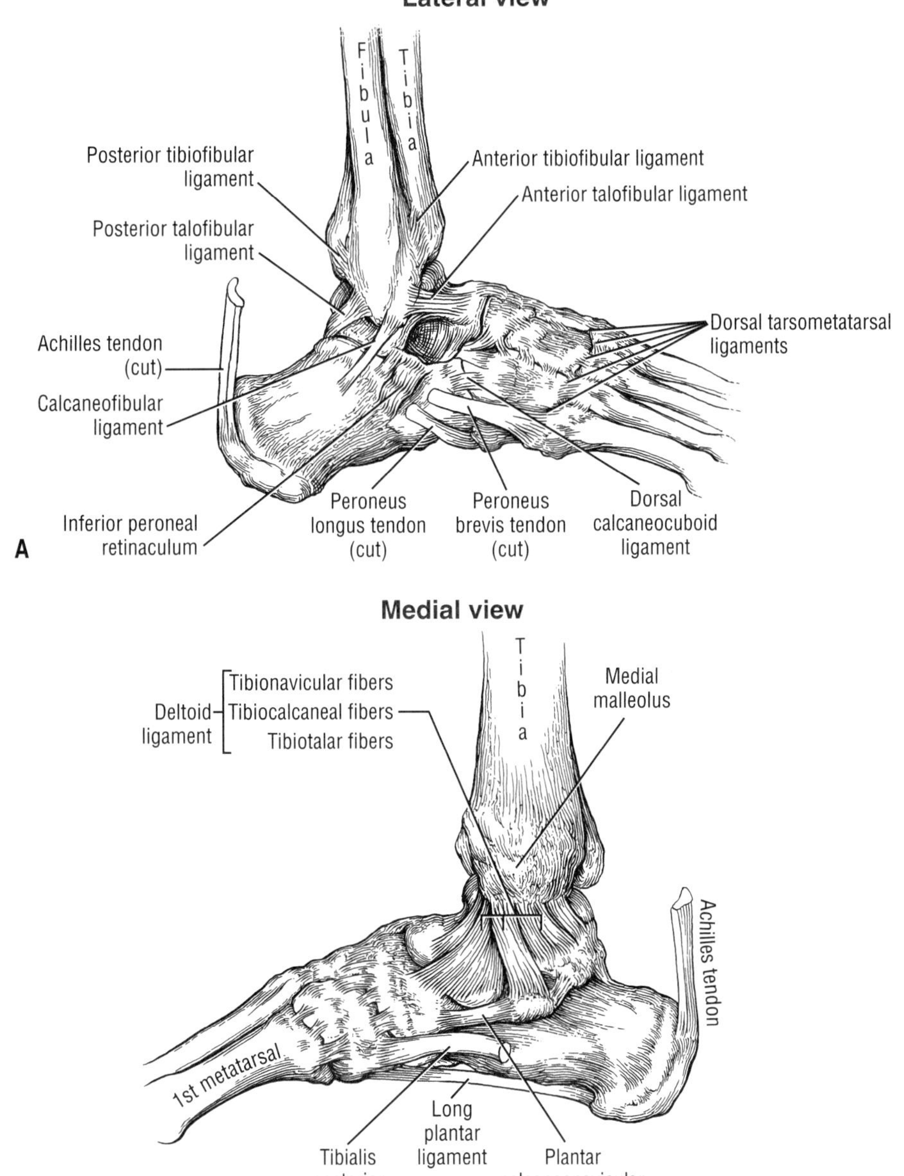

Figure 11-10 Right ankle highlighting the **(A)** lateral collateral and distal tibiofibular ligaments and **(B)** deltoid (medial collateral) ligament. (From Neumann DA: *Kinesiology of the musculoskeletal system: foundations for physical rehabilitation,* St Louis, 2002, Mosby, Figures 14-13 *[B]* and 14-14 *[A]*.)

LIGAMENTS SUPPORTING THE TALOCRURAL JOINT

Structure	Function	Comments
Interosseus membrane	Binds the tibia to the fibula; provides stability to the distal tibiofibular and talocrural joints	Serves as the proximal attachment for numerous muscles of the ankle and foot
Anterior and posterior tibiofibular ligaments	Binds the distal tibiofibular joint, improving stability of the mortise	Injury to these ligaments is often involved with a "high-ankle" sprain
Deltoid ligament	Limits eversion	A triangular-shaped ligament originating off the medial malleolus. The ligament has three sets of fibers: tibionavicular, tibiocalcaneal, and tibiotalar
Lateral collateral ligaments	Limit inversion	Consists of three different ligaments: anterior talofibular, calcaneofibular, and posterior talofibular. The most frequently injured ligament is the anterior talofibular ligament, typically resulting from excessive inversion and plantar flexion

Normal range of motion for dorsiflexion is about 0 to 20 degrees. The 0-degree or neutral position of the foot is determined by a 90-degree angle between the fifth metatarsal and the fibula. The normal range of motion for plantar flexion is 0 to 50 degrees (Figure 11-11).

Dorsiflexion and plantar flexion of the ankle occur about a near medial-lateral axis of rotation that travels through the tips of each malleolus (see Figure 11-11, A). These easily identifiable bony markers allow visualization of the axis, enabling one to understand the function of the muscles that cross this joint. Muscles that course anterior to this medial-lateral axis of rotation perform dorsiflexion, whereas muscles that course posterior to this axis of rotation perform plantar flexion.

The arthrokinematics of the talocrural joint are traditionally based on the convex trochlea of the talus within the fixed concave mortise. This occurs when the foot is off the ground, as the convex trochlea rolls and slides in opposite directions within the mortise. Figure 11-12 highlights the arthrokinematics of dorsiflexion of the talocrural joint. Realize, however, that most of the time the foot is fixed to the ground during the stance phase of walking. In this case, the concavity formed by the mortise rolls and slides in the *same* direction over the convex articular surface of the talus.

Functional Considerations: Most- and Least-Stable Positions of the Talocrural Joint

While walking, maximal dorsiflexion occurs late in stance phase, just before the heel rises off the ground (at about 40% of the gait cycle; see Figure 11-2). Realize that while in the stance phase of walking, the term dorsiflexion describes the position of the *leg relative to the foot.* At this point in the gait cycle the ankle is most stable because most of the collateral ligaments and all plantar flexor muscles are stretched (Figure 11-13, A). The dorsiflexed ankle is further stabilized as the wider, anterior part of the trochlea of the talus becomes wedged into the mortise (Figure 11-13, B). For these reasons the *close-packed* position of the ankle is full dorsiflexion. Such stability is necessary in late stance to prepare for the action of the strongly activated plantar flexor muscles during jumping or the push-off phase of fast walking.

The least stable position of the talocrural joint is full plantar flexion. Full plantar flexion—the *loose-packed* position of the joint—slackens most of the collateral ligaments and all of the plantar flexor muscles. The position of full plantar flexion also causes the mortise (distal tibia and fibula) to "loosen its grip" on the talus; this places the

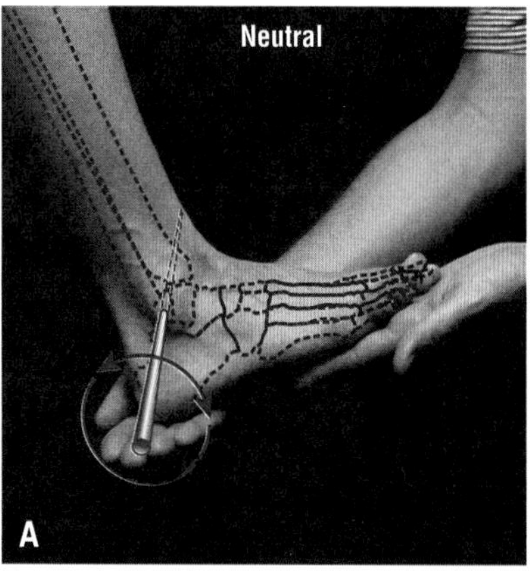

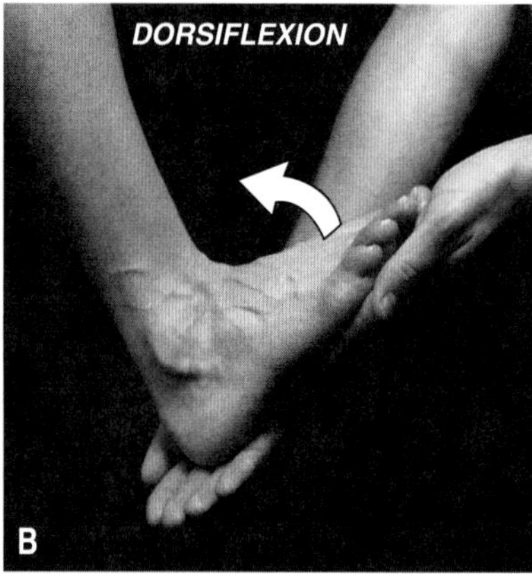

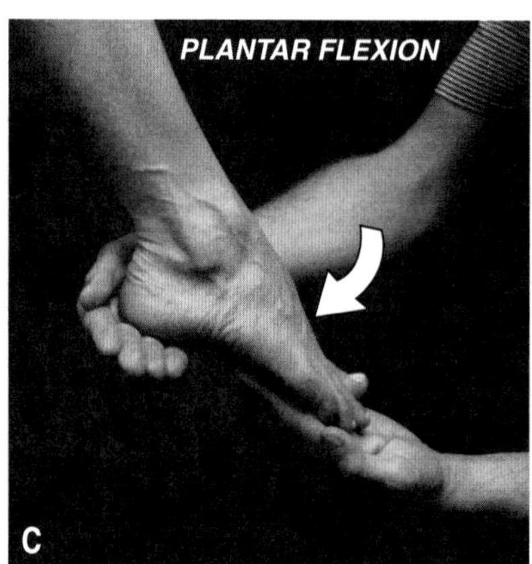

Figure 11-11 Axis of rotation and osteokinematics at the talocrural joint. **A,** Neutral position of the ankle. **B,** Dorsiflexion. **C,** Plantar flexion. (From Neumann DA: *Kinesiology of the musculoskeletal system: foundations for physical rehabilitation,* St Louis, 2002, Mosby, Figure 14-16, *C-E.*)

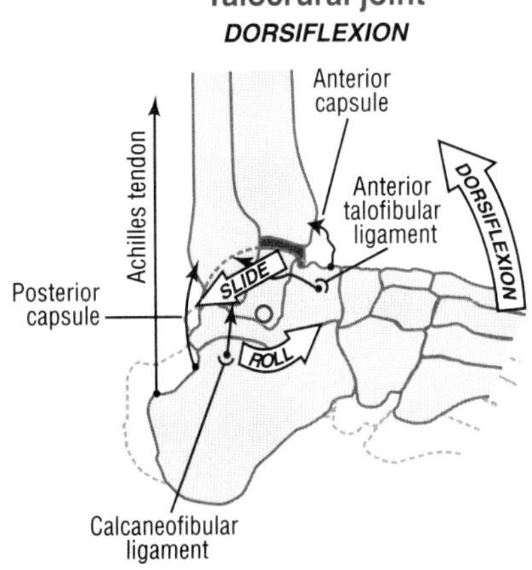

Figure 11-12 Lateral view of the ankle and foot showing the arthrokinematics at the talocrural joint during dorsiflexion. Stretched structures are shown as thin elongated arrows; slackened structures are shown as wavy arrows. (From Neumann DA: *Kinesiology of the musculoskeletal system: foundations for physical rehabilitation,* St Louis, 2002, Mosby, Figure 14-17, *A*.)

narrower width of the top of the talus between the malleoli, thereby releasing tension within the mortise. Weight bearing over a fully plantar flexed ankle, therefore, places the talocrural joint at a relatively unstable position. Wearing high heels, or landing from a jump in a plantar flexed (and usually inverted) position, increases the likelihood of spraining the ankle and injuring the lateral ligaments.

SUBTALAR JOINT

General Features

The subtalar joint is located within the rearfoot (see Figure 11-1). This joint consists of the articulation between the facets on the inferior surface of the talus and the matching facets on the superior surface of the calcaneus. The shape of this joint is specifically designed to allow *frontal and horizontal plane* motions between the foot and lower leg. These motions are essential for adapting to uneven ground surfaces or cutting laterally or medially while walking or running.

Kinematics

The kinematics of the subtalar joint allow the combined motions of inversion/adduction and eversion/abduction of the rearfoot (Figure 11-14). (Recall that these motions are components of supination and pronation, respectively.) To appreciate the components that make up these motions, firmly grasp the calcaneus (heel) and twist it in a side-to-side and rotary fashion. The side-to-side motions are inversion and eversion, which are most often used clinically to evaluate the strength and range of motion of the subtalar joint. The rotary (horizontal plane) motions are adduction and abduction. During subtalar motions, the trochlea of the talus is usually well stabilized within the mortise shape of the talocrural joint.

The motions just described for the subtalar joint involve the calcaneus moving underneath the fixed talus, such as which occurs when the foot is off the ground. More realistically, however, the subtalar joint usually operates in a weight-bearing position, when the calcaneus is fixed against the ground during the stance phase of walking. Because the talus is firmly stabilized within the mortise, subtalar joint motion is most often expressed as a combined movement of both the *talus and the lower leg*, relative to a stationary calcaneus.

Functional Considerations: Subtalar Joint—Critical Kinematic Link between the Leg and Foot

As described above, motion at the subtalar joint is commonly expressed in one of two ways: either when the calcaneus is free, such as during the swing phase, or when it is in firm

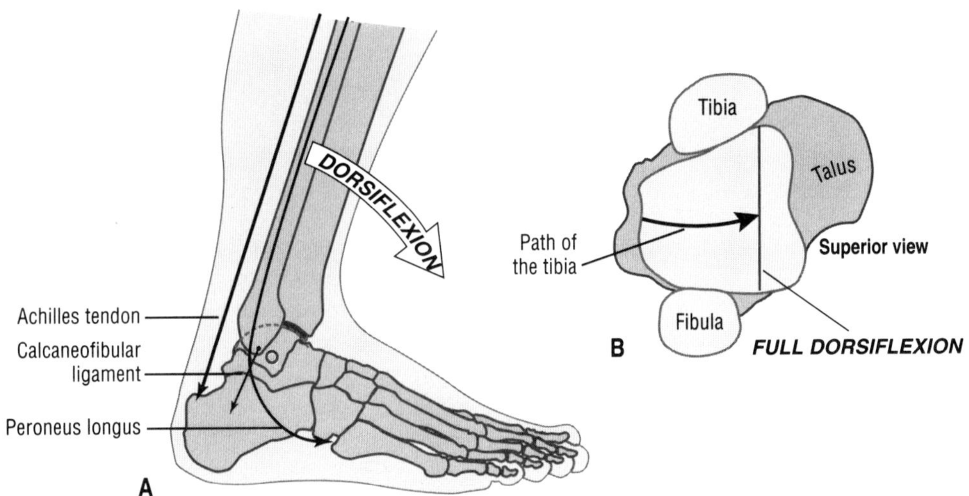

Figure 11-13 Factors that increase the mechanical stability of the fully dorsiflexed talocrural joint. **A,** Increased tension in several connective tissues and muscles, indicated by thin black arrows. **B,** Superior surface of talus is wider anteriorly. Dorsiflexion therefore results in a wedging effect, as the wide anterior portion of the talus becomes pressed into the mortise. (From Neumann DA: *Kinesiology of the musculoskeletal system: foundations for physical rehabilitation,* St Louis, 2002, Mosby, Figure 14-18.)

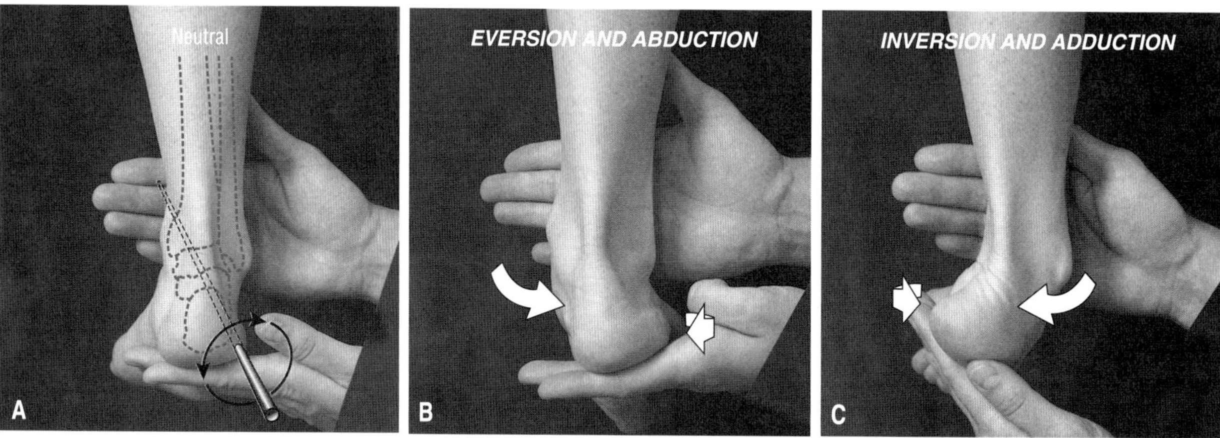

Figure 11-14 Osteokinematics of the subtalar joint. **A,** The axis of rotation and neutral position of the subtalar joint. **B,** Eversion and abduction at the subtalar joint. **C,** Inversion and adduction at the subtalar joint. (From Neumann DA: *Kinesiology of the musculoskeletal system: foundations for physical rehabilitation,* St Louis, 2002, Mosby, Figure 14-20, *C-E.*)

contact with the ground during the stance phase of walking. While in the stance phase the *leg and talus* move as one mechanical unit over the fixed calcaneus. Although the motion at the subtalar joint is small, it is nevertheless important. The subtalar joint allows a dissipation of the relatively slight horizontal and frontal plane rotations of the leg and talus that naturally occur when the lower extremity is in contact with the ground during the stance phase. If the subtalar joint were fused, the leg, talus, and calcaneus would all be forced to move together—following the rotating lower extremity.

The normal subtalar joint is well utilized during walking and running, especially on unlevel terrain. To illustrate, consider the following example: When standing on level ground, the leg and talus are in relative alignment with the calcaneus, as indicated by the red dots across the subtalar joint in Figure 11-15, A. Consider, however, what happens when the foot encounters uneven ground. Figure 11-15, *B*, illustrates the response of the subtalar joint as the medial side of the foot steps on a rock. In this scenario, the calcaneus rotates, resulting in inversion of the subtalar joint. This "righting" mechanism of the foot allows the leg to remain vertical, even while standing or walking on uneven surfaces. If this motion is excessive, however, it may result in a sprain of the lateral ligaments.

In other circumstances it may be necessary that the calcaneus remain firmly planted on the ground, while the leg (and body) cut in medial or lateral directions. As illustrated in Figure 11-15, C, with the calcaneus well fixed, a medially directed movement of the talus and leg can occur as subtalar joint inversion. Realize that, although different bones are moving in Figure 11-15, *B* and C, the final position of the subtalar joint in both scenarios is the same—*inversion*. Without the available motion provided by the subtalar joint, walking on uneven surfaces would be extremely difficult and likely result in loss of balance or injury to the ankle and foot.

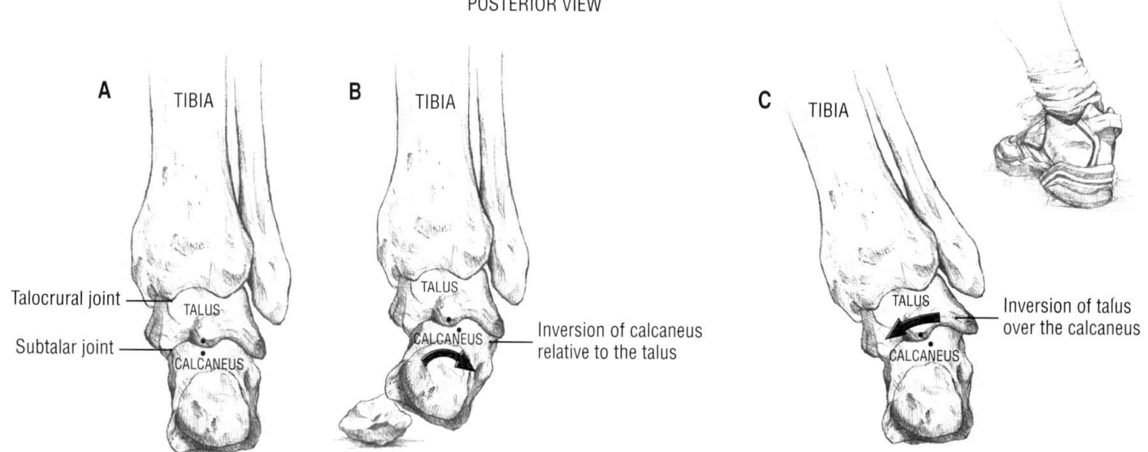

Figure 11-15 Posterior view of the right subtalar joint. **A,** The talus and calcaneus are all in alignment. **B,** The calcaneus rotates into inversion as a result of stepping on a rock. This action allows the leg and talus to remain vertical. **C,** A cutting motion results in the talus and leg rotating medially into inversion over a fixed calcaneus.

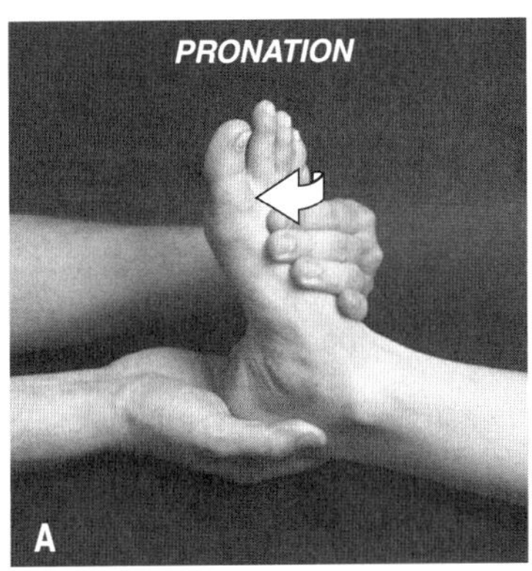

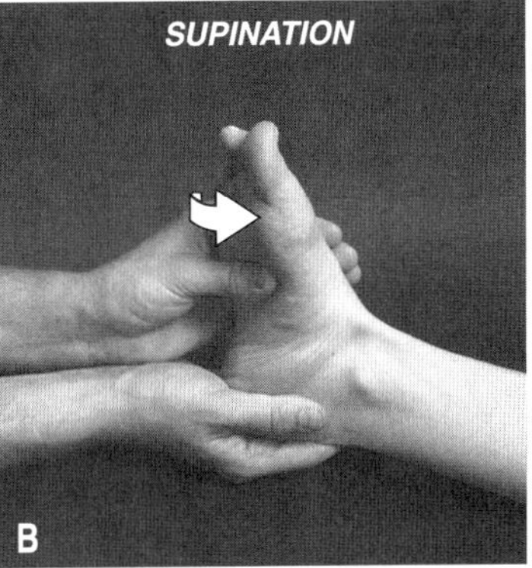

Figure 11-16 Pronation **(A)** and supination **(B)** at the transverse tarsal joint. (From Neumann DA: *Kinesiology of the musculoskeletal system: foundations for physical rehabilitation,* St Louis, 2002, Mosby, Figure 14-25, *D-E.*)

TRANSVERSE TARSAL JOINT

General Features

The transverse tarsal joint separates the rearfoot from the midfoot (see Figure 11-1). This extensive joint consists of two separate articulations: the *talonavicular joint* and the *calcaneocuboid joint*. This pair of joints allows the midfoot to move independently of the rearfoot (i.e., the calcaneus and talus). The most important feature of this articulation, however, is its ability to perform the most *pure form of pronation and supination*. (Recall that pronation has nearly equal elements of eversion, abduction, and dorsiflexion; supination has nearly equal elements of inversion, adduction, and plantar flexion.) Figure 11-16 shows a physical therapist assistant moving a foot through an arc of pronation (Figure 11-16, *A*) and supination (Figure 11-16, *B*).

The oblique motions of pronation and supination at the transverse tarsal joint provide tremendous kinematic versatility to the foot. The midfoot (and attached forefoot) can mold into many positions, allowing the entire foot to conform to many different terrains while walking or running. Often the transverse tarsal joint functions in conjunction with the subtalar joint to control the final components of pronation and supination across the entire foot.

MEDIAL LONGITUDINAL ARCH OF THE FOOT

The *medial longitudinal arch* is the primary shock absorbing structure of the foot. This arch is also known as the "in step" of the foot (Figure 11-17). While standing *statically* (at rest), the height of the medial longitudinal arch is supported mainly by *non-muscular tissues* such as ligaments, joints, and, most importantly, the tough plantar fascia (see red spring in Figure 11-18, *A*). This band of connective tissue extends between the base of the calcaneus and the proximal phalanges. Acting as an elastic truss, the plantar fascia absorbs body weight as it simultaneously supports the height of the medial longitudinal arch. Active muscle forces are generally not required to support the normal arch, at least while standing.

In contrast to the healthy foot depicted in Figure 11-18, *A*, Figure 11-18, *B*, shows a person with a dropped or excessively fallen medial longitudinal arch (see abnormal footprint). This condition, also known as **pes planus,** is often associated with an over-stretched and weakened plantar fascia, as well as an over-pronated subtalar joint. A person with this condition must often rely on active muscle forces produced by intrinsic and extrinsic muscles of the foot to support the arch (shown in red in Figure 11-18, *B*). This overcompensation may eventually overtax these muscles, possibly leading to fatigue, heel spurs, and a number of inflammatory conditions, including plantar fasciitis. Treatments for these conditions often include controlling inflammation, strengthening of the supporting musculature, and recommending a proper arch support. The use of an arch support during rehabilitation may be particularly beneficial because it holds the foot in proper alignment and relieves the overused musculature from its "supporting duties."

While walking, the medial longitudinal arch and local muscles functionally interact as the primary *dynamic* shock

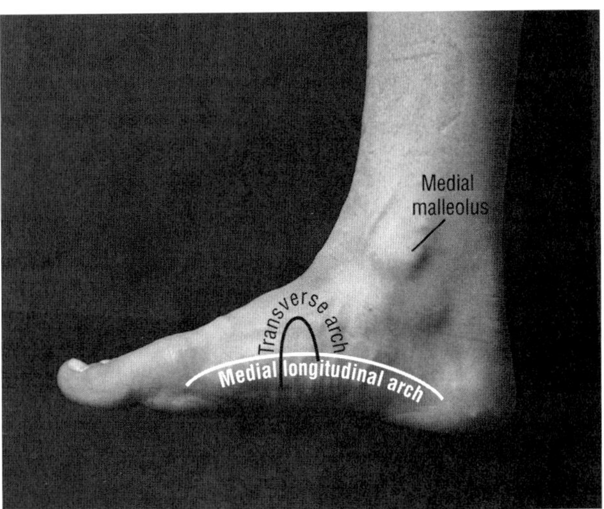

Figure 11-17 The medial side of the foot shows the medial longitudinal arch *(white)* and the transverse arch *(black)*. (From Neumann DA: *Kinesiology of the musculoskeletal system: foundations for physical rehabilitation,* St Louis, 2002, Mosby, Figure 14-26.)

absorbers of the foot. The arch normally lowers (or gives) slightly during the early stance phase, allowing the foot to gradually accept body weight. As part of this mechanism, the subtalar joint (rearfoot) everts slightly. (This can be observed by watching someone walk from behind.) Both the lowering of the arch and slight eversion of the subtalar joint are controlled, in part, through eccentric activation of the invertor muscles, such as the tibialis posterior and tibialis anterior. The eccentric activation protects the foot by providing a *slowed and controlled* decent of the arch. This mechanism provides an excellent example of how eccentric activation of muscle can help protect the underlying bones and joints. This important load acceptance mechanism employed during early stance phase is essential to the health and protection of the foot.

Interestingly, during the later part of the stance phase, the medial longitudinal arch *rises* as the foot prepares for push-off. The raised arch, combined with slight inversion of the subtalar joint and strong activation of intrinsic and extrinsic muscles, converts the foot into a more stable and rigid structure. The foot is now prepared for the strong activation of the plantar flexor muscles required at push-off. A foot with pes planus typically remains in excessive pronation (with a lowered arch) late into stance phase. As a result, the foot remains relatively unstable at a time when more stability is normally required.

Normal arch

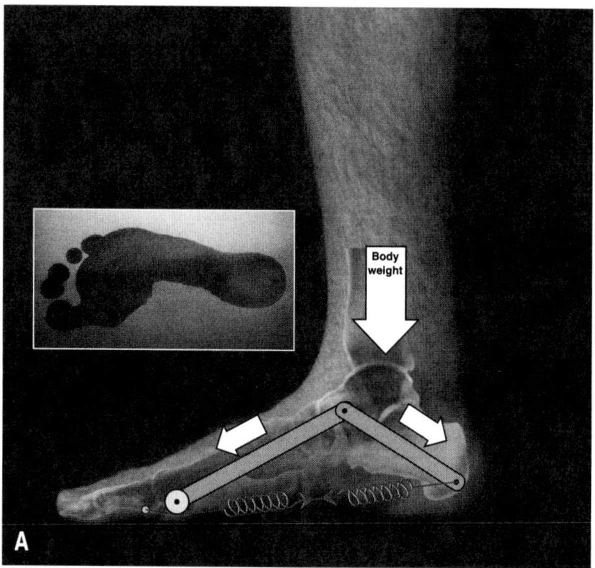

Dropped arch

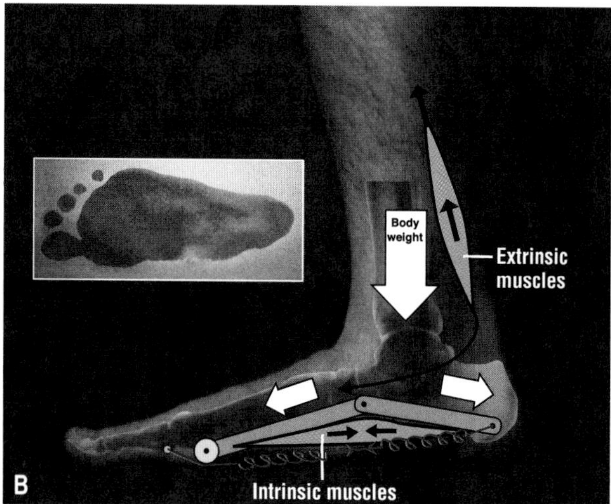

Figure 11-18 Medial views of the foot show a mechanism of accepting body weight while standing. **A,** With a normal medial longitudinal arch, body weight is accepted and absorbed through slight stretch of the plantar fascia—depicted as a red spring. **B,** With an abnormally dropped medial longitudinal arch (pes planus), the over-stretched plantar fascia—depicted as an over-stretched spring—cannot adequately absorb body weight. As a consequence, various intrinsic and extrinsic muscles are required to compensate for the weakened arch. (From Neumann DA: *Kinesiology of the musculoskeletal system: foundations for physical rehabilitation,* St Louis, 2002, Mosby, Figure 14-27.)

Clinical INSIGHT

Pes Cavus

Pes cavus refers to a foot with an abnormally high medial longitudinal arch (Figure 11-19). Although much more rare than pes planus, pes cavus usually results in inadequate dispersion of weight-bearing forces through the foot. Because the foot is more rigid in its arched position, the foot is unable to "give" and weight bearing occurs primarily through the metatarsal heads and calcaneus with minimal shock absorption. This condition is usually non-progressive and generally treated with orthotics or surgery.

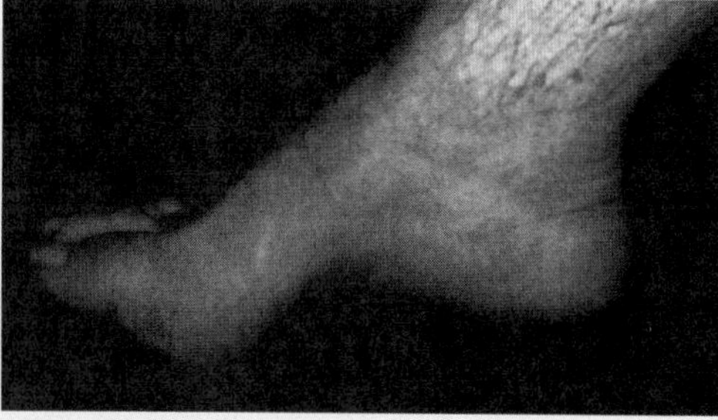

Figure 11-19 Medial view of an individual with pes cavus of the right foot. (From Richardson EG: Neurogenic disorders. In Canale ST, editor: *Campbell's operative orthopaedics*, vol 4, ed 9, St Louis, 1998, Mosby.)

Distal Joints of the Foot

The distal joints of the foot include the tarsometatarsal, metatarsophalangeal, and interphalangeal joints. All of these joints have an important role in walking.

TARSOMETATARSAL JOINTS

The tarsometatarsal joints are composed of the articulations between the bases of the metatarsals and the distal surfaces of the three cuneiforms and the cuboid (Figure 11-20). Marking the junction between the midfoot and the forefoot, these joints serve as the base joints for the rays of the foot. The joints are relatively rigid, except for the first, which allows moderate amounts of dorsiflexion and plantar flexion, coupled with small amounts of inversion and eversion. The first tarsometatarsal joint must give slightly during the stance phase of gait. The second tarsometatarsal joint is the most stable of all the tarsometatarsal joints, primarily because its base is wedged between the medial and lateral cuneiform bones.

METATARSOPHALANGEAL JOINTS

The metatarsophalangeal (MTP) joints are formed between the convex head of the metatarsals and the shallow concavity of the proximal phalanges (see Figure 11-20). The joints allow similar motions as the metacarpophalangeal joints in the hand: extension (dorsiflexion), flexion (plantar flexion), and abduction and adduction. About 60 to 65 degrees of hyperextension are necessary during the push-off phase of walking. This range of motion can be easily verified by looking at your own foot as you stand up on tip-toes.

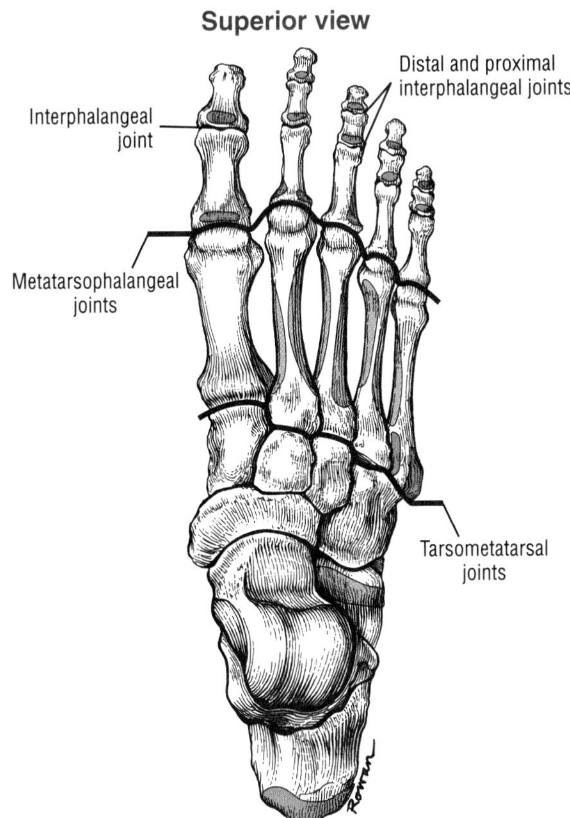

Figure 11-20 Superior view of the right foot highlighting the tarsometatarsal and metatarsophalangeal joints. (From Neumann DA: *Kinesiology of the musculoskeletal system: foundations for physical rehabilitation,* St Louis, 2002, Mosby, Figure 14-4.)

INTERPHALANGEAL JOINTS

As in the fingers, each toe has a proximal interphalangeal (PIP) and distal interphalangeal (DIP) joint, except for the great toe, which has only one interphalangeal joint (see Figure 11-20). Motion at these joints is limited primarily to flexion and extension. Extension is typically limited to the 0-degree or neutral position of the joint.

Table 11-3 summarizes the important kinesiologic features of the proximal and distal joints of the ankle and foot.

Muscle and Joint Interaction

Movements of the ankle and foot are controlled by extrinsic or intrinsic muscles. *Intrinsic* muscles have both proximal and distal attachments within the foot, whereas *extrinsic* muscles have their proximal attachments within the lower leg or distal femur, and distal attachments within the foot. Both sets of muscles provide static control, dynamic thrust, and shock absorption to the distal end of the lower extremity.

Innervation of the Muscles of the Foot and Ankle

The extrinsic muscles are arranged in three compartments within the leg: anterior, lateral, and posterior. Each compartment is innervated by a different nerve, each arising from the sciatic nerve. The large sciatic nerve, which spans the length of the posterior thigh, bifurcates (splits) near the posterior knee into the tibial and common peroneal nerves (Figure 11-21). The tibial nerve continues distally throughout the posterior lower leg (Figure 11-22). The common peroneal nerve courses laterally, wraps around the fibular head, and splits into the superficial peroneal and deep peroneal nerves (see Figure 11-21). The muscles innervated by these nerves are outlined in Boxes 11-1 and 11-2.

Just posterior to the medial malleolus, the tibial nerve bifurcates into the *medial and lateral plantar nerves* (see Figure 11-22). These two nerves innervate all of the intrinsic muscles of the foot, except for the extensor digitorum brevis (which is innervated by the deep branch of the peroneal nerve).

TABLE 11-3 JOINTS OF THE ANKLE AND FOOT: MOVEMENTS, RANGE, AND PLANES OF MOTION

Joint	Primary Movements	Range of Motion	Predominate Plane of Motion	Comments
Talocrural	Dorsiflexion Plantar flexion	0-20 0-60	Sagittal	Considered the "true" ankle joint
Subtalar	Inversion/ adduction and eversion/ abduction	Typically reported in frontal only: Inversion: 0-25 degrees Eversion: 0-12 degrees	Combined frontal and horizontal	While weight bearing, this joint allows non-sagittal motions of the lower leg to occur relative to a fixed calcaneus
Transverse tarsal	Pronation and supination	Triplanar motion: difficult to accurately measure	Oblique plane	Allows the purest of pronation and supination motions
Tarsometatarsal	Dorsiflexion and plantar flexion (primarily at first joint)	Difficult to measure	Sagittal	
Metatarsophalangeal	Flexion Extension	0-35 degrees 0-65 degrees (great toe 0-85 degrees)	Sagittal	Adequate amounts of hyperextension are important during push off
	Adduction Abduction	Limited	Horizontal	Improves balance during walking and standing
Proximal and distal interphalangeal	Flexion Extension	0-70 Limited	Sagittal	Flexion of the toes assists with increasing friction between skin and walking surface; helps grab the earth

BOX 11-1

Innervation of the Extrinsic Muscles of the Ankle and Foot

Deep Peroneal Nerve (see Figure 11-21)
Innervates all muscles in the anterior compartment of the leg. These muscles perform dorsiflexion as one of their primary actions.

- Tibialis anterior
- Extensor digitorum longus
- Extensor hallucis longus
- Peroneus tertius

Superficial Peroneal Nerve (see Figure 11-21)
Innervates the two muscles in the lateral compartment of the leg; both perform plantar flexion and eversion.

- Peroneus longus
- Peroneus brevis

Tibial Nerve (see Figure 11-22)
Innervates all of the muscles in the posterior compartment of the leg. These muscles perform plantar flexion or combined plantar flexion and inversion as their primary actions.

- Gastrocnemius
- Soleus
- Plantaris
- Tibialis posterior
- Flexor digitorum longus
- Flexor hallucis longus

BOX 11-2

Innervation of the Intrinsic Muscles of the Foot

Media Plantar Nerve
- Flexor digitorum brevis
- Abductor hallucis
- Flexor hallucis brevis
- Lumbrical (second toe)

Lateral Plantar Nerve
- Abductor digiti minimi
- Quadratus plantae
- Flexor digiti minimi
- Adductor hallucis
- Plantar interossei
- Dorsal interossei
- Lumbricals (third to fifth toes)

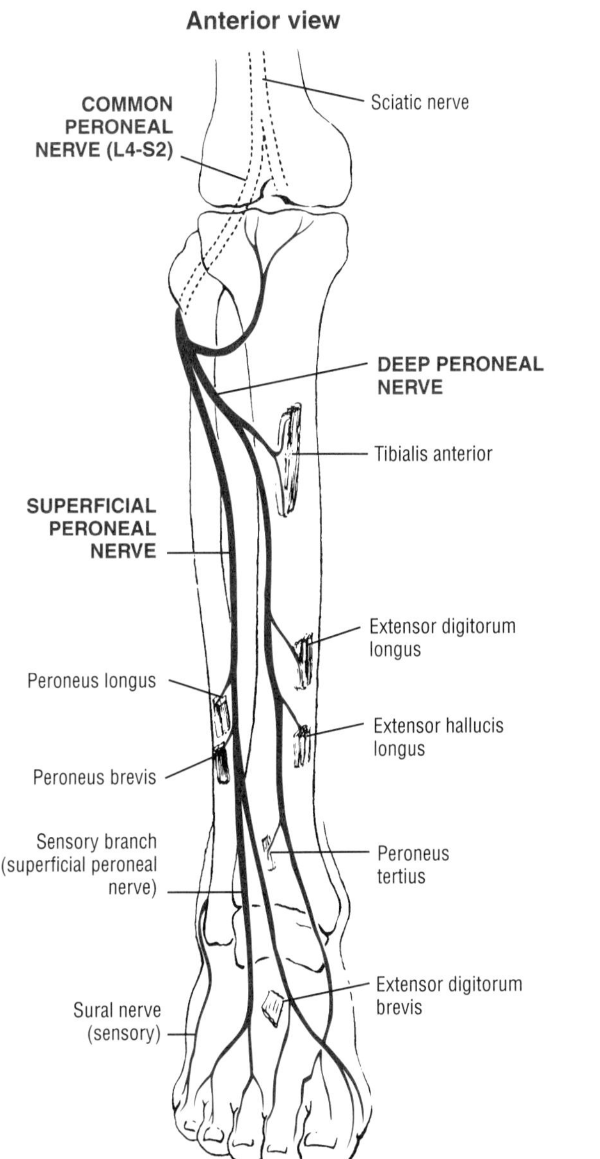

Figure 11-21 The path and innervations of the deep peroneal and superficial peroneal nerves. (Modified from Waxman S: *Correlative neuroanatomy*, ed 24, New York, 2000, Lange Medical Books/McGraw-Hill.)

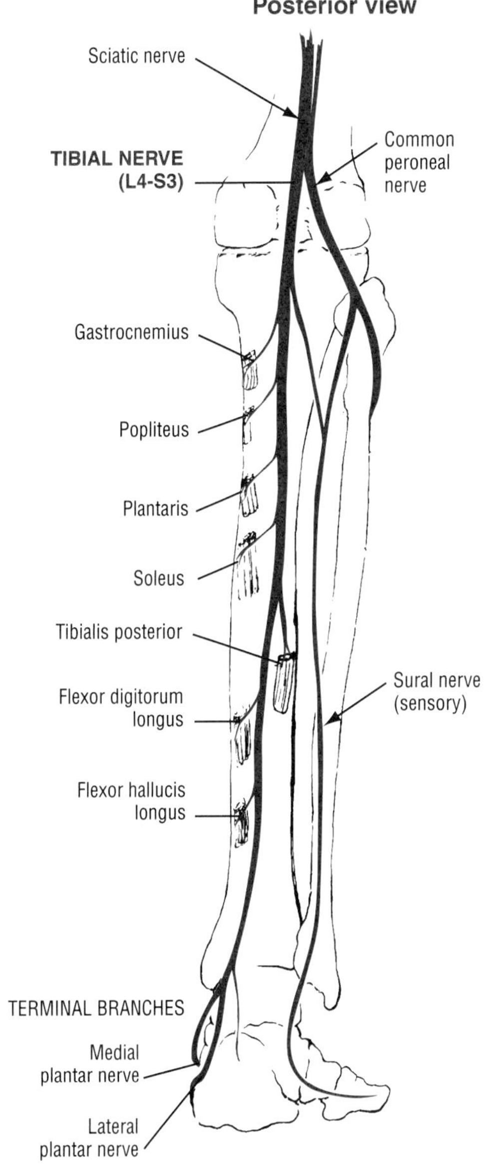

Figure 11-22 The path and innervations of the tibial nerve. Note that the tibial nerve splits into the medial and lateral plantar nerves. (Modified from Waxman S: *Correlative neuroanatomy,* ed 24, New York, 2000, Lange Medical Books/McGraw-Hill.)

Extrinsic Muscles of the Ankle and Foot

Because the extrinsic muscles cross multiple joints and axes of rotation, they possess multiple actions across the foot and ankle. The muscular action of these muscles (like all muscles) is determined by the position of their line of pull relative to the axis of rotation. Figure 11-23 shows the relationship of the extrinsic muscles to the axes of rotation of the talocrural and subtalar joints, indicating their potential actions. (For simplicity, only inversion and eversion actions will be described for the muscles that cross the subtalar joint.) Note that all muscles listed in Figure 11-23 have two actions, shown as either dorsiflexion or plantar flexion at the talocrural joint, and inversion or eversion at the subtalar joint.

ANTERIOR COMPARTMENT MUSCLES

The four muscles of the anterior compartment are the tibialis anterior, extensor digitorum longus, extensor hallucis longus, and the peroneus tertius. As a group, these muscles originate at the proximal tibia, adjacent fibula, and interosseous membrane. All four muscles are innervated by the deep peroneal nerve, and all four perform dorsiflexion as one of their primary actions.

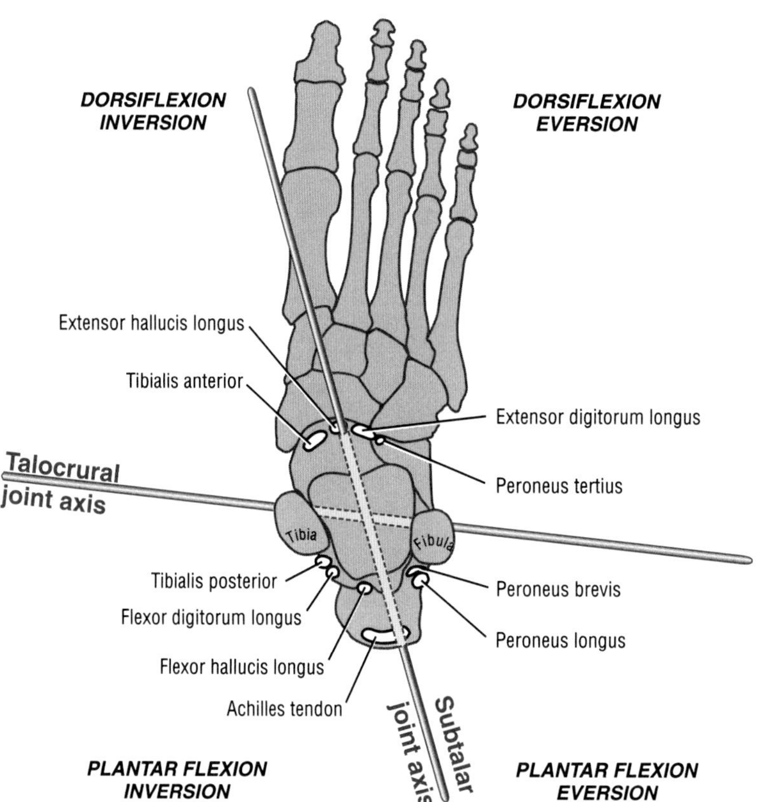

Figure 11-23 The multiple actions of muscles that cross the talocrural and subtalar joints are shown, as viewed from above. The actions of each muscle are based on its position relative to the axis of rotation at each of the two joints. (From Neumann DA: *Kinesiology of the musculoskeletal system: foundations for physical rehabilitation,* St Louis, 2002, Mosby, Figure 14-40.)

ANTERIOR VIEW

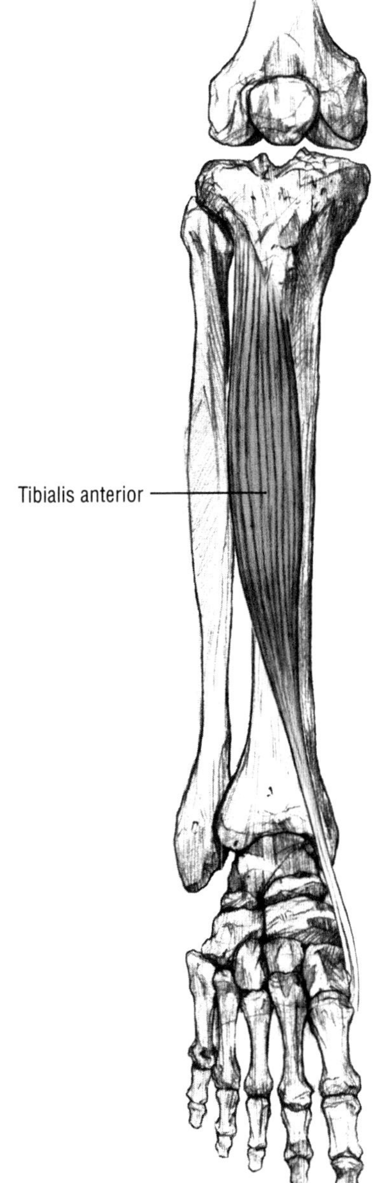

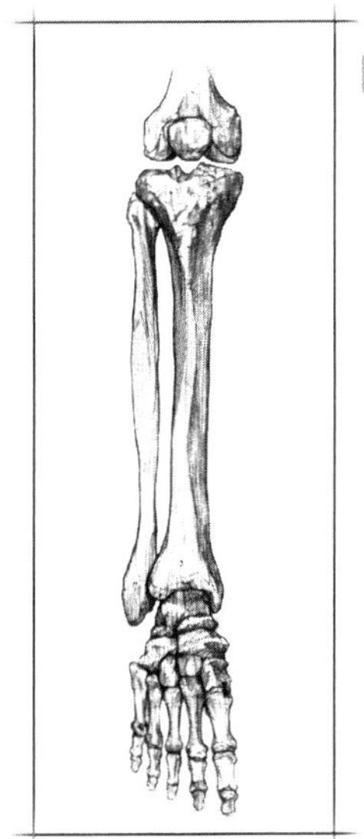

Tibialis Anterior

Proximal Attachment: Proximal two thirds of the lateral surface of the tibia and the interosseous membrane

Distal Attachment: Medial and plantar aspects of the medial cuneiform and the base of the first metatarsal

Innervation: Deep branch of the peroneal nerve

Actions:
- Dorsiflexion
- Inversion

Comments: The tendon of this muscle is easily palpable during combined dorsiflexion and inversion. Paralysis or weakness of this muscle may result in "foot drop" while in the swing phase of gait—this is described in a subsequent section.

ANTERIOR VIEW

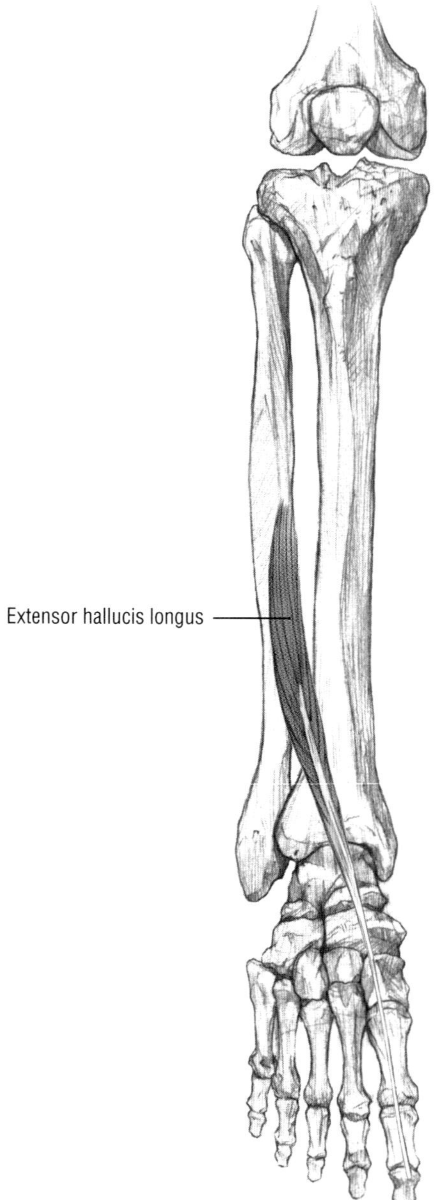

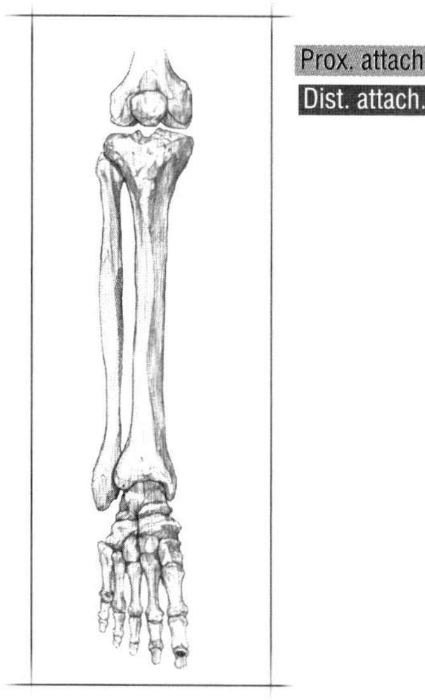

Extensor Hallucis Longus

Proximal Attachment: Middle section of the fibula and adjacent interosseous membrane

Distal Attachment: Dorsal base of the distal phalanx of the great toe

Innervation: Deep branch of the peroneal nerve

Actions:
- Extension of the great toe
- Dorsiflexion

Comments: Because this muscle courses parallel with the axis of rotation at the subtalar joint (see Figure 11-23), it is neither an invertor nor an evertor.

ANTERIOR VIEW

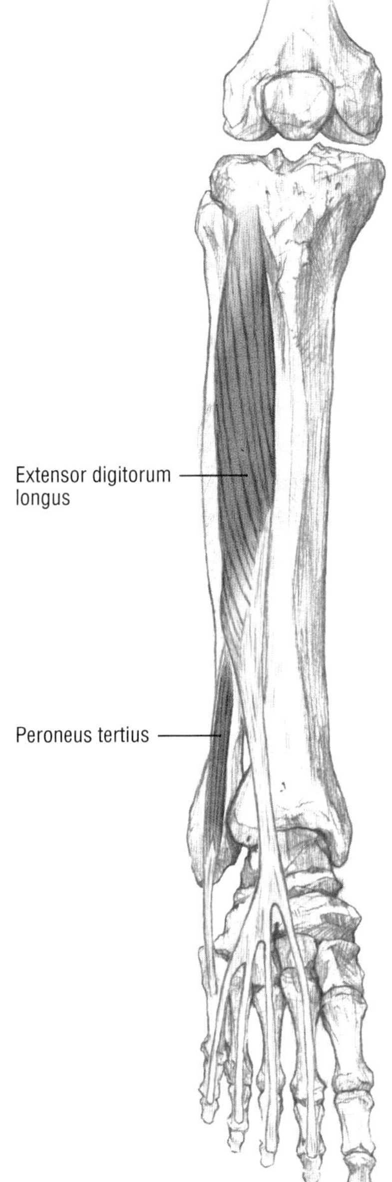

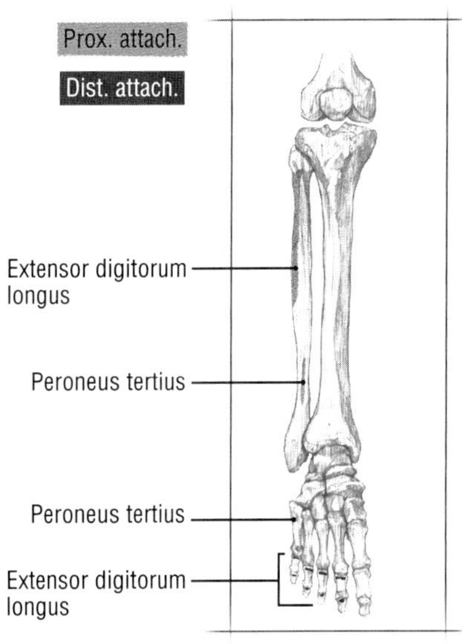

Extensor Digitorum Longus

Proximal Attachment: Lateral condyle of the tibia, proximal two thirds of the medial surface of the fibula and adjacent interosseous membrane

Distal Attachment: Splits into four tendons that attach to the proximal base of the dorsal surface of the middle and distal phalanges

Innervation: Deep branch of the peroneal nerve

Actions:
- Extension of toes 2-5 (MTP, PIP, and DIP joints)
- Dorsiflexion
- Eversion

Comments: The name of this muscle clearly indicates its primary action. Because this muscle crosses the anterior side of the medial-lateral axis of rotation at the talocrural joint, it is also a dorsiflexor of the talocrural joint. Persons with weakened anterior tibialis may compensate by using the force of the extensor digitorum longus to dorsiflex the ankle. Tightness, spasticity, or overuse of this muscle may result in a "claw toe" deformity of toes 2-5 (hyperextension of the MTP and flexion of the PIP and DIP joints).

Continued

Peroneus Tertius

Proximal Attachment: Distal one third of the medial surface of the fibula and adjacent interosseous membrane

Distal Attachment: Dorsal surface of the base of the fifth metatarsal

Innervation: Deep branch of the peroneal nerve

Actions:
- Dorsiflexion
- Eversion

Comments: Strengthening of this muscle is often an important component of treating inversion ankle sprains. Because the peroneus tertius is able to perform both dorsiflexion and eversion, it is perfectly suited to resist plantar flexion and inversion—motions that frequently cause injury to the lateral collateral ligaments, especially the anterior talofibular ligament.

Functional Considerations

Clinical Signs of Weakness of the Dorsiflexor Muscles: "Foot Drop" versus "Foot Slap." The dorsiflexors of the ankle have two important functions during gait. During the swing phase the dorsiflexors contract, elevating the foot to clear the ground. At early stance phase (between heel contact and foot flat), the dorsiflexors are activated eccentrically to slowly lower the sole of the foot to the ground. Injury to the exposed and vulnerable deep peroneal nerve can cause paresis (weakness) or paralysis of the dorsiflexor muscles. Weakness of this muscle group can hamper the mechanics of walking. **Foot drop** describes a condition in which the foot drops into plantar flexion as the leg is advanced during the swing phase of gait. In order to prevent the foot from dragging against the ground, often a high-stepping gait is performed, giving the appearance of the individual stepping over an imaginary obstacle.

If the dorsiflexors are unable to generate sufficient eccentric activation between heel contact and foot flat, the forefoot quickly makes contact with the ground. This impairment is often referred to as *foot slap*, due to the slapping sound that occurs as the sole of the foot rapidly hits the floor.

These conditions associated with weakness of the dorsiflexors are often treated by selectively strengthening these muscles. Orthotics may also be used to hold the foot in relative dorsiflexion to prevent the plantar flexors from becoming over-shortened and tight.

Shin Splints. Shin splints is a common painful condition that may affect the muscles that attach to the medial and posterior sides of the tibia. Although several terms and different pathologies have been associated with this condition, it often involves the dorsiflexor muscles and typically affects runners. During running, the dorsiflexors must shift from concentric activation, as the leg is advanced, to eccentric activation, as the distal foot is lowered immediately following heel strike. If the dorsiflexors are untrained, they may become inflamed through overuse. Excessive pronation of the foot during running or walking may worsen the condition because the dorsiflexors are repeatedly activated in an over-stretched position. For this reason, clinicians often recommend orthotics to support the foot and provide the inflamed dorsiflexor muscles with much-needed rest. Ice, ultrasound, and therapeutic taping are also used to alleviate pain in the inflamed musculature.

LATERAL COMPARTMENT MUSCLES

The two muscles in the lateral compartment of the leg are the peroneus longus and peroneus brevis; both are primary evertors of the foot.

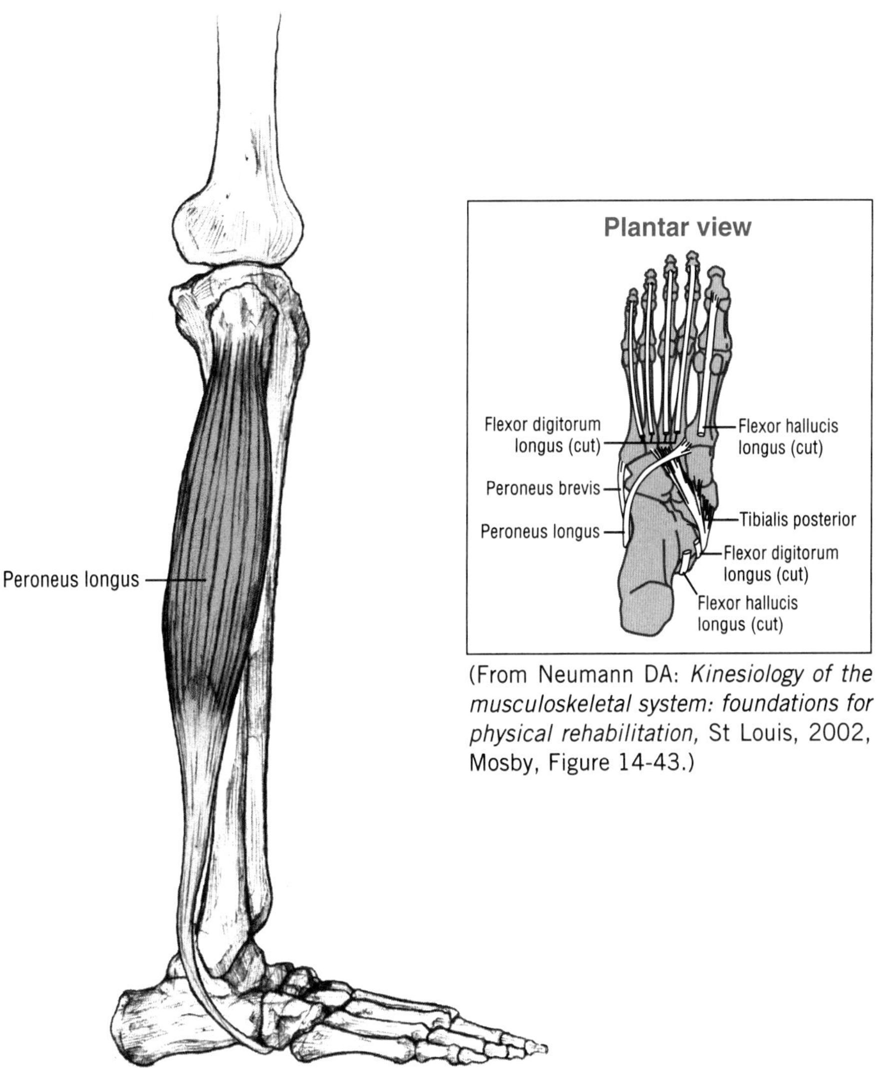

(From Neumann DA: *Kinesiology of the musculoskeletal system: foundations for physical rehabilitation,* St Louis, 2002, Mosby, Figure 14-43.)

Peroneus Longus

Proximal Attachment: Lateral condyle of the tibia; head and proximal two thirds of the lateral surface of the fibula

Distal Attachment: Lateral surface of the medial cuneiform and plantar base of the first metatarsal (see plantar view inset)

Innervation: Superficial branch of the peroneal nerve

Actions:
- Eversion
- Plantar flexion

Comments: The peroneus longus uses the lateral malleolus and a groove in the cuboid as biomechanical pulleys to produce plantar flexion and eversion, respectively. This pulley system is essential to maintaining the muscle's line of force relative to the joints' axes of rotation. Observe that the tendon of this muscle courses *under* the foot to attach to the base of the *first* metatarsal bone.

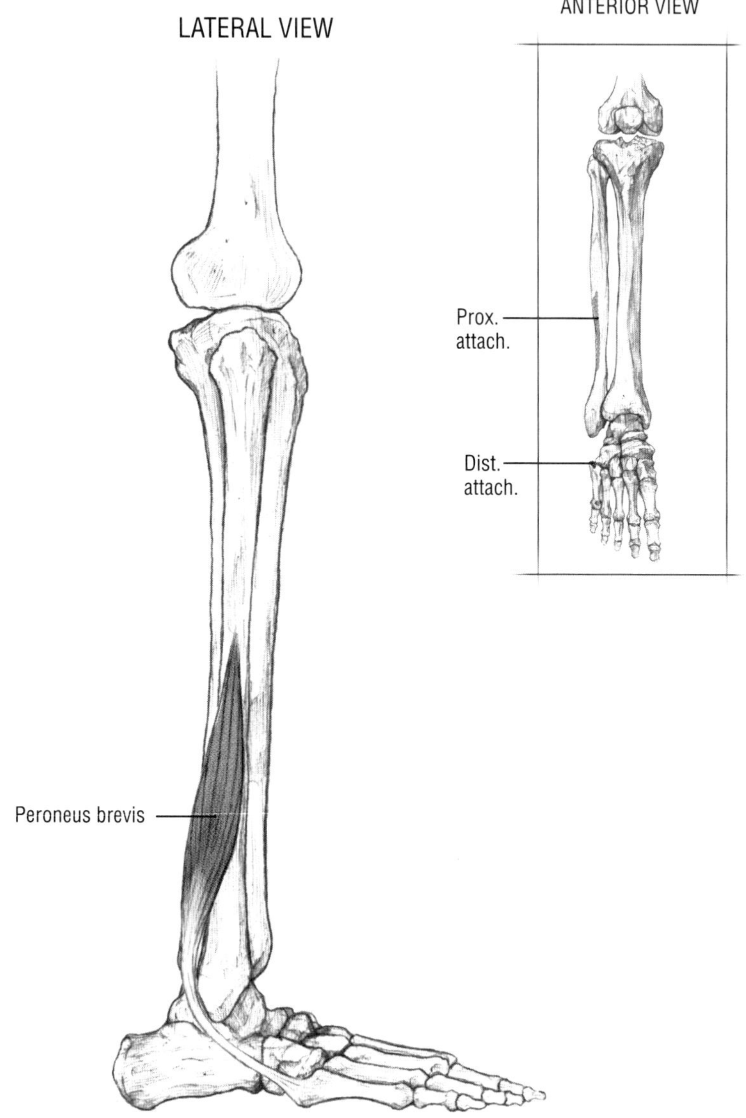

Peroneus Brevis

Proximal Attachment: Distal two thirds of the lateral surface of the fibula

Distal Attachment: Styloid process of the fifth metatarsal

Innervation: Superficial branch of the peroneal nerve

Actions:

- Plantar flexion
- Eversion

Comments: The tendon of the peroneus brevis is frequently involved with an *avulsion fracture* of the styloid process of the fifth metatarsal. This occurs when the tendon and part of the styloid process are torn away from the base of the bone. This injury—often referred to as a dancer's fracture—may occur following a strong contraction of the peroneus brevis in an attempt to "brake" an excessive (and often unexpected) inversion movement at the ankle or foot. This severe inversion ankle injury may also rupture several of the lateral collateral ligaments.

Functional Considerations

The peroneus longus and peroneus brevis muscles provide an important element of lateral stability to the ankle and foot. This lateral stability is particularly evident during late stance phase, as the heel rises in preparation for push-off. At this point in the gait cycle, all the plantar flexors are contracting to propel the body upward and forward. As evident in Figure 11-23, *most plantar flexor muscles are also invertors of the foot.* This situation is normally balanced by a simultaneous contraction of the peroneus longus and brevis—two strong evertor muscles that are also plantar flexors. The important force balance between the invertors and evertors is very evident as one stands up on tip-toes (Figure 11-24). With weakness of the peroneal muscles, the foot is more likely to uncontrollably flip strongly into inversion, possibly resulting in a lateral ankle sprain.

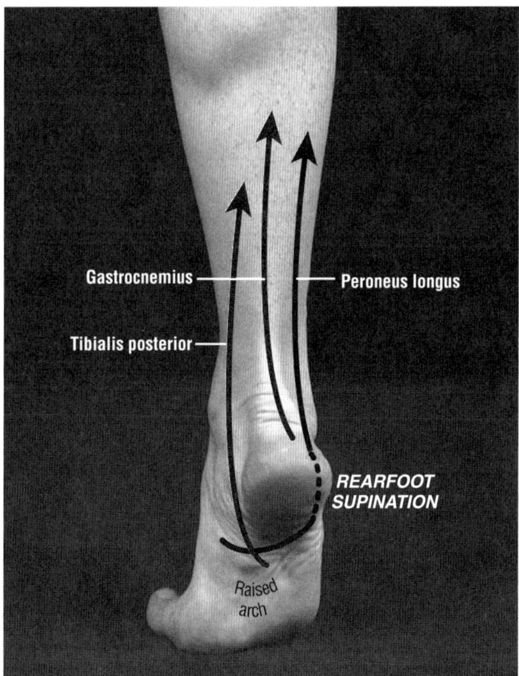

Figure 11-24 The line of force of several plantar flexors while an individual rises up on tip-toes. Note that the peroneus longus *(black)* and tibialis posterior *(red)* form a sling around the midfoot. The peroneus longus plays an important role in offsetting the inversion component of the tibialis posterior muscle. (From Neumann DA: *Kinesiology of the musculoskeletal system: foundations for physical rehabilitation,* St Louis, 2002, Mosby, Figure 14-44.)

POSTERIOR COMPARTMENT MUSCLES

The muscles of the posterior compartment are divided into two groups: superficial and deep. The *superficial group* includes the gastrocnemius, soleus (together known as the **triceps surae**), and plantaris. The *deep group* includes the tibialis posterior, flexor digitorum longus, and flexor hallucis longus. All muscles in the posterior compartment are innervated by the tibial nerve and perform plantar flexion as one of their primary actions.

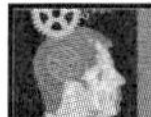

Consider this...

Lateral Ankle Sprains

One of the most common injuries of the lower extremity involves an inversion sprain of the ankle and foot, often associated with damage to the lateral ligaments (Figure 11-25). There are three reasons why the lateral collateral ligaments are sprained far more often than the deltoid (medial) ligaments.

- Size
  The lateral collateral ligaments are relatively thin. The medial collateral ligament is strong, thick, and wide.
- Inversion bias
  The available motion into inversion at the subtalar joint is twice that of eversion. Often weight is placed on the leg with the ankle in too much inversion, such as when landing awkwardly from a jump. This places much of the body's weight over the already stretched lateral ligaments.
- Lack of quick response from the supporting musculature
  Sprains of the lateral ligaments typically occur from excessive inversion. The muscles best designed to protect against excessive inversion sprains are in the peroneal muscles. Unfortunately, however, most inversion sprains occur before these muscles can respond. Strengthening the peroneal muscles is therefore only one component of treating someone with chronic ankle instability. Other treatments involve proprioceptive training, often through the use of a "wobble board," trampoline, or single-leg stance activities. Dynamic balance activities such as walking on uneven or spongy surfaces are also used to help train these muscles to respond—more quickly—to rapid inversion of the ankle and foot.

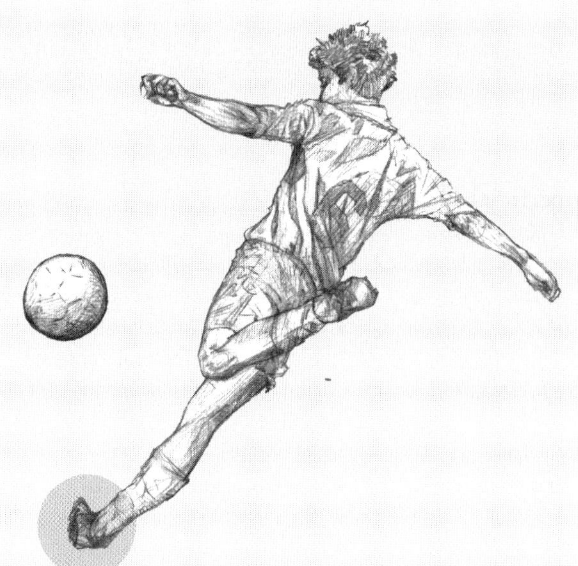

Figure 11-25 Soccer player suffering a right ankle inversion sprain.

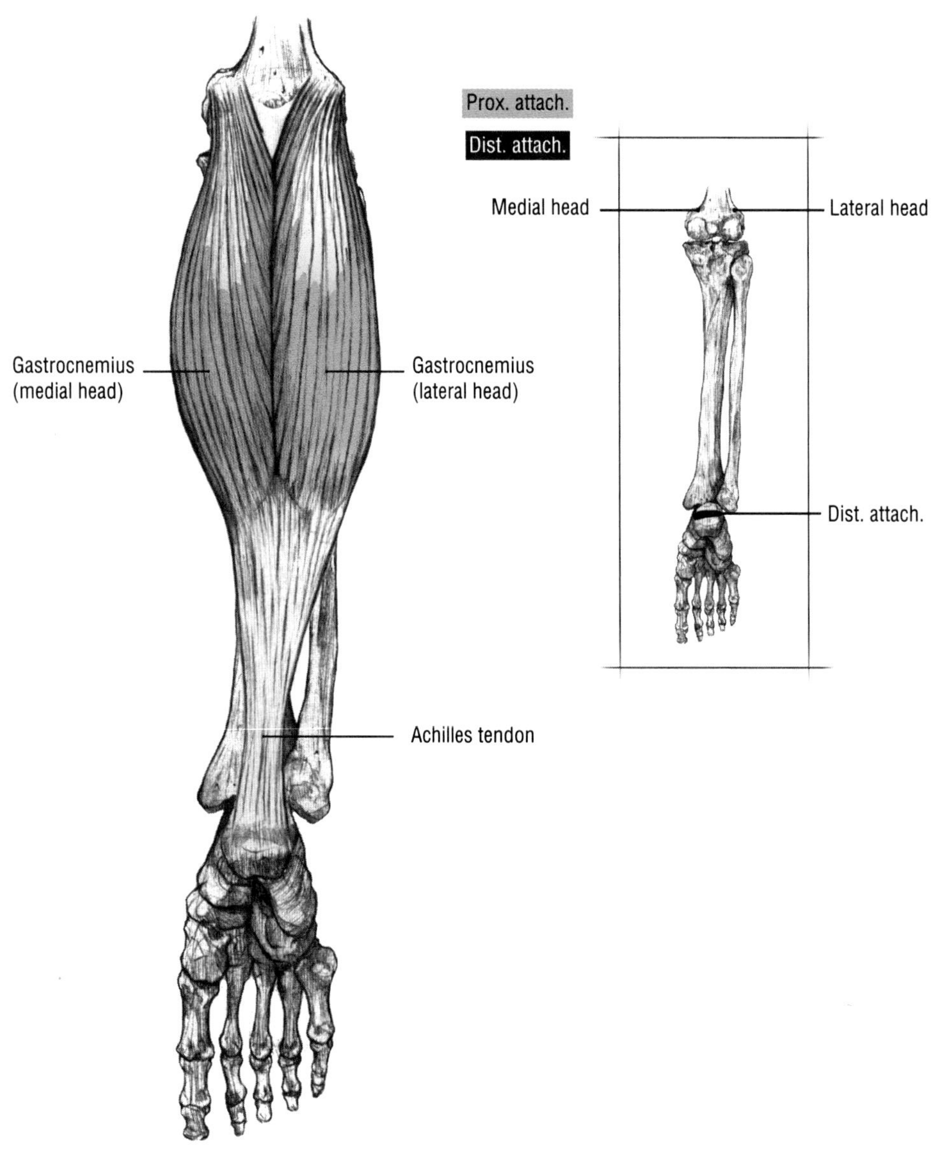

Superficial Group

Gastrocnemius

Proximal Attachments:
- Medial head—the posterior aspect of the medial femoral condyle
- Lateral head—the posterior aspect of the lateral femoral condyle

Distal Attachment: Calcaneal tuberosity via the Achilles tendon

Innervation: Tibial nerve

Actions:
- Plantar flexion
- Flexion of the knee

Comments: The gastrocnemius muscle is able to produce a large plantar flexion torque due to its relatively large cross-sectional area combined with the large internal moment arm provided by the protruding calcaneal tuberosity. A large torque is required to propel the weight of the body upward and forward, such as when running or jumping.

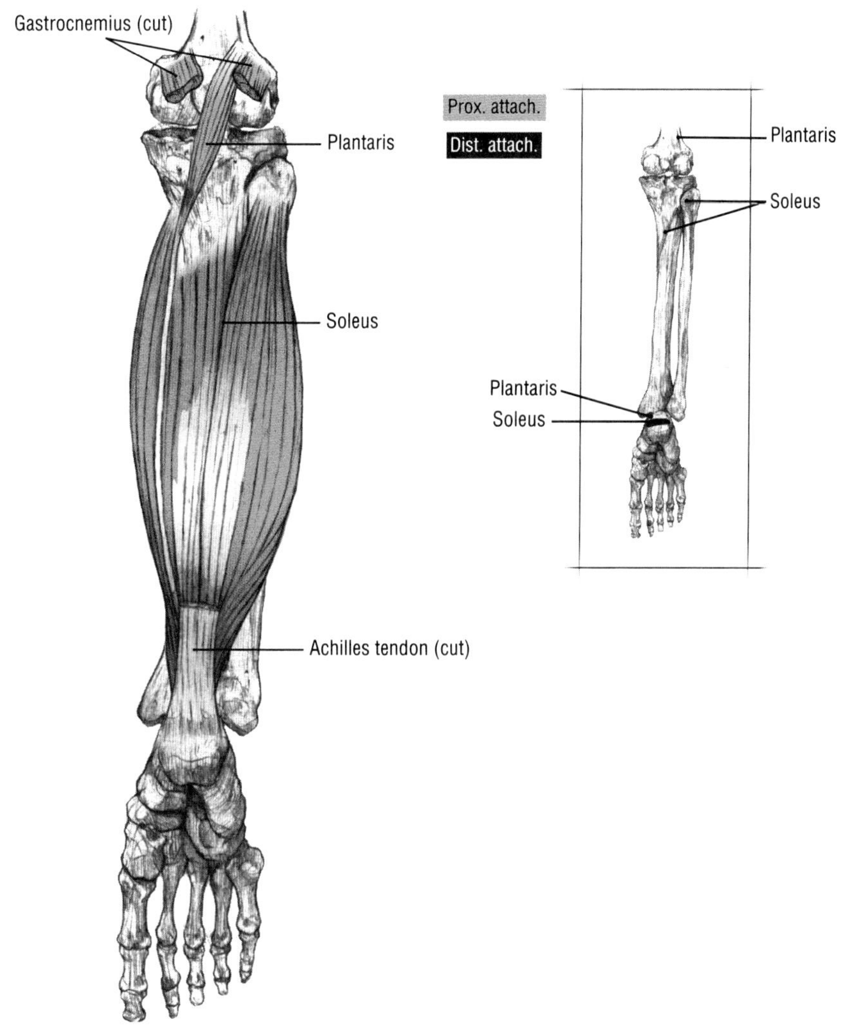

Soleus

Proximal Attachment: Proximal one third of the posterior fibula and fibular head and posterior aspect of the tibia

Distal Attachment: Calcaneal tuberosity via the Achilles tendon

Innervation: Tibial nerve

Action: Plantar flexion

Comments: The gastrocnemius and soleus muscles are typically referred to as the calf muscle group. Conditions may arise where a therapist needs to test the strength of just one of these muscles independently of the other. Knowledge of the different attachments of these two muscles may assist in this process. Assume, for example, that the therapist is interested in testing the plantar flexion strength produced primarily by the soleus muscle. To do this, the therapist may request that the patient perform a maximum effort plantar flexion force with the knee *fully flexed*. The flexed-knee position slackens the two-joint gastrocnemius but does not alter the length of the one-joint soleus. As a consequence, the slackened gastrocnemius is robbed of much of its ability to produce plantar flexion at the ankle. The plantar flexion force measured by the therapist, therefore, is assumed to represent the force produced primarily by the soleus.

Plantaris

Proximal Attachment: Lateral supracondylar line of the femur

Distal Attachment: Medial aspect of the Achilles tendon to insert on the calcaneal tuberosity

Innervation: Tibial nerve

Actions:
- Plantar flexion
- Flexion of the knee

Comments: The small plantaris contributes little to the overall plantar flexion force at the ankle.

Functional Considerations

SOLEUS VERSUS GASTROCNEMIUS: FORM AND FUNCTION. Both the soleus and gastrocnemius provide the primary source of plantar flexion torque to the ankle; however, the design of these muscles permits different specialties.

The soleus is a "pure" plantar flexor, without the ability to flex the knee. This muscle is composed of primarily *slow-twitch muscle fibers*, which make it an ideal choice for activities that require relatively low forces over a long duration, such as standing or controlling postural sway. The gastrocnemius, on the other hand, is composed of more *fast-twitch fibers*, which make it better equipped to perform more explosive activities such as sprinting and jumping. Interestingly, these explosive activities ideally suited for the gastrocnemius combine *ankle plantar flexion with knee extension*. This combination of motions prevents over-shortening of this two-joint muscle—as the gastrocnemius shortens to produce plantar flexion, it is simultaneously stretched across the extending knee. This situation maximizes the muscle's ability to produce an effective force.

BIOMECHANICS OF RAISING UP ON TIP-TOES. The functional strength of a plantar flexor muscle such as the gastrocnemius is often evaluated by requiring a subject to repeatedly rise up on tip-toes. Normally, this is a relatively easy task, even if performed using one leg. The relative ease of this action should be somewhat surprising, given that the entire body must be lifted. The relative ease of standing up on tip-toes is largely due to the large moment arm available to the gastrocnemius. As illustrated in Figure 11-26, upon rising up on the toes, the axis of rotation for the gastrocnemius shifts from the ankle (talocrural joint) to the metatarsophalangeal (MTP) joints. This shift greatly increases the moment arm available to the muscle (see Figure 11-26, B). Also, because the line of body weight falls *between* the axis of rotation and the line of force of the gastrocnemius, the muscle is operating as a *second-class* lever system, similar to the way a wheelbarrow operates. Because the internal moment arm available to the calf muscles (see Figure 11-26, B) is three times longer than the external moment arm available to gravity (see Figure 11-26, C), an individual weighing 180 lb would require only 60 lb of plantar flexion force to rise up on tip-toes. This is a great advantage, but realize that the center of gravity of the body will be elevated only one third the distance that the muscle contracts.

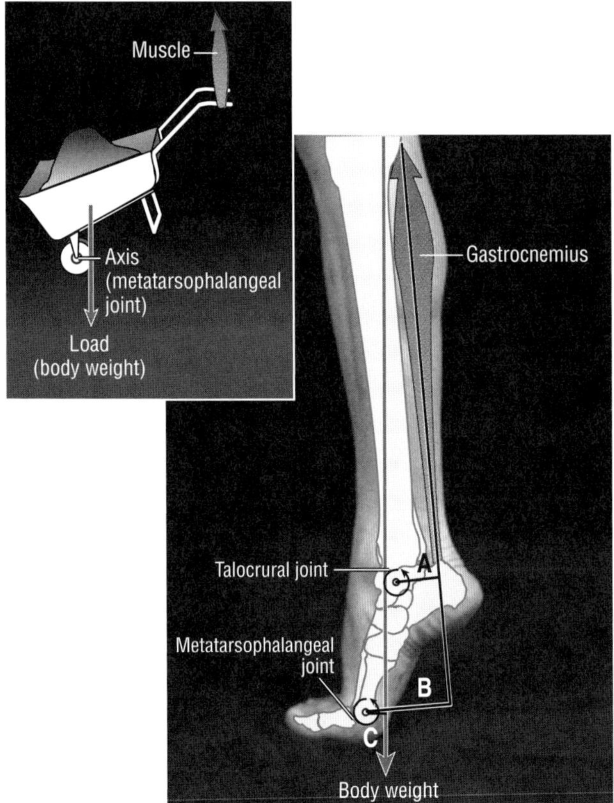

Figure 11-26 A model showing how the biomechanics of rising up on tip-toes is similar to the operation of a wheelbarrow. When standing up on tip-toes, the axis of rotation shifts from the talocrural joint (acting with moment arm marked *A)* to the metatarsophalangeal joints. Once up on tip-toes, the internal moment arm *(B)* available to the gastrocnemius is three times longer than the external moment arm *(C) available* to body weight. (From Neumann DA: *Kinesiology of the musculoskeletal system: foundations for physical rehabilitation,* St Louis, 2002, Mosby, Figure 14-50.)

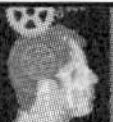

Consider this...

Soleus as a Secondary Extensor of the Knee

The soleus plays an important role as a plantar flexor of the ankle, but also as an important extensor and stabilizer of the knee. With the sole of the foot in firm contact with the ground, activation of the soleus results in closed-chain plantar flexion. This action drives the superior aspect of the tibia (and attached knee) posteriorly, effectively *extending the knee* (Figure 11-27). Persons with weakened quadriceps may be able to use this function of the soleus as an alternative source of knee extension torque.

It is possible, however, that an over-active (spastic) soleus muscle can create excessive (and undesired) extension of the knee while bearing weight through the lower limb. This scenario often occurs in a person who has had a stroke with resulting increased spasticity of the soleus muscles. Over time, the increased activity in this muscle can contribute to *genu recurvatum* (hyperextension of the knee) as weight is placed over the leg.

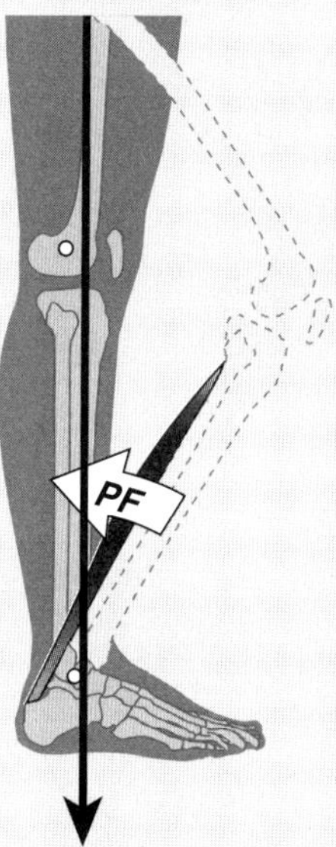

Figure 11-27 With the foot firmly fixed to the ground, activation of the soleus produces extension of the knee. Note that this is a result of closed-chain plantar flexion *(PF)* motion of the ankle. (From Neumann DA: *Kinesiology of the musculoskeletal system: foundations for physical rehabilitation,* St Louis, 2002, Mosby, Figure 14-48.)

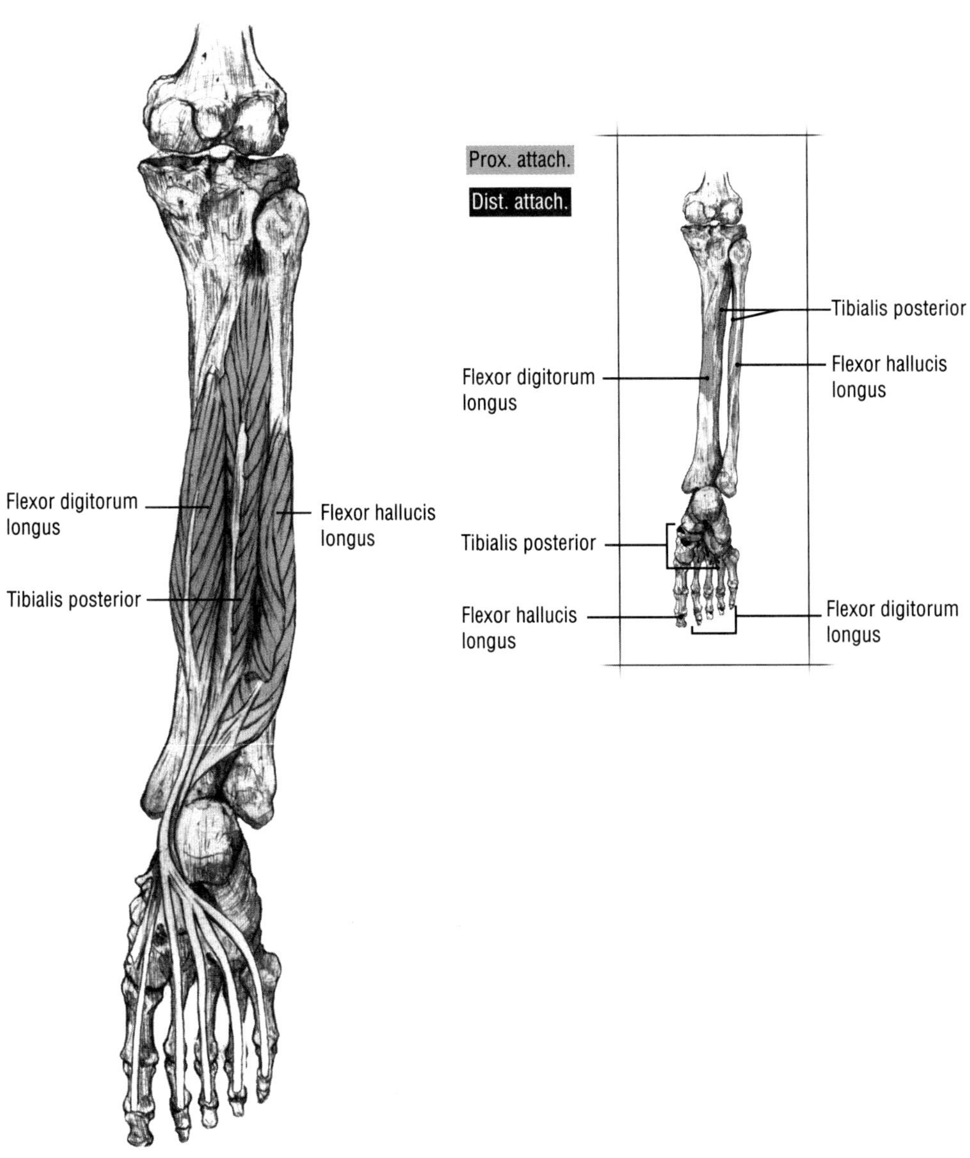

DEEP GROUP

Tibialis Posterior

Proximal Attachment: Proximal two thirds of the posterior aspect of the tibia, fibula, and interosseous membrane

Distal Attachment: Multiple attachments to every tarsal bone except the talus; also attaches to the bases of the second, third, and fourth metatarsals. The most prominent insertion is on the navicular tuberosity.

Innervation: Tibial nerve

Actions:
- Plantar flexion
- Inversion

Comments: The extensive distal attachments and line of pull of the tibialis posterior make this muscle the foot's most effective invertor of the subtalar joint and supinator at the transverse tarsal joint. This muscle force provides essential support to the medial longitudinal arch of the foot. A ruptured tibialis posterior tendon often causes traumatic pes planus (flat foot).

Flexor Hallucis Longus

Proximal Attachment:	Distal two thirds of the posterior fibula
Distal Attachment:	Plantar surface of the base of the distal phalanx of the great toe
Innervation:	Tibial nerve
Actions:	• Flexion of the great toe • Plantar flexion • Inversion
Comments:	During running or jumping, the flexor hallucis longus is highly active during the end stage of push-off, when the great toe is in a position of hyperextension. This force is useful for generating friction between the plantar surfaces of the toes and the walking surface.

Flexor Digitorum Longus

Proximal Attachment:	Posterior surface of the middle one third of the tibia
Distal Attachment:	By four separate tendons to the base of the distal phalanx of the four lesser toes
Innervation:	Tibial nerve
Actions:	• Flexion of toes 2 to 5 • Plantar flexion • Inversion
Comments:	Spasticity or tightness of the flexor digitorum longus may result in a posture of plantar flexion of the ankle, inversion of the foot, and flexion of the toes.

***Clinical* INSIGHT**

"Turf Toe"

"Turf toe" describes an injury that typically results from traumatic hyperextension of the metatarsophalangeal joint of the great toe. As a result of the severe hyperextension, the surrounding capsule may become torn and the base of the great toe becomes swollen and painful. As the name implies, this injury is common to field athletes who commonly perform high-velocity cutting actions such as in soccer, American football, or rugby.

This painful condition is initially treated with rest, ice, and anti-inflammatory drugs. As a measure of protection, an individual with turf toe may be fitted with a rigid plate in the sole of the shoe to prevent unwanted extension of the toes.

Functional Considerations: Role of the Deep Compartment Muscles in Supporting the Medial Longitudinal Arch. The tibialis posterior, flexor hallucis longus, and flexor digitorum longus comprise the deep group of the posterior compartment. These muscles are the primary invertors (or supinators) of the foot. They most often are used eccentrically to resist eversion (or pronation) of the foot during the early stance phase of walking. This function is especially important for the tibialis posterior muscle. In cases of an over-stretched and weakened medial longitudinal arch, the tibialis posterior may become over-worked, eventually resulting in fatigue and painful overuse syndromes.

Intrinsic Muscles of the Foot

In general, the intrinsic muscles of the foot are most active during the push-off phase of walking or running. These muscles contract as a group to help reinforce the relatively raised position of the medial longitudinal arch. This function helps stabilize the foot just at the time the plantar flexor muscles contract for push-off. The relevant anatomic information of the intrinsic muscles is covered in the table below and on pp. 334-336.

DORSUM OF THE FOOT

The dorsum of the foot has just one intrinsic muscle, the extensor digitorum brevis, which performs extension of the toes.

Muscle	Proximal Attachment	Distal Attachment	Actions	Innervation
Extensor digitorum brevis	Dorsal-lateral aspect of the calcaneus, just proximal to the calcaneocuboid joint	Through four separate tendons that blend with the extrinsic extensor tendons coursing to digits 1-4	Extension of the first four toes	Deep branch of the peroneal nerve

PLANTAR ASPECT OF THE FOOT

The intrinsic muscles of the plantar aspect of the foot are organized into four layers (Figure 11-28). The tough plantar fascia covers the outermost layer.

First Layer

The first layer consists of the flexor digitorum brevis, abductor hallucis, and abductor digiti minimi (see Figure 11-28, A).

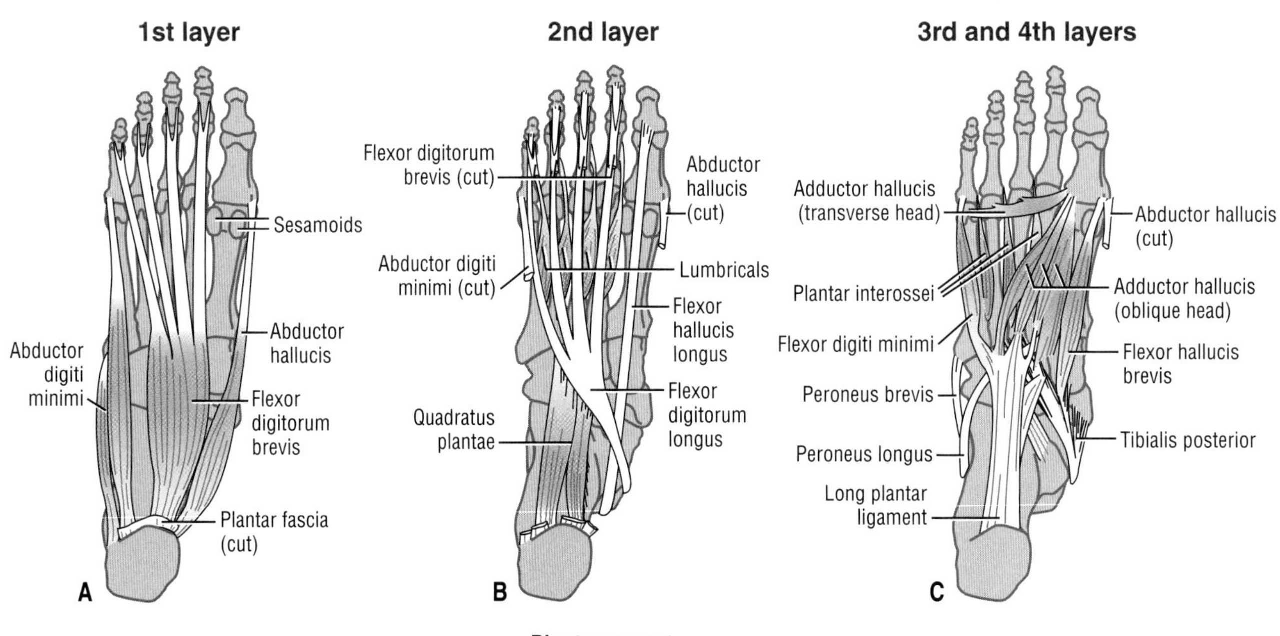

Figure 11-28 The intrinsic muscles of the foot are organized into four layers. **A,** First layer (most superficial); **B,** second layer; and **C,** third and fourth layers (deepest layers). (From Neumann DA: *Kinesiology of the musculoskeletal system: foundations for physical rehabilitation,* St Louis, 2002, Mosby, Figure 14-51.)

Muscle	Proximal Attachment	Distal Attachment	Actions	Innervation
Flexor digitorum brevis	Plantar aspect of the calcaneal tuberosity and plantar fascia	Through 4 tendons to the base of the middle phalanx of the 4 lesser toes	Flexion of the metatarsophalangeal and proximal interphalangeal joints of the 4 lesser toes	Medial plantar nerve
Abductor hallucis	Flexor retinaculum, medial process of the calcaneus, and plantar fascia	Medial side of the base of the proximal phalanx of the great toe (hallux)	Abduction of the great toe	Medial plantar nerve
Abductor digiti minimi	Medial and lateral processes of the calcaneal tuberosity, and base of the fifth metatarsal	Lateral side of the proximal phalanx of the fifth toe	Abduction of the fifth toe	Medial plantar nerve

Second Layer

The second layer consists of the quadratus plantae and the four lumbricals (see Figure 11-28, *B*).

Muscle	Proximal Attachment	Distal Attachment	Actions	Innervation
Quadratus plantae	By two heads to the plantar aspect of the calcaneus	Lateral border of the flexor digitorum longus tendon	Helps to stabilize the tendons of the flexor digitorum longus, preventing them from migrating medially when under force	Lateral plantar nerve
4 Lumbricals	Tendons of the flexor digitorum longus	Dorsal digital expansion of the 4 lesser toes	Flexion of the metatarsophalangeal joints, simultaneously extending the interphalangeal joints	To second toe: medial plantar nerve To third to fifth toes: lateral plantar nerve

Third Layer

The third layer consists of the adductor hallucis, flexor hallucis brevis, and the flexor digiti minimi (see Figure 11-28, C).

Muscle	Proximal Attachment	Distal Attachment	Actions	Innervation
Adductor hallucis	*Oblique head:* Plantar aspect of the base of second through fourth metatarsals and sheath of the peroneus longus tendon *Transverse head:* Off the plantar aspect of the supporting ligaments of the third through fifth MTP joints	Both heads converge to insert on the lateral base of the proximal phalanx of the great toe	Flexion and adduction of the MTP joint of the great toe	Lateral plantar nerve
Flexor hallucis brevis	Plantar surface of the cuboid and lateral cuneiform bones; parts of the tendon of the tibialis posterior	By two heads to the medial and lateral aspects of the base of the proximal phalanx of the great toe (embedded with 2 small sesamoid bones)	MTP flexion of the great toe	Medial plantar nerve
Flexor digiti minimi	Plantar aspect of the base of the fifth metatarsal	Lateral base of the proximal phalanx of the fifth toe	MTP flexion of the fifth toe	Lateral plantar nerve

MTP, Metatarsophalangeal.

Fourth Layer

The fourth layer consists of the dorsal and plantar interossei (see plantar interossei in Figure 11-28, C).

Muscle	Proximal Attachment	Distal Attachment	Actions	Innervation
4 Dorsal interossei	*First:* First and second metatarsals *Second:* Second and third metatarsals *Third:* Third and fourth metatarsals *Fourth:* Fourth and fifth metatarsals	*First:* Medial base of the proximal phalanx of the second toe *Second:* Lateral base of the proximal phalanx of the second toe *Third:* Lateral base of the proximal phalanx of the third toe *Fourth:* Lateral base of the proximal phalanx of the fourth toe	Abduction of toes 2-4	Lateral plantar nerve
3 Plantar interossei	*First:* Medial side of third metatarsal *Second:* Medial side of fourth metatarsal *Third:* Medial side of fifth metatarsal	*First:* Medial side of the proximal phalanx of the third toe *Second:* Medial side of the proximal phalanx of the fourth toe *Third:* Medial side of the proximal phalanx of the fifth toe	Adduction of toes	Lateral plantar nerve

Summary

The structure of the ankle and foot is designed primarily for two functions. First, the foot must be sufficiently pliable during early stance phase in order to absorb the impact of weight bearing, as well as adapt to the shape of the ground. This is accomplished primarily by connective tissues including the muscles that slowly lower the medial longitudinal arch as the foot pronates (everts). This action helps absorb the compressive force of body weight. Secondly, in the mid-to-late stance phases of gait, the foot must be rendered more rigid in order to tolerate the muscular thrust of push-off. The increased stability occurs as the medial longitudinal arch rises and the foot begins to invert (supinate) slightly under the active control of intrinsic and extrinsic muscles.

The unique design and function of the ankle and foot is elegantly expressed primarily during the stance phase of walking. During this time, even though the calcaneus is fixed to the ground, the foot must dissipate the continued rotation and forward progression of the entire lower limb. The function of the ankle and foot is therefore strongly linked to movement and function of the entire lower extremity. Dysfunctions of the hip, knee, or even the back may therefore be associated with problems originating at the ankle or foot. Restoring optimum function of the ankle and foot may consequently be a prerequisite for helping to correct musculoskeletal problems throughout the entire lower limb.

Study Questions

1. The primary motions that occur at the talocrural joint are:
   a. Dorsiflexion and plantar flexion
   b. Inversion and eversion
   c. Adduction and abduction
   d. None of the above
2. The subtalar joint is best described as the articulation between the:
   a. Talus and the distal tibia and fibula
   b. Talus and the cuboid
   c. Talus and the calcaneus
   d. Calcaneus and the navicular
3. The combined action of dorsiflexion, eversion, and abduction is described as __________ of the ankle and foot.
   a. Supination
   b. Pronation
   c. Hyperextension
   d. Varus
4. One of the primary functions of the longitudinal arch is to:
   a. Limit excessive supination of the foot
   b. Help safely absorb weight-bearing forces through the foot
   c. Prevent excessive plantar flexion at the talocrural joint
   d. Prevent excessive flexion at the lateral four metatarsophalangeal joints

5. Inversion and eversion:
   a. Occur about a medial-lateral axis of rotation
   b. Occur about an anterior-posterior axis of rotation
   c. Occur in the frontal plane
   d. A and C
   e. B and C
6. Which of the following joints allows nearly equal amounts of motion in all three planes?
   a. Talocrural
   b. Subtalar
   c. Transverse tarsal
   d. Metatarsophalangeal joint of the great toe
7. A muscle that courses posterior to the medial-lateral axis of rotation of the ankle can be predicted to produce which of the following actions?
   a. Dorsiflexion
   b. Plantar flexion
   c. Inversion
   d. Eversion
8. Which of the following joints is commonly referred to as a "mortise joint"?
   a. Subtalar joint
   b. Transverse tarsal joint
   c. Proximal interphalangeal joints
   d. Talocrural joint
9. Which of the following positions is considered the close-packed, most stable position of the talocrural joint?
   a. Full adduction
   b. Full abduction
   c. Full dorsiflexion
   d. Full plantar flexion
10. The primary motions allowed at the subtalar joint are:
    a. Dorsiflexion and plantar flexion
    b. Inversion and eversion
    c. Abduction and adduction
    d. A and B
    e. B and C
11. A muscle that courses on the medial side of the anterior-posterior axis of rotation can be predicted to produce which of the following motions?
    a. Dorsiflexion
    b. Plantar flexion
    c. Inversion
    d. Eversion
12. Which of the following muscles courses posterior to the medial-lateral axis of rotation of the ankle?
    a. Tibialis anterior
    b. Peroneus brevis
    c. Peroneus tertius
    d. Extensor hallucis longus
    e. A and D
13. Which of the following muscles is *not* considered part of the triceps surae?
    a. Flexor digitorum longus
    b. Gastrocnemius
    c. Soleus
    d. A and B
    e. A and C
14. Pes planus is a condition that is best described as:
    a. Paralysis or paresis of the dorsiflexor muscles
    b. A chronically dropped, or low, medial longitudinal arch of the foot
    c. An abnormal high, or raised, medial longitudinal arch of the foot
    d. A valgus deformation at the metatarsophalangeal joint of the great toe
15. Which of the following nerves innervates most of the muscles that dorsiflex the foot?
    a. Tibial nerve
    b. Deep peroneal nerve
    c. Superficial peroneal nerve
    d. Lateral plantar nerve
16. Injury to the tibial nerve will most likely result in weakness of which of the following actions?
    a. Dorsiflexion
    b. Plantar flexion
    c. Eversion
    d. Extension of digits 1 to 4
17. Foot drop or foot slap would most likely result from weakness of which of the following muscles?
    a. Tibialis anterior and extensor digitorum longus
    b. Peroneus longus and peroneus brevis
    c. Gastrocnemius and soleus
    d. Flexor hallucis longus and tibialis posterior
18. Which of the following muscles has the potential to plantar flex the ankle *and* flex the knee?
    a. Flexor hallucis longus
    b. Soleus
    c. Peroneus tertius
    d. Gastrocnemius
19. Which of the following helps to prevent excessive inversion of the ankle and foot?
    a. The deltoid ligaments
    b. The lateral collateral ligaments of the ankle and foot
    c. Activation of the peroneus tertius
    d. A and C
    e. B and C
20. With the foot firmly fixed to the ground, which of the following muscles can assist with extending the knee?
    a. Extensor hallucis longus
    b. Tibialis anterior
    c. Soleus
    d. Peroneus tertius
21. The tibialis posterior and peroneus longus are similar in which of the following ways?
    a. Both muscles course anterior to the medial-lateral axis of rotation at the ankle
    b. Both muscles perform eversion
    c. Both muscles perform plantar flexion
    d. Both muscles are innervated by the tibial nerve

22. The gastrocnemius and soleus both attach to the calcaneal tuberosity via the Achilles tendon.
    a. True
    b. False
23. The peroneus brevis is innervated by the same nerve that innervates the tibialis posterior.
    a. True
    b. False
24. The talocrural joint is more stable in a position of plantar flexion than a position of dorsiflexion.
    a. True
    b. False
25. One of the primary functions of the plantar fascia is to support the medial longitudinal arch of the foot.
    a. True
    b. False
26. The tibialis anterior can perform dorsiflexion and inversion.
    a. True
    b. False
27. The abductor hallucis, flexor digitorum brevis, and abductor digiti minimi are all intrinsic muscles of the foot.
    a. True
    b. False
28. The tibialis posterior is innervated by the same nerve that innervates the flexor hallucis longus.
    a. True
    b. False
29. The gastrocnemius muscle is maximally elongated in a position of dorsiflexion and full knee flexion.
    a. True
    b. False
30. Inversion and eversion of the foot primarily occur at the talocrural joint.
    a. True
    b. False

ADDITIONAL READINGS

Allen LR, Flemming D, Sanders TG: Turf toe: ligamentous injury of the first metatarsophalangeal joint, *Mil Med* 169(11):xix-xxiv, 2004.

Basmajian JV, Stecko G: The role of muscles in arch support of the foot, *J Bone Joint Surg Am* 45:1184-1190, 1963.

Bass CR, Lucas SR, Salzar RS et al: Failure properties of cervical spinal ligaments under fast strain rate deformations, *Spine* 32(1):E7-E13, 2007.

Beynnon BD, Vacek PM, Murphy D et al: First-time inversion ankle ligament trauma: the effects of sex, level of competition, and sport on the incidence of injury, *Am J Sports Med* 33(10):1485-1491, 2005.

Buchanan KR, Davis I: The relationship between forefoot, midfoot, and rearfoot static alignment in pain-free individuals, *J Orthop Sports Phys Ther* 35(9):559-566, 2005.

Cavanagh PR, Rodgers MM, Iiboshi A: Pressure distribution under symptom-free feet during barefoot standing, *Foot Ankle* 7(5):262-276, 1987.

Colville MR, Marder RA, Boyle JJ et al: Strain measurement in lateral ankle ligaments, *Am J Sports Med* 18(2):196-200, 1990.

Cornwall MW, McPoil TG: Motion of the calcaneus, navicular, and first metatarsal during the stance phase of walking, *J Am Podiatr Med Assoc* 92(2):67-76, 2002.

Esterman A, Pilotto L: Foot shape and its effect on functioning in Royal Australian Air Force recruits. Part 1: Prospective cohort study, *Mil Med* 170(7):623-628, 2005.

Glasoe WM, Yack HJ, Saltzman CL: Anatomy and biomechanics of the first ray, *Phys Ther* 79(9):854-859, 1999.

Hubbard TJ, Hertel J, Sherbondy P: Fibular position in individuals with self-reported chronic ankle instability, *J Orthop Sports Phys Ther* 36(1):3-9, 2006.

Kulig K, Burnfield JM, Reischl S et al: Effect of foot orthoses on tibialis posterior activation in persons with pes planus, *Med Sci Sports Exerc* 37(1):24-29, 2005.

Manoli A, Graham B: The subtle cavus foot, "the underpronator," *Foot Ankle Int* 26(3):256-263, 2005.

McPoil TG, Knecht HG, Schuit D: A survey of foot types in normal females between ages of 18 and 30 years, *J Orthop Sports Phys Ther* 9:406-409, 1988.

Murray MP, Guten GN, Sepic SB et al: Function of the triceps surae during gait. Compensatory mechanisms for unilateral loss, *J Bone Joint Surg Am* 60(4):473-476, 1978.

Piazza SJ. Mechanics of the subtalar joint and its function during walking, *Foot Ankle Clin* 10(3):425-442, 2005.

Powers CM, Maffucci R, Hampton S: Rearfoot posture in subjects with patellofemoral pain, *J Orthop Sports Phys Ther* 22(4):155-160, 1995.

Reischl SF, Powers CM, Rao S et al: Relationship between foot pronation and rotation of the tibia and femur during walking [comment], *Foot Ankle Int* 20(8):513-520, 1999.

Standring S, editor: *Gray's anatomy: the anatomical basis of clinical practice*, St Louis, 2005, Churchill Livingstone.

Tome J, Nawoczenski DA, Flemister A et al: Comparison of foot kinematics between subjects with posterior tibialis tendon dysfunction and healthy controls, *J Orthop Sports Phys Ther* 36(9):635-644, 2006.

Verhagen RA, de KG, van Dijk CN: Long-term follow-up of inversion trauma of the ankle, *Arch Orthop Trauma Surg* 114(2):92-96, 1995.

Vicenzino B, Branjerdporn M, Teys P et al: Initial changes in posterior talar glide and dorsiflexion of the ankle after mobilization with movement in individuals with recurrent ankle sprain, *J Orthop Sports Phys Ther* 36(7):464-471, 2006.

CHAPTER 12

Kinesiology of Human Gait

CHAPTER OUTLINE

OBJECTIVES

- Describe the primary events of the gait cycle.
- Define the common terms used to describe human gait.
- Describe the muscular and joint interactions that occur during heel contact.
- Describe the muscular and joint interactions that occur during foot flat.
- Describe the muscular and joint interactions that occur during mid stance.
- Describe the muscular and joint interactions that occur during heel off and toe off.
- Describe the muscular and joint interactions that occur during early, mid, and terminal swing.
- Define the common terms that are used to describe human gait.
- Explain the role of the hip abductor muscles during the stance phase of gait.
- Describe the common gait deviations, including impairments that may cause the deviations.

KEY TERMS

cadence
double-limb support
early swing
foot flat
gait cycle
heel contact
heel off
mid stance
mid swing
push-off
single-limb support
stance phase
step
step length
step width
stride
stride length
swing phase
terminal swing
toe off
Trendelenburg sign
walking velocity

Gait refers to the manner in which a person walks. Normally, walking is a very efficient biomechanic process, requiring relatively little use of energy. Although the process appears automatic and easy, walking is actually a complex and high-level motor function.

Normal walking requires a healthy body, especially in regard to the nervous and musculoskeletal systems. Injury and pathology within these systems often results in a significant decrease in the ease and efficiency of walking. Without proper rehabilitation, a person's walking

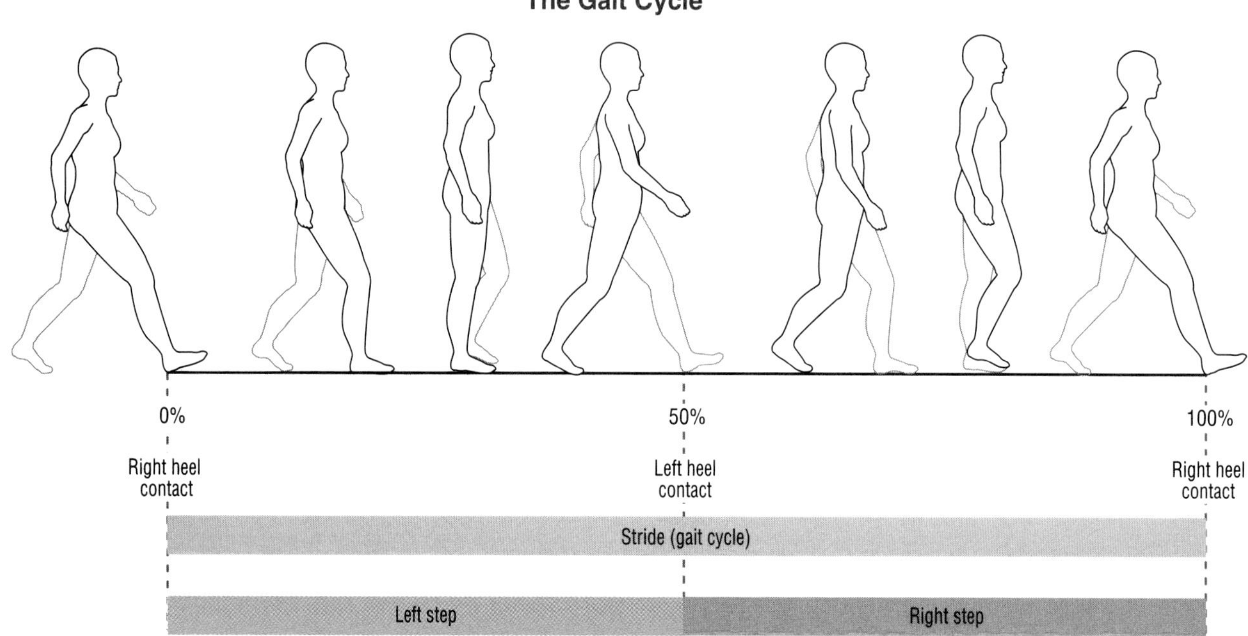

Figure 12-1 Gait cycle from right heel contact to the subsequent right heel contact. (From Neumann DA: *Kinesiology of the musculoskeletal system: foundations for physical rehabilitation,* St Louis, 2002, Mosby, Figure 15-6.)

pattern may be unnecessarily labored and inefficient. An individual may also develop compensatory strategies for walking that can cause tightness or prolonged weakness of muscles. The ability to walk safely often determines how soon a person can return home from a hospital or rehabilitation facility. A significant component of a physical therapy evaluation, therefore, is dedicated to analyzing a patient's gait; this is a pre-requisite to determining the best plan of treatment.

Walking represents the ultimate expression of normal kinesiology of the trunk and lower extremities. This chapter studies the primary kinesiologic features of normal gait, with an emphasis on the muscular activation and ranges of motion typically required at the hip, knee, and ankle. This chapter also examines the kinesiology of abnormal gait. Several common gait deviations are described, with the intention of providing a basis to effectively treat the underlying pathomechanics.

Terminology

The study of gait uses a special set of terminology. Much of this terminology relates to the events that occur within the gait cycle. The **gait cycle** describes all the important events that occur between two successive heel contacts of the same limb (Figure 12-1). Because of the dynamic and continuous nature of walking, the gait cycle is described as occurring between 0% and 100% (Figure 12-2). As shown in Figure 12-2, during the first 60% of the gait cycle the foot remains in contact with the ground; this is known as the **stance phase**. The stance phase is subdivided into five events:

- **Heel contact:** The instant the lower limb contacts the ground (0% of the gait cycle)
- **Foot flat:** The period that the entire plantar aspect of the foot is on the ground (8% of the gait cycle)
- **Mid stance:** The point where the body weight passes directly over the supporting lower extremity (30% of the gait cycle); coincides with a vertically oriented lower leg
- **Heel off:** The instant the heel leaves the ground (40% of the gait cycle)
- **Toe off:** The instant the toe leaves the ground (60% of the gait cycle)

A period referred to as **push-off** is used to describe the combined events of heel off and toe off, when the stance foot is literally "pushing off" toward the next step, typically spanning 40% to 60% of the gait cycle.

In the last 40% of the gait cycle, the limb is off the ground in the **swing phase**. The swing phase is subdivided into three events (see Figure 12-2):

- **Early swing:** The period from toe off to mid swing (60% to 75% of the gait cycle)
- **Mid swing:** The period when the foot of the swing leg passes next to the foot of the stance leg (75% to 85% of the gait cycle). This corresponds to the mid stance phase of the opposite lower extremity.
- **Terminal swing:** The period ranging from mid swing until heel contact (85% to 100% of the gait cycle)

In addition to the terms that define the events within gait cycle, the following terms and concepts are useful in the study of gait (Figure 12-3). Note that the following terms are based on a healthy adult, walking at an average speed. Walking faster or slower causes significant changes in these variables.

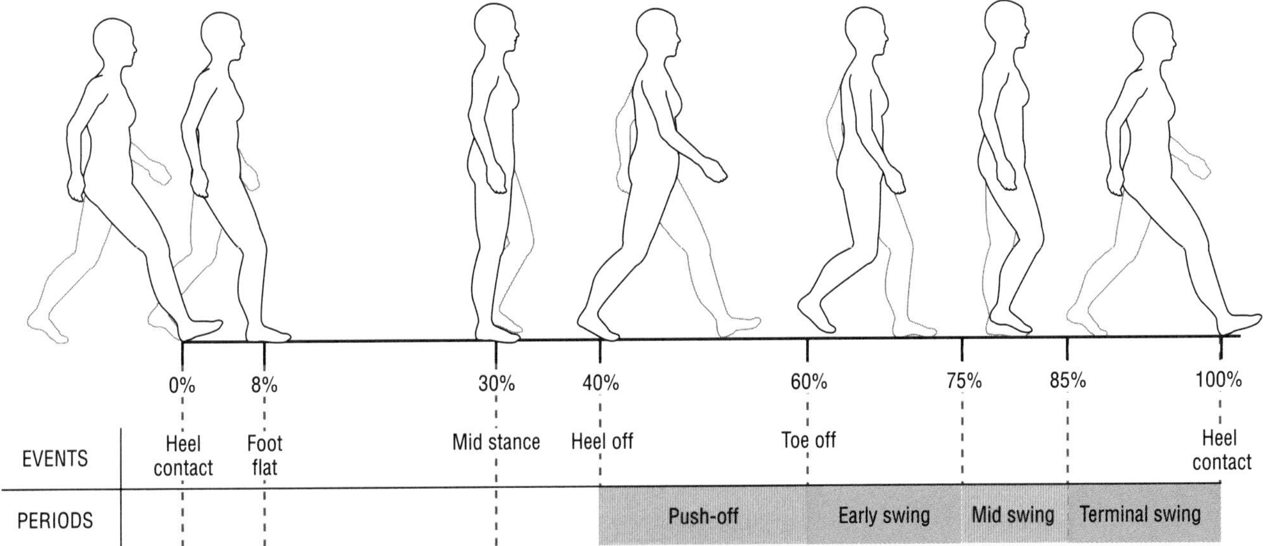

Figure 12-2 Traditional subdivisions of the gait cycle. (From Neumann DA: *Kinesiology of the musculoskeletal system: foundations for physical rehabilitation*, St Louis, 2002, Mosby, Figure 15-11.)

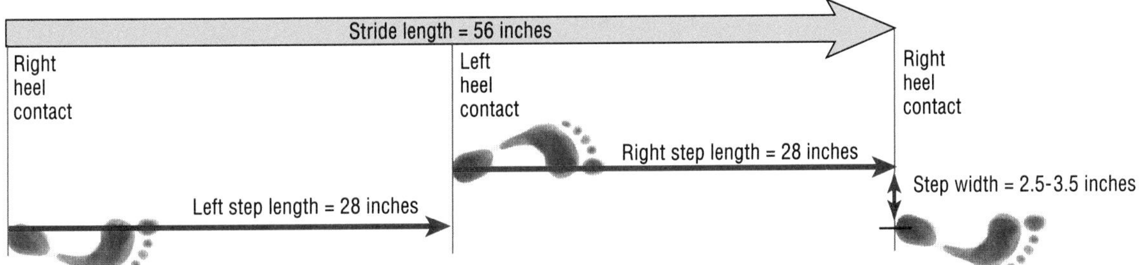

Figure 12-3 Spatial descriptors of gait and their normal values. (From Neumann DA: *Kinesiology of the musculoskeletal system: foundations for physical rehabilitation*, St Louis, 2002, Mosby, Figure 15-7.)

- **Stride:** The events that take place between successive heel contacts of the *same* foot. All events within one stride occur within a gait cycle.
- **Step:** The events that occur between successive heel contacts of *opposite* feet; for example, between left and right heel contacts
- **Step length:** The distance traveled in one step, which, on average, is about 28 inches in the healthy adult
- **Stride length:** The distance traveled in one stride (between two consecutive heel contacts of the same foot); typically 56 inches in the healthy adult
- **Step width:** The distance between the heel centers of two consecutive foot contacts. Normally, this distance is about 3 inches in the healthy adult.
- **Cadence:** The number of steps taken per minute; also called step rate. The average cadence for a healthy adult is 110 steps per minute.
- **Walking velocity:** The speed at which an individual walks. Normal walking velocity is about 3 miles per hour; walking velocity increases by increases in cadence or step length, or both.

Details of the Gait Cycle

As described earlier, the gait cycle is divided into specific events; for example, foot flat, toe off, etc. This section provides the kinesiology unique to these events, with a focus on the muscle activation and joint motion.

Although normal gait involves movement in all three planes, the upcoming discussion focuses on the sagittal plane movements of the hip, knee, and ankle (talocrural) joints. Figure 12-4 shows the sagittal plane range of motion of the hip, knee, and ankle throughout the full gait cycle. This figure should be referred to throughout the following sections. Bear in mind that the discussions below refer to the kinesiology of a typical adult walking on level surfaces at an average speed.

Stance Phase

The stance phase of gait comprises approximately the first 60% of the gait cycle. The five events of the gait cycle are listed in the box on the following page.

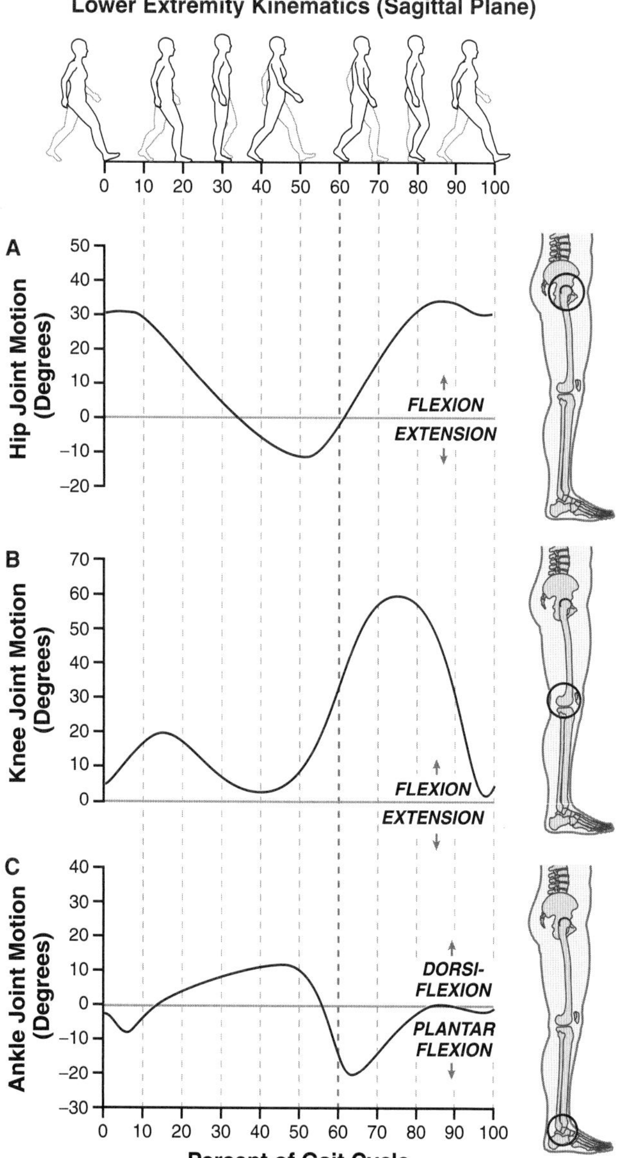

Figure 12-4 Normal sagittal plane ranges of motion at the **(A)** hip, **(B)** knee, and **(C)** ankle during a gait cycle. (From Neumann DA: *Kinesiology of the musculoskeletal system: foundations for physical rehabilitation,* St Louis, 2002, Mosby, Figure 15-15.)

Five Components of Stance Phase

- *Heel contact:* 0% point of the gait cycle
- *Foot flat:* 8% point of the gait cycle
- *Mid stance:* 30% point of the gait cycle
- *Heel off:* 40% point of the gait cycle
- *Toe off:* 60% point of the gait cycle

HEEL CONTACT (0% POINT OF THE GAIT CYCLE)

Heel contact marks the beginning of the gait cycle as the heel contacts or strikes the ground (heel contact is often referred to as heel strike) (Figure 12-5, *left*). At this point in the gait cycle the center of gravity of the body is at its lowest point. At heel contact, the ankle is held in neutral dorsiflexion through isometric activation of the dorsiflexor muscles. As the ankle transitions toward foot flat (the next event), the dorsiflexor muscles (e.g., tibialis anterior) are eccentrically active to lower the ankle into plantar flexion.

The knee is slightly flexed at heel contact as a way to absorb the shock of initial weight bearing. The quadriceps (knee extensors) are eccentrically active to allow a slight give to the flexed knee and prevent the knee from buckling as weight is transferred onto the stance limb.

The hip is in about 30 degrees of flexion. As weight bearing continues, the hip extensor muscles are isometrically active to prevent the trunk from "jackknifing" forward (see Figure 12-5, *left*).

FOOT FLAT (8% POINT OF THE GAIT CYCLE)

Foot flat is defined as the point when the entire plantar surface of the foot is in contact with the ground (see Figure 12-5). This event is often described as the *loading-response phase*. During this time, the muscles and joints of the lower limb assist with shock absorption, as the lower extremity continues to accept increasing amounts of body weight. Immediately following foot flat, the opposite limb begins to leave the ground and enters its early swing phase.

At foot flat, the ankle has just rapidly moved into 5 to 10 degrees of plantar flexion. This motion is controlled through eccentric activation of the dorsiflexor muscles. Immediately following foot flat, the ankle begins to move toward dorsiflexion, as the leg advances forward over the foot. Because the calcaneus is fixed under body weight, dorsiflexion of the ankle in the stance phase occurs as the *lower leg moves over a fixed foot.*

The knee continues to flex to about 15 degrees, acting as a shock-absorbing spring. The knee extensor muscles continue to be active eccentrically, as the hip extensor muscles shift from isometric to slight concentric activation, guiding the hip toward extension (see Figure 12-5, *right*).

MID STANCE (30% POINT OF THE GAIT CYCLE)

Mid stance occurs as the lower leg approaches the vertical position (Figure 12-6, *left*). The leg is in single-limb support, as the other limb is freely swinging forward. The hip and knee are in near extension, as the ankle continues to move into greater dorsiflexion.

At mid stance, the ankle approaches about 5 degrees of dorsiflexion. During this time, the dorsiflexor muscles are *inactive;* instead, the plantar flexor muscles are eccentrically active, controlling the rate at which the lower leg advances (dorsiflexes) forward over the foot. The knee reaches a near-fully extended position. Because the line of gravity falls just anterior to the medial-lateral axis of rotation of the knee, the knee is mechanically locked into extension. Little activation is therefore normally required of the quadriceps at this time. The hip approaches

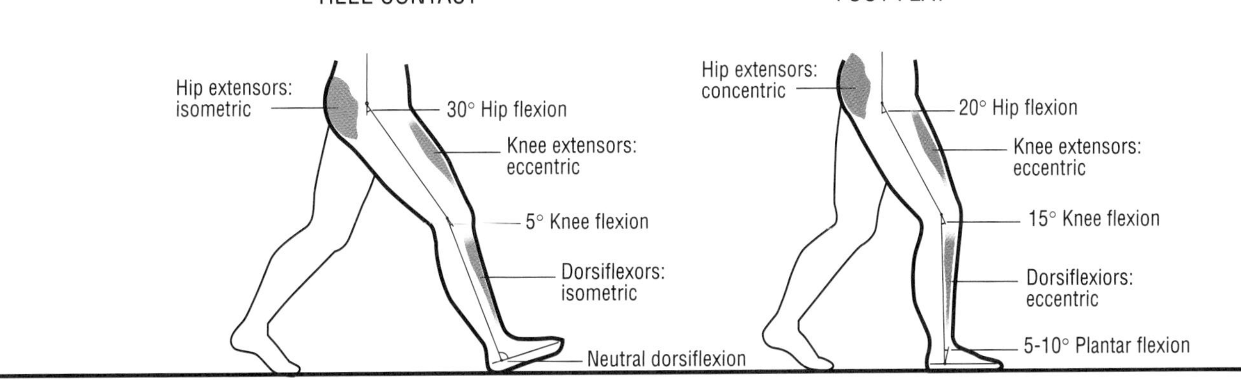

Figure 12-5 Primary muscle and joint actions during the stance phase of a gait cycle: heel contact and foot flat.

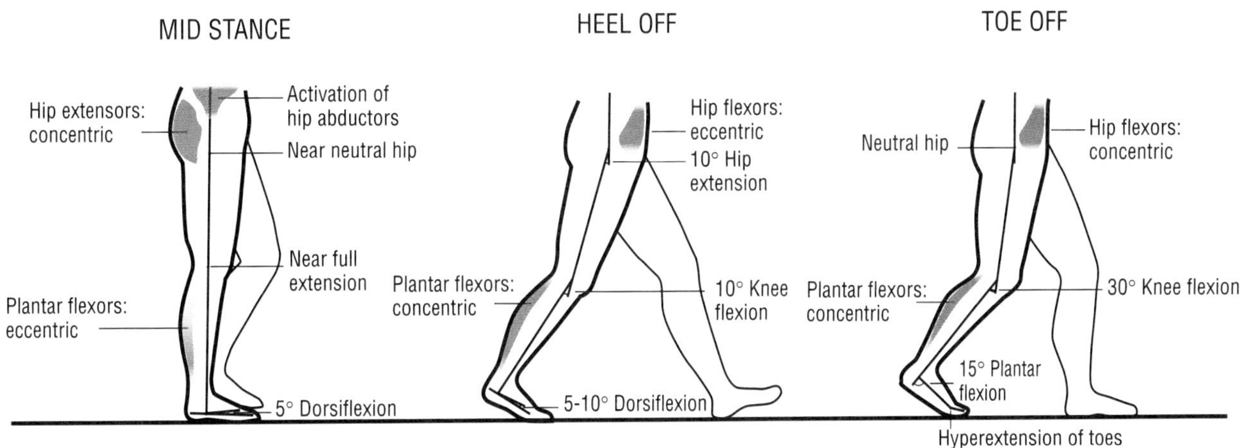

Figure 12-6 Primary muscle and joint actions during the stance phase of a gait cycle: mid stance, heel off, and toe off.

0 degrees of extension. The hip extensors such as the gluteus maximus are only slightly active to help stabilize the hip as the body is propelled forward. This activation is minimal during slow walking on level surfaces, but increases significantly with increasing speed and slope of walking surface.

During mid stance, the stance leg is in single-limb support as the other leg is freely swinging toward the next step. The hip abductor muscles (e.g., gluteus medius) of the stance leg therefore are active to stabilize the hip in the frontal plane, preventing the opposite side of the pelvis from dropping excessively (see Figure 12-6, *left*).

HEEL OFF (40% POINT OF THE GAIT CYCLE)

The events of heel off occur just after mid stance as the lower leg and ankle begin "pushing off" to propel the body upward and forward (see Figure 12-6, *middle*). As the name implies, the heel-off phase begins as the heel breaks contact with the ground.

At the beginning of heel off, the ankle continues to dorsiflex to about 10 degrees. This action stretches the Achilles tendon, which prepares the calf muscles for propulsion. As heel off progresses, the plantar flexor muscles switch their activation from eccentric (to control forward motion of the leg) to concentric. This concentric action produces plantar flexion for propulsion, or push-off.

At heel off, the extended knee prepares to flex, often driven by a short burst of activity from the hamstring muscles. The hip continues to extend to about 10 degrees of extension. Eccentric activation of the hip flexors, in particular the iliopsoas, helps to control the rate and amount of hip extension (see Figure 12-6, *middle*). Tight ligaments of the hip or tight hip flexor muscles will reduce the amount of hip extension at this point in the gait cycle, thereby reducing stride length.

TOE OFF (60% POINT OF THE GAIT CYCLE)

Toe off is the final event of the stance phase of gait (see Figure 12-6, *right*). The events that occur during this period are designed to complete push-off and begin the early swing phase. As the name implies, toe off coincides with the toes leaving the ground. The contralateral leg begins its foot flat phase and begins to accept a greater portion of body weight.

At toe off, the toes are in marked hyperextension at the metatarsophalangeal joints. The ankle continues plantar flexing (to about 15 degrees) through concentric activation of the plantar flexor muscles. The muscular force for push-off is typically shared between the plantar flexors and the hip extensor muscles. Activation of the gastrocnemius and soleus is usually minimal while walking on level surfaces and at a slow speed but increases significantly with increasing speed and incline.

At toe off, the knee is flexed 30 degrees. In the very end of toe-off phase, the slightly extended hip starts to flex due to concentric activation of the hip flexor muscles (see Figure 12-6).

Consider this...

Transition between Single- and Double-Limb Support: The "Balancing Act" of Walking

Within a given stance phase, the body experiences two periods of double-limb support and one period of single-limb support.

During **double-limb support**, both legs are in contact with the ground. This period occurs during the first and last 10% of the stance phase (Figure 12-7). During these periods of walking, the body's center of gravity is at its lowest point. The lower center of gravity combined with bilateral support affords maximum stability to the body as a whole—useful as weight is transferred between limbs.

Conversely, the period of **single-limb support** occurs once every stance phase, approximately between 10% and 50% of the gait cycle (see Figure 12-7). At mid stance phase (the very middle point of single-limb support), the body is supported by only one limb at the same time its center of gravity is highest from the ground. Like trying to balance on a tall unicycle, these two factors reduce the stability of the body as a whole. Fortunately, this period of instability and relative imbalance is short-lived because within less than a half second after mid stance, the contralateral limb strikes the ground, thus reestablishing balance and stability to the body. Walking, therefore, can be viewed as a series of losing and catching one's balance.

Although the process of walking is nearly automatic for the healthy individual, impairments involving the nervous system (such as hemiplegia, ataxia, sensory loss, or spasticity) can significantly hamper walking. Observing an individual ambulating with a neurologic disorder provides good evidence of the numerous complex processes that must occur to produce normal walking.

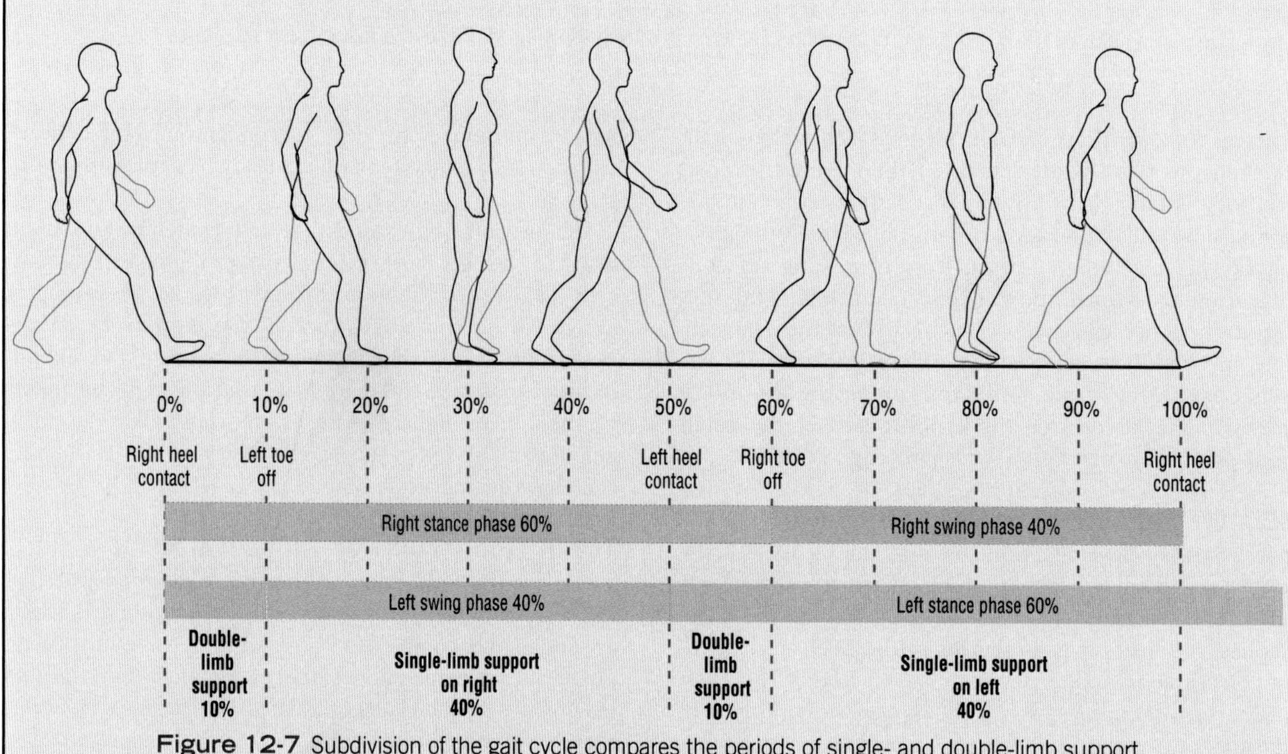

Figure 12-7 Subdivision of the gait cycle compares the periods of single- and double-limb support phases of gait. (From Neumann DA: *Kinesiology of the musculoskeletal system: foundations for physical rehabilitation*, St Louis, 2002, Mosby, Figure 15-10.)

Swing Phase

The swing phase of the gait cycle is subdivided into early swing, mid swing, and terminal swing. Fundamentally, the swing phase advances the leg forward to the next step (Figure 12-8).

> **Three Events of the Swing Phase**
>
> - *Early swing:* occurs between 60% to 65% of gait cycle
> - *Mid swing:* occurs between 75% to 85% of gait cycle
> - *Terminal swing:* occurs between 85% to 100% of gait cycle

EARLY SWING (60% TO 65% OF THE GAIT CYCLE)

During early swing the leg begins to accelerate forward. The plantar-flexed ankle begins to dorsiflex by concentric activation of the dorsiflexor muscles. The dorsiflexing ankle allows the foot to clear the ground as it is advanced forward. The knee continues to flex, largely driven by indirect action of the flexing hip. The hip flexor muscles continue to contract, pulling the extended thigh forward (see Figure 12-8, *left*).

MID SWING (75% TO 85% OF THE GAIT CYCLE)

At mid swing, the contralateral leg is in mid stance, fully supporting the weight of the body. The ankle is held in neutral dorsiflexion via isometric activation of the dorsiflexor muscles (see Figure 12-8, *middle*).

In mid swing, the knee is flexed about 45 to 55 degrees, which helps shorten the functional length of the lower limb to facilitate its advance. The hip approaches about 30 degrees of flexion through concentric activation of the hip flexor muscles.

TERMINAL SWING (85% TO 100% OF THE GAIT CYCLE)

In terminal swing the limb begins to decelerate in preparation for heel contact (see Figure 12-8, *right*). In the final stages of terminal swing, the leg is placed well in front of the body. The ankle dorsiflexors continue their isometric activation, holding the ankle in neutral dorsiflexion and preparing for heel contact.

The knee has moved from a flexed position in mid swing to almost full extension. Interestingly, the hamstrings are active eccentrically to slow the rapidly extending knee. Individuals who lack the ability to activate their hamstrings just before heel contact are prone to injury because the knee is likely to "snap" forcefully into extension at heel strike. The hip flexor muscles, which have powered the leg into nearly 35 degrees of flexion, become inactive in terminal swing. The hip extensor muscles are active eccentrically to decelerate the forward progression of the thigh (see Figure 12-8, *right*).

Summary of the Sagittal Plane Kinesiology of the Gait Cycle

At initial contact, motions at the hip, knee, and ankle (talocrural) joints have functionally elongated the lower extremity. The goal of the action is to maximize stride length. Shortly after heel strike, controlled knee flexion and ankle plantar flexion help to absorb the forces of initial contact. This helps to provide a smooth transition to full weight bearing. The hip and knee then extend, supporting a critical height of the body's center of mass that allows the contralateral leg to advance and clear the ground. During the first half of swing phase, all of the joints of the lower extremity begin to flex, functionally shortening the lower extremity. In terminal swing, the advancing lower extremity is slowed in preparation for the next heel strike.

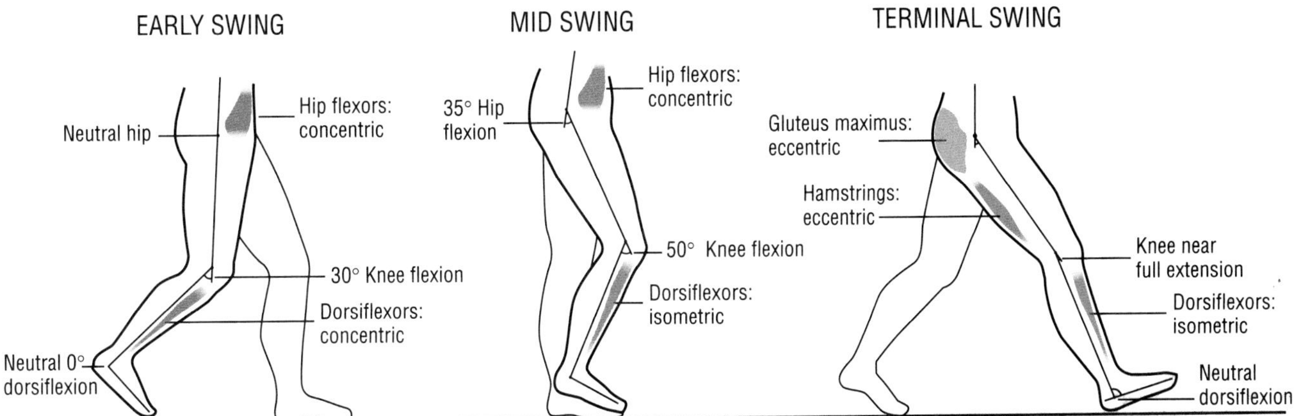

Figure 12-8 Primary muscle and joint actions during the swing phase of a gait cycle: early swing, mid swing, and terminal swing.

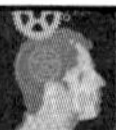

Consider this...

The Ups and Downs of the Gait Cycle

During normal gait, the body bobs up and down, and from side to side. These naturally occurring motions have a purpose. Figure 12-9, *A*, illustrates the natural vertical displacement of the body's center of mass while walking. The lowest part of the gait cycle occurs just after heel contact as weight is transferred onto the stance leg. This lowering action, characterized by flexion of the hip and knee, is a shock-absorbing mechanism. Without the mechanism, the jolt of initial weight bearing may, over time, cause injury to the lower extremity and spine.

The highest part of the gait cycle occurs in mid stance. At this point the stance leg is fully upright, allowing maximal clearance for the swing leg to be advanced.

As well as moving up and down, normal gait includes a natural side-to-side, or lateral, displacement of the center of mass. The lateral displacement, though relatively small, effectively shifts the body's center of mass over the stance leg. As indicated in Figure 12-9, *B*, the largest lateral displacement occurs during mid stance, when the opposite extremity is in full swing.

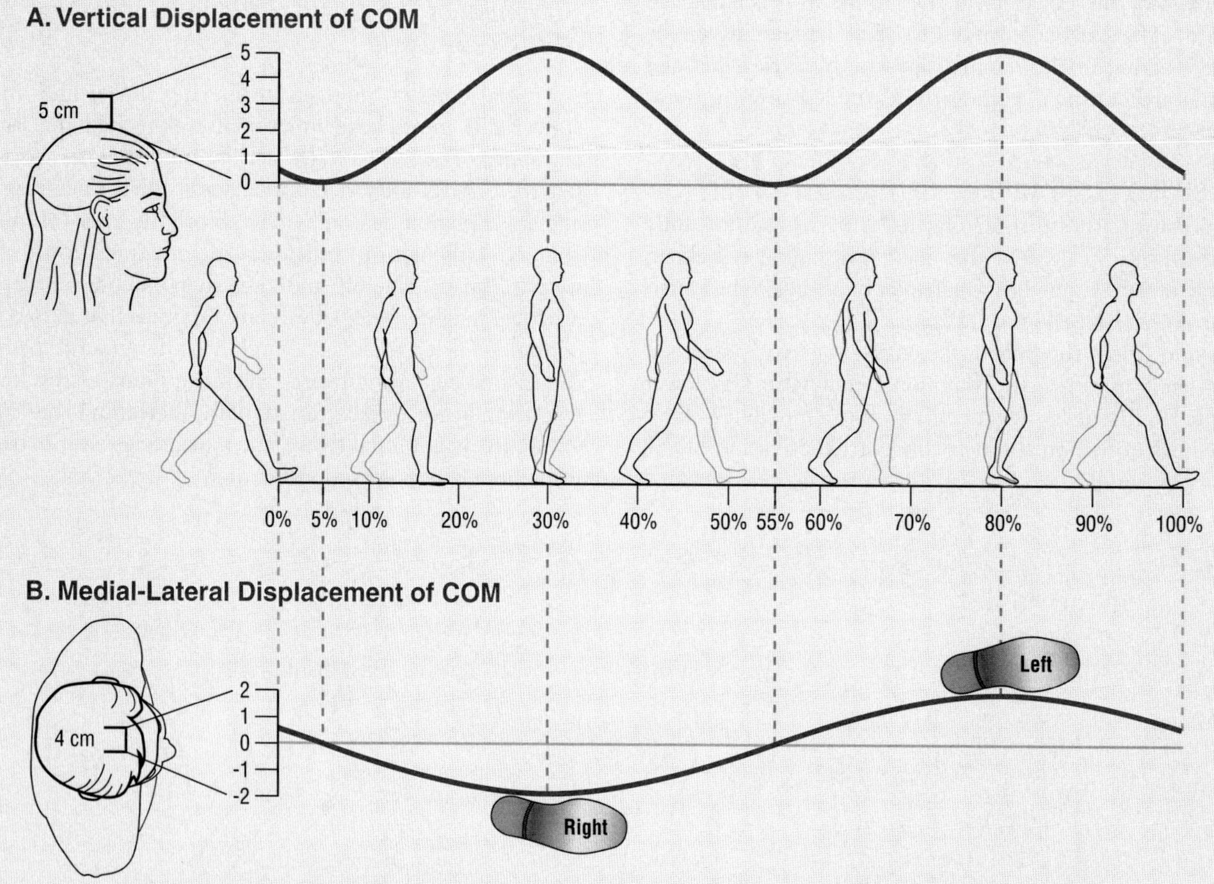

Figure 12-9 Average displacement of the center of mass *(COM)* during gait. **A,** Vertical displacement of the COM. **B,** Medial-lateral displacement of the COM. (From Neumann DA: *Kinesiology of the musculoskeletal system: foundations for physical rehabilitation*, St Louis, 2002, Mosby, Figure 15-13.)

Summary of the Frontal Plane Kinesiology of the Gait Cycle

The hip abductor muscles stabilize the *hip* within the frontal plane during the single-limb support phase of walking. When a given limb enters mid stance, the opposite leg is in its swing phase—not in contact with the ground. Activation of the stance leg's hip abductor muscles normally holds the pelvis level, allowing the swing leg to advance toward the next step. Without sufficient strength of the hip abductor muscles on the stance leg, the opposite side of the pelvis may *drop* excessively under the force of gravity. This abnormal response is known as a positive **Trendelenburg sign** and strongly suggests weakness of the hip abductor muscles.

The *knee* is stabilized in the frontal plane primarily by its bony shape and by tension in the medial and lateral collateral ligaments. This natural stability may be lost through ligamentous injury. A torn medial collateral ligament, for example, may lead to genu valgus, potentially altering normal gait mechanics. Interestingly, instability of the knee may also arise from impairments at the hip or at the foot. For instance, weakness of the hip abductors or excessive pronation of the foot, or both, may produce excessive valgus strain on the knee during the stance phase. Over time, this strain may over-stretch the medial collateral ligament.

While walking, the subtalar and transverse tarsal joints dictate much of the frontal plane kinesiology of the foot. These joints help transform the foot from a pliable platform at early stance to a more rigid platform at late stance. The kinematics of the subtalar joint provides an insight into this transformation. After initial heel contact, the subtalar joint everts (pronates) as the medial longitudinal arch of the foot lowers. These events create a more pliable position of the foot—an essential part of the shock-absorbing mechanism of early stance. At mid to late stance, the subtalar joint moves toward inversion (supination), which resets the height of the medial longitudinal arch. The position of inversion arranges the bones of the foot to their most stable position, forming a rigid lever for push-off.

Summary of the Horizontal Plane Kinesiology of the Gait Cycle

While walking, the horizontal plane movements of the lower extremity are slight and difficult to measure. These motions are, however, very important. The movements are controlled primarily at either end of the lower extremity: proximally by the hip and distally by the subtalar and transverse tarsal joints.

During walking the pelvis rotates in the horizontal plane about a vertical axis of rotation through the hip joint of the stance leg. Consider, for example, rotation of the pelvis as observed from a top view (Figure 12-10). During the stance phase on the right leg, the left side of the pelvis rotates forward, helping to advance the left leg as it swings forward. Fundamentally, from a top view, walking occurs as a series of forward rotations of the "swing side" of the pelvis. Interestingly, because the trunk remains relatively stationary during walking, the lumbar spine must rotate slightly to decouple the rotating pelvis from the thorax.

The horizontal plane rotations of the foot are related to supination and pronation and were described in the previous section.

Superior view: rotation of the pelvis

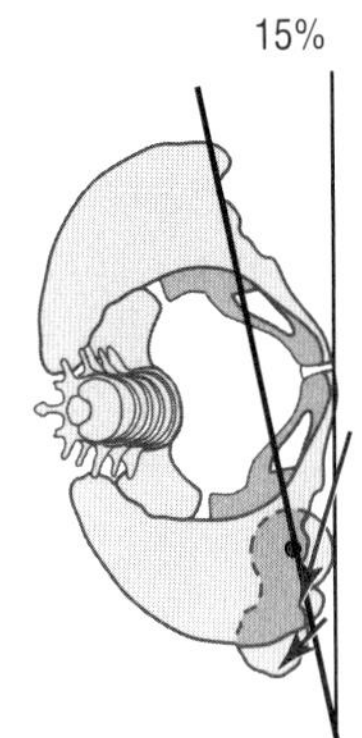

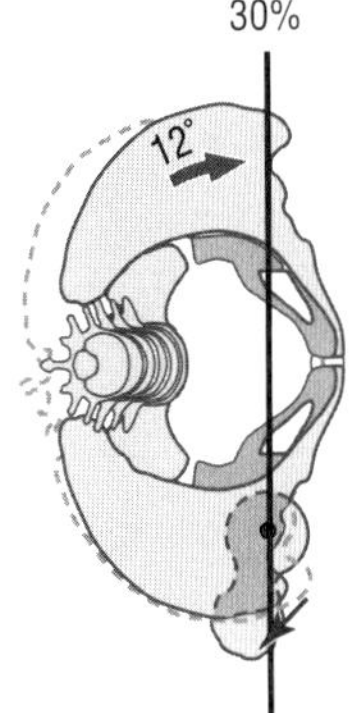

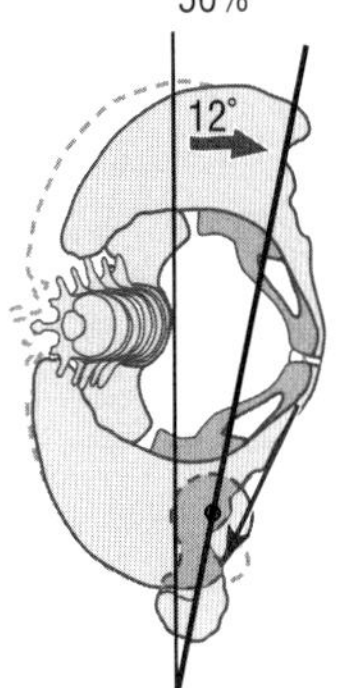

Figure 12-10 Superior view showing the horizontal plane rotation of the pelvis during the 15%, 30%, and 50% points of the gait cycle. These points of the gait cycle coincide with the swing phase of the left lower extremity. The progressive forward rotation of the left side of the pelvis assists with the advancing of the left lower extremity. (From Neumann DA: *Kinesiology of the musculoskeletal system: foundations for physical rehabilitation*, St Louis, 2002, Mosby, Figure 12-39.)

Gait Deviations

Normal walking requires sufficient strength and range of motion of all participating muscles and joints. In addition, adequate sensory feedback (proprioception) and balance is needed to coordinate the movement and posture of the body as a whole. Following injury or pathology, walking can become difficult or, at worst, impossible. Fortunately, the human body is remarkably adaptable. Certain biomechanical compensations performed, often subconsciously, by the patient can provide the necessary forces and range of motion for basic gait. Often patients show a very characteristic *gait deviation* that is associated with either compensation or a consequence of a given impairment. The following section describes the kinesiology of several common gait deviations.

Clinical INSIGHT

Simple Clinical Measurements of Gait

Many sophisticated technologies exist to measure the spatial and temporal aspects of gait. More simple measures can still yield valuable information. Walking speed, for example, can be measured with a stopwatch and a known distance. Step length and step width can be measured by the use of ink marks made by shoes or feet on a roll of paper covering the floor.

Clinically these measurements can be used to help document progress or existing functional limitations. Below are listed some average values used to assess normal gait.

Normal Values for Gait

- *Walking speed:* 3 miles/hour
- *Step rate:* 110 steps/minute (1.87 steps/second)
- *Step length:* 28 inches (72 cm)

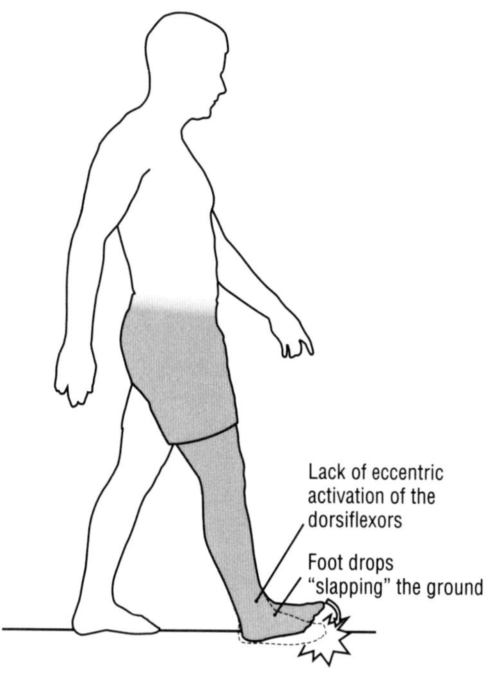

Foot Slap

Impairment:	Weakness of the dorsiflexors; may follow injury to the common peroneal nerve, distal neuropathy, or hemiplegia
Description of Deviation:	Upon heel strike, the foot quickly drops into plantar flexion, producing a slapping sound as the forefoot hits the ground.
Reason for Deviation:	Inability of the dorsiflexor muscles to slowly control plantar flexion

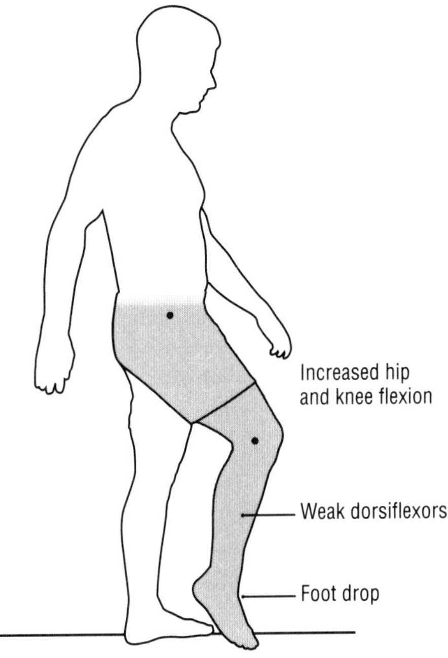

High Stepping Gait

Impairment: Marked weakness of the dorsiflexors, resulting in foot drop

Description of Deviation: Individual appears to be stepping over an imaginary obstacle (hence the term "*high stepping*")

Reason for Deviation: In order to clear the foot from the ground, the hip and knee must be excessively flexed to advance the leg.

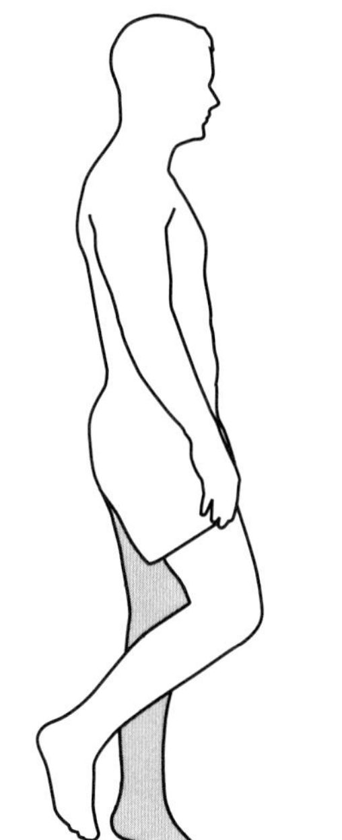

Vaulting Gait

Impairment: Any impairment of the lower extremity that reduces the ability to functionally reduce the length of the advancing limb (e.g., inability to flex the hip or the knee)

Description of Deviation: Individual rises up on the toes of the stance foot *(left leg in figure)* to allow clearance for the contralateral advancing limb

Reason for Deviation: Standing on tip-toes creates extra clearance for the contralateral (long) leg to clear the ground during swing.

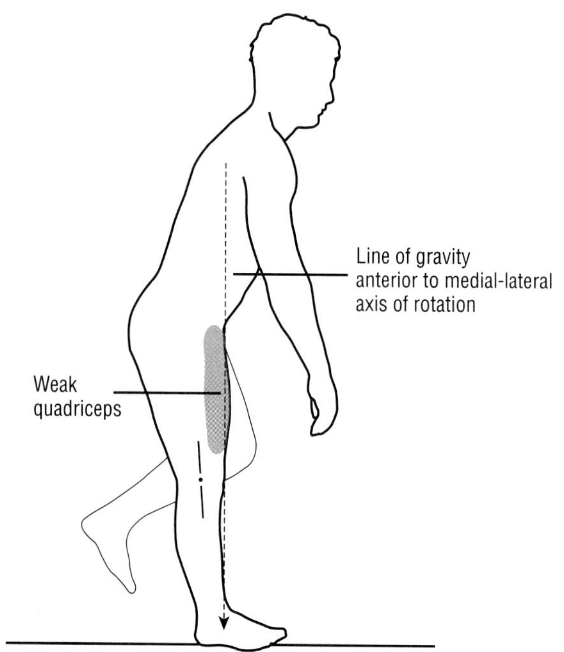

Weak Quadriceps Gait

Impairment:	Weakness or avoidance of activation of the quadriceps muscle
Description of Deviation:	Knee remains fully extended throughout stance; combined with excessive forward lean of the trunk
Reason for Deviation:	Forward lean of the trunk shifts the line of gravity anterior to the medial-lateral axis of the knee. This maneuver mechanically locks the knee in extension, reducing the need for activation of the quadriceps muscle.
Comments:	This gait deviation may stress the posterior capsule of the knee and potentially lead to genu recurvatum.

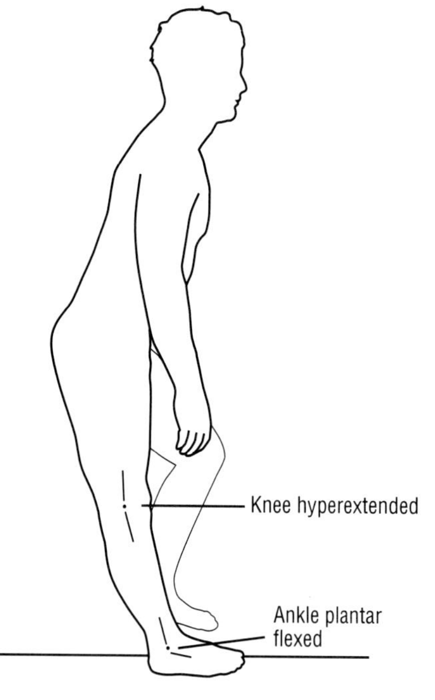

Genu Recurvatum

Impairment (Two Scenarios):	**A:** Long term paralysis of the quadriceps with over-stretched posterior capsule of the knee; may also involve paralysis of the knee flexor muscles **B:** Severe plantar flexion contracture
Description of Deviation:	Excessive hyperextension of the knee during stance phase of gait
Reasons for Deviation:	**A:** Over-stretched posterior capsule of the knee or paralysis of the knee flexor muscles fail to limit knee extension. **B:** With a plantar flexion contracture, the lower leg deviates posteriorly relative to the ankle. This posture forces the knee into hyperextension, eventually over-stretching its posterior capsule.

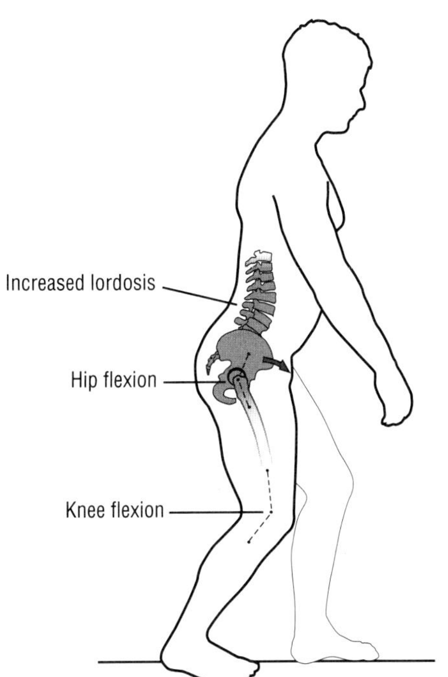

Walking with Hip or Knee Flexion Contracture

Impairment: Hip or knee flexion contracture

- May be associated with several pathologies such as spasticity or tightness of the hip and knee flexor muscles, weakness of hip extensor muscles, pain, or joint limitations due to arthritis

Description of Deviation: Flexed position of the hip and knee during the stance phase of gait

Reason for Deviation: Increased tightness in tissues that normally allow full hip and knee extension

Comments: Often this deviation is associated with increased lumbar lordosis and reduced stride length. This deviation is often referred to as a "crouched gait" when describing the walking pattern of a person with cerebral palsy. In this case the hip flexion contracture is often associated with tightness in the hip adductor and internal rotator muscles.

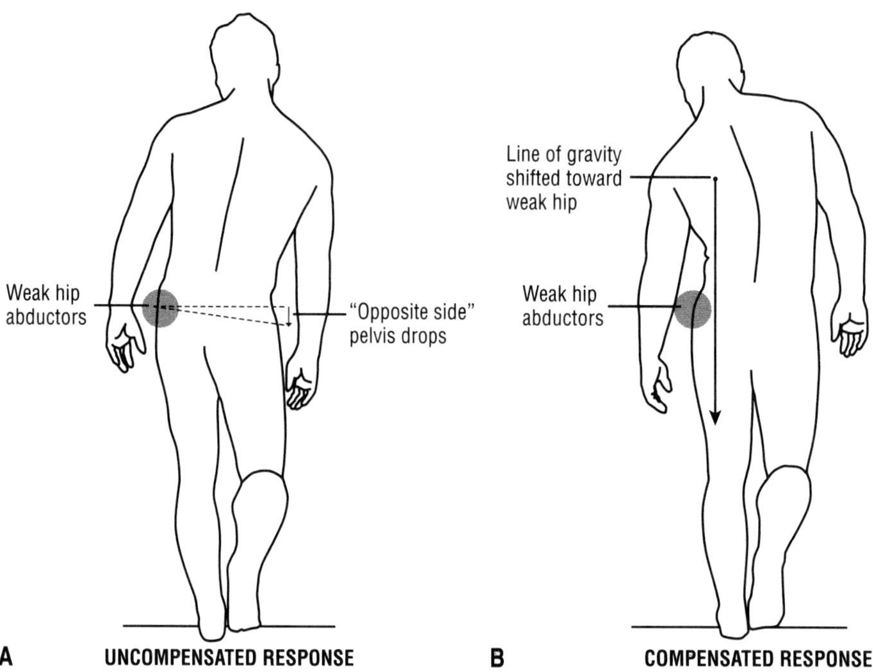

Weak Hip Abductor Gait

Impairment: Weakness of the hip abductor muscles

- May occur secondary to Guillain-Barré syndrome, muscular dystrophy, poliomyelitis, hip pain, arthritis of the hip, obesity, or any condition that reduces activation of hip abductor muscles

Description of Deviation (Two Forms):

- *Uncompensated response*: During single-limb support, the pelvis leans to the side *opposite* the weak hip abductor muscles **(A)**.
- *Compensated response*: During single-limb support, the trunk and pelvis lean to the *same side* as the weak hip abductors **(B)**.

Reason for Deviation:

- *Uncompensated response*: The hip abductors of the stance (left) leg are unable to produce enough force to hold the pelvis level; thus the pelvis (and often trunk) uncontrollably leans to the *opposite* (right) side. This is also referred to as a *positive Trendelenberg sign* **(A)**.
- *Compensated response*: Purposely leaning the pelvis and trunk to the *same* (left) side as the weak hip abductor muscles. This compensation shifts the line of gravity to the left, closer to the axis of rotation of the stance hip. As a consequence, the external torque demands are reduced on the hip, thereby reducing the demands on the weak hip abductor muscles **(B)**.

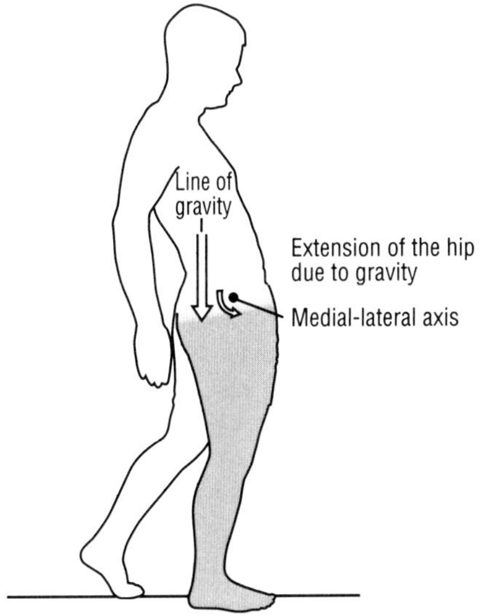

Weak Gluteus Maximus Gait

Impairment: Weakness of the hip extensors, such as gluteus maximus
- Poliomyelitis

Description of Deviation: Backward lean of the trunk during early stance phase of gait

Reason for Deviation: Leaning the trunk posteriorly during the stance phase shifts the body's line of gravity posterior to the hip, reducing the demands of the hip extensor muscles.

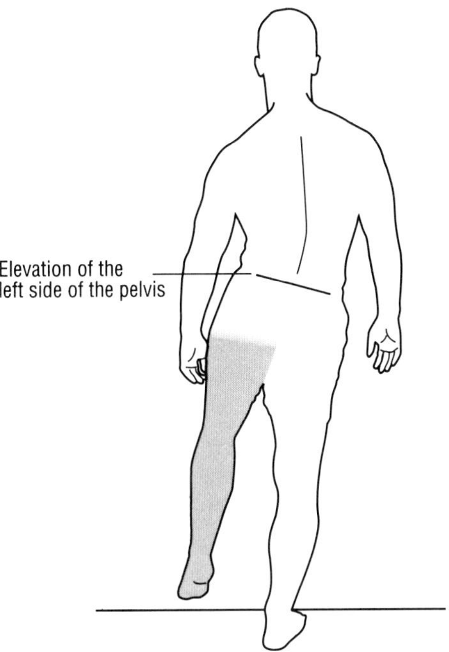

Hip Hiking Gait

Impairment: Inability to functionally shorten the swing leg; for example, weakness of hip flexor muscles

Description of Deviation: Excessive elevation of the pelvis on the side of the swing leg

Reason for Deviation: Elevating, or hiking, the pelvis provides extra clearance for the advancing leg.

Comments: This compensation maneuver often occurs with other maneuvers (for similar reasons) such as circumduction (see p. 354) and vaulting.

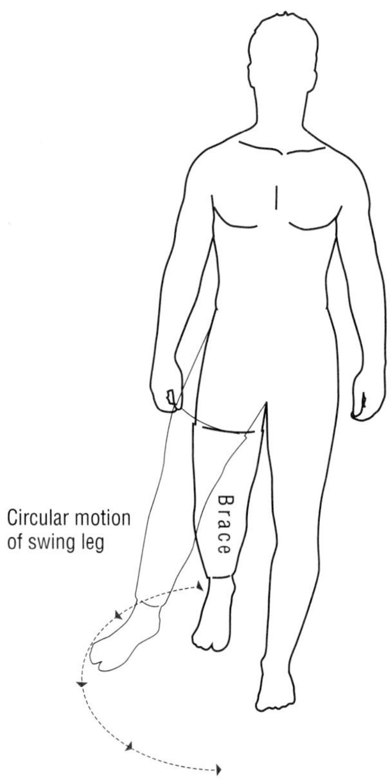

Hip Circumduction

Impairment:	Inability to functionally shorten the swing leg; for example, reduced active or passive hip or knee flexion or as a consequence of wearing a "straight-leg" brace at the knee
Description of Deviation:	Swing leg is advanced in a semicircular arc
Reason for Deviation:	Circumduction creates extra clearance to advance the functionally long leg.
Comments:	This maneuver may place additional demands on the hip abductor muscles to help advance the swing limb.

Summary

Understanding the kinesiology of walking requires a firm understanding of the muscular and joint interactions of the entire lower extremity. This understanding is a vital component of a physical therapy treatment and evaluation. Successful "gait training" usually improves a person's speed, safety, and metabolic efficiency of walking. These variables often dictate an individual's ultimate level of functional independence.

Study Questions

1. Foot slap is a gait deviation most likely due to which of the following impairments?
   a. Contracture or tightness of the hamstrings
   b. Weakness of the quadriceps
   c. Weakness of the dorsiflexor muscles
   d. Weakness of the hip abductor muscles
2. Which of the following is *not* true regarding the heel contact component of a gait cycle?
   a. Heel contact occurs at the beginning (0%) period of the gait cycle.
   b. At heel contact, the ankle is typically held in about 20 degrees of plantar flexion.
   c. At heel contact, the knee is slightly flexed to help absorb the impact of initial weight bearing.
   d. At heel contact, the hip extensor muscles are active to prevent the trunk from jackknifing forward.
3. Which of the following are considered components of the stance phase of a gait cycle?
   a. Heel off
   b. Mid swing
   c. Foot flat
   d. A and C
   e. All of the above
4. At which of the following periods within a gait cycle is the leg in single-limb support?
   a. Heel contact
   b. Foot flat
   c. Mid stance
   d. A and B
   e. All of the above
5. Which of the following events follows the mid-stance period of a gait cycle?
   a. Foot flat
   b. Heel off

c. Toe off
d. Early swing

6. Which of the following best describes the events that occur during terminal swing?
   a. Strong concentric contraction of the plantar flexors to reach the foot forward
   b. Hip and knee both in a fully extended position
   c. Eccentric activation of the hamstrings to decelerate the extending knee
   d. Concentric activation of all the hip extensor muscles
7. Which of the following best describes a weak quadriceps gait deviation?
   a. A fully extended knee throughout stance combined with a forward lean of the trunk to keep the line of gravity anterior to the medial-lateral axis of the knee
   b. Rising up on tip-toes during the stance phase of gait, to clear the swing leg from the ground
   c. Hyperextension of the hip during the swing phase of gait
   d. Excessive flexion of the knees and hips during the stance phase of gait
8. Which of the following is considered an average walking velocity for a healthy adult?
   a. 3 miles per hour
   b. 5 miles per hour
   c. 6 miles per hour
   d. 1 mile per hour
9. Which of the following gait deviations or compensations is most likely used by a person walking with a brace that keeps the knee in extension?
   a. Uncompensated weak hip abductor gait
   b. High stepping gait
   c. Hip circumduction
   d. A and B
   e. All of the above
10. The body's center of gravity is at its highest point during which of the following periods of a gait cycle?
   a. Heel contact
   b. Early swing
   c. Mid stance
   d. Foot flat
11. Which of the following best describes a *vaulting* gait deviation?
   a. Excessive hyperextension of the knee during the stance phase of gait
   b. Flexion of the hip and knee during the stance phase of gait
   c. Rising up on the toes of the stance leg to create extra clearance for the swing leg
   d. Pelvis drops excessively on the side opposite the stance limb
12. Concentric contraction of the hip flexor muscles is most likely to occur during:
   a. Mid stance
   b. Early swing
   c. Foot flat
   d. Terminal swing
13. The hamstrings are activated eccentrically during terminal swing in order to slow the advancing leg.
   a. True
   b. False
14. The periods of double-limb support are considered the least stable portions of a gait cycle.
   a. True
   b. False
15. The subtalar and transverse tarsal joints cooperate to transform the foot into a pliable platform during early stance. This is an essential component of the shock-absorbing mechanism during the transition to full weight bearing.
   a. True
   b. False
16. An individual with a hip flexion contracture of the right leg is likely to display genu recurvatum of the same (right) leg.
   a. True
   b. False
17. The dorsiflexor muscles are isometrically activated during mid swing to prevent the foot from falling into plantar flexion.
   a. True
   b. False
18. The stance phase of gait comprises the first 60% of a gait cycle.
   a. True
   b. False
19. If a person displays a compensated response to left hip abductor weakness, he or she will most likely lean the trunk to the left.
   a. True
   b. False
20. The foot flat portion of a gait cycle typically coincides with a position of double-limb support.
   a. True
   b. False

ADDITIONAL READINGS

Bergmann G, Graichen F, Rohlmann A: Hip joint loading during walking and running, measured in two patients, *J Biomech* 26(8):969-990, 1993.

Besier TF, Lloyd DG, Ackland TR: Muscle activation strategies at the knee during running and cutting maneuver, *Med Sci Sports Exerc* 35(1):119-127, 2003.

Biewener AA, Farley CT, Roberts TJ et al: Muscle mechanical advantage of human walking and running: implications for energy cost, *J Appl Physiol* 97(6):2266-2274, 2004.

Butler RJ, Davis IS, Hamill J: Interaction of arch type and footwear on running mechanics, *Am J Sports Med* 34(12):1998-2005, 2006.

Chan CW, Rudins A: Foot biomechanics during walking and running, *Mayo Clin Proc* 69(5):448-461, 1994.

DeLeo AT, Dierks TA, Ferber R et al: Lower extremity joint coupling during running: a current update, *Clin Biomech (Bristol, Avon)* 19(10):983-991, 2004.

Eng JJ, Pierrynowski MR: The effect of soft foot orthotics on three-dimensional lower-limb kinematics during walking and running, *Phys Ther* 74(9):836-844, 1994.

Ferber R, Davis IM, Williams DS III: Gender differences in lower extremity mechanics during running, *Clin Biomech (Bristol, Avon)* 18(4):350-357, 2003.

Gottschall JS, Kram R: Ground reaction forces during downhill and uphill running, *J Biomech* 38(3):445-452, 2005.

Lees A, Lake M, Klenerman L: Shock absorption during forefoot running and its relationship to medial longitudinal arch height, *Foot Ankle Int* 26(12):1081-1088, 2005.

Mann RA, Moran GT, Dougherty SE: Comparative electromyography of the lower extremity in jogging, running, and sprinting, *Am J Sports Med* 14(6):501-510, 1986.

O'Connor KM, Hamill J: The role of selected extrinsic foot muscles during running, *Clin Biomech (Bristol, Avon)* 19(1):71-77, 2004.

Schache AG, Blanch P, Rath D et al: Three-dimensional angular kinematics of the lumbar spine and pelvis during running, *Hum Move Sci* 21(2):273-293, 2002.

Stackhouse CL, Davis IM, Hamill J: Orthotic intervention in forefoot and rearfoot strike running patterns, *Clin Biomech (Bristol, Avon)* 19(1):64-70, 2004.

Tashman S, Collon D, Anderson K et al: Abnormal rotational knee motion during running after anterior cruciate ligament reconstruction, *Am J Sports Med* 32(4):975-983, 2004.

Tashman S, Kolowich P, Collon D et al: Dynamic function of the ACL-reconstructed knee during running, *Clin Orthop* 454:66-73, 2007.

Taunton JE, Ryan MB, Clement DB et al: A retrospective case-control analysis of 2002 running injuries, *Br J Sports Med* 36(2):95-101, 2002.

Van Den Bogert AJ, Read L, Nigg BM: An analysis of hip joint loading during walking, running, and skiing, *Med Sci Sports Exerc* 31(1):131-142, 1993.

CHAPTER 13

Kinesiology of Mastication and Ventilation

CHAPTER OUTLINE

OBJECTIVES

- Identify the bones and bony features relevant to the temporomandibular joint.
- Describe the capsule and ligament that supports the temporomandibular joint.
- Identify the motions that occur at the temporomandibular joint.
- Describe the muscular and joint interactions involved in opening the mouth.
- Describe the muscular and joint interactions involved in closing the mouth.
- Justify the actions of the primary muscles of the temporomandibular joint through knowledge of the muscles' proximal and distal attachments.
- Explain Boyle's law in reference to the process of inspiration and expiration.
- Compare the mechanics of quiet expiration with forced expiration.
- Cite the primary muscles of inspiration.
- Cite the primary muscles of forced expiration.
- Describe the muscular interactions involved in forced inspiration.
- Describe the muscular interactions involved in forced expiration.
- Explain why accessory muscles of inspiration are often used by an individual with chronic obstructive pulmonary disease.

KEY TERMS

Boyle's law
chronic obstructive pulmonary disease
depression
elevation
expiration
forced expiration
forced inspiration
inspiration
lateral excursion
mastication
protrusion
quiet expiration
retrusion
ventilation

TEMPOROMANDIBULAR JOINT

Mastication is the process of chewing, tearing, and grinding food with the teeth. This process involves an interaction among the muscles of mastication, teeth, tongue, and the pair of temporomandibular joints. The temporomandibular joint, commonly referred to as the TMJ, consists of the articulation between the condyle of the mandible and the mandibular fossa of the temporal bone. Each jaw is equipped with a pair of TMJs, each palpable during jaw movement at a point just anterior to the ear. Any movement of the jaw such as chewing, speaking, and swallowing requires movement of the TMJ. Pathology or trauma involving the TMJ can be extremely painful and debilitating because of the rich sensory innervation to this frequently used joint. Pain originating in the TMJ is often referred to other areas and perceived as headache or neck pain. This chapter highlights the relevant anatomy and kinesiology of the TMJ as a basis for understanding and treating various disorders associated with this joint.

Osteology and Related Structures

The *mandible*, *temporal*, *maxillae*, *zygomatic*, *sphenoid*, and *hyoid* bones are related to the structure and function of the TMJ. Although this text highlights the most important features of these bones, additional anatomic features are included for future reference in Figure 13-1.

Mandible

The mandible, or lower jaw bone, is the largest of the facial bones (Figure 13-2). This highly mobile bone is suspended from the cranium by muscles, ligaments, and the capsule of the TMJ. Many of the important bony landmarks are described as follows.

The *body* is the horizontal portion of the mandible with sockets for the lower 16 adult teeth (see Figure 13-2). The *ramus* projects vertically from the body of the mandible. The *angle* of each mandible provides the attachment for the masseter and medial pterygoid muscles. The *mandibular condyle* is the convex portion of bone arising from the ramus. Each condyle articulates with the concave mandibular fossa of the temporal bone, forming the TMJ (see Figure 13-1). The *coronoid process* is the thin triangular projection of bone arising from the anterior aspect of the ramus. The *mandibular notch* extends between the coronoid process and mandibular condyle (see Figure 13-2).

Temporal Bone

The *mandibular fossa* of the temporal bone articulates with the mandibular condyle, forming the TMJ. The anterior aspect of the mandibular fossa is marked by the *articular*

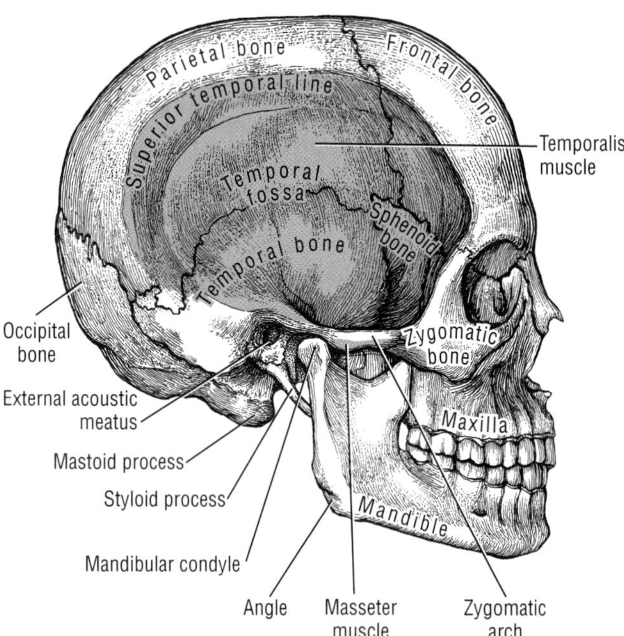

Figure 13-1 Lateral view of the skull with emphasis on bony landmarks associated with the temporomandibular joint. The proximal attachments of the temporalis and masseter muscles are indicated in red. (From Neumann DA: *Kinesiology of the musculoskeletal system: foundations for physical rehabilitation,* St Louis, 2002, Mosby, Figure 11-1.)

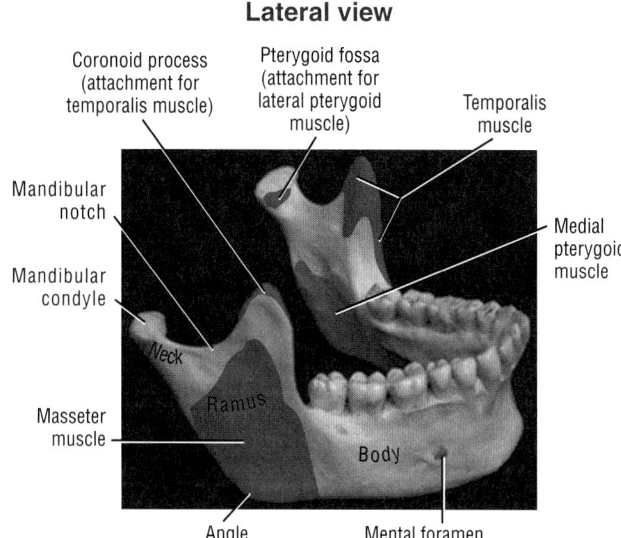

Figure 13-2 A lateral view of the mandible indicating the important bony features; the muscular attachments are indicated in gray. (From Neumann DA: *Kinesiology of the musculoskeletal system: foundations for physical rehabilitation,* St Louis, 2002, Mosby, Figure 11-2.)

eminence (Figure 13-3). Just posterior to the mandibular fossa is the *external auditory meatus*: the external opening for the ear. The *zygomatic process of the temporal bone* projects anteriorly, forming the posterior half of the *zygomatic arch* (see Figure 13-3). The zygomatic arch is formed by the union of the zygomatic process of the temporal bone and the temporal process of the zygomatic bone (cheek bone) (see Figure 13-1). The zygomatic arch serves as the proximal attachment for the masseter muscle. The *temporal fossa* is a slightly depressed area on the side of the skull formed by the union of five different cranial bones (see Figure 13-1).

Maxillae

The right and left maxillae unite to form a single maxilla, or upper jaw. The maxilla is firmly fused to the adjacent bones of the face including the sphenoid, nasal, and zygomatic bones. The inferior aspects of the maxilla contain sockets for the upper teeth (Figure 13-4).

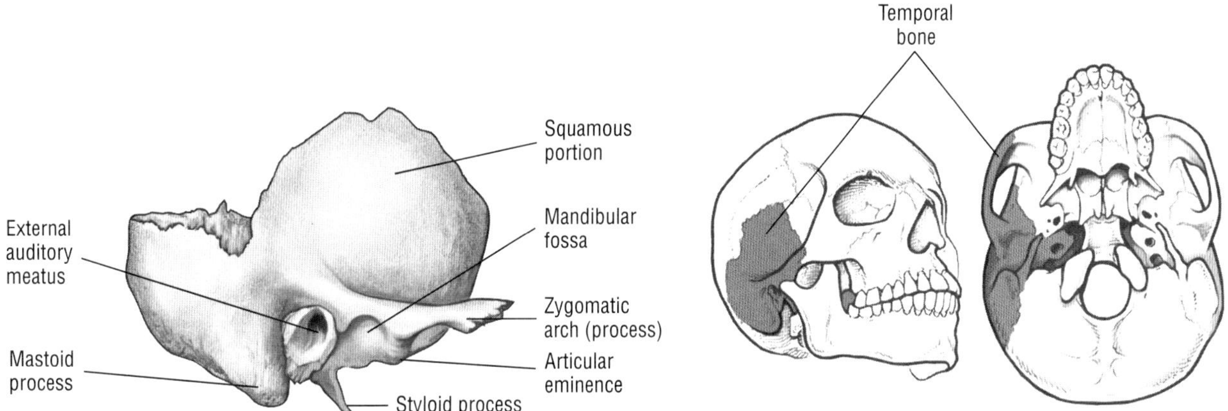

Figure 13-3 The right temporal bone. (From Muscolino JE: *Kinesiology: the skeletal system and muscle function*, St Louis, 2006, Mosby/Elsevier, Figure 4-12, *A* and *B*. Modified from Thibodeau GA, Patton KT: *Anatomy & physiology*, ed 5, St Louis, 2003, Mosby.)

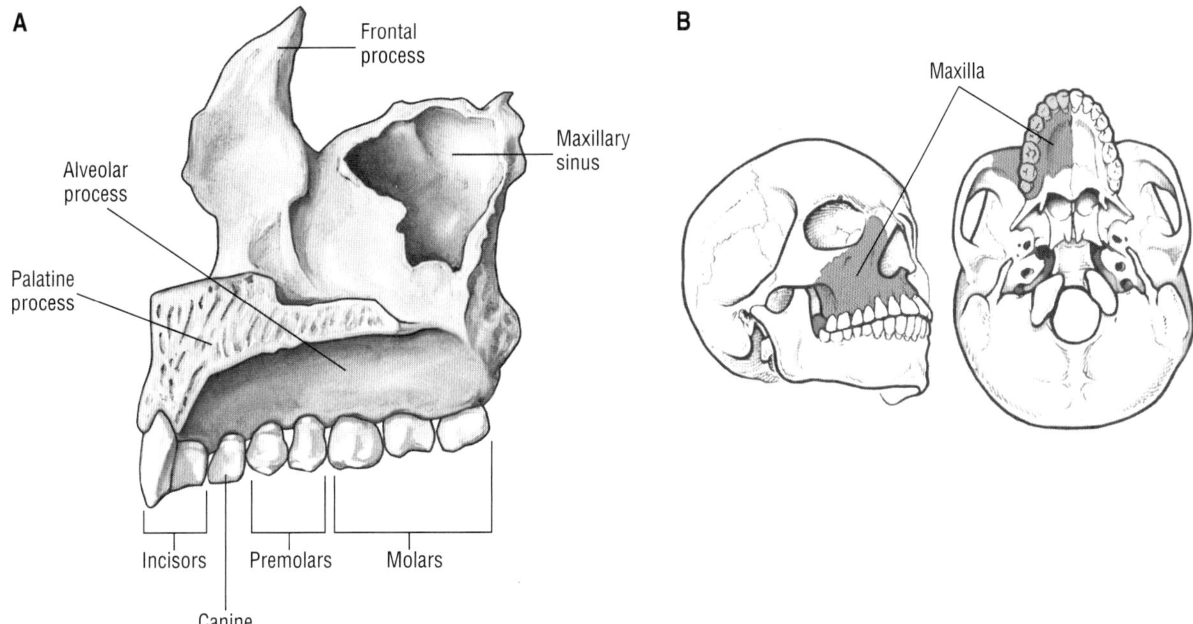

Figure 13-4 **A,** Medial view of the right maxilla. **B,** Lateral and inferior views of the right maxilla. (From Muscolino JE: *Kinesiology: the skeletal system and muscle function*, St Louis, 2006, Mosby, Figure 4-15, *A* and *B*. Modified from Thibodeau GA, Patton KT: *Anatomy & physiology*, ed 5, St Louis, 2003, Mosby.)

Zygomatic Bone

The zygomatic bone forms the cheek region and lateral orbit of the eye (Figure 13-5). As mentioned earlier, the *temporal process of the zygomatic bone* forms the anterior half of the zygomatic arch (see Figure 13-1).

Sphenoid Bone

The sphenoid bone (Figure 13-6) is a single, deep bone that runs transversely across the cranium. The *greater wings* are located on either side of the cranium, just anterior to the temporal bone. Projecting inferiorly are the *medial* and *lateral pterygoid plates* (see Figure 13-6); the lateral plate provides proximal attachments for the medial and lateral pterygoid muscles.

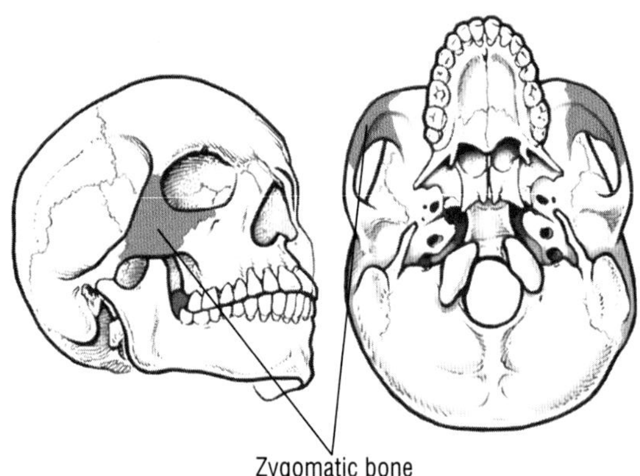

Figure 13-5 Lateral and inferior views of the skull highlighting the right zygomatic bone. (From Muscolino JE: *Kinesiology: the skeletal system and muscle function*, St Louis, 2006, Mosby, Figure 4-15, *E*. Modified from Thibodeau GA, Patton KT: *Anatomy & physiology*, ed 5, St Louis, 2003, Mosby.)

Hyoid Bone

The hyoid bone is located at the base of the throat, just anterior to the third cervical vertebra. The very mobile hyoid serves as an attachment for several muscles involved with moving the tongue, swallowing, and opening the jaw (see Figure 13-11, p. 365).

Supporting Structures

- *Articular Disc*: The articular disc of the TMJ rests between the mandibular condyle and the mandibular fossa of the temporal bone (Figure 13-7, A). This prominent structure consists of dense fibrous connective tissue. The disc provides joint stability, reduces joint contact pressure, and helps safely guide the condyle across the rough articular eminence of the temporal bone.
- *Capsule*: The TMJ is surrounded by a fibrous capsule. Laterally, the capsule thickens and is called the lateral ligament of the TMJ. The capsule and lateral ligament provide stability to the TMJ during chewing motions (Figure 13-7, B).

Kinematics

The primary motions of the TMJ are protrusion and retrusion, lateral excursion, and elevation and depression. All of these motions play an essential role in mastication (chewing).

Protrusion and Retrusion

Protrusion, also referred to as protraction, describes the anterior translation of the mandible (Figure 13-8, A). As

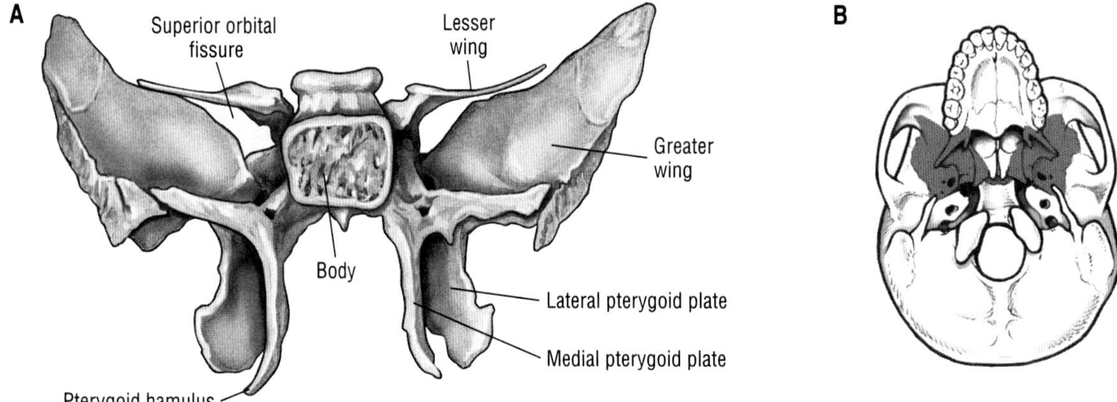

Figure 13-6 A, Posterior view of the sphenoid bone removed from the skull; note the lateral and medial pterygoid plates. **B,** Inferior view of the skull highlighting the sphenoid bone. (From Muscolino JE: *Kinesiology: the skeletal system and muscle function*, St Louis, 2006, Mosby, Figure 4-13, *C*. Modified from Thibodeau GA, Patton KT: *Anatomy & physiology*, ed 5, St Louis, 2003, Mosby.)

will be described, protrusion is an important component of opening the mouth.

Retrusion, also called retraction, is the opposite of protrusion. This motion occurs as the mandible translates posteriorly, an important motion for closing the mouth (Figure 13-8, *B*).

Lateral Excursion

Lateral excursion occurs as the mandible translates side to side (Figure 13-9). This motion is used to grind food between the teeth.

Depression and Elevation

Depression of the mandible *opens* the mouth, whereas **elevation** *closes* the mouth (Figure 13-10). Both motions play a fundamental role in eating, yawning, and talking. The adult mouth can be opened an average of slightly more than 2 inches. This degree of opening is often gauged by the ability to fit three knuckles (proximal interphalangeal joints) into the mouth.

As illustrated in Figure 13-10, A, fully depressing the mandible—opening the mouth—requires extreme anterior translation (protrusion) of each mandibular condyle relative to its mandibular fossa. Normally, the articular disc

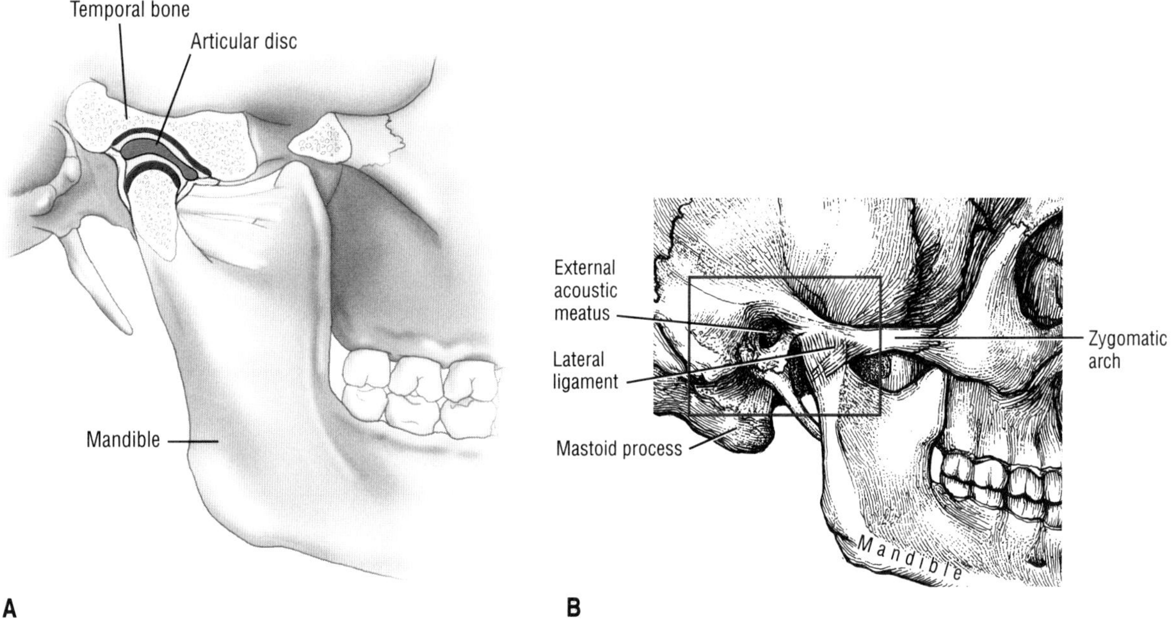

Figure 13-7 A, A sagittal plane cross section of the right temporomandibular joint highlighting the articular disc. **B,** A lateral view of the skull showing the outer portions of the capsule: the lateral ligament of the temporomandibular joint. (**A,** From Muscolino JE: *Kinesiology: the skeletal system and muscle function*, St Louis, 2006, Mosby, Figure 6-20, *A*. **B,** From Neumann DA: *Kinesiology of the musculoskeletal system: foundations for physical rehabilitation,* St Louis, 2002, Mosby, Figure 11-10.)

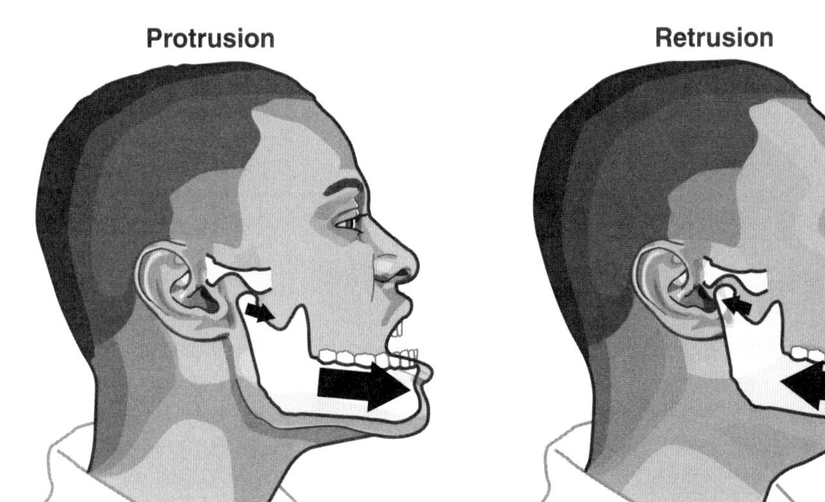

Figure 13-8 Protrusion **(A)** and retrusion **(B)** of the mandible. (From Neumann DA: *Kinesiology of the musculoskeletal system: foundations for physical rehabilitation*, St Louis, 2002, Mosby, Figure 11-12.)

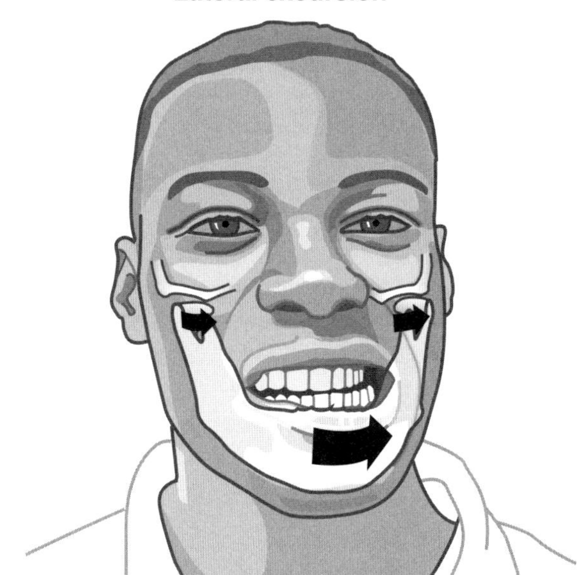

Figure 13-9 Lateral excursion of the mandible. (From Neumann DA: *Kinesiology of the musculoskeletal system: foundations for physical rehabilitation*, St Louis, 2002, Mosby, Figure 11-13.)

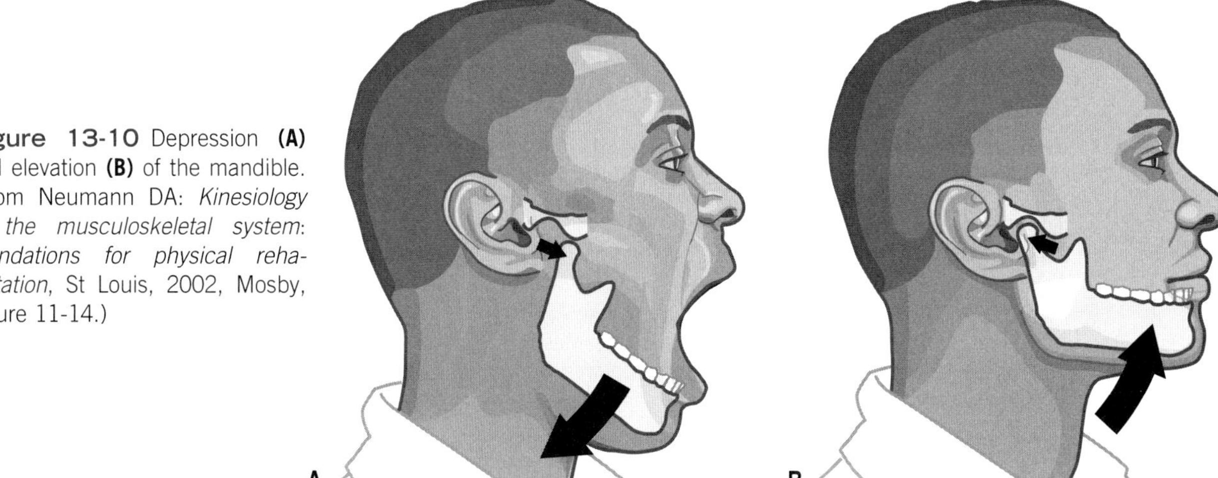

Figure 13-10 Depression **(A)** and elevation **(B)** of the mandible. (From Neumann DA: *Kinesiology of the musculoskeletal system: foundations for physical rehabilitation*, St Louis, 2002, Mosby, Figure 11-14.)

translates anteriorly along with each mandibular condyle, helping to properly guide the motion. The disc is "reseated" into the joint as the mandible is elevated and retrudes (retracts) during closure of the mouth (see Figure 13-10, *B*). In both opening and closing the mouth, the articular disc is essential in minimizing the contact stress between the mandibular condyle and the articular eminence of the temporal bone.

Muscle and Joint Interaction

Muscles of the Temporomandibular Joint

PRIMARY MUSCLES

The primary muscles of the TMJ are the masseter, temporalis, medial pterygoid, and lateral pterygoid. These muscles work together in a relatively complex fashion when opening and closing the mouth; this will be explained in greater detail as the chapter progresses (see Figure 13-12, p. 366).

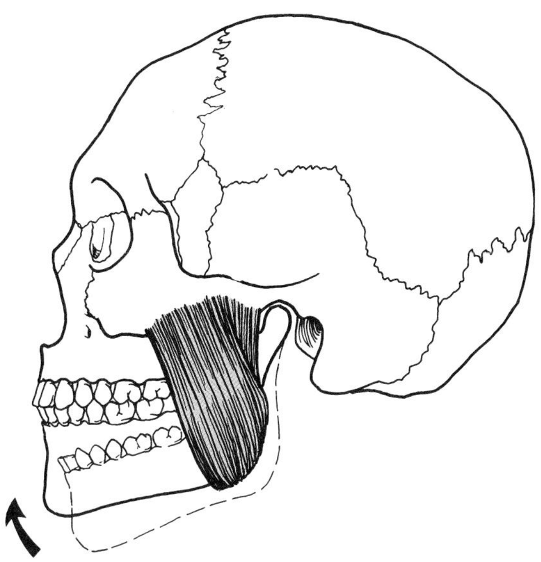

(Modified from Okeson JP: *Management of temporomandibular disorders and occlusion*, ed 5, St Louis, 2003, Mosby, Figure 1-22, *A*.)

Masseter

Proximal Attachment: Zygomatic arch

Distal Attachment: External surface of the mandible, between the angle and coronoid process of the ramus

Innervation: Cranial nerve V

Actions: Bilateral:

- Elevation of the mandible (closing the mouth)

Unilateral:

- Lateral excursion (to ipsilateral side)

Comments: The masseter is a thick, powerful muscle, easily palpable just above the angle of the mandible during a biting motion. Bilateral activation of the masseters elevates the mandible, bringing the teeth together for mastication. The primary function of the masseter is to develop large forces between the molars for effective grinding and crushing of food.

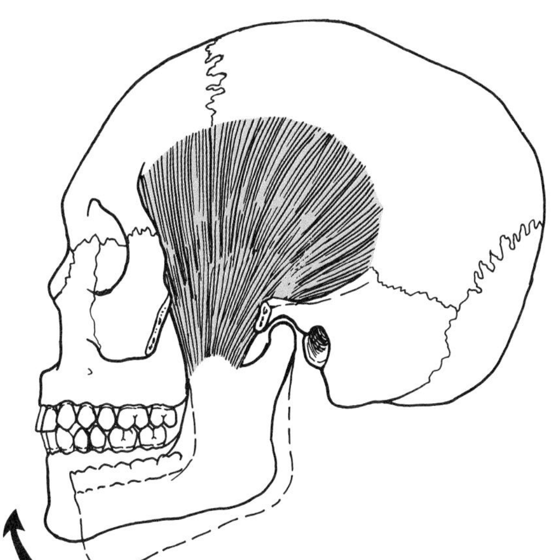

(Modified from Okeson JP: *Management of temporomandibular disorders and occlusion*, ed 5, St Louis, 2003, Mosby, Figure 1-22, *B*.)

Temporalis

Proximal Attachment: Temporal fossa

Distal Attachment: Coronoid process and anterior edge of the ramus of the mandible

Innervation: Cranial nerve V

Actions: Bilateral:

- Elevation of the mandible (closing the mouth)
- Retrusion of the mandible (posterior fibers)

Unilateral:

- Lateral excursion (to ipsilateral side)

Comments: The temporalis is a fan-shaped muscle that fills much of the concavity of the temporal fossa. The temporalis narrows into a broad tendon as it courses distally through a space between the zygomatic arch and the lateral side of the skull. This muscle contributes to both essential kinematic elements of closing the mouth: elevation *and* retrusion of the mandible.

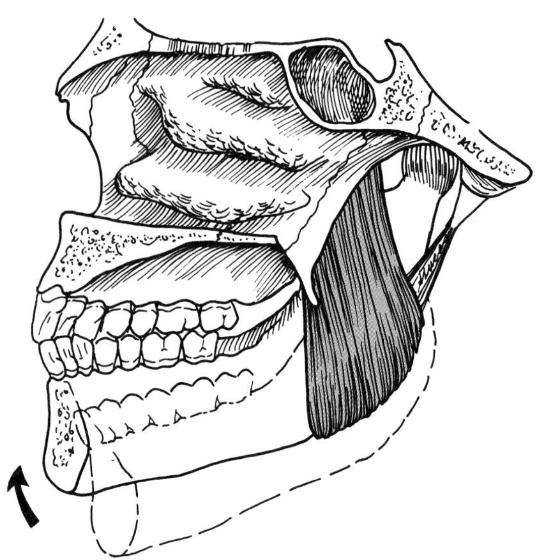

(Modified from Okeson JP: *Management of temporomandibular disorders and occlusion*, ed 6, St Louis, 2008, Mosby, Figure 1-24, *B*.)

Medial Pterygoid

Proximal Attachment: Medial surface of the lateral pterygoid plate

Distal Attachment: Internal surface of the angle and ramus of the mandible

Innervation: Cranial nerve V

Actions: Bilateral:

- Elevation of the mandible (closing the mouth)

Unilateral:

- Lateral excursion (to contralateral side)

Comments: The medial pterygoid and the masseter form a sling around the angle of the mandible. This sling affords a similar and secure line of pull for both muscles, especially useful for biting actions. Simultaneous bilateral contraction of these muscles can produce an average of almost 100 lb of biting force in the healthy adult.

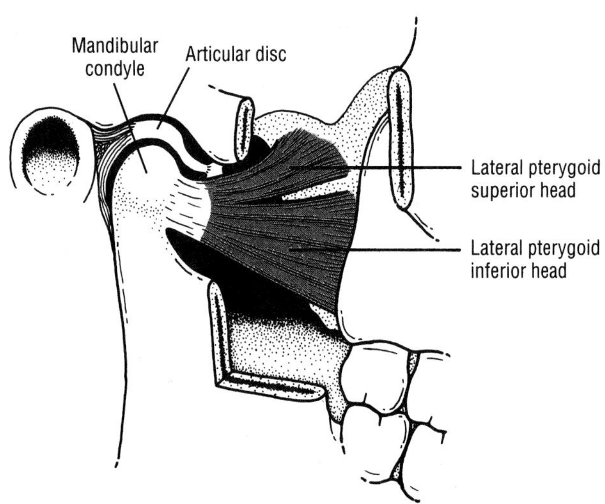

(Modified from Kaplan AS, Assael LA: *Temporomandibular disorders: diagnosis and treatment*, Philadelphia, 1991, Saunders.)

Lateral Pterygoid

Proximal Attachment:

- Superior head: Greater wing of the sphenoid bone
- Inferior head: Lateral surface of the lateral pterygoid plate

Distal Attachment: Near the condyle of the mandible; the superior head also attaches to the articular disc of the TMJ

Innervation: Cranial nerve V

Actions: Bilateral:

- Depression of the mandible (opening the mouth; inferior head only)
- Protrusion of the mandible

Unilateral:

- Lateral excursion (to contralateral side)

Comments: The two heads of the lateral pterygoid help with mandibular protrusion and lateral excursion. The inferior head of the lateral pterygoid is important in the arthrokinematics of *opening* the jaw (further described in the next section). The inferior head pulls the mandible (and articular disc) forward and down, which causes the jaw to swing open and translate forward. Both of these motions are required to widely open the mouth.

The inferior head of the lateral pterygoid is the primary muscle used to open the jaw. Interestingly, the superior head of the lateral pterygoid is most active while forcefully closing the mouth.

SECONDARY MUSCLES

The suprahyoid and infrahyoid muscles are considered secondary muscles of mastication (Figure 13-11). Both groups of muscles are involved with depression of the mandible and subsequent opening of the mouth, movement of the tongue, swallowing, and speaking. The infrahyoid muscles stabilize the hyoid bone so that the suprahyoid muscles have a firm base to assist with depression of the mandible.

The suprahyoid muscles include the digastric, geniohyoid, mylohyoid, and stylohyoid. The first table below provides the attachments and actions of these muscles. The infrahyoid muscles include the omohyoid, sternohyoid, sternothyroid, and thyrohyoid. The second table below provides the attachments and actions of these muscles.

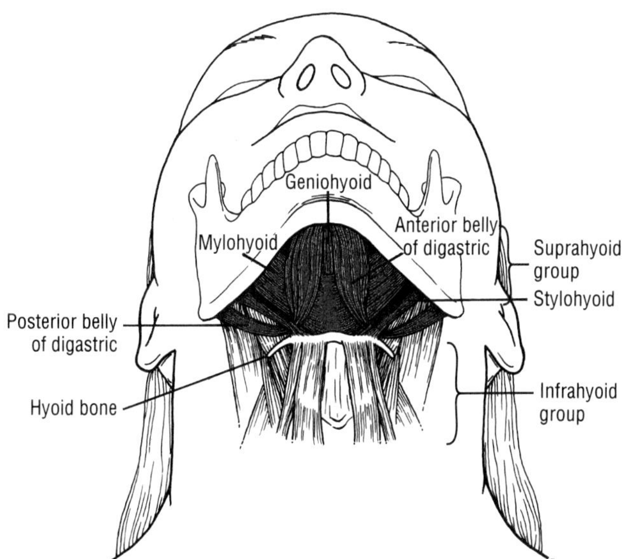

Figure 13-11 The suprahyoid muscles *(red)* and infrahyoid muscles are shown attaching to the hyoid bone. (Modified from Kaplan AS, Assael LA: *Temporomandibular disorders: diagnosis and treatment,* Philadelphia, 1991, Saunders.)

Clinical **INSIGHT**

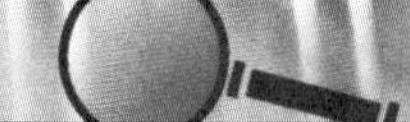

Temporomandibular Disorders

Temporomandibular disorder (TMD) is a broad and often vague term that defines a number of clinical problems that involve the masticatory system. TMDs are typically associated with a dysfunction of the joint, disc, and surrounding musculature. Muscular dysfunctions typically respond more favorably to conservative treatment than pathology involving the disc. In addition to pain during movement, the signs and symptoms include clicking, popping, or locking of the joint; reduce bite force; tension headaches; and limited opening of the mouth.

Many of the common conservative treatments for TMD are listed below:

- Exercise and postural correction
- Biofeedback/relaxation procedures
- Use of cold or heat
- Patient education
- Joint mobilization
- Ultrasound
- Behavioral modification
- Intra-oral appliances (splints)

SUPRAHYOID MUSCLES

Muscle	Proximal Attachment	Distal Attachment	Actions
Digastric	*Anterior belly*: Internal surface of the body of the mandible *Posterior belly*: Mastoid process	Hyoid bone	Depression of mandible
Geniohyoid	Midline of the internal surface of the body of the mandible	Hyoid bone	Depression of mandible
Mylohyoid	Internal surface of the body of the mandible	Hyoid bone	Depression of mandible
Stylohyoid	Styloid process of the temporal bone	Hyoid bone	Depression of mandible

INFRAHYOID MUSCLES

Muscle	Proximal Attachment	Distal Attachment	Actions
Omohyoid	Superior border of the scapula, near scapular notch	Hyoid bone	Stabilize hyoid bone
Sternohyoid	Manubrium of the sternum and medial clavicle	Hyoid bone	Stabilize hyoid bone
Sternothyroid	Manubrium of the sternum	Thyroid cartilage	Stabilize hyoid bone*
Thyrohyoid	Thyroid cartilage	Hyoid bone	Stabilize hyoid bone

*Indirect action by stabilizing the thyroid cartilage for the thyrohyoid muscle.

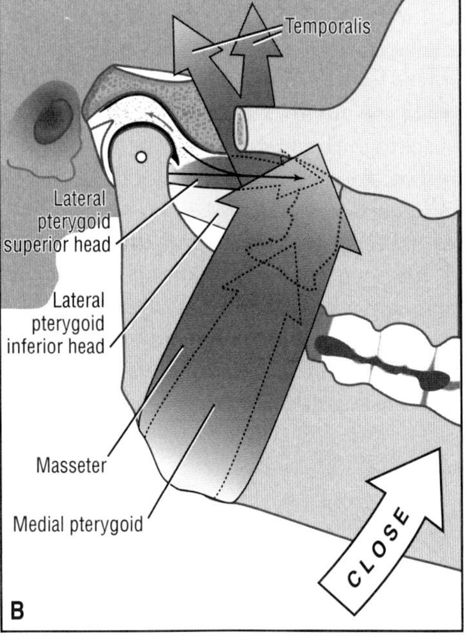

Figure 13-12 The muscle and joint interaction while **(A)** opening the mouth and **(B)** closing the mouth. (From Neumann DA: *Kinesiology of the musculoskeletal system: foundations for physical rehabilitation,* St Louis, 2002, Mosby, Figure 11-22.)

Functional Considerations

Summary of Opening the Mouth. Widely opening the mouth occurs primarily through contraction of the inferior head of the lateral pterygoid. The suprahyoid muscles and gravity assist with this action. As depicted in Figure 13-12, A, opening of the mouth involves depression of the mandible, combined with forward translation (protrusion) of the mandibular condyle. The lateral pterygoid (inferior head) controls the anterior translation component, whereas the suprahyoid muscles produce depression of the mandible.

Summary of Closing the Mouth. Forcefully closing the mouth such as when biting or chewing involves strong forces from the masseter, medial pterygoid, and temporalis muscles. As illustrated in Figure 13-12, *B,* closing the mouth involves mandibular elevation and retrusion. The superior head of the lateral pterygoid is most active while closing the mouth, which helps guide the reseating of the disc within the joint. Interestingly, only the tendon of the *superior head* has firm attachments to the articular disc.

During opening and closing the mouth, the position of the articular disc plays an important role in the smoothness of the action. The lateral ligament and lateral pterygoid (superior head) guide the disc's movement to ensure optimal alignment of the TMJ. Asynchronized or asymmetric motions between the disc and TMJ often cause pain and a clicking sound or, in more extreme cases, locking of the jaw.

Summary of Lateral Excursion. Lateral excursion, or lateral deviation, is a primary component of mastication, as food is ground between the teeth. This motion primarily involves an interaction of all four primary muscles of mastication. For example, lateral excursion to the left primarily involves activation of the left temporalis and masseter, and activation of the right medial and lateral pterygoid muscles (Figure 13-13).

Summary

Speaking, swallowing, and chewing are essential functions based on a properly functioning TMJ. Various orthopedic injuries or disorders affect the TMJ and can have a profound impact on the level of a person's function. Clinicians who understand the anatomy and kinesiology of the TMJ can more adeptly formulate treatment plans and modify exercise programs to help treat TMJ disorders.

VENTILATION

Ventilation is the mechanical process by which air is inhaled and exhaled through the lungs. The mechanics of ventilation are based on an interaction between the muscles and joints of the axial skeleton. This section provides a brief overview of the kinesiology of ventilation.

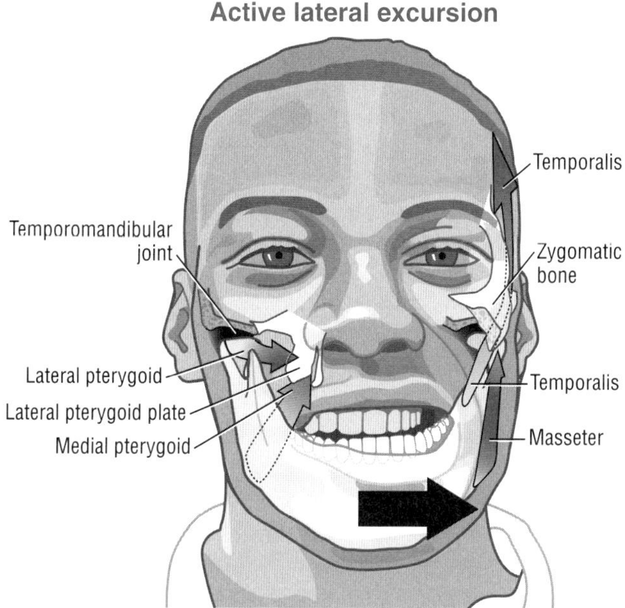

Figure 13-13 The muscular interaction involved in performing left lateral excursion of the mandible. (From Neumann DA: *Kinesiology of the musculoskeletal system: foundations for physical rehabilitation,* St Louis, 2002, Mosby, Figure 11-18.)

Ventilation allows for the exchange of oxygen and carbon dioxide between the lungs and the blood. This process ultimately drives the physiology of activated muscles that move and stabilize the joints of the body.

The relative intensity of ventilation can be described as quiet or forced. In the healthy population, *quiet ventilation* occurs during relatively sedentary activities—those with low metabolic demands. In contrast, *forced ventilation* occurs during strenuous activities that require rapid and large exchanges of air, such as when exercising or in the presence of some respiratory diseases.

Lung Volumes

Figure 13-14 shows the lung volumes and capacities in the normal adult. As depicted, the *total lung capacity* is about 5½ liters of air; however, most of this capacity is not used during normal breathing. *Tidal volume* is defined as the volume of air moved in and out of the lungs during each ventilation cycle. At rest, an adult's tidal volume is about ½ liter (or only about 10% of total lung volume). The *inspiratory reserve volume* is the amount of air that can be taken into the lungs (above the tidal volume) upon **forced inspiration**. The *expiratory reserve volume* is the amount of air that can be pushed out of the lungs (beyond the tidal volume) upon **forced expiration**. *Vital capacity* is the total volume of air that can be moved in and out of the lungs.

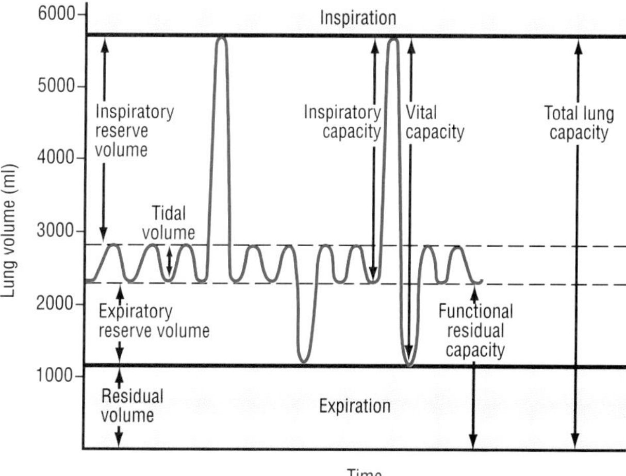

Figure 13-14 The lung volumes and capacities in the normal adult. (From Guyton AC, Hall JE: *Textbook of medical physiology,* ed 10, Philadelphia, 2000, Saunders.)

Inspiration and Expiration

Ventilation is described as consisting of two main events: inspiration and expiration. **Inspiration** is the process of drawing air into the lungs, whereas **expiration** is the process of pushing air out of the lungs. Most of the physics behind inspiration and expiration is based on **Boyle's law**, which states that the volume and pressure of a gas are inversely proportional. For example, *increasing the volume* of a container filled with a gas (such as air) spontaneously *reduces the pressure* within the container. (This relationship is considered inversely proportional because as one variable increases the other one automatically decreases.) This reduced pressure creates a suction effect that attempts to draw air in from outside the container. Relating this analogy to human ventilation, during inspiration, the rib cage—or thorax—expands while the dome of the diaphragm muscle drops. These two factors *increase* the intrathoracic volume, which, in turn, *decreases* the pressure within the lungs (interpleural space). As pictured in Figure 13-15, *A*, these mechanics are similar to that of a syringe pulling air or liquid into its shaft. As the plunger of the syringe is pulled outward, air or fluid is sucked inward. Similarly, as the thorax is expanded during ventilation, the reduced pressure draws air into the lungs through the trachea (Figure 13-15, *B*).

Expiration is the process of exhaling air from the lungs into the environment. In order to push air out of the lungs, the ribcage and enclosed lungs constrict, thereby increasing the pressure within the lungs; this forces the air outward. **Quiet expiration** is normally a passive process that does *not* depend on muscular activation. The decrease in intrathoracic volume is caused by the natural elastic recoil of the lungs, thorax, and connective tissues of stretched inspiratory muscles, similar to the way air is pushed out of an untied (and inflated) balloon. Forced expiration, however, involves active contraction of expiratory muscles such as the abdominals (see Figure 13-16, p. 370). This process occurs commonly while coughing, sneezing, or forcefully exhaling such as when blowing out candles.

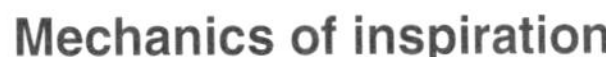

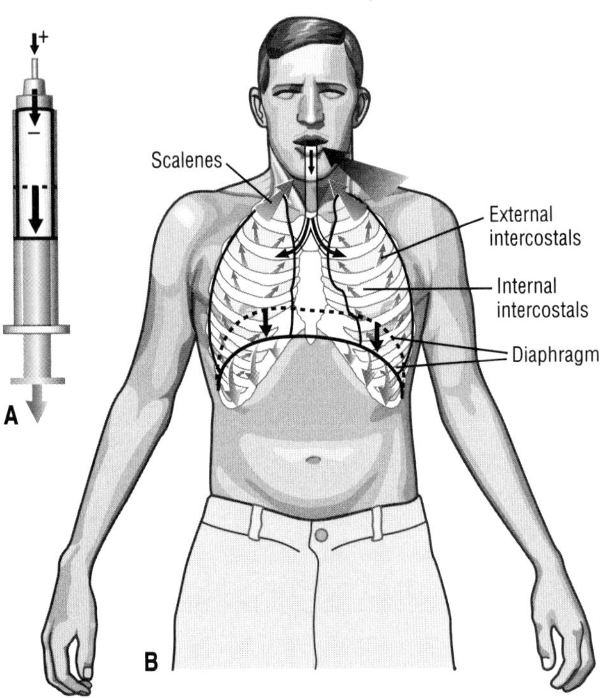

Figure 13-15 The muscular mechanics of inspiration. This analogy shows Boyle's law: **A,** Pulling the plunger outward increases the volume within the shaft and draws air inward. **B,** Contraction of the primary muscles of inspiration increases intrathoracic volume and pulls air *into* the lungs. (From Neumann DA: *Kinesiology of the musculoskeletal system: foundations for physical rehabilitation*, St Louis, 2002, Mosby, Figure 11-24.)

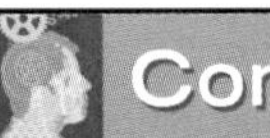

The Ins and Outs of Breathing

Inspiration is an active process, typically involving numerous muscles. In order to reduce the pressure within the lungs, the intrathoracic volume must increase. This typically occurs in three ways: (1) elevation of the ribs, (2) elevation and forward expansion of the sternum, and (3) increasing the vertical diameter of the thorax—caused by contraction of the diaphragm. Therefore any muscle that contributes to one or more of these actions is considered a muscle of inspiration.

As mentioned earlier, quiet expiration is primarily a passive process, but forced expiration requires muscular force to constrict the thorax and thereby decrease intrathoracic volume. Therefore any muscle that assists with (1) depression of the ribs, (2) depression and pulling in on the sternum, or (3) decreasing the vertical diameter of the thorax is considered a muscle of forced expiration.

Muscle Actions during Ventilation

Muscles of Inspiration

The primary muscles of inspiration are the diaphragm, scalenes, and intercostals. These muscles are considered primary because they are active during all intensities of breathing.

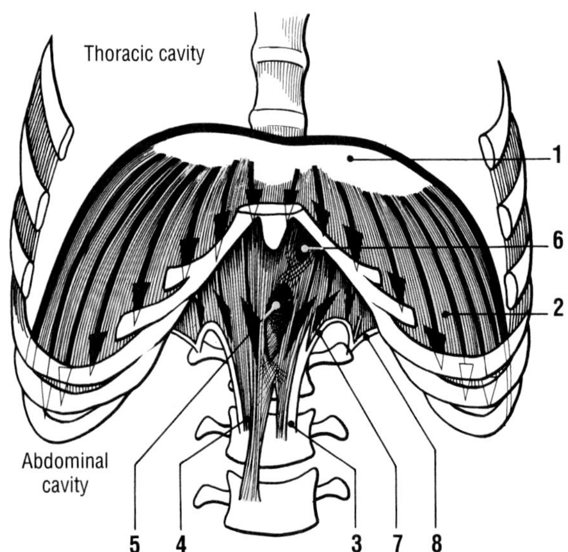

The action of the diaphragm during inspiration. *1,* Central tendon; *2,* muscle fibers (costal part); *3,* left crus; *4,* right crus; *5,* opening for the aorta; *6,* opening for the esophagus; *7,* part of the psoas muscle; and *8,* part of the quadratus lumborum muscle. (Modified from Kapandji IA: *The physiology of joints*, vol 3, New York, 1974, Churchill Livingstone.)

Diaphragm

Inferior Attachments:
- Costal part: Inner surfaces of the cartilages and adjacent bony regions of ribs 6 to 12
- Sternal part: Posterior side of the xiphoid process
- Lumbar part: Bodies of L1-L3 through two distinct tendinous attachments called the left and right crus

Superior Attachment: Central tendon near the dome of the diaphragm

Innervation: Phrenic nerve (C3-C5)

Actions: Primary muscle of inspiration

Comments: The diaphragm is the most important and efficient muscle of inspiration, performing 70% to 80% of the work. The efficiency reflects the muscle's ability to expand the intrathoracic volume in three diameters: vertical, medial-lateral, and anterior-posterior.

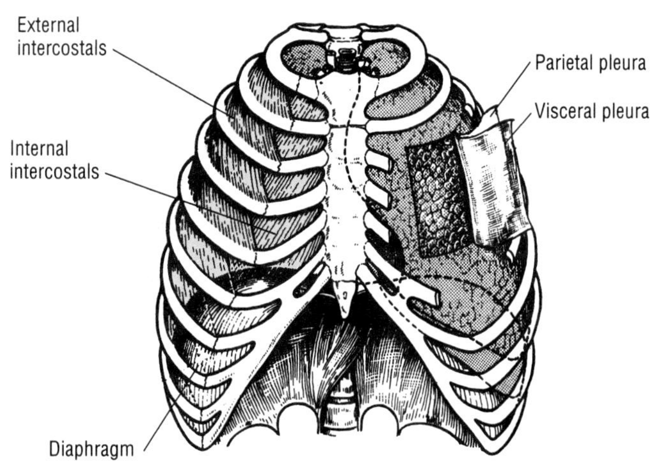

The bony housing of the thorax is shown highlighting the external and internal intercostals. (Modified from McNaught AB, Callander R: *Illustrated physiology*, New York, 1975, Churchill Livingstone.)

External Intercostals

Attachments: Eleven per side; each muscle arises from the inferior border of a rib and inserts on the upper border of the rib below

Innervation: Intercostal nerves (T2-12)

Action: Assist with inspiration by elevating ribs and thereby expanding the thorax

Comments: The external intercostals can expand the thorax by elevating the ribs. Note that these muscles course in an oblique direction, similar to that of the (abdominal) external obliques.

Internal Intercostals

Attachments: Eleven per side, each muscle arises from the upper border of a rib and inserts on the lower border of the rib above. Note that these muscles are deep to the external intercostals, and the fibers run in a nearly perpendicular direction to that of the external intercostals, similar to that of the (abdominal) internal obliques.

Innervation: Intercostal nerves (T2-12)

Action: Assist with force expiration by depressing the ribs

Comments: Although typically described as muscles of forced expiration, the internal intercostals have also been shown to be active during inspiration. The precise action of both the internal and external intercostals is still unclear. It is agreed, however, that both sets of muscles help stabilize the intercostal spaces, thereby preventing the thoracic wall from being sucked (pulled) inward during inspiration.

SCALENES

The anterior, middle, and posterior scalenes attach between the cervical spine and the upper two ribs (see the image associated with the section Scalenes on p. 208 in Chapter 8). With the cervical spine stabilized, bilateral contraction of these muscles can assist with inspiration by elevating the upper ribs. Although the scalenes are active along with the diaphragm during every inspiration cycle, hypertrophy of these muscles typically indicates labored breathing, often a symptom of a respiratory disorder.

Clinical INSIGHT

Diaphragm: The "Workhorse" of Inspiration

The diaphragm is the most important muscle of inspiration. As illustrated in the figure on p. 368 the diaphragm is a dome-shaped muscle that forms the floor of the thoracic cavity. Contraction of the diaphragm pulls the dome downward, quickly increasing intrathoracic volume. Unlike other inspiratory muscles, contraction of the diaphragm significantly increases intrathoracic volume by expanding the height, width, and depth of the thorax.

Spinal cord injuries at or above the C3 or C4 level result in partial or complete paralysis of the diaphragm (recall the diaphragm is innervated by the phrenic nerve that is formed by nerve roots C3-C5). Without artificial means of ventilation, a person suffering paralysis of the diaphragm may likely die. In order to live, these individuals must be equipped with a machine that performs mechanical ventilation. Such machines assist with inspiration by pushing controlled amounts of air into the lungs, often through a tube placed directly into the trachea (via a tracheostomy). Careful medical attention is required to prevent infection. Rehabilitation of these patients involves educating the caregiver on how to effectively operate the mechanical ventilator, appropriately respond to inadequate ventilation, and prevent infection and buildup of secretions within the upper respiratory tract.

Clinical INSIGHT

Chronic Obstructive Pulmonary Disease

Chronic obstructive pulmonary disease (COPD) is a disorder that typically incorporates three components: (1) chronic bronchitis, (2) emphysema, and (3) asthma. This disease is often associated with many years of smoking. Symptoms of COPD include chronic inflammation and narrowing of the bronchioles, chronic cough, and mucus-filled airways, with over-distention and destruction of the alveolar walls. A significant complication of COPD is the loss of the natural elastic recoil within the lungs and collapse of the bronchioles. As a result, air remains trapped in the lungs at the end of quiet or forced expiration. This complication is called hyperinflation of the lungs and often gives a person suffering from COPD a barrel-chested appearance.

Persons with COPD often depend on accessory muscles to assist the primary muscles of inspiration. Even at rest, ventilation can be labored. Accessory muscles of inspiration such as the sternocleidomastoid and pectoralis minor often contract to elevate the ribs and sternum to assist with inspiration.

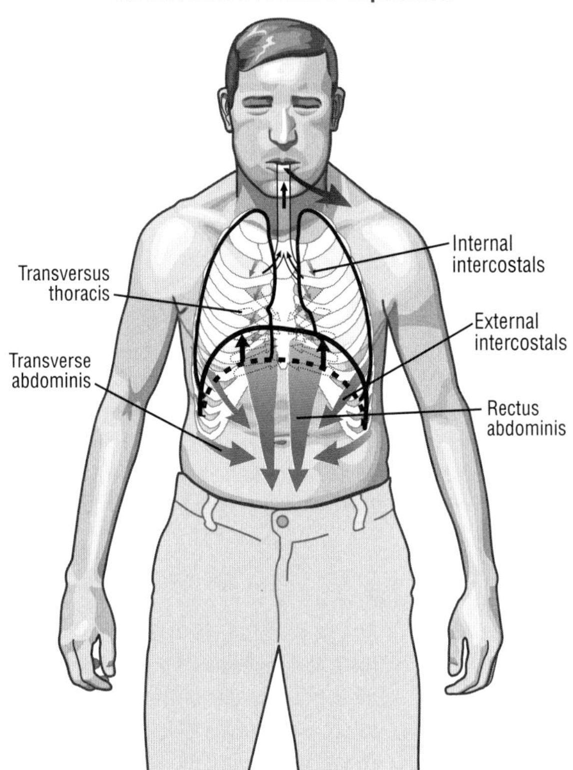

Figure 13-16 The muscular interaction involved with forced expiration. Contraction of the abdominals and internal intercostal muscles are shown contracting in red. The transversus thoracis (not described in text) is also capable of pushing air out of the lungs. The passive recoil of the diaphragm is indicated by the pair of thick, black vertical arrows. (From Neumann DA: *Kinesiology of the musculoskeletal system: foundations for physical rehabilitation*, St Louis, 2002, Mosby, Figure 11-30.)

Muscles of Forced Expiration

As described above, quiet expiration is normally a passive process, driven primarily by the elastic recoil of the thorax, lungs, and relaxing diaphragm. During forced expiration, such as when coughing or vigorously exhaling after running, active muscle contraction is required to rapidly reduce intrathoracic volume (Figure 13-16). Muscles of forced expiration include the four abdominal muscles and, at times, the internal intercostals.

The abdominal muscles include the rectus abdominis, external and internal obliques, and the transverse abdominis (see the images associated with these four major muscle groups on pp. 213-214 in Chapter 8). These four muscles produce forced expiration by flexing the trunk and also depressing the ribs. Also, these muscles compress the abdominal wall and contents, which increases intra-abdominal pressure. As a result, the relaxed diaphragm is pushed upward, decreasing intrathoracic volume and forcing air out of the lungs.

FUNCTIONAL CONSIDERATIONS: ABDOMINAL MUSCLE CONTROL DURING FORCED EXPIRATION

Forced expiration is driven primarily by the abdominal muscles. Adequate control over these muscles is important for physiologic functions such as coughing and adequately responding to a gag reflex. Both of these functions are vital to health and safety. Coughing or vigorously clearing the throat is a natural way to remove secretions from the lungs, thereby reducing the likelihood of infection. A strong contraction of the abdominals is also used to dislodge objects lodged in the trachea (e.g., when choking on a piece of food).

Persons with weakened or paralyzed abdominal muscles must learn alternative methods of coughing or have others manually assist with this function. Consider, for example, a person with complete spinal cord injury at the T4 level resulting in complete paralysis of the lower extremities and abdominal muscles. Clinicians must take care to educate this patient and caregivers on the importance of effective airway clearance and techniques for a manually assisted cough.

Summary

An extraordinarily large number of muscles and joints interact during ventilation. The actions of many different muscles can produce similar effects on changing intrathoracic volume, therefore allowing inspiration and expiration. This redundancy provides for an adaptable and responsive system—a necessity considering the complexity and simultaneous demands placed on the muscles involved with the vital process of ventilation.

Study Questions

1. Which of the following terms best describes anterior translation of the jaw?
   a. Lateral excursion
   b. Elevation
   c. Protrusion
   d. Retrusion
2. Which of the following bones forms the upper jaw?
   a. Mandible
   b. Maxillae
   c. Sphenoid
   d. Temporal
3. Which of the following muscles is primarily involved with *opening* the mouth?
   a. Temporalis
   b. Masseter
   c. Medial pterygoid
   d. Lateral pterygoid (inferior head)
   e. A and B
4. Widely opening the mouth requires __________ of the mandibular condyle.
   a. Anterior translation (protrusion)
   b. Posterior translation (retrusion)
   c. Little movement
   d. Lateral excursion
5. Activation of the right medial pterygoid and right lateral pterygoid will cause:
   a. Lateral excursion of the mandible to the right
   b. Lateral excursion of the mandible to the left
   c. Simultaneous activation of the infrahyoid muscles
   d. The hyoid bone to drop 1 to 2 inches toward the sternum
6. Which of the following muscles attaches proximally to the zygomatic arch?
   a. Medial pterygoid
   b. Lateral pterygoid
   c. Masseter
   d. Temporalis
7. Which of the following bones make up the lower jaw?
   a. Sphenoid
   b. Mandible
   c. Maxillae
   d. Zygomatic
8. The total volume of air that can be moved in and out of the lungs on maximal forced inspiration and maximal forced expiration is called:
   a. Tidal volume
   b. Vital capacity
   c. Expiratory reserve volume
   d. Inspiratory reserve volume
9. Which of the following is considered the most important muscle of inspiration?
   a. Internal intercostals
   b. Diaphragm
   c. Scalenes
   d. External intercostals
10. Persons with chronic obstructive pulmonary disease (COPD) often have a barrel-chested appearance because:
    a. Air becomes trapped in the lungs at the end of quiet or forced expiration
    b. Of significant hypertrophy of the abdominal obliques
    c. Of excessive calcium buildup within the rib cage
    d. Of paralysis of the diaphragm
11. According to Boyle's law, as the volume of a system increases:
    a. The pressure within that system increases proportionally
    b. The pressure within that system decreases proportionally
    c. The pressure within that system remains constant
12. The scalenes are able to assist with inspiration:
    a. By depressing the upper ribs and superior aspect of the sternum
    b. By elevating upper ribs and sternum
    c. By depressing the lower ribs and lower aspect of the sternum
    d. By lowering the floor of the thoracic cavity
13. Which of the following statements is true?
    a. Quiet expiration is primarily driven by the elastic recoil of the ribs and surrounding connective tissues.
    b. Forced expiration involves active contraction of the abdominal muscles.
    c. Any muscle that increases intrathoracic volume can be considered a muscle of inspiration.
    d. A and B
    e. All of the above
14. Expiration is the result of a decrease in intrathoracic volume.
    a. True
    b. False
15. The temporalis muscle is primarily involved with depression of the mandible.
    a. True
    b. False
16. Contraction of the diaphragm expands intrathoracic volume in three diameters: vertical, medial-lateral, and anterior-posterior.
    a. True
    b. False
17. The volume of air moved in and out of the lungs during each ventilation cycle is called the tidal volume.
    a. True
    b. False
18. Retrusion describes an anterior translation of the mandible.
    a. True
    b. False
19. The masseter, medial pterygoid, and temporalis muscles are all involved with the action of closing the mouth.
    a. True
    b. False

20. Reduction of the intrathoracic volume will cause air to be drawn into the lungs.
    a. True
    b. False

ADDITIONAL READINGS

Baba K, Haketa T, Sasaki Y et al: Association between masseter muscle activity levels recorded during sleep and signs and symptoms of temporomandibular disorders in healthy young adults, *J Orofac Pain* 9(3):226-231, 2005.

Bettinelli D, Kays C, Bailliart O et al: Effect of gravity on chest wall mechanics, *J Appl Physiol* 92(2):709-716, 2002.

Bhutada MK: Functions of the lateral pterygoid muscle, *Ann R Australas Coll Dent Surg* 17:68-69, 2004.

Bravetti P, Membre H, Haddioui AE et al: Histological study of the human temporo-mandibular joint and its surrounding muscles, *Surg Radiol Anat* 26(5):371-378, 2004.

Budzinska K, Supinski G, DiMarco AF: Inspiratory action of separate external and parasternal intercostal muscle contraction, *J Appl Physiol* 67(4):1395-1400, 1989.

Cala SJ, Kenyon CM, Lee A et al: Respiratory ultrasonography of human parasternal intercostal muscle in vivo, *Ultrasound Med Biol* 24(3):313-326, 1998.

Campbell EJ: The role of the scalene and sternomastoid muscles in breathing in normal subjects; an electromyographic study, *J Anat* 89(3):378-386, 1955.

Chandu A, Suvinen TI, Reade PC et al: Electromyographic activity of frontalis and sternocleidomastoid muscles in patients with temporomandibular disorders, *J Oral Rehabil* 32(8):571-576, 2005.

Chaves TC, Grossi DB, de Oliveira AS et al: Correlation between signs of temporomandibular (TMD) and cervical spine (CSD) disorders in asthmatic children, *J Clin Pediatr Dent* 29(4):287-292, 2005.

Christo JE, Bennett S, Wilkinson TM et al: Discal attachments of the human temporomandibular joint, *Aust Dent J* 50(3):152-160, 2005.

Clanton TL, Diaz PT: Clinical assessment of the respiratory muscles, *Phys Ther* 75(11):983-995, 1995.

De Laat A, Meuleman H, Stevens A et al: Correlation between cervical spine and temporomandibular disorders, *Clin Oral Investig* 2(2):54-57, 1998.

De Troyer A: Relationship between neural drive and mechanical effect in the respiratory system, *Adv Exp Med Biol* 508:507-514, 2002.

De Troyer A, Gorman RB, Gandevia SC: Distribution of inspiratory drive to the external intercostal muscles in humans, *J Physiol (Lond)* 546(Pt 3):943-954, 2003.

De Troyer A, Kelly S, Zin WA: Mechanical action of the intercostal muscles on the ribs, *Science* 220(4592):87-88, 1983.

De Troyer A, Estenne M: Coordination between rib cage muscles and diaphragm during quiet breathing in humans, *J Appl Physiol Respir Environ Exerc Physiol* 57(3):899-906, 1984.

De Troyer A, Estenne M: Functional anatomy of the respiratory muscles, *Clin Chest Med* 9(2):175-193, 1988.

DiMarco AF, Romaniuk JR, Supinski GS: Action of the intercostal muscles on the rib cage, *Respir Physiol* 82(3):295-306, 1990.

Estenne M, Yernault JC, De TA: Rib cage and diaphragm-abdomen compliance in humans: effects of age and posture, *J Appl Physiol* 59(6):1842-1848, 1985.

Finucane KE, Panizza JA, Singh B: Efficiency of the normal human diaphragm with hyperinflation, *J Appl Physiol* 99(4):1402-1411, 2005.

Goldman JM, Rose LS, Williams SJ et al: Effect of abdominal binders on breathing in tetraplegic patients, *Thorax* 41(12): 940-945, 1986.

Goldstein DF, Kraus SL, Williams WB et al: Influence of cervical posture on mandibular movement, *J Prosthet Dent* 52(3):421-426, 1984.

Goodheart G: Applied kinesiology in dysfunction of the temporomandibular joint, *Dent Clin North Am* 27(3):613-630, 1983.

Han JN, Gayan-Ramirez G, Dekhuijzen R et al: Respiratory function of the rib cage muscles, *Eur Respir J* 6(5):722-728, 1993.

Helms CA, Katzberg RW, Dolwick MF: *Internal derangements of the temporomandibular joint*, San Francisco, 1983, Radiology Research and Education Foundation.

Herb K, Cho S, Stiles MA: Temporomandibular joint pain and dysfunction, *Curr Pain Headache Reports* 10(6):408-414, 2006.

Iglarsh ZA, Snyder-Mackler L: Temporomandibular joint and the cervical spine. In Richardson JV, Iglarsh ZA, editors: *Clinical orthopaedic physical therapy*, Philadelphia, 1994, Saunders.

Katzberg RW, Westesson PL: *Diagnosis of the temporomandibular joint*, Philadelphia, 1993, Saunders.

Krumpe PE, Knudson RJ, Parsons G et al: The aging respiratory system, *Clin Geriatr Med* 1(1):143-175, 1985.

Loring SH, De Troyer A: Actions of the respiratory muscles. In Roussos C, Macklem PT, editors: *The thorax*, New York, 1985, Marcel Dekker.

Naeije M, Hofman N: Biomechanics of the human temporomandibular joint during chewing, *J Dent Res* 82(7):528-531, 2003.

Okeson JP: *Management of temporomandibular disorders and occlusion*, ed 6, St Louis, 2008, Mosby.

Osborn JW: The disc of the human temporomandibular joint: design, function and failure, *J Oral Rehabil* 12(4):279-293, 1985.

Rauhala K, Oikarinen KS, Raustia AM: Role of temporomandibular disorders (TMD) in facial pain: occlusion, muscle and TMJ pain, *Cranio* 17(4):254-261, 1999.

Rocabado M: Arthrokinematics of the temporomandibular joint, *Dent Clin North Am* 27(3):573-594, 1983.

Sindelar BJ, Herring SW: Soft tissue mechanics of the temporomandibular joint, *Cells Tissues Organs* 180(1):36-43, 2005.

Stamm T, Hohoff A, Van MA et al: On the three-dimensional physiological position of the temporomandibular joint, *J Orofac Orthop* 65(4):280-289, 2004.

Takazakura R, Takahashi M, Nitta N et al: Diaphragmatic motion in the sitting and supine positions: healthy subject study using a vertically open magnetic resonance system, *J Magn Reson Imaging* 19(5):605-609, 2004.

Verges S, Notter D, Spengler CM: Influence of diaphragm and rib cage muscle fatigue on breathing during endurance exercise, *Respir Physiol Neurobiol* 154(3):431-442, 2006.

Whitelaw WA, Ford GT, Rimmer KP et al: Intercostal muscles are used during rotation of the thorax in humans, *J Appl Physiol* 72(5):1940-1944, 1992.

Answer Key for Study Questions

Chapter 1

1. e
2. c
3. b
4. d
5. b
6. d
7. c
8. b
9. c
10. b
11. b
12. b
13. a
14. a
15. d
16. c
17. a
18. e
19. a
20. a
21. a
22. a
23. b
24. b
25. b
26. a
27. b
28. a
29. b
30. b

Chapter 2

1. b
2. c
3. c
4. c
5. b
6. b
7. e
8. b
9. a
10. b
11. a
12. b
13. b
14. a
15. d
16. c
17. d
18. a
19. b
20. c

Chapter 3

1. e
2. b
3. c
4. c
5. a
6. b
7. d
8. d
9. b
10. b
11. a
12. a
13. b
14. a
15. b
16. a
17. b
18. a
19. b
20. a

Chapter 4

1. b
2. d
3. b
4. c
5. b
6. a
7. b
8. c
9. c
10. d
11. c
12. d
13. e
14. d
15. b
16. a
17. b
18. b
19. c
20. e
21. a
22. a
23. b
24. b
25. a
26. a
27. b
28. a
29. a
30. a

Chapter 5

1. d
2. c
3. b
4. a
5. e
6. b
7. a
8. e
9. e
10. b
11. a
12. b
13. c
14. c
15. b
16. c
17. c
18. b
19. b
20. a
21. a
22. b
23. a
24. b
25. a
26. b

27. b
28. a
29. a
30. a

Chapter 6

1. c
2. b
3. b
4. a
5. b
6. b
7. a
8. c
9. c
10. c
11. a
12. c
13. a
14. a
15. a
16. b
17. a
18. b
19. a
20. a

Chapter 7

1. d
2. d
3. b
4. e
5. c
6. e
7. c
8. b
9. c
10. a
11. a
12. a
13. a
14. a
15. b
16. b
17. a
18. a
19. a
20. a

Chapter 8

1. a
2. b
3. a
4. d
5. b
6. c
7. c
8. a
9. b
10. c
11. d
12. b
13. d
14. d
15. e
16. a
17. a
18. c
19. c
20. b
21. c
22. a
23. b
24. a
25. b
26. b
27. a
28. b
29. b
30. b
31. a

Chapter 9

1. b
2. c
3. a
4. a
5. b
6. d
7. e
8. c
9. b
10. a
11. e
12. b
13. a
14. c
15. b
16. b
17. d
18. a
19. d
20. c
21. a
22. a
23. b
24. a
25. a
26. b
27. a
28. b
29. b
30. b

Chapter 10

1. d
2. b
3. d
4. a
5. c
6. b
7. c
8. c
9. d
10. b
11. d
12. b
13. b
14. c
15. e
16. c
17. c
18. b
19. c
20. d
21. a
22. c
23. a
24. b
25. a
26. b
27. a
28. a
29. a
30. b

Chapter 11

1. a
2. c
3. b
4. b
5. e
6. c
7. b
8. d
9. c
10. e
11. c
12. b
13. a
14. b
15. b
16. b
17. a
18. d

19. e
20. c
21. c
22. a
23. b
24. b
25. a
26. a
27. a
28. a
29. b
30. b

Chapter 12

1. c
2. b
3. d
4. c
5. b
6. c
7. a
8. a
9. c
10. c
11. c
12. b
13. a
14. b
15. a
16. b
17. a
18. a
19. a
20. a

Chapter 13

1. c
2. b
3. d
4. a
5. b
6. c
7. b
8. b
9. b
10. a
11. b
12. b
13. e
14. a
15. b
16. a
17. a
18. b
19. a
20. b

Glossary

abduction: movement of a body segment *away* from the midline, typically occurring in the frontal plane.

actin-myosin cross bridge: the dynamic interaction between two muscle proteins (actin and myosin), essential to the mechanics of muscle contraction.

active movements: movements of the body produced volitionally by muscular activation.

actively efficient: most optimal activation pattern of a multi-articular muscle, occurring as the muscle simultaneously shortens across one joint and lengthens across the other.

actively insufficient: the reduced strength of an active movement caused by an over-shortening of the agonist multi-articular muscle.

adduction: movement of a body segment *toward* the midline, typically occurring in the frontal plane.

agonist: the muscle or muscle group that is most directly involved with the execution of a particular movement.

amphiarthrosis: a type of joint often located in the midline of the body; formed primarily by fibrocartilage and hyaline cartilage (e.g., the intervertebral body joints of the spine).

anatomic position: the standard body position used as a reference for describing the location of all body parts and movements.

angle of inclination: the frontal plane angle created between the femoral neck and the shaft of the femur; typically 125 degrees.

antagonist: the muscle or muscle group that produces the actions *opposite* that of an agonist muscle (e.g., the triceps are antagonists to the biceps).

anterior: the front, or toward the front of the body.

anterior pelvic tilt: the action of tilting the superior aspect of the pelvis anteriorly while holding the trunk upright. This motion creates a short arc, pelvic-on-femoral (hip) flexion motion that is naturally accompanied by an increasing lumbar lordosis.

anterior spondylolisthesis: anterior displacement of one vertebra relative to another; most commonly between L5 and S1.

appendicular skeleton: the bones of the appendages, or extremities—all the bones of the upper extremity including the scapula and clavicle and all the bones of the lower extremity including the pelvis.

arthritis: a degenerative joint disease resulting from the deterioration of the bones and cartilage that compose the affected joints.

arthrokinematics: the motions that occur *between* the articular surfaces of a joint: roll, slide, and spin.

articular cartilage: connective tissue that lines the articular surfaces of synovial joints; serves as a shock-absorbing mechanism between bones.

avascular necrosis: death or degeneration of bone resulting from a lack of blood supply to the affected bones.

axial skeleton: the central, bony axis of the body, consisting of the skull, hyoid bone, sternum, ribs, and vertebral column including the sacrum and coccyx.

axis of rotation: an imaginary line extending through a joint about which rotation occurs; the pivot point for joint motion.

Boyle's law: a principle of physics stating that the volume and pressure of a gas (including air) are inversely proportional.

cadence: the number of steps taken per minute; also called step rate.

cancellous bone: a porous (spongy) bone that typically comprises its internal aspect.

carpal tunnel: the space between the flexor retinaculum of the wrist and the carpal bones. This tunnel allows passage of the median nerve and nine tendons from the flexor digitorum superficialis, flexor digitorum profundus, and flexor pollicis longus.

carpal tunnel syndrome: pain or paresthesia of the hand over the sensory distribution of the median nerve, resulting from compression of the median nerve within the carpal tunnel. Most often this condition is caused by repetitive and extreme movements of the wrist.

cauda equina: a set of peripheral nerves located within the vertebral canal within the lumbosacral region.

caudal: toward the inferior aspect of the body.

center of mass: the point at the exact center of an object's mass (also referred to as the center of gravity).

cephalad: toward the head or superior aspect of the body.

chronic obstructive pulmonary disease: a chronic lung disease that combines emphysema, asthma, or chronic bronchitis; characterized by chronic airway obstruction, decreased elastic recoil of the lungs, and chronic over-inflation of the lungs.

circumduction: circular motion of a body segment through two or more planes.

closed-chain motion: a motion that occurs as a result of the proximal bony segment of a joint moving about a relatively fixed distal segment.

close-packed position: unique position within most joints of the body where the articular surfaces are most congruent and the ligaments are maximally taut.

co-contraction: typically describes the condition when the agonist and antagonist muscles are simultaneously and isometrically active, often to provide stability to a joint.

Colles' fracture: fracture of the distal radius near the radial styloid process.

compression force: a force that presses two or more objects together, such as joint surfaces.

concentric activation: a type of muscle activation that results in contraction or shortening of the muscle.

congruency: optimal fit between two surfaces; typically used to describe the optimal fit of a joint that is in its close-packed position.

contracture: abnormal shortening or stiffening of a muscle or connective tissue typically resulting in postural abnormalities and reduced range of motion.

core stabilization exercises: a group of exercises or techniques designed to improve the stability of the muscles in the vertebral column or trunk, or both.

cortical (compact) bone: a relatively dense type of bone that typically lines its external aspect.

counternutation: a slight motion that normally occurs at the sacroiliac joint, defined by posterior rotation of the sacrum relative to the ilium.

coxa valga: an abnormally *increased* angle of inclination of the proximal femur; diagnosis is made when the frontal plane angle between the femoral neck and the medial aspect of the shaft of the femur is much *greater than* 125 degrees.

coxa vara: an abnormally decreased angle of inclination of the proximal femur; diagnosis is made when the frontal plane angle between the femoral neck and the medial aspect of the shaft of the femur is much *less than* 125 degrees.

cross-sectional area: a measure of the thickness of a muscle. The larger a muscle's cross-sectional area, the larger its maximal potential to produce an active force.

cubitus valgus: the normal frontal plane angle formed between the humerus and medial aspect of the forearm; usually measures 15 degrees; often referred to as the "carrying angle."

cubitus varus: an abnormal frontal plane angle formed between the humerus and medial aspect of the forearm; often defined when the angle is much less than 15 degrees or when the forearm deviates toward the midline.

deep: toward the "core" or inside of the body.

degrees of freedom: the number of independent planes of movement allowed at a joint. A joint can have up to 3 degrees of freedom.

depression: inferior translation of a body segment.

diaphysis: the central shaft of a bone.

diarthrosis: an articulation between two or more bones that contains a fluid-filled joint cavity, such as the shoulder and hip; also called a synovial joint.

distal: away from the torso or midline of the body.

distal attachment: refers to a muscle or ligament's most distal attachment to a bone (frequently contrasted with proximal attachment). The distal attachment of a muscle is also called its insertion.

dorsal: the posterior surface of the body or body segment.

dorsiflexion: describes a sagittal plane motion of the ankle or foot in which the dorsum of the foot is drawn upward toward the tibia (shin).

double-limb support: the part of the gait cycle in which both feet are in contact with the ground.

downward rotation: motion of the scapula in which the glenoid fossa moves from an upward rotated position to a downward rotated position. This motion occurs naturally as the shoulder is adducted or extended from an elevated position.

dynamic stabilization: stabilization of a particular *moving* bone or body segment.

early swing: the part of the gait cycle when the leg is in the beginning period of its forward (swinging) motion.

eccentric activation: a muscle produces an active force while it simultaneously lengthens.

elevation: upward motion of a bony segment; typically used in reference to the mandible (jaw) elevating to close the mouth, or elevation of the scapula on the thorax.

end feel: an assessment of the feel of a joint as it reaches its terminal range of motion.

endomysium: the tissue surrounding each muscle fiber; composed of a relatively dense meshwork of collagen fibrils that help transfer contractile force to the tendon.

endosteum: a membrane that lines the surface of the medullary canal of bone.

epimysium: the connective tissue that surrounds the outer layer or "belly" of a muscle.

epiphyses: the expanded portions of bone that arise from the diaphysis (shaft); each long bone has a proximal and distal epiphysis.

eversion: a frontal plane motion of the foot in which a point on its plantar aspect rotates laterally.

excessive cubitus valgus: an abnormal frontal plane angle formed between the humerus and the medial aspect of the forearm that is markedly greater than 15 degrees. Normal cubitus valgus of the elbow typically measures 15 degrees.

excessive genu valgum: a frontal plane angle of the knee (measured laterally) that is less than 170 degrees, giving an individual a "knock-kneed" appearance.

excursion: the change of a muscle's length; typically referring to how much a muscle is lengthened or shortened during a specific motion.

expiration: the process of exhaling air from the lungs.

extension: a sagittal plane motion of one bone as it approaches the extensor surface of another.

extensor lag: the inability of the quadriceps to complete the last 15 to 20 degrees of active knee extension; typically due to pain, swelling, and inflammation.

extensor mechanism: connective tissue located on the dorsal surfaces of the digits; allows a way that the extrinsic and intrinsic muscles of the hand can simultaneously extend the interphalangeal joints.

external force: a push or pull produced by sources located outside the body. These typically include gravity or physical contact applied against the body.

external moment arm: the distance between the axis of rotation of a joint and the perpendicular intersection of an external force.

external rotation: horizontal or transverse plane motion of a bony segment that results in the anterior surface of the bone rotating *away* from the midline.

external torque: torque generated from external forces, such as gravity.

facet joint orientation: the spatial orientation of the facet (apophyseal) joints within the vertebral column; usually indicates the dominant motion within the vertebral region.

fasciculus: a bundle of muscle fibers.

flexion: a sagittal plane motion of one bone as it approaches the flexor surface of another.

foot drop: a gait deviation, typically due to weakness of the dorsiflexors, resulting in unwanted "dropping" of the foot during the swing phase of gait.

foot flat: a subdivision of the stance phase of the gait cycle when the plantar aspect of the foot is completely in contact with the ground.

force: a push or pull that produces, arrests, or modifies a motion.

force-couple: an action at a joint that occurs when two or more muscles produce forces in different linear directions but produce a torque in the same rotary direction.

forced expiration: exhaling air from the lungs as a result of active contraction of expiratory muscles such as the abdominals.

forced inspiration: the process of forcefully inhaling air into the lungs.

frontal plane: divides the body into front and back sections. Most abduction and adduction motions occur in the frontal plane.

gait cycle: the sequence of events taking place between successive heel contacts of the same foot.

genu recurvatum: marked hyperextension of the knee.

genu valgum: the normal frontal plane angle formed between the femur and lateral aspect of the lower leg. With the knee extended, this angle is about 170 to 175 degrees (i.e., the leg deviates away from the midline about 5 to 10 degrees). Excessive genu valgum gives a knock-kneed appearance.

genu varum: an abnormal frontal plane angle formed between the femur and lateral aspect of the lower leg. With the knee extended, this angle is greater than 180 degrees (i.e., the lower leg deviates toward the midline about 5 to 10 degrees). Genu varum gives a bowlegged appearance.

heel contact: a subdivision of the stance phase of the gait cycle when the heel makes contact with the ground.

heel off: a subdivision of the stance phase of the gait cycle when the heel breaks contact with the ground.

herniated nucleus pulposus: a pathologic condition in which the nucleus pulposus migrates through cracks in the annulus fibrosis of an intervertebral disc. This is often referred to as a bulging or slipped disc.

hip drop: a gait deviation in which one side of the pelvis inadvertently lowers during the swing phase of gait.

hip hiking: a gait compensation in which one side of the pelvis is elevated (hiked) to help clear the swing leg from the ground.

horizontal abduction: a motion of the shoulder that describes the arms being drawn *posteriorly* in the horizontal plane with the shoulders held in 90 degrees of abduction. Frequently referred to as horizontal extension.

horizontal adduction: a motion of the shoulder that describes the arms being drawn *anteriorly* in the horizontal plane with the shoulders held in 90 degrees of abduction. Frequently referred to as horizontal flexion.

horizontal (transverse) plane: divides the body into upper and lower sections. Most rotational movements such as internal and external rotation of the shoulder or hip and rotation of the trunk occur in the horizontal plane. Also called transverse plane.

hypertrophy: an increase in muscle mass.

impingement: abnormal and excessive contact between two components of the musculoskeletal system. This term often describes shoulder impingement, a pathologic condition that occurs as the humerus collides with the undersurface of the acromion of the scapula during shoulder abduction.

inferior: below, or toward the feet.

insertion: the distal attachment of a muscle or ligament.

inspiration: the process of inhaling air into the lungs.

internal force: a force that is generated from within the body.

internal moment arm: the distance between the axis of rotation of a joint and the perpendicular intersection of an internal force.

internal rotation: horizontal or transverse plane motion of a bony segment that results in the anterior surface of the bone rotating *toward* the midline.

internal torque: torque generated from internal forces such as muscle.

inversion: a frontal plane motion of the foot in which a point on its plantar aspect rotates medially.

isometric activation: an active force produced by muscle while it remains at a constant length.

joint reaction force: the compressive force between the articular surfaces of a joint; most often the result of muscular activation.

kinematics: branch of mechanics that describes the *motion* of a body without regard to the forces or torques that may produce the motion.

kinesiology: the study of human movement.

kinetics: branch of mechanics that describes the effect of *forces* acting on the body.

kyphosis: a normal sagittal plane curvature of the vertebral column; convex posteriorly and concave anteriorly. The thoracic and sacral regions of a normal spine display kyphotic curves.

lateral: away from the midline of the body or body segment.

lateral epicondylitis: inflammatory condition involving the proximal attachment of the wrist extensor muscles; also called tennis elbow. Referred to as lateral epicondylalgia when pain is present without inflammation.

lateral excursion: a side-to-side (lateral) motion of a bony segment; typically refers to movement of the jaw laterally, such as when grinding food with the teeth.

lateral tracking of the patella: describes an excessively lateral path of the patella during flexion and extension of the knee. Although a mild amount of lateral tracking is common, an excessive amount is considered pathologic.

leverage: the relative moment arm length possessed by a particular force.

line of gravity: the direction of the gravitational pull on a body.

line of pull: the direction of a muscle's force.

lordosis: a normal sagittal plane curvature of the spine; concave posteriorly and convex anteriorly. The cervical and lumbar regions of a normal spine display lordotic curves.

manual muscle test: manually resistive test performed to assess the strength of a particular muscle or muscle group.

mastication: the process of chewing, tearing, and grinding food with the teeth.

medial: toward the midline.

medial longitudinal arch: the arch of the foot that creates its characteristic concave medial in-step.

medullary canal: the central hollow tube within the diaphysis of a long bone.

mid stance: a subdivision of the stance phase of the gait cycle when the leg is in a vertical position. Mid-stance phase on one limb normally corresponds with mid-swing phase on the other limb.

mid swing: a subdivision of the swing phase when the leg is in the middle period of its forward (swinging) motion.

midline: an imaginary line that courses vertically through the exact middle of the body.

moment arm: the distance between the axis of rotation of a joint and the perpendicular intersection of a force.

mortise: describes the shape of the talocrural joint of the ankle. The articulation of the talus and the distal tibia and fibula resembles a carpenter's mortise joint.

muscle belly: the body of a muscle; composes the bulk of an individual muscle.

muscle fiber: an individual cell with multiple nuclei that contains all of the contractile elements of muscle.

muscular substitution: an action performed by muscles other than those that would normally produce a particular action.

myofibril: contains contractile proteins within a sarcomere.

neutral spine: a vertebral column that displays or maintains its natural curvatures: lordosis of the cervical and lumbar regions and kyphosis of the thoracic and sacral regions.

normal anteversion: the normal twist or torsion of the long axis of the femurs. Normal anteversion is 15 degrees.

nutation: A slight motion that normally occurs at the sacroiliac joint, defined by anterior rotation of the sacrum relative to the ilium.

open-chain motion: the motion that occurs as a result of the distal bony segment of a joint moving about a relatively fixed proximal segment.

opposition: the ability to touch the thumb precisely to the tips of the other four digits.

origin: the proximal attachment of a muscle or ligament.

osteokinematics: the motion of bones relative to the three cardinal planes.

palmar: referring to the anterior aspect or palm of the hand.

passive insufficiency: the reduced strength and range of motion of an active movement caused by overstretching of an antagonistic multi-articular muscle.

passive movements: movements of a particular body segment produced by a force other than muscle activation.

passive range of motion: the amount of bony motion at a joint that is independent of muscle activation.

perimysium: connective tissue that surrounds individual muscle fasciculi.

periosteum: a thin, tough membrane that covers the external surface of bones.

pes anserinus: the collective insertion of the semitendinosus, gracilis, and sartorius muscles to the proximal-medial region of the tibia.

pes cavus: an abnormally high or raised medial longitudinal arch of the foot.

pes planus: an abnormally low medial longitudinal arch of the foot. Also referred to as flatfoot.

plantar: the sole or bottom of the foot.

plantar flexion: the sagittal plane of motion where the foot moves downward, such as when stepping on the accelerator pedal of a car.

posterior: the back, or toward the back of the body.

posterior pelvic tilt: the action of tilting the superior aspect of the pelvis posteriorly while holding the trunk upright. This motion creates a short arc, pelvic-on-femoral (hip) extension movement that is naturally accompanied by a decreasing lumbar lordosis.

pronation: describes the forearm motion involved with turning the palms downward. Also describes a motion of the foot that results from the combined movements of dorsiflexion, eversion, and abduction.

prone: describes the position of lying face down.

protraction: translation or rotation of a bone or body segment generally in an *anterior* direction, typically in the horizontal plane.

protrusion: anterior translation (protraction) of the mandible (jaw).

proximal: toward the torso or midpoint of the body.

proximal attachment: refers to a muscle or ligament's most proximal attachment to a bone (frequently contrasted with its distal attachment). The proximal attachment of a muscle is also called its origin.

push-off: a generic term that describes the final subdivisions of the stance phase of the gait cycle related with propulsion (toe off and heel off).

Q-angle (quadriceps angle): a clinical measurement that quantifies the overall line of force of the quadriceps muscle relative to the patellar tendon.

quiet expiration: exhalation of air from the lungs, driven by the passive elastic recoil of lungs, surrounding muscles, and connective tissues. Normally, quiet expiration does not require active muscle force.

quiet inspiration: inhalation of air into the lungs at rest.

radial deviation: motion of the wrist in which the hand moves laterally in the frontal plane, toward the radius.

reposition: motion that returns the fully opposed thumb to the anatomic position.

resultant force: a summation of the effects of multiple force vectors.

retraction: translation or rotation of a bone or body segment generally in a *posterior* direction, typically in the horizontal plane.

retrusion: posterior translation (retraction) of the mandible (jaw).

reverse action: a muscular action that causes the proximal segment of a joint to move toward the relatively fixed distal segment.

roll: an arthrokinematic term describing when multiple points of one rotating articular surface contact multiple points of another articular surface.

rotation: the arc of movement of a body segment about an axis of rotation.

rotator cuff: a group of four shoulder muscles—supraspinatus, infraspinatus, teres minor, and subscapularis—that surround and help to stabilize the glenohumeral joint.

sagittal plane: divides the body into left and right halves. Typically, flexion and extension movements occur in the sagittal plane.

sarcomere: the basic contractile unit of muscle fiber. Each sarcomere is composed of two main protein filaments—actin and myosin—which are the main structures responsible for muscular contraction.

scapulohumeral rhythm: the natural ratio or rhythm that exists between the humerus and the scapula during abduction of the shoulder; specifically, for every 2 degrees of glenohumeral abduction, the scapula simultaneously and upwardly rotates 1 degree.

scoliosis: abnormal frontal and horizontal plane curvatures within the vertebral column.

screw-home mechanism: a locking mechanism of the knee created as the joint externally rotates slightly in conjunction with full extension.

segmental stabilization: a type of exercise designed to stabilize individual segments of the vertebral column.

single-limb support: the portion of the gait cycle in which the body is supported by only one leg.

slide: an arthrokinematic term describing when a single point on one articular surface contacts multiple points on another articular surface.

sliding filament theory: a theory of muscular contraction in which active force is generated as actin filaments slide past the myosin filaments, resulting in contraction of an individual sarcomere.

spin: an arthrokinematic term describing when one articular surface rotates on a single point on another articular surface (like a toy top).

spinal nerve: the union of a ventral and dorsal nerve root containing motor and sensory fibers, respectively.

stabilizer: a muscle that functions to fixate a particular bony segment.

stance phase: phase of gait when the leg is in contact with the ground; occupies the first 60% of the entire gait cycle.

static stability: stabilization of a particular bone or body segment that results in no or very little movement.

stenosis: a narrowing; typically referring to the vertebral canal or intervertebral foramen.

step: the period between successive heel contacts of opposite feet.

step length: the distance between successive heel contacts of opposite feet.

step width: the distance between the heel centers of two consecutive foot contacts. Normally, this distance is about 3 inches in the healthy adult.

stride: the period between successive heel contacts of the same foot; also defined as one gait cycle.

stride length: the distance traveled in one stride (between two consecutive heel contacts of the same foot).

subluxation: an incomplete or partial dislocation of a joint.

superficial: toward the external surface of the body.

superior: above.

supination: describes the forearm motion involved with turning the palms upward. Also describes a motion of the foot that results from the combined movements of plantar flexion, inversion, and adduction.

supine: describes the position of lying face up.

swing phase: phase of gait when the leg is *not* in contact with the ground, but advancing forward; occupies the last 40% of the gait cycle.

synarthrosis: a type of joint that allows little to no movement. Examples include the sutures of the skull and the distal tibiofibular joint.

synergists: muscles that work together to perform a particular action.

tenodesis: passive motion produced at one joint caused by the stretching of a multi-articular muscle across another joint. For example, stretching the long finger flexors across the extended wrist results in passive flexion of the fingers.

terminal swing: a subdivision of the swing phase when the leg is in the end period of its forward (swinging) motion (just before heel-contact phase).

thoracic outlet syndrome: compression of the brachial plexus and/or subclavian vessels as they exit the thorax. This condition often results in tingling and numbness of the upper extremity.

toe off: a subdivision of the stance phase of the gait cycle when the toes break contact with the ground.

torque (or moment): the rotary equivalent to a force—defined by the product of a force times its moment arm.

translation: linear motion in which all parts of a body move parallel to and in the same direction as every other point in the body.

Trendelenburg sign: a Trendelenburg test is performed to evaluate the functional strength of the hip abductor muscles. The patient is asked to stand on one leg as the therapist notes the position of the pelvis. A *positive Trendelenburg sign* occurs if the pelvis drops to the side of the lifted leg—away from the tested muscle. This response indicates weakness of the hip abductor muscles on the stance limb. A *negative Trendelenburg sign* occurs if the pelvis remains level as the leg is lifted. This response indicates normal functional strength of the hip abductor muscles on the stance limb.

triceps surae: name given to the muscles that compose the majority of the calf: the gastrocnemius and soleus muscles.

ulnar deviation: motion of the wrist in the frontal plane that the hand moves medially, toward the ulna.

ulnar drift: significant abnormal ulnar deviation of the fingers; often the result of chronic rheumatoid arthritis.

upward rotation: motion of the scapula in which the glenoid fossa moves upward. This motion occurs naturally as the shoulder is abducted or flexed.

valgus: the distal bony segment of a joint (or bone) projects *laterally* relative to the proximal segment of the joint.

varus: the distal bony segment of a joint (or bone) projects *medially* relative to the proximal segment of the joint.

vector: a quantity such as velocity or force that is completely specified by its magnitude and direction.

ventilation: the mechanical process by which air is inhaled and exhaled through the lungs.

walking velocity: the speed at which an individual walks. Normal walking velocity is about 3 miles per hour.

winging: abnormal condition of the scapula in which the medial border flares away from the rib cage, giving the appearance of a bird's wing. Typically, this is an indication of weakness of the serratus anterior muscle.

Wolff's law: the premise that bone is laid down in areas of high stress and reabsorbed in areas of low stress.

INDEX

Page numbers followed by f indicate figures; b, boxes; and t, tables.